Indian Head Massage

3rd edition

Helen McGuinness

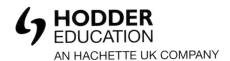

HODDER
EDUCATION
AN HACHETTE UK COMPANY

Orders: please contact Bookpoint Ltd, 130 Milton Park, Abingdon, Oxon OX14 4SB.
Telephone: (44) 01235 827720. Fax: (44) 01235 400454. Lines are open from
9.00–5.00, Monday to Saturday, with a 24 hour message answering service.
You can also order through our website www.hoddereducation.co.uk.

British Library Cataloguing in Publication Data
A catalogue record for this title is available from the British Library

ISBN: 978 0 340 94604 6

First Published 2007
Impression number   10 9 8 7 6 5 4 3
Year   2012 2011 2010 2009

Typeset by Pantek Arts Ltd, Maidstone, Kent
Printed in Dubai for Hodder Education, an Hachette UK Company,
338 Euston Road, London NW1 3BH

Contents

Acknowledgements vi

Preface vii

Chapter 1 Introduction to Indian Head Massage 1

Chapter 2 Essential Anatomy and Physiology for Indian Head Massage 16

Chapter 3 Conditions Affecting the Head, Neck and Shoulders 88

Chapter 4 Consultation for Indian Head Massage 105

Chapter 5 Indian Head Massage Case Studies 121

Chapter 6 Indian Head Massage Techniques 130

Chapter 7 Stress Management 193

Chapter 8 Health, Safety, Security and Employment Standards 216

Chapter 9 Promotion and Marketing 247

Frequently Asked Questions 265

Resources 267

Glossary 271

Index 278

Acknowledgements

I would like to acknowledge and thank the following people for their support in the development of the 3rd edition of this book:

My husband Mark for his considerable help and contributions (especially with the web resources), for his constant love and support, and especially for inspiring and encouraging me to write this book; to our beautiful daughter Grace for being so patient whilst I was writing; my parents Roy and Val for their positive encouragement and constant belief in my abilities; my dear friend Dee Chase for her valuable contributions and for her support and encouragement throughout the writing of this book; Dr Nathan Moss for his invaluable advice for Chapter 3 – Conditions Affecting the Head, Neck and Shoulders; The Maharishi Ayurvedic Centre in Lancashire for their kind permission to use references and information on the ingredients of their hair oils; and finally all the Indian Head Massage students and staff at the Holistic Training Centre who have encouraged me to write this book, especially our PA Lorna, who kindly helped me to type up the crosswords.

The publishers would like to thank the following individuals and institutions for permission to reproduce copyright material:

Fig. 1.1 © Luca Tettoni/Corbis; fig. 1.2 © Around the World in a Viewfinder/Alamy; fig. 2.4, 2.5, 2.8, 2.14, 2.16, 2.18 Dr. P. Marazzi/Science Photo Library; fig. 2.6 Dr. Chris Hale/Science Photo Library; fig. 2.7, 2.12 Wellcome Trust Medical Photographic Library; fig. 2.9 CNRI/Science Photo Library ; fig. 2.10 Biophoto Associates/Science Photo Library; fig. 2.11 BSIP/Science Photo Library; fig. 2.13 Science Photo Library; fig. 2.15 J.F. Wilson/Science Photo Library; fig. 2.17 CNRI/Science Photo Library.

Commissioned photographs © by Carl Drury.
With thanks to our model Minna, and to Images Model Agency.

Preface

Originally existing as a family tradition in its country of origin, Indian Head Massage has developed from being a technique mainly practised on the head by family members to become a comprehensive holistic therapy skill that addresses the widespread problems of stress in the Western world.

This book is designed for those undertaking a professional qualification in Indian Head Massage and addresses all the skills and knowledge required for commercial practice and competency in the workplace.

Indian Head Massage has grown in popularity since the latter part of the 1990s to become an integral part of Holistic and Beauty Therapy Course programmes in further education colleges and private training establishments.

Since the second edition of this book was published in 2004, I am delighted to see the popularity of this skill area has grown further and that Indian Head Massage has become a skill much in demand, both here and abroad.

The third edition of the book, published in 2007, benefits from a unique accompanying CD-ROM which will give students a number of resources to help make their learning of the subject fun and stimulating, and will also help them generate sufficient evidence to reach a competent level for commercial practice.

Helen McGuinness

1 Introduction to Indian Head Massage

Massage has always been an important feature of Indian family life. Indian Head Massage is a treatment that has evolved from traditional techniques that have been practised in India as part of a family ritual for thousands of years.

By the end of this chapter you will be able to relate the following to your work as a holistic therapist:

- The basic principles of Ayurveda.
- The history and development of Indian Head Massage as a holistic therapy.
- The benefits and effects of Indian Head Massage.

The History and Development of Indian Head Massage

The traditional art of Indian Head Massage is based on the ancient system of medicine known as Ayurveda, which has been practised in India for thousands of years.

Ayurveda

Ayurveda is recorded as India's oldest healing system. The word 'Ayurveda' comes from Sanskrit and means the 'science of life and longevity'. The Ayurvedic approach to health is the

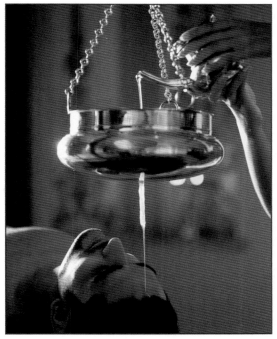

Fig 1.1 Ayurvedic treatment

balance of body, mind and spirit, and the promotion of long life and recommends the use of massage together with diet, herbs, cleansing, yoga, meditation and exercise.

The ancient texts say that the human lifespan should be around 100 years, and that all those years should be lived in total health, physically and emotionally. The whole aim of Ayurveda is in prevention, and in the promotion of positive health, beauty and long life.

The early Ayurvedic texts dating back nearly 4,000 years, feature massage and the principles of holistic treatment, in that health results from harmony within one's self. The Ayur-Veda, a sacred book among Hindus, written around 1800 BC included massage amongst its Ayurvedic principles. The Hindus used techniques, preserved in the Sanskrit texts 2,500 years ago, which detail the underlying principles of Ayurveda in maintaining balance in the body.

Ayurvedic Principles

The Ayurvedic view of health is in physical, emotional and spiritual well-being. The purpose of Ayurveda is to nourish the 'root of life' in order to help keep ourselves healthy and happy.

The Ayurvedic principle identifies three main 'roots of life', or three main principles in nature itself. These three principles, or doshas, are known in Ayurveda as **vata**, **pitta** and **kapha**. Everyone has a unique natural balance of these three principles, and if that balance is maintained in our everyday lives we will be healthy and happy. If the balance is disturbed then problems may develop.

The Five Elements

In Ayurveda, a person is seen as a unique individual made up of five primary elements: **ether** (space), **air**, **fire**, **water** and **earth**. When any of these elements are imbalanced in the environment, they will have an influence on how an individual feels. The foods we eat and the weather are just two of the influences on these elements.

The Ayurvedic principle shows how the five subtle elements are projected through the five senses.

- Through the sense of hearing the element space is generated.
- Through touch the air element arises.
- The fire element is projected by the sense of sight.
- Water and earth arise from the senses of taste and smell respectively.

The five elements make up the basic elements of life, and they form the building blocks of the universe.

Space (ether): represents expansion/contraction

Expansion of consciousness is space. We need space to live, and our body's cells contain spaces.

Air: represents movement/direction

The movement of consciousness determines the direction in which change of position in space takes place. The course of action causes subtle activities and movements within space. According to Ayurvedic perspective, this is the air principle.

Fire: represents transformation/heat

Where there is movement, there is friction, which creates heat. Therefore the third manifestation of consciousness is fire, the principle of heat. The solar plexus is the seat of fire, and this fire principle regulates body temperature. Fire is also responsible for digestion, absorption and assimilation.

Water: represents balance/cold

Due to the heat of fire, consciousness melts into water. According to chemistry, water is H_2O, but according to Ayurveda, water is liquefaction of consciousness. Water exists in the body in many different forms, such as plasma, cytoplasm, serum, saliva and nasal secretion. Water is necessary for nutrition and to maintain the water/electrolyte balance in the body.

Earth: represents crystallization

The next manifestation of consciousness is the earth element. Due to the heat of the fire and water, there is crystallization. According to Ayurveda, earth molecules are nothing but crystallization of consciousness. In the human body all solid structures (hard, firm and compact tissues) are derived from the earth element (e.g. bones, cartilage, nails, hair, teeth and skin).

Even in a single cell:

- the cell membrane is earth
- the cellular vacuoles are space
- cytoplasm is water
- nucleic acid and all chemical components of the cell are fire
- movement of the cell is air.

While each individual is a composite of the five primary elements, certain elements are seen to have an ability to create various physiological functions.

The elements with ether and air in dominance combine to form vata, which governs the principle of movement and therefore can be seen as the force which directs nerve impulses, circulation, respiration and elimination.

The elements with fire and water in dominance combine to form pitta, which is responsible for the process of transformation or metabolism. The transformation of foods into nutrition is an example of pitta function.

It is predominantly the elements of water and earth which combine to form kapha, which is responsible for growth. It also offers protection, for example, in the form of cerebral-spinal fluid, which protects the brain and spinal column. The mucosal lining of the stomach is another example of the kapha dosha protecting the tissues.

The Ayurvedic Perspective

In the Ayurvedic philosophy, the most fundamental aspect of life is in one's inner self, which operates through the five senses to create the five subtle elements that make up the life-giving doshas.

The Ayurvedic view of health is in physical, emotional and spiritual well-being and that health is maintained by the balance of the three subtle life-giving forces or doshas: vata, pitta and kapha.

Each of the three doshas has a role to play in the body and each dosha possesses individual qualities.

- **Vata** is the driving force, and relates mainly to the nervous system and the body's energy centre.
- **Pitta** is fire and relates to metabolism, digestion, enzymes, acid and bile.
- **Kapha** is related to water in the mucous membranes, phlegm, moisture, fat and lymphatics.

The Sub-doshas

Each of the three doshas has a subdivision of five aspects, known as sub-doshas, each one controlling a function or system of the body. These are useful to know, as they can indicate which dosha is unbalanced.

The Importance of *Prana*

The secret of Ayurveda lies in *prana*, the vital force (pra = before and ana = breath). In Ayurveda strong *prana* is the source of good health.

There are five major *pranas* in the human body to support all movement and bodily functions. The five *pranas* are normally called vayus. The descriptions of the *pranas* outlined below are not definitive, as they interrelate to each other and are very complex in their movements.

Prana vayu

This is the 'inward moving' air that is located in the head and the heart. It controls thinking, inhalation, emotions, sensory functioning, memory and receiving the cosmic *prana* from the sun (hot or solar *prana*). It provides the basic energy that moves us in life.

Apana vayu

This is the 'downward moving' air seated in the colon. It controls all the processes of elimination including urine, sweat, menstruation, orgasm and defecation. The apana receives cosmic *prana* from the earth and moon (cool or lunar *prana*). It also rules the elimination of negative emotions and provides mental stability. It is the basis of our immune system and when disturbed is the cause of most diseases.

Udana vayu

This is the 'upward moving' air located in the throat. It controls speech, connects us to the solar and lunar forces (sky and earth; masculine and feminine) and is responsible for spiritual development. Udana controls psychic powers and controls creative expression.

Samana vayu

This is known as the 'equalising or balancing air'. It is seated in the navel and controls the digestive system and harmonises the *prana* and apana vayus. Samana also governs the digestion of air, emotions and feeling. It is hot and solar in nature.

Vyana vayu

This is called the 'pervading' or 'outward moving' air. It is seated in the heart and yet pervades the whole body. It unites the other *pranas* and the tissues and controls nerve and muscle action. It holds the body together and is responsible for all circulation in the body; food, blood and emotions. Vyana provides strength and stability to the body.

Profile of the Dosha Vata

Vata is a combination of the elements air and ether. Vata is the driving force, and relates mainly to the nervous system and the body's energy centre. It is responsible for all movements of the body, mind and senses and the process of elimination. Vata may be dry, light, cold, mobile, active, clear, astringent and dispersing. Due to the dry quality, a person with excess vata will tend to have dry hair, dry skin, a dry colon and a tendency towards constipation.

> **KEY NOTE**
> A unique characteristic of vata is dryness.

Due to the light quality (opposite of heavy) the vata person will tend to have a light body frame, light muscles, light fat and be thin and/or underweight.

Due to the cold quality, the vata person will have cold hands, cold feet and poor circulation.

Due to the mobile quality, vata people are very active. They like jogging and jumping and don't like sitting in one place for very long.

Vata Sub-dosha Profile

In general vata controls all movement in the body and mind, and is related directly to the nervous system. Vata creates dryness in the body when too high and sluggishness when too low. Together with pitta it controls the hormonal function. The other two doshas are inert without vata.

The five subdivisions that controls various aspects of vata are:

1. *Prana* **vayu** controls inhalation, the other four vayus, the five senses, thinking, health and proper growth.
   Indications of imbalance: loss of senses, anxiety and worry, insomnia, dryness, emaciation, disease in general.

2. **Apana vayu** controls elimination, sexual function, menstruation, downwards movements in the body and disease.
   Indications of imbalance: constipation, menstrual problems, dryness, urinary problems, generally all diseases are involved.

3. **Samana vayu** controls movement of the digestive system, the solar plexus and balances the *prana* and apana vayus.
   Indications of imbalance: upset digestion, indigestion, diarrhoea, and malabsorption of nutrients, dryness.

4. **Udan vayu** controls exhalation, speech and the upward movements in the body, growth as a child.
   Indications of imbalance: problems with speech and the throat, weakness of will, general fatigue, lack of enthusiasm.

> **KEY NOTE**
> **Restoring balance to the dosha vata**
> When vata is balanced, mind and body are integrated and all movements flow with ease. When out of balance, thoughts can become disturbed by fear, anxiety and panic; inspiration disappears and forgetfulness may set in. Body aches/pains and constipation may also occur.
> To balance vata it is best to get plenty of rest, eat nourishing foods, slow down, keep warm and have an Indian Head Massage with an oil that has properties to help balance vata.

5. Vyana vayu pervades the whole body as the nervous system, yet it controls heart function and circulation of blood.

Indications of imbalance: arthritis, nervousness, poor circulation, poor motor reflexes, problems with the joints, bone disorders, nervous disorders.

Profile of the Dosha Pitta

Pitta is a combination of the elements fire and water. Pitta is fire and relates to metabolism, digestion, enzymes, acid and bile. It is responsible for heat, metabolism and energy production and digestive functions of the body. The unique characteristics of pitta are heat, sharp, light, liquid, sour, oily and spreading qualities.

Due to the heat characteristic, the pitta person will tend to have a strong appetite and warm skin. The body temperature is a little higher than the vata person. Due to the oily characteristics, a pitta person can have oily skin, but also be sensitive. They have warm, soft skin. Because pitta is light, pitta people are moderate in body frame.

KEY NOTE
A unique characteristic of pitta is heat.

Pitta Sub-dosha Profile

In general pitta is responsible for all metabolic processes. Pitta enables us to digest thoughts, feelings or food. Pitta controls all the heat disorders and relates to the fiery organs in the body and the blood. Together with vata it controls the hormonal function.

Low pitta will cause the whole metabolism to slow down and usually goes with high kapha. Excess pitta causes all kinds of heat-related disorders and inflammations.

The five subdivisions that control various aspects of pitta are:

1. **Alochaka pitta** controls the ability to see and the digestion of what we see.

   Indications of imbalance: eye problems and difficulties in digesting what we see.

2. **Sadaka pitta** controls functions of the heart and the digestion of thoughts and emotions.

   Indications of imbalance: heart failure, repressed emotions and feelings, excessive anger or unprocessed feelings.

3. **Pachaka pitta** controls stomach digestion.

   Indications of imbalance: ulcers, heartburn, cravings, indigestion.

4. **Ranjaka pitta** controls liver/gall bladder digestion.

   Indications of imbalance: anger, irritability, hostility, excessive bile, liver disorders, skin problems, toxic blood, anaemia.

5. **Bhrajaka pitta** controls metabolism of the skin.

   Indications of imbalance: all skin problems, acne, inflammation of the skin.

KEY NOTE
Restoring balance to the dosha pitta
When pitta is balanced, you will feel content, cheerful, warm-hearted and have great physical energy. Imbalance

of pitta may cause feelings of anger, resentment, jealousy, aggression or obsession, and can lead to physical ailments such as heartburn, cystitis, diarrhoea, skin rashes, fever, as well as excess hunger and thirst.

To help balance pitta it is best to avoid pressure, eat foods of a cooling nature, schedule for rest to avoid overworking (and overheating) and have an Indian Head Massage with an oil that has properties to help balance pitta.

Profile of the Dosha Kapha

Kapha is a combination of the elements earth and water. Kapha is related to water in the mucous membranes, phlegm, moisture, fat and lymphatics. It is responsible for physical stability, proper body structure and fluid balance.

The characteristics of kapha are heaviness, slowness, cool, oily, dense, thick, static and cloudy qualities. Kapha is sweet and salty. Due to the heavy quality, kapha people have a slower metabolism and digestion, and have a tendency to put on weight. Because kapha is cool, kapha people have a cool, clammy skin.

> **KEY NOTE**
>
> A unique characteristic of kapha is heaviness.

Kapha Sub-dosha Profile

In general kapha is responsible for the stability of our body and mind. It is the principal cohesion of mind and body. Flexibility and growth are controlled by kapha; moisture and fluid retention are maintained by kapha.

When kapha is too high it restricts vata and subdues pitta, thereby creating congestion on all levels. When kapha is too low it results in dryness and ungrounded thoughts and actions.

1. **Tarpaka kapha** controls fluids in the head, the sinuses and cerebral fluids.
   Indications of imbalance: sinus problems, headaches, loss of smell.

2. **Bodhaka kapha** controls taste and the cravings of taste, digestion and saliva.
   Indications of imbalance: overeating and cravings for sweets, loss of taste, congestion in the throat and mouth areas.

3. **Avalambaka kapha** controls lubrication and the fluids around the heart, lungs and upper back.
   Indications of imbalance: congestion in the lungs or heart, stiffness in the back and upper spine, lethargy.

> **KEY NOTE**
>
> **Restoring balance to the dosha kapha**
>
> When kapha is balanced you will feel strong, even-tempered, kind, compassionate, slow to anger and unflappable. Imbalance of kapha may cause sluggishness, lethargy, depression. Physical complaints such as colds, coughs, allergies, asthma, sinusitis may also occur.
>
> To help balance kapha it is best to eat lightly, exercise more and have an Indian Head Massage with an oil that has properties to help balance kapha.

4. **Kledaka kapha:** controls the lubrication of the digestive processes, maintains a balance with the pitta's bile, provides mental lubrication.

   Indications of imbalance: bloated stomach, slow or congested digestion, excess mucus.

5. **Slesaka kapha** controls the lubrication of the joints in the body and aids in all movements.

   Indications of imbalance: swollen joints, stiff joints, painful movements.

Balance and Harmony of the Three Doshas

When the three doshas are well harmonised and balanced, good health and well-being will result. However, when there is imbalance or disharmony in the elements it can lead to various types of ailments.

The Ayurvedic concept of physical health revolves around the three doshas and the primary purpose is to maintain them in a balanced state to prevent disease and disharmony. This theory is not unique to Indian medicine; the yin and yang theory in Chinese medicine and the Hippocratic theory in Greek medicine are also very similar.

Each individual is made up of unique proportions of vata, pitta and kapha. The ratio of the doshas varies for each individual and Ayurveda sees each person as a special combination, which accounts for our diversity. Each individual's constitution is determined by the state of their parents' doshas at the time of conception: at birth a person has the balance of the three doshas that is right for them. Life and all its forces and influences can cause the doshas to become unbalanced, which can lead to ill health.

Ayurveda offers a model for seeing each person as a unique make-up of the three doshas and designs a treatment protocol to specifically address an individual's health challenges.

When any of the doshas become accumulated, Ayurveda will suggest specific lifestyle and nutritional guidelines to assist the individual in reducing the dosha that has become excessive. Also herbal medicines will be suggested to cure the imbalance and diseases.

Understanding the main principle of Ayurveda offers an explanation as to why people respond differently to a treatment or diet and why individuals with the same disease may require different treatments and medication.

> ## ACTIVITY
>
> The Ayurvedic principle of life shows us how to identify our own natural balance of doshas, and then how to keep them in balance.
>
> Go to **www.whatsyourdosha.com** for a free questionnaire to help establish your own dosha profile and those of your clients.

Massage in Indian Family Life

Traditionally, massage has been an important feature of family life across the generations. In Indian traditions, it is believed that massage preserves the body's life force and energy, and is the most powerful way of relaxing and rejuvenating the body.

In India, it is customary for babies to be massaged every day from birth and to be massaged continually until they are 3 years old. This encourages the bonding process, keeps baby healthy and happy and helps create a secure family environment. From the age of 6, children are taught to show love and respect by sharing a massage with family members.

It is considered compulsory for a bride and groom to receive a massage with chemicals and oils before marriage.

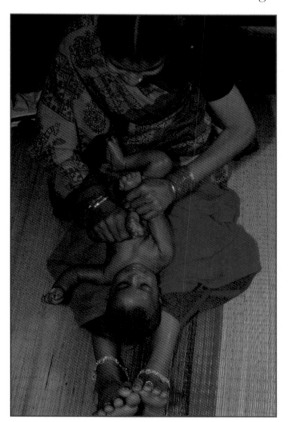

Fig 1.2 Massage in Indian family life

This ceremonial massage is considered to help relax the bride and groom, give them stamina and psychic strength, as well as promote health and fertility.

It is also tradition to massage expectant mothers to help them cope with the physical and emotional demands of labour; massage is applied daily for a minimum of 40 days after the birth. Weekly massage is a family event in India and for the majority continues throughout life to old age.

The Indian Head Massage techniques practised today have evolved from traditional rituals of Indian family grooming. Over generations, Indian women have been taught by their mothers to massage different oils such as coconut, sesame, olive, almond, herbal oils, buttermilk, mustard oil and henna into their scalp in order to maintain their hair in a beautiful condition.

Barbers have developed a more stimulating and invigorating head massage known as 'champi' to incorporate into their daily treatments, which leaves their clients feeling revitalised and alert. In India their particular techniques are passed down through the generations from barber father to barber son.

The tradition of Indian Head Massage has therefore been passed down through the family generations, as Indian women have been taught the tradition of hair massage and grooming from their mothers, and barbers' sons have learnt techniques from their fathers. Head massage forms an integral part of family life and is often a ritual that is not only carried out at home within families, but is commonly seen being performed on street corners, beaches and marketplaces.

Indian Head Massage in the Western World

Despite its existence on the Indian subcontinent for thousands of years, Indian Head Massage has only recently started to gain popularity in the West. Though Indian Head Massage was originally designed for use on the head only, today it has been westernised to include other parts of the body vulnerable to stress, such as the shoulders, upper arms and neck.

It is important to realise that there is a relationship between the head, neck, shoulders and upper arms and by incorporating these parts the treatment becomes more of a stress management treatment than a treatment designed to stimulate the head and improve the hair growth and condition.

Although the techniques are applied to the upper part of the body only (shoulders, upper arms, neck and head), collectively they represent a de-stressing programme for the whole body. Indian Head Massage has therefore become a primary form of stress management treatment in the western world.

Clients seeking relief from stress and tension often find Indian Head Massage a convenient form of treatment to receive in that:

a) there is no need to undress

b) it is quick and effective in terms of results

c) it may be performed anywhere, due to its portable nature.

Therapists find Indian Head Massage a convenient form of treatment to offer in that:

a) no special resources are needed

b) the techniques used are quick and effective

c) clients with special needs (a heavily pregnant client, or a client in a wheelchair) may receive treatment with the minimum fuss.

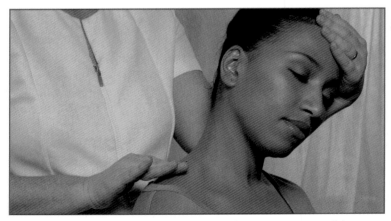

Fig 1.3 Indian Head Massage in the western world

The Future of Indian Head Massage

Today Indian Head Massage is one of the fastest growing holistic therapies. In 1996 and in response to market demand for the skill, Indian Head Massage was first formalised into a Diploma qualification by VTCT (Vocational Training Charitable Trust). Other Awarding Bodies such as ITEC (International Therapy Education Council), CIBTAC (Confederation of International Beauty Therapy and Cosmetology) and City and Guilds have also developed qualifications in this field.

Indian Head Massage has now been incorporated into the National Occupational Standards for both **Hairdressing and Beauty Therapy at Level III**. This is a significant development in that what was previously a variable form of treatment passed down through Indian families has become a professional qualification with national and international standards in the health and beauty industry.

Indian Head Massage is now available in hairdressing and beauty salons, spas, health farms, health clinics, in the workplace, at airports, on airlines, at conferences and exhibitions, on cruise liners and in private practice.

The diversity of practice of Indian Head Massage is due to both its versatility and accessibility. Despite its diversity of development, there is still a significant potential for the practice of Indian Head Massage to be widened in the market. Being a portable skill *and* the perfect antidote to stress and tension, Indian Head Massage is beneficial to all members of the community (young to elderly).

A relatively untapped area of potential is in the corporate market. The treatment can be tailored to be performed within a lunch break, and marketed as a stress management tool and preventative health care therapy. Stress-related issues are responsible for around 60 per cent of the 67 million working days lost each year, according to recent figures from the Health and Safety Executive. The development of Indian Head Massage in the workplace can help to reduce the harmful effects of stress on the workplace, whilst energising and motivating the workforce.

The Effects and Benefits of Indian Head Massage

Although the techniques involved in Indian Head Massage involve only the upper part of the body, the potential benefits are widespread. It can be said that Indian Head Massage is a truly holistic therapy in that it has many physiological and psychological benefits; many clients comment on the fact that they feel as if their whole body is balanced after the treatment.

Effects	Benefits
Increase in blood flow to the head, neck and shoulders	■ Nourishes the tissues and encourages healing ■ Improves the circulation; the delivery of oxygen and nutrients is improved via the arterial circulation and the removal of waste is hastened via the venous flow ■ Dilates the blood vessels helping them to work more efficiently ■ Helps to temporarily decrease blood pressure, due to the dilation of capillaries
Increased lymphatic flow to the head, neck and shoulders	■ Aids the elimination of accumulated toxins and waste products ■ Reduces oedema ■ Stimulates immunity, due to an increase in white blood cells
Relaxes the muscle and nerve fibres of the head, neck and shoulders	■ Relieves muscular tension, soreness and fatigue ■ Increases flexibility ■ Improves muscle tone, balance and posture ■ Can help to relieve tension headaches and aches and pains
Reduces spasms, restrictions and adhesions in the muscle fibres	■ Relieves pain and discomfort ■ Improves joint mobility
Decreases inflammation in the tissues, reducing any thickening of the connective tissue	■ Pain relief ■ Reduces stress placed on bones and joints
Decreases stimulation of the sympathetic nervous system	■ Slows down and deepens breathing ■ Slows down the heart and pulse rate ■ Helps reduce blood pressure ■ Reduces stress and anxiety
Stimulates the parasympathetic nervous system	■ Helps promote rest, relaxation, and sleep ■ Reduction of stress

Effects	Benefits
Stimulates the release of endorphins from the brain	■ Helps relieve pain ■ Helps relieve emotional stress and repressed feelings ■ Elevates the mood ■ Helps relieve anxiety and depression
Deepens external respiration, and increases rate of internal respiration	■ Improves lung capacity ■ Relaxes tightness in the respiratory muscles ■ Increased blood and lymphatic flow helps eliminate toxins more efficiently
Improves circulation and nutrition to the skin and the hair	■ Encourages cell regeneration ■ Increases desquamation (shedding of dead skin cells) ■ Improved elasticity of the skin
Increases sebum production	■ Helps to increase the skin's suppleness and resistance to infection
Promotes vasodilation of the surface capillaries in the skin	■ Helps improve the skin's colour
Increases circulation to the scalp	■ Promotes healthy hair growth ■ Increases desquamation (shedding of dead skin cells) ■ Helps improve the condition of the hair
Increases the supply of oxygen to the brain	■ Helps relieve mental fatigue ■ Promotes clearer thinking ■ Improves concentration ■ Helps increase productivity
Relaxes and soothes tense eye muscles	■ Helps relieve tired eyes and eyestrain ■ Brightens the eyes
Encourages the release of stagnant energy and restores the energy flow to the body	■ Creates a feeling of balance and calm

Self-Assessment Questions

1 Indian Head Massage has evolved from

   a   Sanskrit texts dating from 2,500 years ago

   b   the sacred book of Ayur-Veda dating from 1800 BC

   c   an Indian family tradition

   d   the ancient system of Indian medicine, Ayurveda

2 The Ayurvedic principle is that health is maintained by

   a   having a regular Indian Head Massage

   b   balancing of the three doshas

   c   eating the correct diet

   d   using special oils on the hair

3 In Ayurveda the five elements that make up an individual are

   a   ether, air, food, water and earth

   b   ether, air, fire, water and earth

   c   earth, water, fire, wind and space

   d   earth, cells, fire, water and space

4 In Ayurveda, which of the following is a unique characteristic of the dosha kapha?

   a   dry

   b   light

   c   rough

   d   heavy

5 One of the unique characteristics of the dosha pitta is

   a   cold

   b   heat

   c   dry

   d   soft

6 Which of the following statements is *true* in relation to the dosha vata?

   a   vata is a combination of the elements fire and water

   b   vata is responsible for physical stability and fluid balance

   c   vata is the driving force and is responsible for all movements of the mind, body, senses and the process of elimination

   d   excess vata causes heat-related disorders

7 Which of the following statements is *incorrect*?

a   imbalances in the doshas can lead to ill health

b   each individual is made of the same proportions of vata, pitta and kapha

c   life and all its forces and influences can cause the doshas to become unbalanced

d   each individual's constitution is determined by the state of their parents' doshas at the time of conception

8 Which of the following statements is *incorrect*?

a   Indian Head Massage helps reduce stress and anxiety

b   Indian Head Massage decreases the release of endorphins from the brain

c   Indian Head Massage increases the blood flow to the head, neck and shoulders

d   Indian Head Massage helps relieve tired eyes and eyestrain

2 Essential Anatomy and Physiology for Indian Head Massage

It is important for a holistic therapist to have a knowledge of essential anatomy and physiology in order to carry out treatments safely and effectively and understand the physiological effects of Indian Head Massage on the body. This chapter is devoted to the anatomy and physiology relevant to Indian Head Massage.

By the end of this chapter you will be able to relate the following knowledge to your practice in Indian Head Massage.

- The structure and functions of the skin and hair.

- Diseases and disorders in relation to skin and hair.

- The structure of bone.

- The bones of the head, neck, shoulders, thorax and upper limbs.

- The structure and function of muscle.

- Muscles of the head, neck, upper back, shoulder and upper limbs.

- The blood flow relating to the head and neck.

- The lymphatic drainage of the head and neck.

- The nerve supply to the head and neck.

- The mechanism of respiration.

The Skin

The skin is the largest organ of the body and provides the therapeutic foundation for treatment. Providing more than just an external covering, the skin is a highly sensitive boundary between our bodies and the environment. A thorough knowledge of the structure and functions of the skin will help the therapist to treat clients more effectively.

Functions of the Skin

The skin has several important functions:

Protection

- The skin acts as a physical barrier, protecting the underlying tissues from abrasion. Keratin, a protein found in the skin, provides protection by waterproofing the skin's surface, helping to keep water in and out.

- The skin also provides limited protection from ultraviolet radiation through specialised cells called melanocytes found in the basal cell layer of the epidermis.

- The skin's acidic secretions (sweat and sebum), known as the acid mantle, act as an barrier against foreign agents such as bacteria and viruses.

- Fat cells in the subcutaneous layer of the skin help protect bones and major organs from injury.

Sensation

The skin is like an extension of the nervous system in that it receives stimuli such as pressure, pain and temperature from the external environment and brings this information to the central nervous system.

Heat regulation

The skin helps to regulate the body's temperature at 37°C.

- When the body is losing too much heat, the blood capillaries near the skin's surface constrict to keep warmth in and closer to major organs.

- When the body is too warm, the blood capillaries dilate to allow more blood to flow near the surface in order to cool the body.

- The sweat glands help to cool the body down through the production of sweat.

Excretion

The skin functions as a minor excretory system, eliminating waste through perspiration. The eccrine glands produce sweat, which helps to remove waste materials such as urea, uric acid, ammonia and lactic acid from the skin.

Secretion

The specialised glands in the skin called the sebaceous glands secrete the oily substance sebum which lubricates the skin's surface, keeping it soft and pliable.

Storage

The skin acts as a storage depot for fat and water. About 15 per cent of the body's fluids are stored in the subcutaneous layer.

Absorption

The skin has limited absorption properties. Fat-soluble substances such as oxygen, carbon dioxide, fat-soluble vitamins and steroids can be absorbed by the epidermis, as can small amounts of water.

Vitamin D production

Located in the skin are molecules that are converted by the ultraviolet rays in sunlight to vitamin D. The vitamin D produced is then absorbed into the blood vessels and used by the body for the maintenance of bones and the absorption of calcium and phosphorus in the diet.

Structure of the Skin

Each person's skin varies in its colour, texture and condition. A client's skin can reflect their physiological as well as psychological state, and it is through touch that therapists can help to evaluate this information. Physiological signs of the skin may be shown by the client's colour and circulation, whereas psychological status may be reflected by muscular tightness.

There are two main layers of the skin:

- the **epidermis** which is the outer thinner layer
- the **dermis** which is the inner thicker layer.

Below the dermis is the **subcutaneous layer** which attaches to organs and tissues.

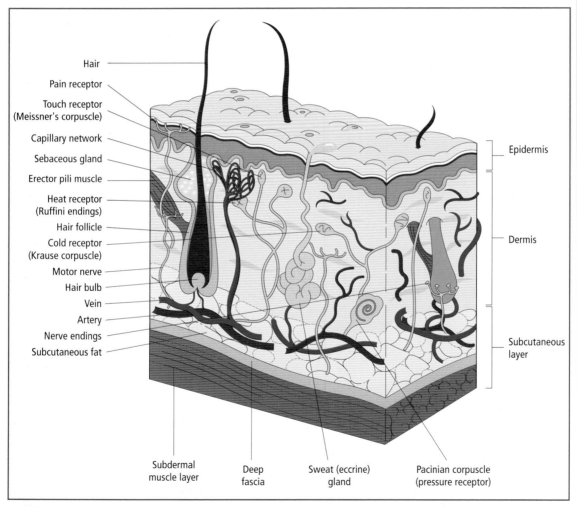

Fig 2.1 Cross section of the skin

The epidermis

The epidermis is the most superficial layer of the skin and consists of five layers of cells:

- the horny layer (stratum corneum, the outermost layer)
- the clear layer (stratum lucidum)
- the granular layer (stratum granulosum)
- the prickle cell layer (stratum spinosum)
- the basal cell layer (stratum germinativum, the innermost layer).

The three outer layers (horny, clear and granular) consist of dead cells as a result of the process known as keratinisation. The cells in the very outermost layer are dead and scaly and are constantly being rubbed away by friction. The inner two layers are composed of living cells. The epidermis does not have a system of blood vessels, therefore all nutrients pass into its cells from blood vessels in the deeper dermis.

The basal cell layer (stratum germinativum)

This is the deepest of the five layers. It consists of a single layer of column cells on a base membrane which separates the epidermis from the dermis. In this layer new epidermal cells are constantly being reproduced. These new cells move upwards through the different epidermal layers before being discarded into the horny layer. New column cells formed by division push adjacent cells towards the skin's surface. At intervals between the column cells are the large star-shaped cells called melanocytes which form the pigment melanin, the skin's main colouring agent.

Prickle cell layer (stratum spinosum)

This is known as the prickle cell layer because each of the rounded cells contained within it has short projections which make contact with the neighbouring cells and give them a prickly appearance. The living cells of this layer are capable of dividing by the process known as mitosis.

Granular layer (stratum granulosum)

This layer consists of flattened cells containing a number of granules which are involved in the hardening of cells through **keratinisation**. Keratinisation is the process that cells undergo when they change from living cells with a nucleus to dead cells without a nucleus. This layer links the living cells of the epidermis to the dead cells above.

Clear layer (stratum lucidum)

This layer consists of transparent cells which permit light to pass through. It consists of three or four rows of flat dead cells which are completely filled with keratin; they have no nuclei as these have degenerated through the keratinisation process. The clear layer of the epidermis is thought to form a barrier zone which controls the movement of water through the skin. This layer is very shallow in facial skin, but thick on the soles of the feet and the palms of the hands, and is generally absent in hairy skin.

Horny layer (stratum corneum)

This is the most superficial outer layer, consisting of dead, flattened, keratinised cells. The cells of the horny layer form a waterproof covering for the skin and help to prevent the penetration of bacteria. This outer layer of dead cells is continually being shed; this process is known as desquamation.

Cell regeneration

Cell regeneration occurs in the epidermis by the process mitosis (cell division). It takes approximately a month for a new cell to complete its journey from the basal cell layer where it is **reproduced**, through the granular layer where it becomes **keratinised**, to the horny layer where it is **desquamated**.

The dermis

The **dermis** lies below the epidermis and is the deeper layer of the skin. Its key functions are to provide nourishment to the epidermis and to give a supporting framework to the tissues. The dermis has two layers: a superficial papillary layer and a deeper reticular layer.

The superficial papillary layer is made up of fatty connective tissue and is connected to the underside of the epidermis by cone-shaped projections called **dermal papillae** which contain nerve endings and a network of blood and lymphatic capillaries.

The deeper reticular layer is formed of tough fibrous connective tissue which contains the following:

- collagen fibres which help to give the skin strength and resilience
- elastic fibres which help to give the skin elasticity
- reticular fibres which help to support and hold all structures in place.

Cells present in the dermis include:

- mast cells which secrete histamine (involved in allergies) causing dilation of blood vessels to bring blood to the area
- phagocytic cells which are white blood cells that are able to travel around the dermis destroying foreign matter and bacteria
- fibroblasts which are cells that help form new fibrous tissue.

Blood supply

Unlike the epidermis, an abundant supply of blood vessels run through the dermis and the subcutaneous layer.

Arteries carry oxygenated blood to the skin via arterioles and these enter the dermis from below and branch into a

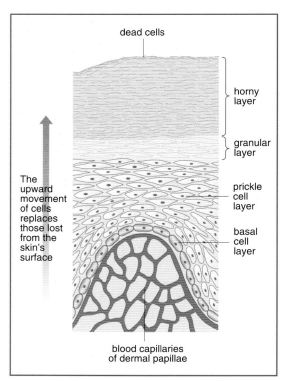

Fig 2.2 Cell regeneration of the epidermis

network of capillaries around active or growing structures. These **capillary networks** form in the dermal papillae to provide the basal cell layer of the epidermis with food and oxygen. They also surround the sweat glands and erector pili muscles, two appendages of the skin.

The capillary networks drain into venules, small veins which carry the deoxygenated blood away from the skin and remove waste products. The dermis is therefore well supplied with capillary blood vessels to bring nutrients and oxygen to the germinating cells in the basal cell layer of the epidermis and to remove waste products from them.

Lymphatic vessels

There are numerous lymphatic vessels in the dermis. They form a network in the dermis facilitating the removal of waste from the skin's tissue. The lymphatic vessels in the skin generally follow the course of veins and are found around the dermal papillae, glands and hair follicles.

Nerves

There is a wide distribution of nerves throughout the dermis. Most nerves in the skin are sensory, which send signals to the brain and are sensitive to heat, cold, pain, pressure and touch. The dermis also has motor nerves which relay impulses to the brain and are responsible for the dilation and constriction of blood vessels, the secretion of perspiration from the sweat glands and the contraction of the erector pili muscles attached to hair follicles.

The subcutaneous layer

This is a thick layer of connective tissue found below the dermis. The type of tissue found in this layer (areolar and adipose) help support delicate structures such as blood vessels and nerve endings.

The subcutaneous layer contains the same collagen and elastin fibres as the dermis and contains the major arteries and veins which supply the skin and form a network throughout the dermis. The fat cells contained within this layer help to insulate the body by reducing heat loss.

Below the subcutaneous layer lies the subdermal muscle layer.

Appendages of the Skin

The appendages are accessory structures that lie in the dermis of the skin and project on to the surface through the epidermis. These include the hair, the erector pili muscle and the sweat and sebaceous glands.

Hair

Hair is an appendage of the skin which grows from a sac-like depression in the epidermis called a hair follicle. Hair grows all over the body, with the exception of the palms of the hands and the soles of the feet.

The primary function of a hair is in physical protection. For example, the hair on the scalp provides partial shading from the sun's rays, and the hairs in the nostrils, eyelashes and eyebrows provide protection from foreign particles.

The structure of a hair

The hair is composed mainly of the protein keratin and is therefore a dead structure.

Longitudinally the hair is divided into three parts:

- **hair shaft** – the part of the hair that lies above the surface of the skin
- **hair root** – the part of the hair which is found below the skin
- **hair bulb** – the enlarged part at the base of the hair root.

Internally the hair has three layers which all develop from the matrix, which is the active growing part of the hair:

- **cuticle:** the outer layer, made up of transparent protective scales which overlap one another. The cuticle protects the cortex and gives the hair its elasticity
- **cortex:** the middle layer, made up of tightly packed keratinised cells containing the pigment melanin, which gives the hair its colour. The cortex helps to give strength to the hair
- **medulla:** the inner layer, made up of loosely connected keratinised cells and tiny air spaces. This layer of the hair determines the sheen and colour of the hair due to the reflection of light through the air spaces.

Hair growth

Hair growth originates from the central area of the hair bulb, the matrix, which is the active growing area where the hair cells divide and reproduce. The living cells produced in the matrix are then pushed upwards from their source of nutrition and are converted to keratin to produce a hair that eventually projects from the open end of the follicle.

The growth cycle of the hair

Hair has a growth pattern which ranges from approximately four to five months for an eyelash hair to approximately four to seven years for a scalp hair.

At the end of each hair's lifespan, the root of the hair separates from its matrix and remains in the follicle until it falls out, or is pulled out. The follicle then shrinks and enters a period of rest. Following its rest period, the follicle will either degenerate completely or enlarge to form a new hair bulb and produce another hair.

Hair colour

Hair colour is due to the presence of melanin in the cortex and medulla of the hair shaft. In addition to the standard black colour, the melanocytes in the hair bulb produce two colour variations of melanin, brown and yellow. Blond, light coloured and red has a high proportion of the yellow variant. Brown and black hair possesses more of the brown and black melanin.

> **KEY NOTE**
> Hair turns grey when the melanocytes in the hair bulb stop producing melanin.

Erector pili muscle

This is a small smooth muscle, attached at an angle to the base of a hair follicle, which serves to make the hair stand erect in response to cold.

Sweat glands

There are two types of sweat glands; the majority are called eccrine glands which are simple coiled tubular glands that open directly on to the surface of the skin. There are several million of them distributed over the surface of the skin although they are most numerous in the palms of the hands and the soles of the

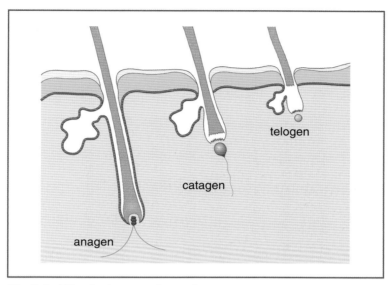

Fig 2.3 The hair growth cycle

feet. Their function is to regulate body temperature and help eliminate waste products. Their active secretion sweat is under the control of the sympathetic nervous system.

The other type of sweat glands are called apocrine glands; these are connected with hair follicles and are only found in the genital and underarm regions. They produce a fatty secretion; breakdown of this secretion by bacteria leads to body odour.

Sebaceous glands

These glands are found all over the body, except for the soles of the feet and the palms of the hands. They are more numerous on the scalp, face, chest and back.

Sebaceous glands commonly open into a hair follicle but some open on to the skin's surface. They produce an oily substance called sebum which contains fats, cholesterol and cellular debris. Sebum coats the surface of the skin and the hair shafts where it prevents excess water loss, lubricates and softens the horny layer of the epidermis and softens the hair.

KEY NOTE

Indian Head Massage can help to bring about an improvement in a client's skin and hair condition over a period of time. The increased circulation to the skin can increase cell nutrition and regeneration, as well as increase elimination of waste from the skin's tissues. Dead keratinised cells which are blocking the pores of the skin can be loosened by massage and the blood supply can flow more freely to feed the skin and hair with nutrients.

Indian Head Massage can also help to increase the production of sebum from the sebaceous glands, helping to lubricate the skin and hair and improve its condition.

Glossary of Useful Terms

Allergic reaction

A disorder in which the body becomes hypersensitive to a particular allergen. When irritated by an allergen, the body produces histamine in the skin as part of the body's defence or immune system.

The effects of different allergens are diverse and they affect different tissues and organs. For instance, certain cosmetics and chemicals can cause rashes and irritation in the skin; certain allergens such as pollen fur, feathers, mould and dust can cause asthma and hay fever. If severe, allergies may result in anaphylactic shock

Comedone

A collection of sebum, keratinised cells and wastes which accumulate in the entrance of a hair follicle. It may be open or closed. An open comedone is a 'blackhead' contained within the follicle, whereas a closed comedone is a 'whitehead', trapped underneath the skin's surface.

Cyst

An abnormal sac containing liquid or a semi-solid substance. Most cysts are harmless.

Erythema

Reddening of the skin due to the dilation of blood capillaries in the dermis just below the epidermis.

Fissure

A crack in the epidermis exposing the dermis.

Keloid

An overgrowth of an existing scar which grows much larger than the original wound. The surface may be smooth, shiny or ridged. The onset is gradual and is due to an accumulation or increase in collagen in the immediate area. The colour varies from red, fading to pink and white.

Lesion

A zone of tissue with impaired function, as a result of damage by disease or wounding.

Macule

A small flat patch of increased pigmentation or discolouration, for example a freckle.

Milia

Sebum trapped in a blind duct with no surface opening. Usually found around the eye area. They appear as pearly, white, hard nodules under the skin.

Mole

Moles are also known as a pigmented naevi. They appear as round, smooth lumps on the surface of the skin. They may be flat or raised and vary in size and colour from pink to brown or black. They may have hairs growing out of them.

Naevus

A mass of dilated capillaries. May be pigmented as in a birthmark.

Papule

Small raised elevation on the skin, less than 1 cm in diameter, which may be red in colour. Often develops into a pustule.

Pustule

Small raised elevation on the skin which contains pus.

Skin tag

Small growth of fibrous tissue, which stands up from the skin and is sometimes pigmented (black or brown).

Scar

A mark left on the skin after a wound has healed. Scars are formed from replacement tissue. Depending on the type and extent of damage, the scar may be raised (hypertrophic), rough and pitted (ice pick), or fibrous and lumpy (keloid). Scar tissue may appear smooth and shiny or form a depression in the surface.

Telangiecstasis

This is a term for dilated capillaries, where there is persistent vasodilation of capillaries in the skin. Usually caused by extremes of temperature and overstimulation of the tissues, although sensitive and fair skins are more susceptible to this condition.

Tumour

A tumour is formed by an overgrowth of cells and almost every type of cell in the epidermis and dermis is capable of benign or malignant overgrowth. Tumours are lumpy and even when they cannot be seen, they can be felt underneath the surface of the skin.

Ulcer

A break or open sore in the skin extending to all its layers.

Vesicles

Small sac-like blisters. A bulla is a vesicle larger than 0.5cm and is commonly called a blister.

Wart

Well-defined benign tumour which varies in size and shape. See viral infections of the skin on page 27.

Weal

A raised area of skin, containing fluid, which is white in the centre with a red edge, commonly seen in the condition urticaria.

Disorders of the Sebaceous Gland

Acne vulgaris

A common inflammatory disorder of the sebaceous glands which leads to the overproduction of sebum. It involves the face, back and chest and is characterised by the presence of comedones, papules, and in more severe cases cysts and scars. Acne vulgaris is primarily androgen induced and appears most frequently at puberty and usually persists for a considerable period of time.

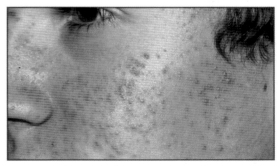

Fig 2.4 Acne vulgaris

Rosacea

A chronic inflammatory disease of the face in which the skin appears abnormally red. The condition is gradual and begins with flushing of the cheeks and nose and as the condition progresses it may become pustular. Aggravating factors include hot, spicy foods, hot drinks, alcohol, menopause, the elements and stress.

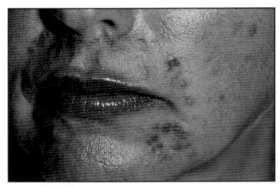

Fig 2.5 Rosacea

Sebaceous cyst

A round, nodular lesion with a smooth shiny surface, which develops from a sebaceous gland. They are usually found on the face, neck, scalp and back. They are situated in the dermis and vary in size from 5 to 50 mm. The cause is unknown.

Seborrhoea

This condition is defined as an excessive secretion of sebum by the sebaceous glands. The glands are enlarged and the skin appears greasy, especially on the nose and the centre zone of the face. The condition may develop into acne vulgaris and is common at puberty, lasting for a few years.

Disorders of the Sweat Glands

Hyperhidrosis

Excessive production of sweat affecting the hands, feet and underarms.

Bacterial Infections

Boil

A boil begins as a small inflamed nodule which forms a pocket of bacteria around the base of a hair follicle or a break in the skin. Local injury or lowered constitutional resistance may encourage the development of boils.

Conjunctivitis

This is a bacterial infection following irritation of the conjunctiva of the eye. In this condition the inner eyelid and eyeball appear red and sore and there may be a pus-like discharge from the eye. The infection spreads by contact with the secretions from the eye of the infected person.

Folliculitis

This is a bacterial infection and appears as a small pustule at the base of a hair follicle. There is redness, swelling and pain around the hair follicle.

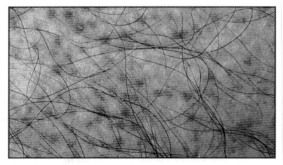

Fig 2.6 Folliculitis

Sycosis barbae

Sycosis barbae is a chronic folliculitis in which there are pustules in the hair follicles and inflammation of the surrounding skin area. Folliculitis is characterised by burning and itching, with pain on manipulation of the hair. Chronic, persistent infection results in spread to the surrounding skin which becomes red and crusted, resembling eczema. The upper lip is particularly susceptible in patients who suffer from chronic nasal discharge from sinusitis or hay fever.

Impetigo

A superficial contagious inflammatory disease caused by streptococcal and staphylococcal bacteria. It is commonly seen on the face and around the ears and features include weeping blisters which dry to form honey coloured crusts. (The bacteria are easily transmitted by dirty fingernails and towels.)

Stye

Acute inflammation of a gland at the base of an eyelash, caused by bacterial infection. The gland becomes hard and tender and a pus-filled cyst develops at the centre.

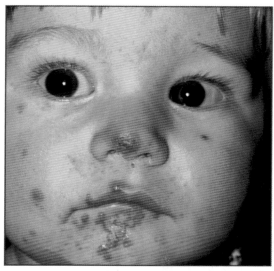

Fig 2.8 Impetigo

Viral Infections of the Skin

Herpes simplex (cold sores)

Herpes simplex is normally found on the face and around the lips. It begins as an itching sensation, followed by erythema and a group of small blisters; which then weep and form crusts. This condition will generally persist for approximately two or three weeks. It will recur at times of stress, ill health or exposure to sunlight.

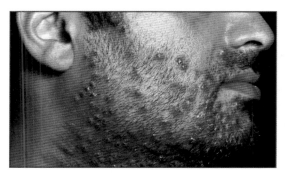

Fig 2.7 Sycosis barbae

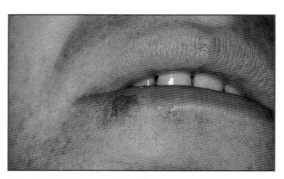

Fig 2.9 Herpes simplex

Herpes zoster (shingles)

Infection along the sensory nerves due to the virus that causes chicken pox. Lesions resemble herpes simplex with erythema and blisters along the lines of the nerves. Areas affected are mostly on the back or upper chest wall. This condition is very painful due to acute inflammation of one or more of the peripheral nerves. Severe pain may persist at the site of shingles for months or even years after the apparent healing of the skin.

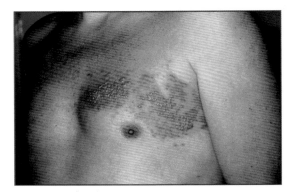

Fig 2.10 Herpes zoster

Warts

A wart is a benign growth on the skin caused by infection with the human papilloma virus.

- Plane warts are smooth in texture with a flat top and are usually found on the face, forehead, back of hands and the front of the knees.

- Plantar warts or verrucae occur on the soles of the feet. These warts are often grey and the centre frequently has pinpoint black spots.

Fungal Infections of the Skin

Ringworm

A fungal infection of the skin, which begins as small red papules that gradually increase in size to form a ring. Affected areas on the body vary in severity from mild scaling to inflamed itchy areas.

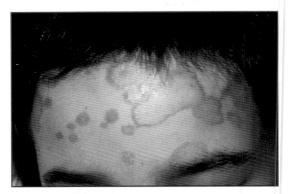

Fig 2.11 Ringworm

Tinea barbae (ringworm of the beard)

Tinea barbae is the name used for fungal infection of the beard and moustache areas. It is less common than *tinea capitis*

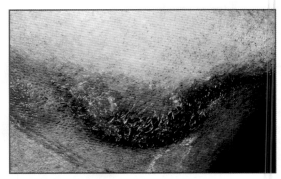

Fig 2.12 Tinea barbae

and generally affects only adult men. The skin is usually very inflamed with red lumpy areas, pustules and crusting around the hairs. The hairs can be pulled out easily. Surprisingly, it is not excessively itchy or painful.

The cause of tinea barbae is most often an animal fungus, originating from cattle or horses. It most often affects farmers and is due to direct contact with an infected animal. It is rarely passed from one person to another.

Tinea capitis (ringworm of the scalp)

This appears as painless, round, hairless patches on the scalp. Itching may be present and the lesion may appear red and scaly.

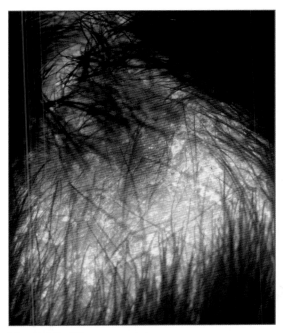

Fig 2.13 Tinea capitis

Tinea pedis (athlete's foot)

This is a highly contagious condition which is easily transmitted in damp, moist conditions such as swimming pools, saunas and showers. Athlete's foot appears as flaking skin between the toes which becomes soft and soggy. The skin may also split and the soles of the feet may occasionally be affected.

Infestation Disorders of the Skin

Pediculosis (lice)

This condition is commonly known as 'lice' and is a contagious parasitic infection, where the lice live off blood sucked from the skin. Head lice are frequently seen in young children and if not dealt with quickly, may lead to a secondary infection as a result of scratching (impetigo). The eggs of head lice (nits) may be found in the hair; these are pale grey or brown oval structures found on the hair shaft close to the scalp. The scalp may appear red and raw due to scratching.

Body lice are rarely seen. They will occur on an individual with poor personal hygiene and live and reproduce in seams and fibres of clothing, feeding off the skin. Lesions may appear as papules, scabs and in severe cases pigmented dry, scaly skin. Secondary bacterial infection is often present. A client affected by body lice will complain of itching, especially in the shoulder, back and buttock areas.

Scabies

A contagious parasitic skin condition, caused by the female mite who burrows into the horny layer of the skin where she lays her eggs. The first noticeable symptom of this condition is severe itching which worsens at night; papules, pustules and crusted lesions may also develop.

Common sites for this infestation are the ulnar borders of the hand, the palms and between the fingers and toes. Other sites include the axillary folds, buttocks, the breasts in the female and the external genitalia in the male.

Pigmentation Disorders

Albinism

A condition in which there is an inherited absence of pigmentation in the skin, hair and eyes, resulting in white hair, pink skin and eyes. The pink colour is produced by underlying blood vessels which are normally masked by pigment. Other clinical signs of this condition include poor eyesight and sensitivity to light.

Chloasma

This is a pigmentation disorder which presents with irregular areas of increased pigmentation, usually on the face. It commonly occurs during pregnancy and sometimes when taking the contraceptive pill, due to stimulation of melanin by the female hormone oestrogen.

Lentigo

Also known as 'liver spots', these are flat dark patches of pigmentation which are found mainly in the elderly on skin exposed to light.

Vitiligo

This condition presents with areas of the skin which lack pigmentation due to the basal cell layer of the epidermis no longer producing melanin. The cause of vitiligo is unknown.

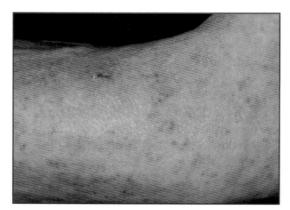

Fig 2.14 Scabies

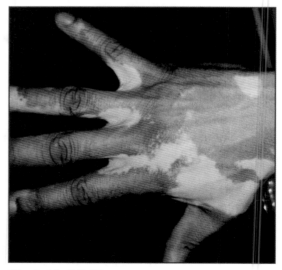

Fig 2.15 Vitiligo

Naevi

Portwine stain

Also known as a 'deep capillary naevus'. Present at birth and may vary in colour from pale pink to deep purple. Has an irregular shape, but is not raised above the skin's surface. Usually found on the face, but may also appear on other areas of the body.

Spider naevi

A collection of dilated capillaries which radiate from a central papule. Often appear during pregnancy or as the result from 'picking a spot'.

Strawberry mark

Usually develops before or shortly after a baby is born, but fades and disappears spontaneously before the child reaches the age of ten. It is raised above the skin's surface.

Hypertrophic Disorders

Malignant melanoma

A malignant melanoma is a deeply pigmented mole which is life threatening if it is not recognised and treated promptly. Its main characteristic is a blue-black nodule which increases in size, shape and colour and is most commonly found on the head, neck and trunk. Over exposure to strong sunlight is a major cause and its incidence is increased in young people with fair skins.

Rodent ulcer

This is a malignant tumour, which starts off as a slow growing pearly nodule, often at the site of a previous skin injury. As the nodule enlarges the centre ulcerates and refuses to heal. The centre becomes depressed and the rolled edges become translucent, revealing many tiny blood vessels. Rodent ulcers do not disappear and if left untreated may invade the underlying bone. *This is the most common form of skin cancer.*

Squamous cell carcinoma

This is a malignant tumour which arises from the prickle cell layer of the epidermis. It is hard and warty and eventually develops a 'heaped-up, cauliflower appearance'. It is most frequently seen in elderly people.

Inflammatory Skin Conditions

Contact dermatitis

Dermatitis literally means 'inflammation of the skin'. Contact dermatitis is caused by a primary irritant which causes the skin to become red, dry and inflamed. Substances which are likely to cause this reaction include acids, alkalis, solvent, perfumes, lanolin, detergent and nickels. There may be skin infection as well.

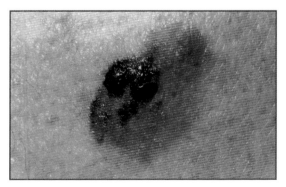

Fig 2.16 Malignant melanoma

Eczema

A mild to chronic inflammatory skin condition characterised by itchiness, redness and the presence of small blisters that may be dry or weep, if the surface is scratched. It can cause scaly and thickened skin, mainly at flexures, for example the cubital area of the elbows and the back of the knees.

Eczema is not contagious; the cause may be genetic or due to internal and external influences.

Psoriasis

A chronic inflammatory skin condition. Psoriasis may be recognised as the development of well-defined red plaques, varying in size and shape, covered by white or silvery scales. Any area of the body may be affected by psoriasis but the most commonly affected sites are the face, elbows, knees, nails, chest and abdomen. It can also affect the scalp, the joints and the nails.

Psoriais is aggravated by stress and trauma but is improved by exposure to sunlight.

Seborrhoeic dermatitis

This is a mild to chronic inflammatory disease of those hairy areas that are well supplied with sebaceous glands. Common sites are the scalp, face, axilla, and the groin. The skin may appear to have a grey tinge or may be dirty yellow in colour. Clinical signs include slight redness, scaling and dandruff in the eyebrows.

Pityriasis simplex capitis (dandruff)

'Dandruff' is a popular collective name signifying a scaly flaking scalp condition. Pityriasis simplex capitis is a non-inflammatory scalp condition which presents as exfoliation of the stratum corneum (outer layer of epidermal cells).

Urticaria

Also known as hives. In this condition lesions appear rapidly and disappear within minutes or gradually over a number of hours. The clinical signs are development of red weals which may later become white. The area becomes itchy or may sting.

There are a number of causes of urticaria, some of which are an allergic reaction to, for example, foods like strawberries, shellfish, or to penicillin, house dust or pet fur. Other causes include stress and sensitivity to light, heat or cold.

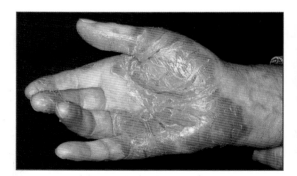

Fig 2.17 Eczema

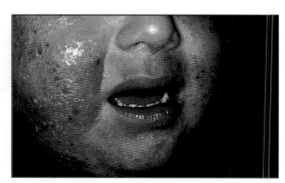

Fig 2.18 Psoriasis

Factors Affecting The Skin

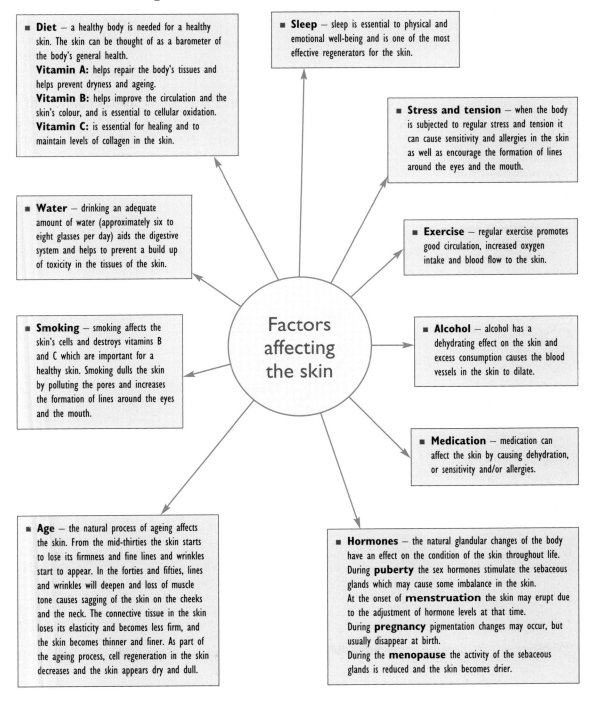

- **Diet** – a healthy body is needed for a healthy skin. The skin can be thought of as a barometer of the body's general health.
  Vitamin A: helps repair the body's tissues and helps prevent dryness and ageing.
  Vitamin B: helps improve the circulation and the skin's colour, and is essential to cellular oxidation.
  Vitamin C: is essential for healing and to maintain levels of collagen in the skin.

- **Sleep** – sleep is essential to physical and emotional well-being and is one of the most effective regenerators for the skin.

- **Stress and tension** – when the body is subjected to regular stress and tension it can cause sensitivity and allergies in the skin as well as encourage the formation of lines around the eyes and the mouth.

- **Water** – drinking an adequate amount of water (approximately six to eight glasses per day) aids the digestive system and helps to prevent a build up of toxicity in the tissues of the skin.

- **Exercise** – regular exercise promotes good circulation, increased oxygen intake and blood flow to the skin.

- **Smoking** – smoking affects the skin's cells and destroys vitamins B and C which are important for a healthy skin. Smoking dulls the skin by polluting the pores and increases the formation of lines around the eyes and the mouth.

- **Alcohol** – alcohol has a dehydrating effect on the skin and excess consumption causes the blood vessels in the skin to dilate.

- **Medication** – medication can affect the skin by causing dehydration, or sensitivity and/or allergies.

Factors affecting the skin

- **Age** – the natural process of ageing affects the skin. From the mid-thirties the skin starts to lose its firmness and fine lines and wrinkles start to appear. In the forties and fifties, lines and wrinkles will deepen and loss of muscle tone causes sagging of the skin on the cheeks and the neck. The connective tissue in the skin loses its elasticity and becomes less firm, and the skin becomes thinner and finer. As part of the ageing process, cell regeneration in the skin decreases and the skin appears dry and dull.

- **Hormones** – the natural glandular changes of the body have an effect on the condition of the skin throughout life. During **puberty** the sex hormones stimulate the sebaceous glands which may cause some imbalance in the skin. At the onset of **menstruation** the skin may erupt due to the adjustment of hormone levels at that time. During **pregnancy** pigmentation changes may occur, but usually disappear at birth. During the **menopause** the activity of the sebaceous glands is reduced and the skin becomes drier.

Factors Affecting Hair Growth

The way our hair looks has a great impact on the way we feel. Shiny lustrous hair is synonymous with good health and vitality. Factors such as diet, age and hormones directly determine its appearance.

- **Diet** — health of the hair comes from within and therefore a poor diet can affect the condition of the hair. For healthy hair, it is important to have a diet rich in protein, essential fatty acids, and essential vitamins and minerals.
  Vitamin B complex and **Vitamin C** to help provide nourishment for hair follicles.
  Minerals such as iron, sulphur and zinc can help the hair if the important mineral content of the hair is missing and the hair is dull in appearance.
  Vitamin B5 is important to help relieve stress in the hair.
  Vitamin A is useful for a dry and scaly scalp.

- **Medication** — medication can affect the hair by drying the skin which in turn blocks the follicles with dead keratinised cells, blocking the circulation to the scalp.

- **Hormonal influences** — the hair is often affected by hormonal changes occurring in the body such as puberty, pregnancy and the menopause.
  Hair can become more greasy during **menstruation**.
  Hair may become dry due to a **thyroid** problem or there may be a temporary hair loss during **pregnancy** (especially after delivery).
  A drop in oestrogen during the **menopause** can have a profound effect on the hair, causing it to become dry, coarse and brittle.

Factors affecting hair growth

- **Illness** — prolonged illness and stress can cause both hair loss and greying, due to the fact that the body is starved of essential nutrients and cell metabolism is slowed down due to infection and/or disease.

- **Allergies** — reaction to products used on the hair and scalp may cause sensitisation of the scalp and this can affect the circulation of blood to the hair. Some clients may develop dandruff in response to sensitisation of hair products.

- **Over processing** — perming and dyeing the hair can alter the shaft of the hair often making it dry and brittle. Frequent use of shampoos full of detergents and chemicals can also dry out the scalp.

- **Stress and tension** — tension in the scalp can reduce the circulation of oxygen and starve the hair root of nutrients needed for healthy growth. Stress can also cause hair loss and premature greying.

The Skeleton

The skeleton is the structure and framework on which other body systems depend for support and protection and is therefore the physical foundation of the body. The main functions of the skeleton are to provide a means of protection, support and attachment for muscles. The skeleton is very important to a therapist as it provides landmarks for locating muscles.

The Structure of Bone

Bone is one of the hardest types of connective tissue in the body, and when fully developed is composed of water, calcium salts and organic matter. Bone tissue is living tissue made from special cells called osteoblasts. There are two main types of bone tissue: compact and cancellous. All bones have both types of tissue, the amount being dependent on the type of bone.

Compact (dense) bone

This is the hard portion of the bone that makes up the main shaft of the long bones and the outer layer of other bones. It protects spongy bone and provides a firm framework for the bone and the body.

Cancellous (spongy) bone

In contrast, this is lighter in weight than compact bone. It has an open sponge-like appearance, and is found at the ends of long bones or at the centre of other bones.

The Development of Bone

The process of bone development is called ossification. This process begins in the embryo near the end of the second month, and is not complete until about the twenty-fifth year of life.

Types of bone

Bones are classified according to their shape. The classifications are long bones, short bones, flat bones, irregular bones and sesamoid bones.

Long bones

Long bones have a long shaft (a diaphysis) and one or more endings, or swellings, (epiphysis). Smooth hyaline cartilage covers the articular surfaces of the shaft endings. Between the diaphysis and epiphysis of growing bone is a flat plate of hyaline cartilage called the epiphyseal cartilage or growth plate. This is the site of bone growth, and as fast as this cartilage grows it is turned into bone, allowing the bone to continue to grow in length.

KEY NOTE

Children's bones are more flexible as their bodies contain more cartilage and soft bone cells because complete calcification has not yet taken place. In older adults the opposite is true as bone cells outnumber cartilage cells and the bone becomes more brittle due to the fact it contains more minerals and fewer blood vessels. This explains why elderly people's bones are more prone to fracture and slower to heal.

Short bones

These bones are generally cube-shaped, with their lengths and widths being roughly equal. The bones of the wrist and the ankle are examples of short bones.

Flat bones

Flat bones are plate-like structures with broad surfaces. Examples include the ribs and the scapulae.

Irregular bones

Irregular bones have a variety of shapes. Examples include the vertebrae and some of the facial bones.

Sesamoid bones

These are small, rounded bones that are embedded in a tendon.

The areas treated with Indian Head Massage include the upper back, shoulders, neck, upper arms and head. These parts are discussed to give the therapist a knowledge of the anatomy of the treatment area.

Vertebrae

The spine, which provides a central axis to the body, consists of 33 individual irregular bones called vertebrae.

The spine is made up of the following:

- 7 cervical vertebrae – bones in the neck
- 12 thoracic vertebrae – bones of the mid spine
- 5 lumbar vertebrae – bones of the lower back
- 5 sacral vertebrae – fused to form sacrum
- 4 coccygeal vertebrae – fused to form coccyx or tail bone.

Vertebrae of the neck

The neck comprises seven bones known as the cervical vertebrae. Although they are the smallest vertebrae in the spine, their bone tissue is denser than those in any other region of the vertebral column.

The top two cervical vertebrae are named C1 and C2.

- **C1** is called the **atlas** and is the bone that sits at the top of the vertebral column embedded in the base of the skull. The atlas supports and balances the head. Sliding joints on either side of the atlas allow the head to move up and down.

- **C2** is called the **axis** and has a peg-like hook that fits into a notch in the atlas. The ring and peg structure of the atlas and axis allows for movement of the head from side to side.

The transverse processes of the cervical vertebrae are distinctive in that they have transverse foramina (or holes) which serve as passageways for arteries leading to the brain.

The spinous processes of the second through to the fifth cervical vertebrae are uniquely forked to provide attachment for the elaborate lattice of muscles of the neck. The spinous process of the seventh cervical vertebrae is longer and can be felt through the skin as it protrudes beyond the other cervical spines.

Vertebrae of the mid spine

There are 12 thoracic vertebrae of the mid spine and these lie in the thorax where they articulate with the ribs. These vertebrae lie flatter and downwards to allow for muscular attachment of the large muscle groups of the back.

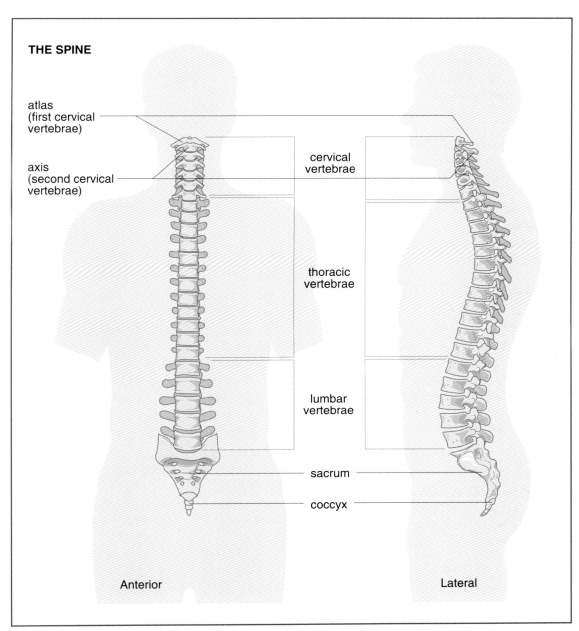

THE SPINE

atlas
(first cervical
vertebrae)

axis
(second cervical
vertebrae)

cervical
vertebrae

thoracic
vertebrae

lumbar
vertebrae

sacrum

coccyx

Anterior

Lateral

Fig 2.19 Vertebrae of the spine

Vertebrae of the lower back

There are five vertebrae that lie in the lower back and they are much larger than the vertebrae above them as they are designed to support body weight.

Sacrum

The sacrum is made up of five fused vertebrae that form a flat triangular-shaped bone lying between the pelvic bones.

Coccyx

The coccyx is made of four coccygeal vertebrae fused together.

The Thoracic Cavity

This is the area of the body enclosed by the ribs, providing protection for the heart and lungs.

Essential bones found in the thoracic cavity include:

- the sternum
- the ribs
- 12 thoracic vertebrae.

The sternum

This is commonly referred to as the breast bone and is a flat bone lying just beneath the skin in the centre of the chest.

The sternum is divided into three parts:

- the manubrium, the top section
- the main body, the middle section
- the xiphoid process, the bottom section.

The top section of the sternum articulates with the clavicle and the first rib. The middle section articulates with the costal cartilages that link the ribs to the sternum. The bottom section provides a point of attachment for the muscles of the diaphragm and the abdominal wall.

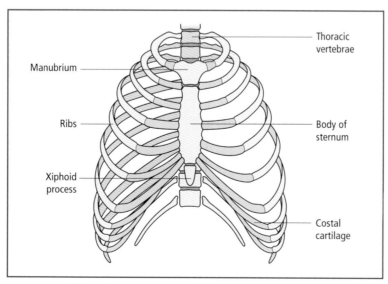

Fig 2.20 The thoracic cavity

The ribs

There are 12 pairs of ribs. They articulate with the thoracic vertebrae posteriorly. Anteriorly, the first ten pairs attach to the sternum via the costal cartilages, the first seven directly (known as the true ribs), the remaining three indirectly (known as the false ribs). The last two ribs have no anterior attachment and are called the floating ribs.

The Bones of the Shoulders

The shoulder girdle connects the upper limbs with the thorax and consists of four bones:

- two clavicles
- two scapulae.

The **clavicle** forms the anterior part of the shoulder girdle. It is a long slender bone with a double curve which is located at the base of the neck and runs horizontally between the sternum and the shoulders. It articulates with the sternum at its medial end and the scapula at its lateral end. The clavicle acts as a brace for the scapula, helping to hold the shoulders in place.

The **scapulae** form the posterior part of the shoulder girdle and are located on either side of the upper back. The scapula is a large flat bone, triangular in outline, which articulates with the clavicle and the humerus. The scapula has several prominent processes that serve as attachments for muscles and ligaments. The combined action of scapula, clavicle, humerus and associated muscles allows for a considerable amount of movement of the shoulder and upper limbs.

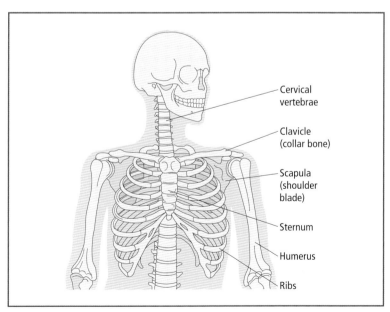

Cervical vertebrae

Clavicle (collar bone)

Scapula (shoulder blade)

Sternum

Humerus

Ribs

Fig 2.21 Bones of the neck, chest and shoulder girdle

Bones of the Upper Limb

The upper limb consists of the following bones:

- humerus
- radius
- ulna
- carpals
- metacarpals
- phalanges.

Humerus

The humerus is the long bone of the upper arm. The head of the humerus

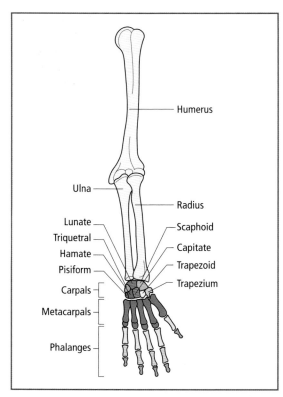

Fig 2.22 Bones of the upper limb

articulates with the scapula, forming the shoulder joint. The distal end of the bone articulates with the radius and ulna to form the elbow joint.

The radius and ulna

The ulna and radius are the long bones of the forearm. The two bones are bound together by a fibrous ring, which allows a rotating movement in which the bones pass over each other. The ulna is the bone of the little finger side and is the longer of the two forearm bones. The radius is situated on the thumb side of the forearm. The joint between the ulna and the radius permits a movement called pronation. This is when the radius moves obliquely across the ulna so that the thumb side of the hand is closest to the body. The movement called supination takes the thumb side of the hand to the lateral side. The radius and the ulna articulate with the humerus at the elbow and the carpal bones at the wrist.

The wrist and hand

Carpals

The wrist consists of eight small bones of irregular size which are collectively called carpals. They fit closely together and are held in place by ligaments. The carpals are arranged in two groups of four; those of the upper row articulate with the ulna and the radius and the lower row articulates with the metacarpals. The upper row nearest the forearm consists of the scaphoid, lunate, triquetral and pisiform; the lower row consists of the trapezium, trapezoid, capitate and hamate.

Metacarpals

There are five long metacarpal bones in the palm of the hand; their proximal ends articulate with the wrist bones and the distal ends articulate with the finger bones.

Phalanges

There are fourteen phalanges, which are the finger bones, two of which are in the thumb or pollex and three in each of the other digits.

Bones of the Skull

The skull rests upon the upper end of the vertebral column and weighs around eleven pounds! It consists of twenty-two bones; eight bones that make up the cranium and fourteen forming the facial skeleton. The cranium encloses and protects the brain and provides a surface attachment for various muscles of the skull.

The eight bones of the cranium are as follows:

- One **frontal*** bone forms the anterior part of the roof of the skull, the forehead and the upper part of the orbits or eye sockets. Within the frontal bones are the two frontal sinuses, one above each eye near the midline.

- Two **parietal*** bones form the upper sides of the skull and the back of the roof of the skull.

- Two **temporal*** bones form the sides of the skull below the parietal and above and around the ears. The temporal bone contributes to part of the cheekbone via the zygomatic arch (formed by the zygomatic and temporal bones). Located behind the ear and below the line of the temporal bones are the mastoid processes to which the sternomastoid muscles of the neck are attached.

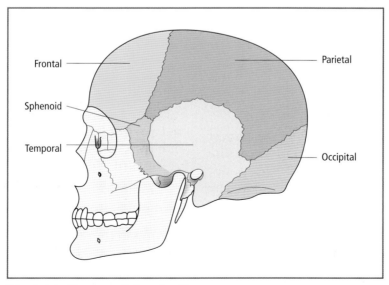

Fig 2.23 Bones of the skull

■ One **sphenoid** bone which is located in front of the temporal bone and serves as a bridge between the cranium and the facial bones. It articulates with the frontal, temporal, occipital and ethmoid bones.

■ One **ethmoid** bone which forms part of the wall of the orbit, the roof of the nasal cavity and part of the nasal septum.

■ The **occipital*** bone which forms the back of the skull.

*These bones are considered to be the primary bones of the skull.

> **KEY NOTE**
> There are many openings present in the bones of the skull which act as passages for blood vessels and nerves entering and leaving the cranial cavity. For instance, there is a large opening at the base of the skull called the foramen magnum through which the spinal cord and blood vessels pass to and from the brain.

Bones of the face

There are 14 facial bones in total and these are mainly in pairs, one on either side of the face:

■ two **maxillae*** – these are the largest bones of the face and they form the upper jaw and support the upper teeth. An important part of the maxillae are the maxillary sinuses which open into the nasal cavity.

■ one **mandible*** – this is the only moveable bone of the skull and forms the lower jaw and supports the lower teeth.

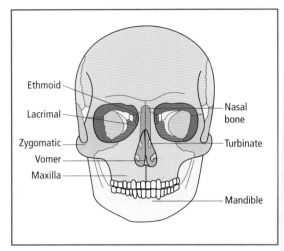

Fig 2.24 Bones of the face

■ two **zygomatic*** – these are the most prominent of the facial bones and they form the cheekbones.

■ two **nasal** – these small bones form the bridge of the nose.

■ two **lacrimal** – these are the smallest of the facial bones and are located close to the medial part of the orbital cavity.

■ two **turbinate** – these are layers of bone located on either side of the outer walls of the nasal cavities.

■ one **vomer** – this is a single bone at the back of the nasal septum.

■ two **palatine** – these are L-shaped bones which form the anterior part of the roof of the mouth.

*These bones are considered to be the primary bones of the face.

The sinuses

There are four pairs of air-containing spaces in the skull and face called the sinuses. The function of the sinuses is to

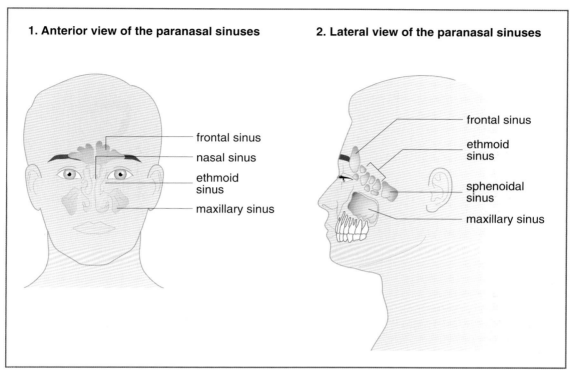

1. Anterior view of the paranasal sinuses

frontal sinus
nasal sinus
ethmoid sinus
maxillary sinus

2. Lateral view of the paranasal sinuses

frontal sinus
ethmoid sinus
sphenoidal sinus
maxillary sinus

Fig 2.25 The sinuses

lighten the head, provide mucus and act as a resonance chamber for sound. The pairs of sinuses are named according to the facial bones by which they are located. They are the frontal sinuses, the sphenoidal sinuses, the ethmoidal sinuses, and the maxillary sinuses (which are the largest).

KEY NOTE

Indian Head Massage can help to make parts of the skeletal system such as the shoulders and neck more mobile by reducing restrictions in the joints, muscles and their fascia.

The Muscular System

There are over 600 skeletal or voluntary muscles in the body that collectively help to create body movement, stabilise joints and maintain body posture. Some skeletal muscles lie superficially, while those layered beneath them are known as deep muscles.

The Functions of the Muscular System

The muscular system consists largely of skeletal muscle tissue which covers the bones on the outside and connective tissue which attaches muscles to the bones of the skeleton. Muscles, along with connective tissue, help to give the body its contoured shape.

The muscular system has three main functions:

- movement
- maintenance of posture
- the production of heat.

Muscle Tissue

Muscle tissue makes up about 50 per cent of your total body weight and is composed of:

- 20 per cent protein
- 75 per cent water
- 5 per cent mineral salts, glycogen and fat.

There are three types of muscle tissue in the body:

1 **Skeletal** or **voluntary** muscle tissue which is primarily attached to bone.

2 **Cardiac** muscle tissue which is found in the walls of the heart.

3 **Smooth** or **involuntary** muscle tissue which is found inside the digestive and urinary tracts, as well as in the walls of blood vessels.

All three types of muscle tissue differ in their structure and functions and the degree of control the nervous system has upon them.

Voluntary muscle tissue

Voluntary muscle tissue is made up of bands of elastic or contractile tissue bound together in bundles and enclosed by a connective tissue sheath which protects the muscle and helps to give it a contoured shape.

Voluntary or skeletal muscle tissue has very little intercellular tissue; it consists almost entirely of muscle fibres held together by fibrous connective tissue and penetrated by numerous tiny blood vessels and nerves. The long slender fibres that make up muscle cells vary in size; some are around 30 cm in length, whereas others are microscopic.

Each muscle fibre is enclosed in an individual wrapping of fine connective tissue called the endomysium. These are wrapped together in bundles, known as fasciculi, covered by the perimysium (fibrous sheath), and are then gathered to form the muscle belly (main part of the muscle) with its own sheath – the fascia epimysium.

The relatively inelastic parts of each of the muscles are tendons, and these are usually made up of the continuation of the endomysium and perimysium.

Each muscle fibre is made up of even thinner fibres called myofibrils. These consist of long strands of microfilaments, made up of two different types of protein strands called actin and myosin. It is the arrangement of actin and myosin filaments which gives the skeletal muscle its striated or striped appearance when viewed under a microscope.

Muscle fibre contraction results from a sliding movement within the myofibrils in which actin and myosin filaments merge. Voluntary muscle works intimately with the nervous system and will therefore only contract if a stimulus is applied to it via a motor nerve. Each muscle fibre receives its own nerve impulse so that fine

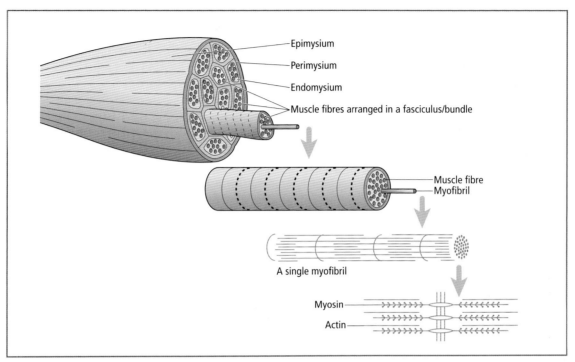

Epimysium
Perimysium
Endomysium
Muscle fibres arranged in a fasciculus/bundle
Muscle fibre
Myofibril
A single myofibril
Myosin
Actin

Fig 2.26 The structure of voluntary muscle tissue

and varied motions are possible. Voluntary muscles also have their own small stored supply of glycogen which is used as fuel for energy. Voluntary muscle tissue differs from other types of muscle tissue in that the muscles tire easily and need regular exercise.

Cardiac muscle

Cardiac muscle is a specialised type of involuntary muscle tissue found only in the walls of the heart. Forming the bulk of the wall of each heart chamber, cardiac muscle contracts rhythmically and continuously to provide the pumping action necessary to maintain a relatively consistent flow of blood throughout the body.

Cardiac muscle resembles voluntary muscle tissue in that it is striated due to the actin and myosin filaments. However, it differs in that it:

■ is branched in structure

■ has intercalated discs between each cardiac muscle cell. These form strong junctions to assist in the rapid transmission of impulses throughout an entire section of the heart, rather than in bundles.

The contraction of the heart is automatic; the stimulus to contract is stimulated from a specialised area of muscle in the heart called the sinoatrial (SA) node, which controls the heart

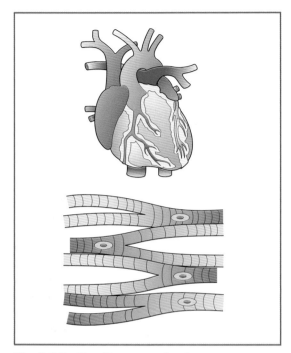

Fig 2.27 Cardiac muscle tissue

rate. As the heart has to alter its force of contraction due to regional requirements, its contraction is regulated not only by nerves, but also by hormones. For example, adrenaline in the blood can speed up contractions.

Smooth muscle

Smooth muscle is also known as involuntary muscle, as it is not under the control of the conscious part of the brain. It is found in the walls of hollow organs such as the stomach, intestines, bladder, uterus and in blood vessels.

The main characteristics of smooth muscle are:

- the muscle cells are spindle-shaped and tapered at both ends

- each muscle cell contains one centrally located oval-shaped nucleus.

Smooth muscle has no striations due to the different arrangement of the protein filaments, actin and myosin, which are attached at their ends to the cell's plasma membrane.

The muscle fibres of smooth muscle are adapted for long, sustained contraction and therefore consume very little energy. One of the special features of smooth muscle is that it can stretch and shorten to a greater extent and still maintain its contractile function. Smooth muscle will contract or relax in response to nerve impulses, stretching or hormones.

Smooth muscle, like voluntary muscle has muscle tone and this is important in areas such as the intestines where the walls have to maintain a steady pressure on the contents.

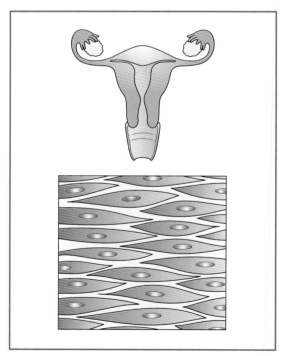

Fig 2.28 Smooth/involuntary muscle tissue

Muscle tone

Even in a relaxed muscle, a few muscle fibres remain contracted to give the muscle a certain degree of firmness. At any given time, a small number of motor units in a muscle are stimulated to contract and cause tension in the muscle rather than full contraction and movement, whilst the others remain relaxed. This state of partial contraction of a muscle is known as muscle tone and is important for maintaining body posture. The group of motor units functioning in this way change periodically so that muscle tone is maintained without fatigue.

KEY NOTE

An increase in the size and diameter of muscle fibres, usually caused by exercise and weight lifting, leads to a condition called hypertrophy.

KEY NOTE

Muscle tone will vary from person to person and will largely depend on the amount of exercise undertaken.
Muscles with good tone have a better blood supply as their blood vessels will not be inhibited by fat.

Good muscle tone may be recognised by the muscles appearing firm and rounded. Poor muscle tone may be recognised by the muscles appearing loose and flattened.

Muscles with less than the normal degree of tone are said to be flaccid and when the muscle tone is greater than normal the muscles become spastic and rigid.

Detailed below are the main muscles involved in Indian Head Massage.

Muscles of the Scalp

Muscle	Position	Attachments	Action	Key Note
Occipitalis	back of the head	to the occipital bone and skin of the scalp	moves the scalp backwards	occipitalis is united to the frontalis muscle by a broad tendon which covers the skull like a cap
Frontalis	front of the skull and across width of forehead	to the skin of eyebrows and the frontal bone at the hairline	wrinkles the forehead and raises the eyebrows	used when expressing surprise
Temporalis	at the sides of the skull above and in front of the ear	to the temporal bone and to the upper part of the mandible	raises the lower jaw when chewing	becomes overtight and painful when there is excessive tension in the jaw

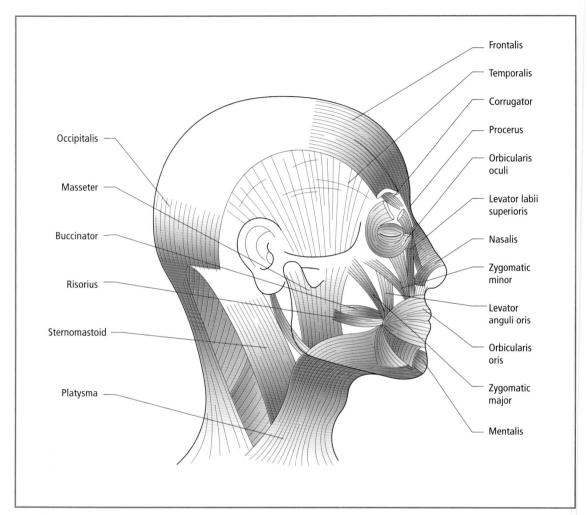

Fig 2.29 Muscles of the head and neck

Muscles of the Head and Neck

Muscle	Position	Attachments	Action	Key Note
Sternomastoid	lies obliquely across each side of the neck	extends from the clavicle and sternum at one end to the mastoid process of the temporal bone (at the back of the ear)	together they flex the neck (pull chin down towards chest); singly they rotate the head to the opposite side.	tends to go into spasm when the head is consistently turned to one side, or pointing downwards, as in working on the telephone and at a desk
Platysma	covers the anterior surface of the neck	extends from chest (upper part of pectoralis major and deltoid) up either side of the neck to the chin	depresses the lower jaw and lower lip	used when yawning and when creating a pouting expression
Orbicularis oculi	circular muscle that surrounds the eye, situated in the subcutaneous tissue of the eyelid	attached to the outer orbits of the eyes, and the skin of the upper and lower eyelids	closes the eye	used when blinking or winking; it also compresses the lacrimal gland, aiding the flow of tears
Orbicularis oris	circular muscle surrounding the mouth	to the maxilla, mandible, lips and the buccinator muscle	closes the mouth	used when shaping the lips for speech and when kissing; it also contracts when tense, as the lips tend to tighten
Corrugator	between the eyebrows	to the frontalis muscle and the inner edge of the eyebrow	brings the eyebrows together	used when frowning
Procerus	in-between the eyebrows	to the nasal bones and the frontalis muscle	draws the eyebrows inwards	contraction creates a puzzled expression
Nasalis	sides of the nose	to the maxillae bones and the nostrils	dilates and compresses the nostrils	used when blowing the nose

▶

Muscle	Position	Attachments	Action	Key Note
Zygomatic major and minor	in the cheek region	from the zygomatic bone to the angle of the mouth	draws angle of mouth upwards and laterally	used when laughing
Levator labii superiorus	towards the inner cheek beside the nose	from upper jaw to the skin at the corners of the mouth and upper lip	raises the upper lip and corner of the mouth	used to create a snarling expression
Risorius	lies horizontally on the cheek, joining at the corners of the mouth	attaches to the zygomatic bone at one end, and the skin of the corner of the mouth at the other end	pulls corner of mouth sideways and upwards	used to create a grinning expression
Buccinator	main muscle in the cheek	attaches to both upper and lower jaw, from the bones of the jaw to the angle of the mouth	compresses the cheek	used when blowing up a balloon or when using a wind instrument
Mentalis	on the chin	attaches to the lower jaw and the skin of lower lip	elevates the lower lip and wrinkles skin of chin	used when expressing displeasure and when pouting
Masseter	thick flattened muscles, over the outer part of the cheek and jaw	from the zygomatic arch to the mandible	raises the jaw and exerts pressure on the teeth when chewing	holds a lot of tension and can be felt just in front of the ear when the teeth are clenched
Triangularis	below the corners of the mouth	from the lower jaw to the skin and muscles of the corner of the mouth	draws the corners of the mouth downwards	used to create an expression of sadness

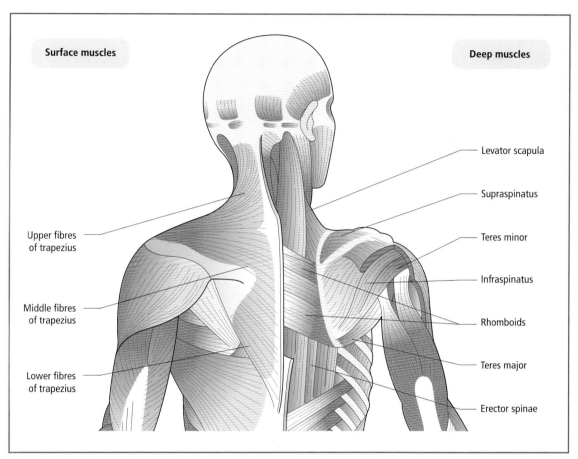

Surface muscles

Deep muscles

Levator scapula

Supraspinatus

Upper fibres
of trapezius

Teres minor

Infraspinatus

Middle fibres
of trapezius

Rhomboids

Teres major

Lower fibres
of trapezius

Erector spinae

Fig 2.30 Muscles of the back and shoulders

Muscles of the Back and Shoulders

Muscle	Position	Attachments	Action	Key Note
Erector spinae	three bands of muscle that lie in the groove between the vertebral column and the ribs	attaches to the sacrum and the iliac crest of pelvis at one end, then to the ribs and the transverse and spinous processes of the vertebrae, and finally to the occipital bone at the other end	extension, lateral (side) flexion and rotation of the vertebral column	a very important postural muscle as it helps to extend the spine
Trapezius	large triangular-shaped muscle in the upper back; fibres are arranged in three groups: upper, middle and lower	extends horizontally from the base of the skull, and the cervical and thoracic vertebrae to the scapula	upper fibres raise the shoulders; middle fibres pull the scapula towards the spine; lower fibres draw the shoulders downwards	commonly holds a lot of upper body tension, causing discomfort and restrictions in the neck and the shoulders
Levator scapula	long strap-like muscle that runs almost vertically through the neck	from the scapula to the cervical vertebrae of the neck	elevates and adducts the scapula (draws the scapula towards spine)	tends to become very tight, which affects the mobility of the neck and the shoulder
Rhomboids	between the scapulae	to the upper thoracic vertebrae at one end and the medial border of the scapula at the other end	adduct the scapula (draw the scapula towards the spine)	often very tight, resulting in aching and soreness in-between the scapulae
Supraspinatus	in the depression above the spine (top ridge) of the scapula	attaches to the spine of the scapula at one end and the humerus at the other end	abducts the humerus (draws the arm away from the body)	often becomes fatigued when working for prolonged periods at a desk or computer, or when driving

Muscle	Position	Attachments	Action	Key Note
Infraspinatus	below the spine of the scapula	attaches to the middle two-thirds of the scapula at one end and the top of the humerus at the other	rotates the humerus laterally (outwards)	tension here can affect the range of mobility in the shoulder
Teres major	across the bottom lateral (outer) edge of the scapula	attaches to the bottom lateral edge of the scapula at one end and the back of the humerus at the other end	adducts and medially (inwardly) rotates humerus	tension here can restrict the mobility of the shoulder and upper arm
Teres minor	across the lateral edge of the scapula, above teres major	attaches to the lateral edge of the scapula, above teres major at one end, and into the top of the posterior of the humerus at the other end	rotates humerus laterally (outwards)	tension here can restrict the mobility of the shoulder and upper arm

Muscles of the Upper Limbs

Muscle	Position	Attachments	Action	Key Note
Deltoid	caps the top of the humerus and the shoulder	attaches to the clavicle and the spine of the scapula at one end and to the side of the humerus at the other	abducts the arm (draws the arm away from the body), draws the arm backwards and forwards	tends to hold upper body tension and will often go into spasm, along with the trapezius muscle
Biceps	anterior (front) of the upper arm	attaches to the scapula at one end and the radius and flexor muscles of the forearm at the other end	flexes the forearm	becomes tight when the body assumes a tension posture (hunched shoulders and arms, elbows hugged tight against the body)

▶

Muscle	Position	Attachments	Action	Key Note
Triceps	posterior (back) of the humerus	attaches to the posterior of the humerus and the outer edge of the scapula at one end, to the ulna below the elbow at the other end	extension (straightens) the forearm	becomes tight when the body assumes a tension posture (hunched shoulders and arms, elbows hugged tight against the body)

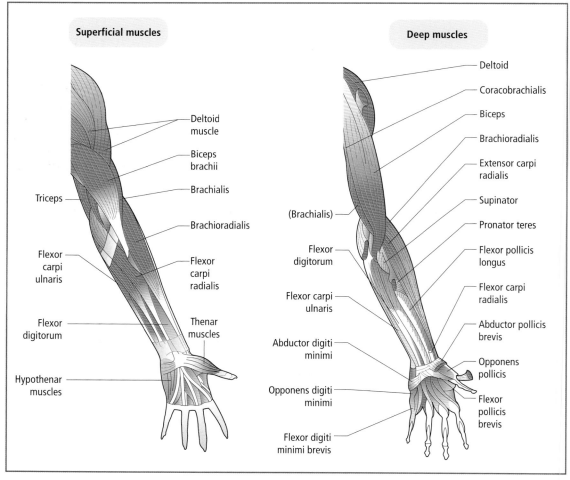

Fig 2.31 Muscles of the upper limbs (anterior)

Flexors of the Forearm

Muscle	Position	Attachments	Action	Key Note
Brachio-radialis	siutated on the radial side of the forearm	attaches to the distal end of the humerus at one end and the radius at the other end	flexes forearm at the elbow	sometimes nicknamed the 'hitchhiker muscle' for its characteritsic action of flexing the forearm in a position halfway between full pronation and full supination
Flexor carpi radialis	extends along the radial side of the anterior of the forearm	from the medial end of the humerus to radial side of forearm and the base of the second and third metacarpals	flexion of the wrist	any of the flexor muscles in the forearm can become easily inflamed due to excess pressure and overwork, a common example being using a keyboard for extended periods of time
Flexor carpi ulnaris	extends along the ulnar side of the anterior of the forearm	from the medial end of the humerus to the pisiform and hamate carpal bones and the base of the fifth metacarpal	flexion of the wrist	see above
Flexor carpi digitorum	extends across the anterior of the radius and ulna	extends from the medial end of the humerus, the anterior of the ulna and radius, to the anterior surfaces of the second to the fifth fingers	flexion of the fingers	see above

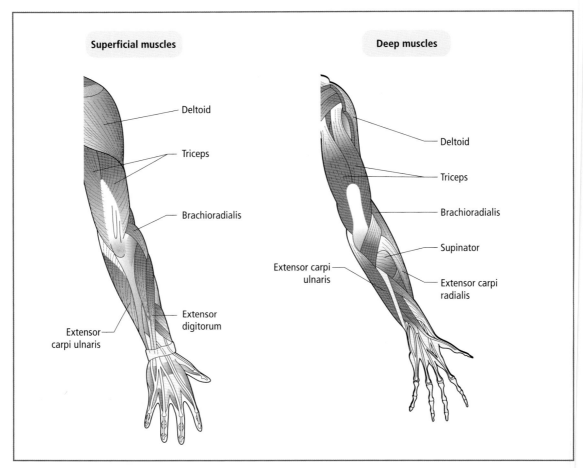

Fig 2.32 Muscles of the upper limbs (posterior)

Extensors of the Forearm

Muscle	Position	Attachments	Action	Key Note
Extensor carpi radialis	extends along the radial side of the posterior of the forearm	from above the lateral end of the humerus to the posterior of the base of the second metacarpal	extension of the wrist	any of the extensor muscles in the forearm can become easily inflamed due to excess pressure and overwork, a common example being using a keyboard for extended periods of time

Muscle	Position	Attachments	Action	Key Note
Extensor carpi ulnaris	extends along the ulnar side of the posterior of the forearm	from above the lateral end of the humerus to the ulna and the posterior side of the base of the fifth metacarpal	extension of the wrist	see above
Extensor digitorum	along the lateral side of the posterior of the forearm	from the lateral end of the humerus to the second to fifth phalanges	extension of the fingers	see above

Muscles of the Hand

Muscle	Position	Action
Thenar eminence	an eminence of soft tissue located on the radial side of the palm of the hand; there are three muscles of the thenar eminence: ■ abductor pollicis brevis ■ flexor pollicis brevis ■ opponens pollicis	all three muscles move the thumb
Hypothenar eminence	an eminence of soft tissue located on the ulnar side of the palm of the hand; there are three muscles of the hypothenar eminence: ■ abductor digiti minimi manus ■ flexor digiti minimi manus ■ opponens digiti minimi	all three muscles move the little finger

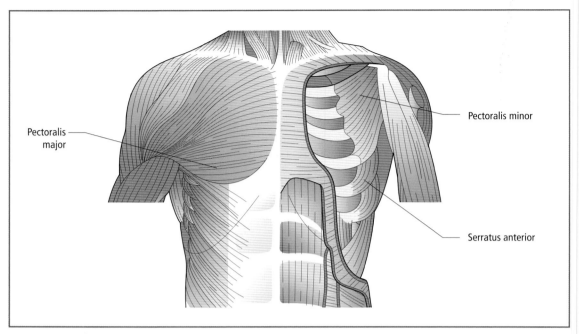

Fig 2.33 Muscles of the chest

Muscles of the Chest

Muscle	Position	Attachments	Action	Key Note
Pectoralis major	covers the front of the upper chest	attaches to the clavicle and sternum at one end and to the humerus at the other end	adducts the arm, medially (inwardly) rotates arm	tightness in the pectoralis major may cause constriction of the chest and result in postural distortions (rounded shoulders)
Pectoralis minor	thin strap-like muscle that lies beneath the pectoralis major muscle	from the upper ribs at one end to the scapula at the other end	draws the shoulder downwards and forwards	Tightness in the pectoralis minor may cause constriction of the chest and result in postural distortions (rounded shoulders)

Muscle	Position	Attachments	Action	Key Note
Serratus anterior	situated on the side of the chest/ ribcage	attaches to the outer surface of the upper eighth or ninth rib at one end to the inner surface of the scapula, along the medial edge nearest the spine	pulls the scapula downwards and forwards	can be affected by chest problems and breathing difficulties

KEY NOTE

Muscular tension is often a sign of emotional as well as physical stress. Indian Head Massage can help to relieve pain from tight, sore muscles as well as relieve muscular fatigue, by increasing blood flow which increases the amount of oxygen and nutrition into the muscles and encourages elimination of waste, absorbing the products of fatigue.

Posture

Posture is a measure of balance and body alignment, and is the maintenance of strength and tone of the body's muscles against gravity. Good posture is said to be when the maximum efficiency of the body is maintained with the minimum effort. When evaluating posture, an imaginary line is drawn vertically through the body and called the centre of gravity line. From the front or back this line should divide the body into two symmetrical halves:

- with feet together the ankles and knees should touch
- the hips should be the same height
- the shoulders should be level

- the sternum and vertebral column should run down the centre of the body in line with the centre of gravity line
- the head should be erect and not tilted to one side.

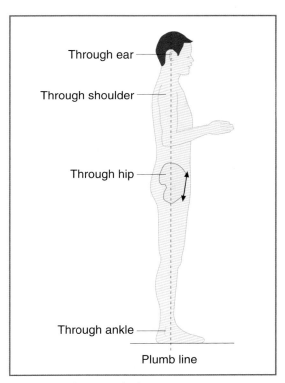

Fig 2.34 Postural alignment

Posture varies considerably in individuals and is influenced by factors such as body frame size, heredity, occupation, habits and personality. Additional factors which may also affect posture include clothing, shoes and furniture.

Good posture is important as it:

- allows a full range of movement
- improves physical appearance
- keeps muscle action to a minimum, thereby conserving energy and reducing fatigue
- reduces the susceptibility of injuries
- aids the body's systems to function efficiently.

Postural defects

Lordosis

This is an abnormally increased inward curvature of the lumbar spine. In this condition the pelvis tilts forward and as the back is hollow the abdomen and buttocks protrude, and the knees may be hyperextended. Typical problems associated with this condition are tightening of the back muscles followed by a weakening of the abdominal muscles. Because of the anterior tilt of the pelvis, hamstring problems are common. An increase in weight or pregnancy may cause or exacerbate this condition.

Kyphosis

This is an abnormally increased outward curvature of the thoracic spine. In this condition the back appears round as the shoulders point forward and the head moves forward. A tightening of the pectoral muscles is common in this condition.

Scoliosis

This is a lateral curvature of the vertebral column, which may be to the left or right side. Evident signs of this condition include unequal leg length, distortion of the ribcage, unequal position of the hips or shoulders and curvature of the spine (usually in the thoracic region).

Poor posture may have the following effects on the body:

- produce alterations in body function and movement
- waste energy
- increase fatigue

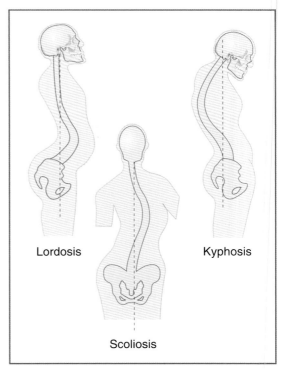

Fig 2.35 Postural defects

- increase the risk of backache and headaches
- impair breathing
- increase the risk of muscular, ligament or joint injury
- affect circulation
- affect digestion
- give a poor physical appearance.

Blood

Blood is the fluid tissue or medium in which all materials are transported to and from individual cells in the body. Blood is therefore the chief transport system of the body.

The Percentage Composition of Blood

Fifty-five per cent of blood is fluid or plasma, which is a clear, pale yellow slightly alkaline fluid:

- 91 per cent of plasma is water
- 9 per cent remaining consists of dissolved blood proteins, waste, digested food materials, mineral salts and hormones.

Forty-five per cent of blood is made up of the blood cells: erythrocytes, leucocytes and thrombocytes.

Functions of Blood

There are four main functions of blood:

- transport
- defence
- regulation
- clotting.

Transport

Blood is the primary transport medium for a variety of substances that travel throughout the body.

- Oxygen is carried from the lungs to the cells of the body in red blood cells.
- Carbon dioxide is carried from the body's cells to the lungs.
- Nutrients such as glucose, amino acids, vitamins and minerals are carried from the small intestine to the cells of the body.
- Cellular wastes such as water, carbon dioxide, lactic acid and urea are carried in the blood to be excreted.
- Hormones, which are internal secretions that help to control important body processes, are transported by the blood to target organs.

KEY NOTE

Red blood cells are called erythrocytes and they contain the red protein pigment haemoglobin that combines with oxygen to form oxyhaemoglobin. The pigment haemoglobin assists the function of the erythrocyte in transporting oxygen from the lungs to the body's cells and carrying carbon dioxide away.

Defence

White blood cells are collectively called leucocytes and they play a major role in combating disease and fighting infection.

KEY NOTE

White blood cells are known as phagocytes as they have the ability to engulf and ingest micro-organisms which invade the body and cause disease. Specialised white blood cells called lymphocytes produce antibodies to protect the body against infection.

Regulation

Blood helps to regulate the body's temperature by absorbing large quantities of heat produced by the liver and the muscles; this is then transported around the body to help to maintain a constant internal temperature. Blood also helps to regulate the body's pH balance.

Clotting

If the skin becomes damaged, specialised blood cells called thrombocytes clot to prevent the body from losing too much blood and to prevent the entry of bacteria.

KEY NOTE

Thrombocytes are also known as platelets. These are small fragments of cells and are the smallest cellular elements of the blood. They are formed in bone marrow and are disc-shaped with no nucleus.

Blood Vessels

Blood flows round the body due to the pumping action of the heart and is carried in vessels known as arteries, veins and capillaries.

Key factors about blood vessels

Arteries

- Arteries carry blood away from the heart.
- Blood is carried under high pressure.
- Arteries have thick muscular and elastic walls to withstand pressure.
- Arteries have no valves, except at the base of the pulmonary artery, where they leave the heart.
- Arteries carry oxygenated blood (except the pulmonary artery to the lungs).
- Arteries are generally deep-seated, except where they cross over a pulse spot.
- Arteries give rise to small blood vessels called arterioles which deliver blood to the capillaries.

Veins

- Veins carry blood towards the heart.
- Blood is carried under low pressure.
- Vein walls are thinner and less muscular.
- Veins have valves at intervals to prevent the backflow of blood.
- Veins carry deoxygenated blood (except the pulmonary veins from the lungs).

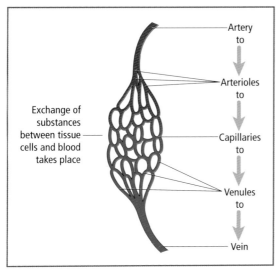

Artery
to

Arterioles
to

Capillaries
to

Venules
to

Vein

Exchange of
substances
between tissue
cells and blood
takes place

Fig 2.36 Blood flow from an artery to a vein

- Veins are generally superficial, not deep-seated.
- Veins form finer blood vessels called venules which continue from capillaries.

KEY NOTE

Both arteries and veins have three layers (external, middle and internal layers) but because an artery must contain the pressure of blood pumped from the heart, its walls are thicker and more elastic.

Capillaries

- Capillaries are the smallest vessels.
- Capillaries unite arterioles and venules, forming a network in the tissues.

- The wall of a capillary vessel is only a single layer of cells thick. It is therefore sufficiently thin to allow the process of diffusion of dissolved substances to and from the tissues to occur.
- Capillaries have no valves.
- Blood is carried under low pressure, but higher than in veins.
- Capillaries are responsible for supplying the cells and tissues with nutrients.

KEY NOTE

The key function of a capillary is to permit the exchange of nutrients and waste between the blood and tissue cells. Substances such as oxygen, vitamins, minerals and amino acids pass through to the tissue fluid to nourish the nearby cells, and substances such as carbon dioxide and waste are passed out of the cell. This exchange of nutrients can only occur through the semipermeable membrane of a capillary, as the walls of arteries and veins are too thick.

Oxygenated blood flowing through the arteries appears bright red in colour due to the oxygen pigment haemoglobin; as it moves through capillaries it offloads some of its oxygen and picks up carbon dioxide. This explains why the blood in veins appears darker.

The Circulatory System

The circulatory system comprises blood, the heart and the vast network of circulatory vessels known as arteries, veins and capillaries. The primary function of the circulatory system is transportation. Within the cardiovascular system there are two circuits: the pulmonary circulation and the systemic circulation.

The pulmonary circulation brings deoxygenated blood from the right ventricle of the heart to the alveoli of the lungs to release carbon dioxide and to regain oxygen. Oxygenated blood returns to the left atrium of the heart and moves into the systemic circuit with the contraction of the left ventricle.

The systemic circuit carries oxygenated blood around the body via the body's main artery: the aorta. On leaving the left ventricle the aorta emerges from the top of the heart. It passes superiorly for a short distance as the ascending aorta and curves to form the arch of the aorta before it passes inferiorly as the descending aorta.

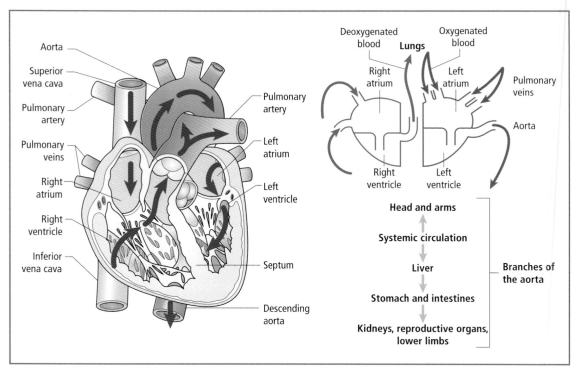

Fig 2.37 Blood circulation/the heart

The Blood Flow to the Head and Neck

As the aorta emerges from the heart it subdivides to form the main trunk called the brachiocephalic trunk which splits and forms:

■ the common carotid artery which supplies oxygenated blood to the head, face and neck and

■ the subclavian artery which supplies blood to the shoulders, chest wall, arms back and central nervous system.

The arterial blood supply to the head and neck

Blood is supplied to parts within the neck, head and brain through branches of the subclavian and common carotid arteries.

The common carotid artery extends from the brachiocephalic trunk and extends on each side of the neck and divides at the level of the larynx into two branches:

■ the internal carotid artery

■ the external carotid artery.

The **internal carotid artery** passes through the temporal bone of the skull to supply oxygenated blood to the brain, eyes, forehead and part of the nose.

The **external carotid artery** is divided into branches (facial, temporal and occipital arteries) which supply the skin and muscles of the face, side and back of the head respectively. This vessel also supplies more superficial structures of the head and neck; these include the salivary glands, scalp, teeth, nose, throat, tongue and thyroid gland.

The **vertebral arteries** are a main division of the subclavian artery. They arise from the subclavian arteries in the base of the neck near the tip of the lungs. They pass upwards through the openings

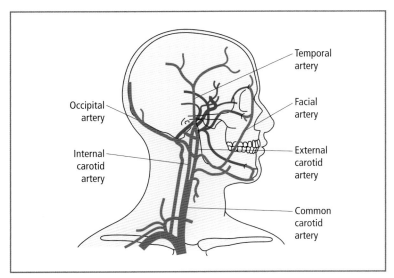

Fig 2.38 Arterial blood supply to the head and neck

(foramina) of transverse processes of the cervical vertebrae and unite to form a single basilar artery. The basilar artery then terminates by dividing into two posterior cerebral arteries that supply the occipital and temporal lobes of the cerebrum.

Venous drainage from the head and neck

The majority of blood draining from the head is passed into three pairs of veins: the external jugular veins, the internal jugular veins and the vertebral veins. Within the brain all veins lead to the internal jugular veins.

The **external jugular vein** is smaller than the internal jugular and lies superficial to it. It receives blood from superficial regions of the face, scalp and neck. The external jugular veins descend on either side of the neck, passing over the sternomastoid muscles and beneath the platysma. They empty into the right and left subclavian veins in the base of the neck.

The **internal jugular veins** form the major venous drainage of the head and neck and are deep veins that parallel the common carotid artery. They collect deoxygenated blood from the brain, passing downwards through the neck beside the common carotid arteries and joining the subclavian veins.

The **vertebral veins** descend from the transverse openings (or foramina) of the cervical vertebrae and enter the subclavian veins. The vertebral veins drain deep structures of the neck, such as the vertebrae and muscles.

KEY NOTE

Indian Head Massage can help to enhance the circulation of blood and hence increase cell nutrition and elimination of cellular waste to and from the head and neck. The improved circulation to the head also helps to refresh the brain, helping relieve stress, tension and fatigue.

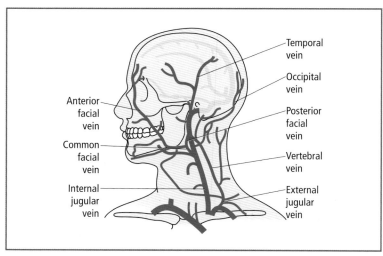

Fig 2.39 Venous drainage from the head and neck

The Lymphatic System

The lymphatic system is a one-way drainage system in that it removes excess fluid from the body's tissues and returns it to the circulatory system. It is also important in helping the body to fight infection.

Lymphatic vessels form a network of tubes that extend all over the body. The smallest of the vessels, lymphatic capillaries, end blindly in the body's tissues. Here they collect a liquid called lymph which leaks out of the body capillaries and accumulates in the tissues. Once collected, lymph flows in one direction along progressively larger lymphatic vessels. Along the network of lymphatic vessels are lymphatic nodes which filter bacteria and micro-organisms from the lymph as it passes through them. The cleansed lymph is then collected by two main lymphatic ducts (the thoracic and the right lymphatic ducts) which empty the lymph into the bloodstream.

The lymphatic system therefore returns the excess fluid which accumulates in the body's tissues back into the bloodstream, while at the same time filtering micro-organisms and releasing antibodies to help the body to fight infection.

What is Lymph?

Lymph is a transparent, colourless, watery liquid which is derived from tissue fluid and is contained within lymphatic vessels. It resembles blood plasma in composition, except that it has a lower concentration of plasma proteins. This is because some large protein molecules are unable to filter through the cells forming the capillary walls so they remain in blood plasma. Lymph contains only one type of cell: these are called lymphocytes.

How is Lymph Formed?

As blood is distributed to the tissues, some of the plasma escapes from the capillaries and flows around the tissue cells, delivering nutrients such as oxygen and water to the cell and picking up cellular waste such as urea and carbon dioxide. Once the plasma is outside the capillary and is bathing the tissue cells, it becomes tissue fluid.

Some of the tissue fluid passes back into the capillary walls to return to the blood stream via the veins, and some is collected by lymphatic vessels where it becomes lymph.

The Connection between Blood and Lymph

The lymphatic system is often referred to as a secondary circulatory system as it consists of a network of vessels that assist the blood in returning fluid from the tissues back to the heart. In this way, the lymphatic system is a complementary system for the circulatory system. After draining the tissues of excess fluid, the lymphatic system returns this fluid to the cardiovascular system. This helps to maintain blood volume, blood pressure and prevent oedema.

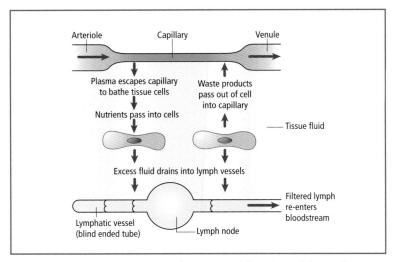

Fig 2.40 The connection between blood and lymph

Structure of the Lymphatic System

The lymphatic system contains the following structures:

- lymphatic capillaries
- lymphatic vessels
- lymphatic nodes
- lymphatic collecting ducts.

Lymphatic capillaries

Lymphatic vessels commence as lymphatic capillaries in the tissue spaces of the body as minute, blind-end tubes, as the lymphatic system is a one-way circulatory pathway. The walls of the lymphatic capillaries are like those of the blood capillaries in that they are a single-cell-layer thick to make it possible for tissue fluid to enter them. However, they are permeable to substances of larger molecular size than those of the blood capillaries.

The lymphatic capillaries mirror the blood capillaries and form a network in the tissues, draining away excess fluid and waste products from the tissue spaces of the body. Once the tissue fluid enters a lymphatic capillary it becomes lymph and is gathered up into larger lymphatic vessels.

KEY NOTE

The movement of lymph throughout the lymphatic system is known as lymphatic drainage and it begins in the lymphatic capillaries. The movement of lymph out of the tissue spaces and into the lymphatic capillaries is assisted by the pressure exerted by the compression of skeletal muscles. This explains why techniques such as Indian Head Massage are an effective way of draining lymph.

Lymphatic vessels

Lymphatic vessels are similar to veins in that they have thin collapsible walls and their role is to transport fluid (lymph) along its circulatory pathway. They have a considerable number of valves which help to keep the lymph flowing in the right direction and prevent backflow. Superficial lymphatic vessels tend to follow the course of veins by draining the skin, whereas the deeper lymphatic vessels tend to follow the course of arteries and drain the internal structures of the body.

KEY NOTE

As the lymphatic system lacks a pump, lymphatic vessels have to make use of contracting muscles to assist the movement of lymph. Therefore, lymphatic flow is at its greatest during exercise due to the increased contraction of muscle.

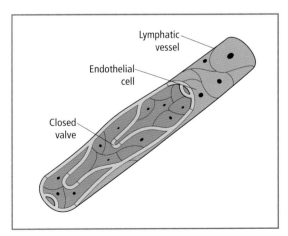

Fig 2.41 A lymph vessel

The lymphatic vessels carry the lymph towards the heart under steady pressure and about two to four litres of lymph pass into the venous system every day. Once lymph has passed through the lymph vessels it drains into at least one lymphatic node before returning to the blood circulatory system.

Lymphatic nodes

At intervals along the lymphatic vessels lymphatic nodes occur. A lymphatic node is an oval- or bean-shaped structure, covered by a capsule of connective tissue. It is made up of lymphatic tissue and is divided into two regions: an outer cortex and an inner medulla.

There are more than 100 lymphatic nodes, placed strategically along the course of lymphatic vessels. They vary in size between 1 to 25 mm in length and are massed in groups; some are superficial and lie just under the skin, whereas others are deeply seated and are found near arteries and veins.

Each lymphatic node receives lymph from several afferent lymphatic vessels and blood from small arterioles and capillaries. Valves of the afferent lymphatic vessels open towards the node; therefore lymph in these vessels can only move towards the node. Lymph flows slowly through the node, moving from the cortex to the medulla, and leaves through an efferent vessel which opens away from the node.

- The afferent vessels enter a lymphatic node.

- The efferent vessels drain lymph from a node.

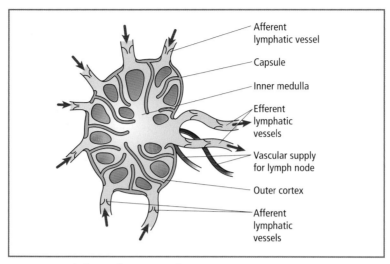

Fig 2.42 A lymphatic node

The function of a lymphatic node is to act as a filter to remove or trap any micro-organisms, cell debris, or harmful substances which may cause infection, so that when lymph enters the blood, it has been cleared of any foreign matter. When lymph enters a node, it comes into contact with two specialised types of leucocytes:

- **Macrophages** – these are phagocytic in action. They engulf and destroy dead cells, bacteria and foreign material in the lymph.

- **Lymphocytes** – these are reproduced wthin the lymphatic nodes and can neutralise invading bacteria and produce chemicals and antibodies to help fight disease.

Once filtered, the lymph leaves the node by one or two efferent vessels, which open away from the node. Lymphatic nodes occur in chains, so that the efferent vessel of one node becomes the afferent vessel of the next node in the pathway of lymph flow. Lymph drains through at least one lymphatic node then passes into two main collecting ducts before it is returned to the blood.

KEY NOTE

If an area of the body becomes inflamed or otherwise diseased, the nearby lymph nodes will swell up and become tender, indicating that they are actively fighting the infection.

Lymphatic ducts

From each chain of lymphatic nodes, the efferent lymph vessels combine to form lymphatic trunks which empty into two main ducts: the thoracic and the right lymphatic ducts. These ducts collect lymph from the whole body and return it to the blood via the subclavian veins.

The thoracic duct

This is the main collecting duct of the lymphatic system. It is the largest lymphatic vessel in the body and extends from the second lumbar vertebra up through the thorax to the root of the neck. The thoracic duct collects lymph from the left side of the head and neck, the left arm, the lower limbs and abdomen, and drains into the left subclavian vein to return the fluid to the bloodstream

The right lymphatic duct

This duct is very short in length. It lies in the root of the neck and collects lymph from the right side of the head and neck and the right arm, and drains into the right subclavian vein, to return the fluid to the bloodstream.

Lymphatic Drainage of the Head and Neck

The main groups of lymphatic nodes relating to the head and neck are given below:

Name of Lymphatic Node	Position	Areas lymph is drained from
Cervical (deep)	deep within the neck, located along the path of the larger blood vessels (carotid artery and internal jugular vein)	the larynx, oesophagus, posterior of the scalp and neck, superficial part of chest and arm
Cervical (superficial)	located at the side of the neck, over the sternomastoid muscle	the lower part of the ear and the cheek region
Submandibular	beneath the mandible	chin, lips, nose, cheeks and tongue
Occipital	at the base of the skull	back of scalp and the upper part of the neck
Mastoid (post-auricular)	behind the ear in the region of the mastoid process	the skin of the ear and the temporal region of the scalp
Parotid	at the angle of the jaw	nose, eyelids and ear

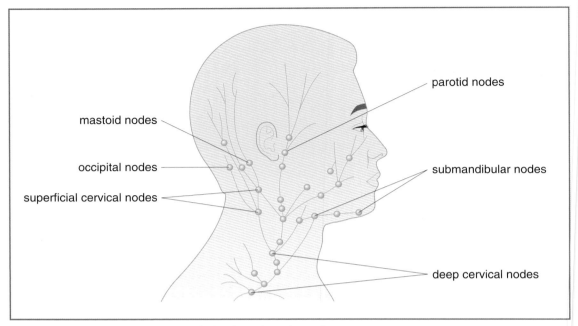

Fig 2.43 Lymphatic nodes of the head and neck

The Nervous System

The nervous system comprises the brain, spinal cord and nerves (neurones) which together form a communication network to coordinate the various actions of the body.

The nervous system works on the same principle as a computer in that it receives information, processes the information and produces an output. The information received reaches the brain from the sensory organs and internal organs; the information is then processed within the brain. The output is through the action of organs, muscles or glands.

The nervous system contains billions of interconnecting neurones which are designed to transmit nerve impulses.

There are three types of neurones:

- **Sensory neurones** receive stimuli from sensory organs and receptors and transmit the impulse to the spinal cord and brain. Sensations transmitted by sensory neurones include heat, cold, pain, taste, smell, sight and hearing.

- **Motor neurones** conduct impulses away from the brain and the spinal cord to muscles and glands to stimulate them into carrying out their activities.

- **Association (mixed) neurones** link sensory and motor neurones, helping to form the complex pathways that enable the brain to interpret incoming sensory messages, decide what should be done and send out instructions in response in order to keep the body functioning properly.

KEY NOTE

It is important for therapists to have a basic knowledge of the nervous system to understand its effects, in relation to Indian Head Massage, of inducing relaxation and minimising pain.

Clients will experience the effects of massage on their muscle tension via the sensory nerves in their muscles. Techniques used in Indian Head Massage help clients to become aware of specific areas of tension and can thereby initiate relaxation and reduce the unconscious motor message (of tension) to the muscles.

The nervous system has two main parts:

- the **central nervous system** (the main control system), consisting of the brain and the spinal cord

- the **peripheral nervous system**, consisting of 31 pairs of spinal nerves, 12 pairs of cranial nerves and the autonomic nervous system.

The Central Nervous System

The brain

The brain is an extremely complex mass of nervous tissue lying within the skull. It is the main communication centre of the nervous system and its function is

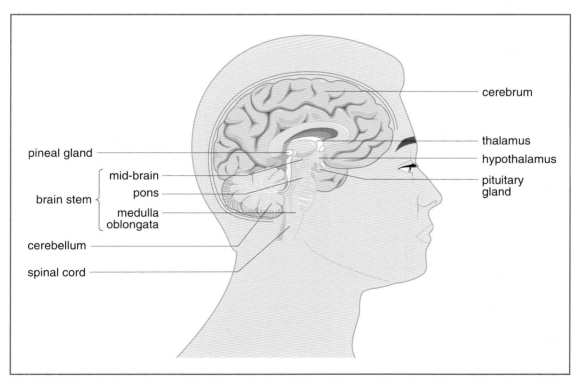

Fig 2.44 The brain

to coordinate the nerve stimuli received and effect the correct responses.

The main parts of the brain include:

The cerebrum

This is the largest portion of the brain and makes up the front and top part of the brain. It is divided into two large cerebral hemispheres. The outer layer of the cerebrum is called the cerebral cortex and is the region where the main functions of the cerebrum are carried out. The cortex is concerned with all forms of conscious activity: sensations such as vision, touch, hearing, taste and smell; control of voluntary movements; reasoning; emotion; and memory.

The cortex of each cerebral hemisphere has a number of functional areas:

- **Sensory areas**: these receive impulses from sensory organs all over the body; there are separate sensory areas for vision, hearing, touch, taste and smell.

- **Motor areas**: these areas have motor connections through motor nerve fibres with voluntary muscles all over the body.

- **Association areas**: in these areas association takes place between information from the sensory areas and remembered information from past experiences. Conscious thought then takes place and decisions are made which often result in conscious motor activity controlled by motor areas.

The brain requires a continuous supply of glucose and oxygen as it is unable to store glycogen, unlike the liver and muscles.

The thalamus

This is a relay and interpretation centre for all sensory impulses, except olfaction.

The hypothalamus

This small structure governs many important homeostatic functions. It regulates the autonomic nervous system and the endocrine system by governing the pituitary gland. It controls hunger, thirst, temperature regulation, anger, aggression, hormones, sexual behaviour, sleep patterns and consciousness.

The pituitary gland

This is a small body situated beneath the hypothalamus in a bony cavity at the base of the skull. It is known as the master endocrine gland as its hormones control and stimulate other glands to produce their hormones.

The pineal gland

This is a small mass of nerve tissue attached by a stalk in the central part of the brain. It is located deep between the cerebral hemispheres, where it is attached to the upper portion of the thalamus.

The pineal gland secretes a hormone called melatonin, which is involved in the regulation of circadian rhythms, patterns of repeated activity that are associated with the environmental cycles of day and night such as sleep/wake rhythms. The pineal gland is also thought to influence the mood.

The cerebellum

The cerebellum is a cauliflower-shaped structure located at the posterior of the cranium, below the cerebrum. The cerebellum is concerned with muscle tone, the coordination of skeletal muscles and balance.

The brain stem contains three main structures:

- **The mid-brain**: this contains the main nerve pathways connecting the cerebrum and the lower nervous system as well as certain visual and auditory reflexes that coordinate head and eye movements with things seen and heard.

- **The pons**: this is below the mid-brain and it relays messages from the cerebral cortex to the spinal cord.

- **The medulla oblongata**: this is often considered the most vital part of the brain. It is an enlarged continuation of the spinal cord and connects the brain with the spinal cord. Control centres within the medulla oblongata include for those for the heart, lungs and intestines.

The spinal cord

The spinal cord is an extension of the brain stem, extending from an opening at the base of the skull down to the second lumbar vertebra. Its function is to relay impulses to and from the brain. Sensory tracts conduct impulses to the brain and motor tracts conduct impulses from the brain.

The peripheral nervous system

This is the communication pathway connecting the central nervous system to the rest of the body.

It consists of the following.

Thirty-one pairs of spinal nerves

The spinal nerves pass out of the spinal cord and each has two thin branches which link it with the autonomic nervous system. Spinal nerves receive sensory

KEY NOTE

Within the spinal cord there are two pathways for sensory information to reach the brain.

The **fast** pathway transmits impulses rapidly and relates to receptors sensitive to light pressure, vibration and touch.

The **slow** pathway transmits information about pain, temperature and pressure.

When the fast pathway is activated (i.e. through massage to the skin), the pain pathway in inhibited, as pleasant sensations from the massage arrive at the brain before the pain sensation, thereby helping to displace the awareness of pain.

impulses from the body and transmit motor signals to specific regions of the body, thereby providing two-way communication between the central nervous system and the body.

Each of the spinal nerves is numbered and named according to the level of the spinal column from which they emerge. There are:

- eight cervical
- twelve thoracic
- five lumbar
- five sacral
- one coccygeal.

Each spinal nerve is divided into several branches, forming a network of nerves or plexuses which supply different parts of the body.

- The **cervical plexuses** of the neck supply the skin and muscles of the head, neck, and upper region of the shoulders.

- The **brachial plexuses** supply the skin and muscles of the arm, shoulder and upper chest.

- The **lumbar plexuses** supply the front and sides of the abdominal wall and part of the thigh.

- The **sacral plexuses** at the base of the abdomen supply the skin and muscles and organs of the pelvis.

- The **coccygeal plexus** supplies the skin in the area of the coccyx and the muscles of the pelvic floor.

Twelve pairs of cranial nerves

The cranial nerves lead to and from the brain and control feeling and function of the various parts of the head and face, including the muscles, eyes, ears and nose. Some of the nerves are mixed, containing both motor and sensory nerves, while others are either sensory or motor.

- **Olfactory** a sensory nerve of olfaction (smell).

- **Optic** a sensory nerve of vision.

- **Oculomotor** a mixed nerve that innervates both internal and external muscles of the eye and a muscle of the upper eyelid.

- **Trochlear** the smallest of the cranial nerves and is a motor nerve that innervates the superior oblique muscle of the eyeball that helps you look upwards.

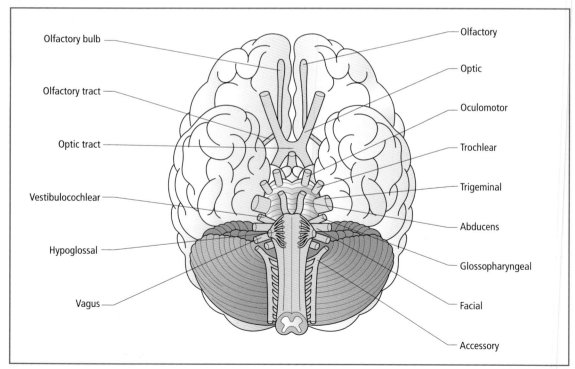

Fig 2.45 Cranial nerves

- **V – Trigeminal** a mixed nerve (containing motor and sensory nerves) that conducts impulses to and from several areas in the face and neck. It also controls the muscles of mastication (the masseter, the temporalis and the pterygoids). It has three main branches – ophthalmic, maxillary and mandibular.

  The opthalmic branch carries sensations from the eye, nasal cavity, skin of the forehead, upper eyelid, eyebrow and part of the nose.

  The maxillary branch carries sensations from the lower eyelid, upper lip, gums, teeth, cheek, nose, palate and part of the pharynx.

  The mandibular branch carries sensations from the lower gums, teeth, lips, palate and part of the tongue.

- **VI – Abducens** a mixed nerve that innervates only the lateral rectus muscle of the eye, which helps you look to the side.

- **VII – Facial** a mixed nerve that conducts impulses to and from several areas in the face and neck. The sensory branches are associated with the taste receptors on the tongue and the motor fibres transmit impulses to the muscles of facial expression.

- **VIII – Vestibulocochlear** a sensory nerve that transmits impulses generated by auditory stimuli and stimuli related to equilibrium, balance and movement.

- **IX – Glossopharyngeal** a mixed nerve that innervates structures in the mouth and throat. It supplies motor fibres to part of the pharynx and to the parotid salivary glands and sensory fibres to the posterior third of the tongue and the soft palate.

- **X – Vagus** this nerve is unlike the other cranial nerves in that it has branches to numerous organs in the thorax and abdomen as well as the neck. It supplies motor nerve fibres to the muscles of swallowing and motor nerve fibres to the heart and organs of the chest cavity. Sensory fibres carry impulses from the organs of the abdominal cavity and the sensation of taste from the mouth.

- **XI – Accessory** functions primarily as a motor nerve, innervating muscles in the neck and upper back (such as the trapezius and the sternomastoid), as well as muscles of the palate, pharynx and larynx.

- **Hypoglossal** a motor nerve that innervates the muscles of the tongue.

The autonomic nervous system

The part of the nervous system that controls the automatic body activities of smooth and cardiac muscle and the activities of glands. It is divided into the sympathetic and parasympathetic divisions, which possess complementary responses.

The sympathetic system

The activity of the sympathetic system is to prepare the body for expending energy and dealing with emergency situations.

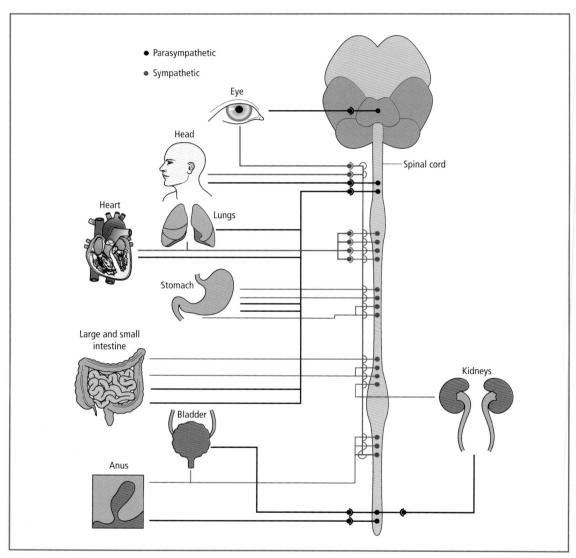

Fig 2.46 The autonomic nervous system

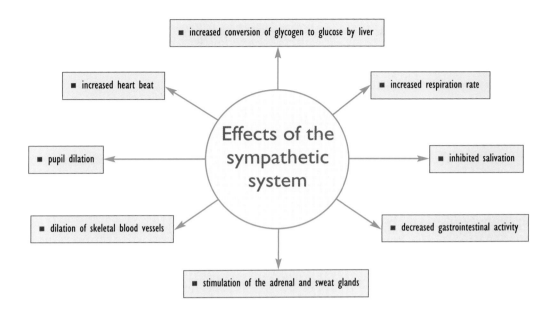

The parasympathetic system

The parasympathetic nervous system balances the action of the sympathetic division by working to conserve energy and create the conditions needed for rest and sleep.

Effects of the parasympathetic activity include:

- resting heart rate
- resting respiratory rate
- constriction of skeletal blood vessels
- increased gastro-intestinal activity
- pupil construction
- stimulated salivation.

KEY NOTE

The sympathetic nervous system is activated at times of anger, fright, anxiety or any type of emotional upset, whether real or imagined. The relaxing effects of an Indian Head Massage can help to *decrease* the effects of the sympathetic nervous system, whilst *stimulating* parasympathetic activity to promote relaxation and reduce stress levels. It can also help to reduce stress hormones such as cortisol by activating the relaxation process.

Indian Head Massage is also thought to increase serotonin levels which can help to decrease stress levels and depression.

Respiration

Oxygen is needed by every cell of the body for survival and delivery. Respiration is the process by which the living cells of the body receive a constant supply of oxygen and remove carbon dioxide and other gases. The respiratory system consists of the nose, the pharynx, the larynx, the trachea, the bronchi and the lungs which provide the passageway for air in and out of the body.

During inhalation air is drawn in through the nose, pharynx, trachea and bronchi and into the lungs. Inside the lungs each bronchus divides to form a tree of tubes called bronchioles which progressively decrease in diameter and end in microscopic air sacs called alveoli. Oxygen from the inhaled air that reaches the alveoli diffuses through the alveolar walls and into the surrounding blood capillaries. This oxygen-rich blood is carried first to the heart and is then pumped to cells throughout the body. Carbon dioxide diffuses out of the blood into the alveoli and is removed from the body during exhalation.

The Mechanism of Respiration

The mechanism of respiration is the means by which air is drawn in and out of the lungs and is an active process where the muscles of respiration contract to increase the volume of the thoracic cavity.

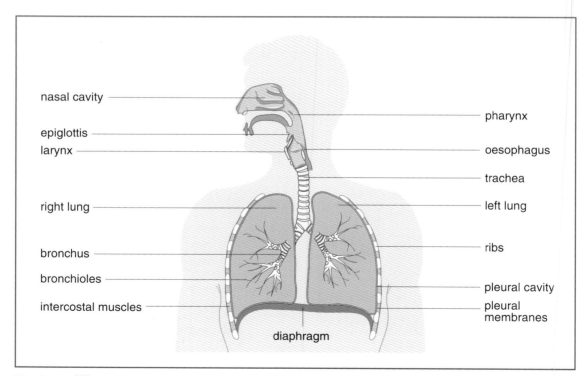

nasal cavity

pharynx

epiglottis
larynx

oesophagus

trachea

right lung

left lung

bronchus

ribs

bronchioles

pleural cavity

intercostal muscles

pleural membranes

diaphragm

Fig 2.47 The respiratory tract

Rib movements in breathing

Inhaling

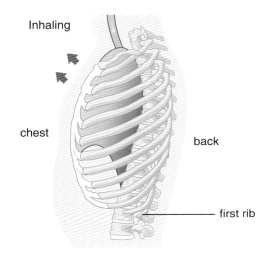

chest   back

first rib

Exhaling

lungs

chest   back

Inhaling. The diaphragm and intercostal muscles contract, pulling the ribs upward. This increases the volume of the chest cavity, drawing air into the lungs.

Exhaling. The contracted muscles relax, the ribs fall slightly and decrease the volume of the chest. Air is forced out of the lungs.

How the diaphragm works

Inhaling

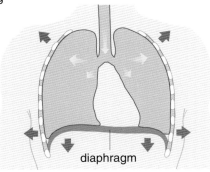

diaphragm

Exhaling

diaphragm

Inhaling. As the rib cage expands *(arrows, above)*, the diaphragm contracts and flattens downwards, enlarging the chest cavity.

Exhaling. The diaphragm relaxes and is pressed up by the abdominal organs, returning to its dome shape. The chest narrows, driving air out of the lungs.

Fig 2.48 The mechanism of respiration

The major muscle of respiration is the diaphragm. During inspiration the diaphragm contracts and flattens, increasing the volume of the thoracic cavity and is responsible for 75 per cent of air movement into the lungs. The external intercostals are also involved in respiration and upon contraction they increase the depth of the thoracic cavity by pulling the ribs upwards and outwards. The external intercostal muscles are responsible for bringing approximately 25 per cent of the volume of air into the lungs.

The combined contraction of the diaphragm and the external intercostals increases the thoracic cavity, which decreases the pressure inside the thorax so that air from outside the body is pulled into the lungs.

Other accessory muscles which assist in inspiration include the sternomastoid, serratus anterior, pectoralis minor, pectoralis major and the scalene muscles in the neck.

During normal respiration the process of expiration is passive and is brought about by the relaxation of the diaphragm and the external intercostal muscles. This increases the internal pressure inside the thorax so that air is pushed out of the lungs. In forced expiration, the process of expiration becomes active and is assisted by muscles such as the internal intercostals which help to depress the ribs. Abdominal muscles such as the external and internal obliques, rectus abdominus and the transversus abdominus help to compress the abdomen and force the diaphragm upwards, thus assisting expiration.

KEY NOTE

Breathing affects both our physiological and psychological state. By freeing tight respiratory muscles, Indian Head Massage can help to increase the vital capacity and function of the lungs.

Self-Assessment Questions

1 In which of the following layers are epidermal cells constantly being reproduced?

   a   horny layer

   b   granular layer

   c   clear layer

   d   basal cell layer

2 Which is the thinnest layer of the skin?

   a   dermis

   b   epidermis

   c   subcutaneous layer

   d   subdermal layer

3 Hair growth occurs from the

   a   cuticle

   b   cortex

   c   medulla

   d   matrix

4 Hair grows from a sac-like depression called the

   a   hair shaft

   b   hair root

   c   hair follicle

   d   hair bulb

5 Hair colour is due to the presence of melanin in which parts of the hair shaft?

   a   cortex and medulla

   b   cuticle and cortex

   c   cuticle and medulla

   d   medulla only

6 The sebaceous glands produce an oily substance called

   a   sweat

   b   lactic acid

   c   sebum

   d   keratin

7 Which lies beneath the subcutaneous layer of the skin?

   a   papillary layer

   b   reticular layer

   c   clear layer

   d   subdermal muscle layer

8 Which of the following is *not* a function of the skin?

   a   protection

   b   heat regulation

   c   fight infection

   d   absorption

9 Which of the following is a fungal infection of the skin?

a   impetigo

b   herpes simplex

c   ringworm

d   scabies

10 How many bones are located in the neck?

a   8

b   10

c   12

d   7

11 The bone forming the posterior part of the shoulder girdle is the

a   clavicle

b   scapula

c   sternum

d   manubrium

12 The long bone of the upper arm is the

a   radius

b   ulna

c   humerus

d   scaphoid

13 The bones forming the wrist are called the

a   metacarpals

b   tarsals

c   carpals

d   metatarsals

14 A bone of the skull that forms the sides of the skull above and around the ears is called the

a   frontal bone

b   temporal bone

c   occipital bone

d   ethmoid bone

15 The bone of the face that forms the lower jaw is called the

a   maxilla

b   zygomatic

c   mandible

d   lacrimal

16 The muscle that extends from the chest, up the sides of the neck to the chin is called the

a   pectoralis major

b   occipitalis

c   temporalis

d   platsyma

17 The fan-shaped muscle on the side of the skull, above and in front of the ear, is called the

a   occipitalis

b   buccinator

c   mentalis

d   temporalis

18 The muscle that surrounds the eye is called

a   orbicularis oris

b   risorius

c   masseter

d   orbicularis oculi

19 The action of the risorius muscle is to

a   raise the corner of the mouth

b   close the mouth

c   draw end corners of the mouth laterally

d   elevate the lower lip

20 The action of the sternomastoid muscle is to

a   depress the mandible

b   extend the head

c   elevate and retract the lower jaw

d   turn the head to one side

21 The action of the buccinator muscle is to

  a   raise the lower jaw

  b   compress the cheek

  c   elevate and retract the lower jaw

  d   elevate the lower lip

22 The muscles that extend along the radial side of the forearm are the

  a   flexors

  b   extensors

  c   hypothenar eminence

  d   thenar eminence

23 The function of an artery is to

  a   carry oxygenated blood

  b   carry deoxygenated blood

  c   prevent backflow of blood

  d   carry blood under low pressure

24 The name of the blood vessels that are responsible for supplying oxygenated blood to the head and neck is

  a   the brachiocephalic arteries

  b   the subclavian arteries

  c   the jugular veins

  d   the carotid arteries

25 The name of the blood vessels responsible for draining deoxygenated blood from the head and neck is

  a   the jugular veins

  b   the superior vena cava

  c   the brachiocephalic veins

  d   the vertebral veins

26 The name of the structure that carries lymph towards the heart under steady pressure is a

  a   lymphatic capillary

  b   lymphatic node

  c   lymphatic vessel

  d   lymphatic duct

27 The lymph nodes that drain lymph from the back of the scalp and the upper part of the neck are called

    a   submandibular nodes

    b   deep cervical nodes

    c   occipital nodes

    d   parotid nodes

28 The lymph nodes that drain lymph from the larynx, oesophagus, posterior of the scalp and neck, and superficial part of the chest and arm are called

    a   superficial cervical nodes

    b   mastoid nodes

    c   deep cervical nodes

    d   occipital nodes

29 The central nervous system consists of

    a   the sympathetic and parasympathetic nervous systems

    b   the facial and spinal nerves

    c   the brain and the spinal cord

    d   the autonomic nervous system

30 Which of the following is *not* an effect of the sympathetic nervous system?

    a   pupil dilation

    b   increased gastrointestinal activity

    c   dilation of skeletal blood vessels

    d   increased heartbeat

31 The process of inspiration is brought about by

    a   the combined relaxation of the diaphragm and the internal intercostal muscles

    b   the combined contraction of the diaphragm and the external intercostal muscles

    c   the combined relaxation of the diaphragm and the external intercostal muscles

    d   the combined contraction of the diaphragm and the internal intercostal muscles

3 Conditions Affecting the Head, Neck and Shoulders

A considerable increase in stress levels in sophisticated present-day life has led to a great deal of interest in holistic therapies such as Indian Head Massage, which continues to grow in popularity. More and more people are seeking the benefits of an Indian Head Massage treatment to help improve their emotional and physical well-being.

Therapists practising Indian Head Massage need to be knowledgeable within the sphere of their chosen therapy, but also be sufficiently familiar with conditions affecting the head, neck and shoulders in order to design a safe and effective treatment plan that is adapted to the client's needs.

By the end of this chapter, you will be able to relate the following to your practical work:

- Knowledge of common conditions of the head, neck and shoulders.

- The cautions, recommendations and restrictions involved in treatment applications.

This knowledge will help to empower therapists to make an informed decision as to a suitable treatment plan that is within safe and ethical medical guidelines. It is very important that a therapist never diagnoses a client's medical condition, and refers the client to their GP before any form of treatment is commenced.

KEY NOTE

It should be noted that while the information given reflects an accurate representation of the condition in generic terms, all clients will vary in the severity of their condition. Each client should be individually assessed as to their condition at the time of the proposed treatment and reassessed on subsequent treatments. The guidelines given are meant as a general guide and thus therapists are encouraged to seek further clarification of a client's medical condition from the GP and from the client themselves.

Alopecia

A term used to describe temporary baldness or severe hair loss which may follow illness, shock, a period of extreme stress, or may be the side effect of drug therapy (for example, chemotherapy). It is important to distinguish temporary baldness from male pattern baldness, which is progressive and permanent and is unlikely to be helped by therapies such as Indian Head Massage.

Patchy hair loss, or alopecia areata, is a relatively common disorder. The onset is fairly sudden and presents with a round or oval bald area; the loss of hair may be complete or so-called 'exclamation mark hairs' may be seen in the bald patches or at the edges. Occasionally the scalp is erythematous (red) in the part affected. The skin itself is not scaly, unlike the bald areas seen in fungal infection of the scalp. In alopecia areata there may be one or several bald patches. The most frequent course for alopecia areata to take is for the hair to regrow after a period of time (frequently two to three months). When regrowth occurs, the hair is often white but usually repigments in time.

Cautions, Restrictions and Recommendations

- Concentrate on massaging the scalp to increase the local circulation, using almond or coconut oil.
- Wrap a warm towel round the head after the treatment to help aid the absorption.
- Encourage the client to use the oils and massage the scalp at home twice a week, leaving the oils to absorb for about two hours before shampooing.
- Advise the client of the importance of dietary requirements for healthy hair (adequate protein and essential fatty acids to promote healthy growth, and vitamin B complex and vitamin C to provide nourishment for the hair follicles; vitamin B5 helps to relieve stress).

Angina

Pain in the left side of the chest and usually radiating to the left arm. Caused by insufficient blood to the heart muscle, usually on exertion or excitement. The pain is often described as constricting or suffocating, and can last for a few seconds or moments. The patient may become pale and sweaty. This condition indicates ischaemic heart disease.

Cautions, Restrictions and Recommendations

- Stress predisposes an angina attack; Indian Head Massage can help to reduce stress levels by reducing the activity of the sympathetic nervous system.
- As sudden exposure to extreme heat or cold can bring on an attack, keep the client warm and avoid extreme fluctuations in temperature.
- It is important that clients have their necessary medications with them when they attend for treatment, in the event of an emergency.

Ankylosing spondylitis

A systemic joint disease characterised by inflammation of the intervertebral disc spaces, costovertebral and sacroiliac joints. Fibrosis, calcification, ossification and stiffening of joints are common and the spine becomes rigid. Typically, a client will complain of persistent or intermittent lower back pain. Kyphosis is present when the thoracic or cervical regions of the spine are affected and the weight of the head compresses the vertebrae and bends the spine forward. This condition can cause muscular atrophy, loss of balance and falls. Typically, ankylosing spondylitis affects young male adults.

Cautions, Restrictions and Recommendations

- Position the client according to individual comfort – extra cushioning and support may be required.

- Avoid forcibly mobilising ankylosed joints, and in the case of cervical spondylitis avoid hyperextending the neck.

- Gentle massage may be very beneficial and the heat generated may help to ease the pain.

- Advise the client to do breathing exercises regularly in order to help mobilise the thorax.

Anxiety

This can be defined as fear of the unknown, but as an illness it can vary from a mild form to panic attacks and severe phobias that can be disabling socially, psychologically and, at times, physically. It presents with a feeling of dread that something serious is likely to happen and is associated with palpitations, rapid breathing, sweaty hands, tremor (shakiness), dry mouth and general pains in the muscles. It can present with similar features of mild to moderate depression of the agitated type. The causes of anxiety can be related to personality with some genetic and behavioural predisposition, or a traumatic experience or physical illness, for example, hyperthyroidism.

Cautions, Restrictions and Recommendations

- Clients are likely to present with various symptoms and therefore a thorough assessment is required.

- Indian Head Massage and relaxation exercises are likely to be a valuable source of help and support.

- Clients with anxiety are more likely to become emotionally dependent on their therapist and may need to be referred to another professional for help.

Arthritis: Osteoarthritis

A joint disease characterised by the breakdown of articular cartilage, growth of bony spikes, swelling of the surrounding synovial membrane and stiffness and tenderness of the joint. Is also known as degenerative arthritis. It is common in the elderly and takes a progressive course. This condition involves varying degrees of joint pain, stiffness, limitation of movement, joint instability and deformity. It commonly affects the weight-bearing joints: the hips, knees, the lumbar and cervical vertebrae.

Cautions, Restrictions and Recommendations

- Passive and gentle friction movements around the joint may be beneficial where there is minimal pain, but excessive movement may cause joint pain and damage.

- Gentle massage may help with muscle spasms, joint stiffness and muscle atrophy.

- Always ask the client to demonstrate the range of movement possible in their shoulder and their neck; this will guide you as to the limitations of treatment possible.

Arthritis: Rheumatoid

Chronic inflammation of peripheral joints, resulting in pain, stiffness and potential damage to joints. It can cause severe disability. Joint swellings and rheumatoid nodules are tender.

Cautions, Restrictions and Recommendations

- Although Indian Head Massage cannot cure arthritis, it can help to prevent its progress through relaxation and reduction of discomfort.

- In the early stages of diagnosis, clients should be encouraged to have treatment in order to maintain the range of joint movements and help prevent contractures.

- In the acute stage, avoid massaging but encourage passive movement of the affected joints. In the chronic-stage treatments, massage movements can help to reduce the thickening that occurs in and around the articular cartilage.

- Always ensure there is no pain and that care is taken when gently mobilising a joint.

- Treatment is generally of shorter duration as clients may be taking painkillers and be unable to give adequate feedback.

Asthma

A condition in which there are attacks of shortness of breath and difficulty in breathing caused by spasm or swelling of the bronchial tubes, in turn caused by hypersensitivity to allergens such as the pollens of various plants, grass, flowers, pet hair, dust mites and various proteins in foodstuffs such as shellfish, eggs and milk. Asthma may be exacerbated by exercise, anxiety, stress or smoking. It runs in families and can be associated with hayfever and eczema.

Cautions, Restrictions and Recommendations

- Indian Head Massage is ideally suited as a treatment for asthma sufferers as clients are seated in an upright position.

- Always obtain a detailed history during the consultation stage, specifically the triggers that bring on an attack. If the client has a history of allergies then ensure that the client is not allergic to any preparations or substances you may be proposing to use.

- Relaxation provided by the treatment in conjunction with deep breathing exercises can help to reduce bronchiospasm and should be encouraged.

- It is advisable for the client to have their required medications handy, in the event of an attack.

Bell's Palsy

A disorder of the 7th cranial nerve (facial nerve) that results in paralysis on one side of the face. The disorder usually comes on suddenly and is commonly caused by inflammation around the facial nerve as it travels from the brain to the exterior. It may be caused by pressure on the nerve caused by tumours, injury to the nerve, infection of the meninges or inner ear, or dental surgery. Diabetes, pregnancy and hypertension are other causes.

The condition may present with a drooping of the mouth on the affected side caused by flaccid paralysis of the facial muscles and there may be difficulty in puckering the lips because of paralysis of the orbicularis oris muscle. Taste may be diminished or lost if the nerve proximal to the branch which carries taste sensations has been affected. The condition also presents with the individual having difficulty in closing the eye tightly and creasing the forehead. The buccinator muscle is also affected, which prevents the client from puffing the cheeks and is the cause of food getting caught between the teeth and cheeks. There is also excessive tearing from the affected eye. Pain may be present near the angle of the jaw and behind the ear. Eighty to ninety per cent of individuals recover spontaneously and completely in around one to eight weeks. Corticosteroids may be used to reduce the inflammation of the nerve.

Cautions, Restrictions and Recommendations

- Be aware that cold and chills are known to trigger Bell's palsy.

- Use light strokes in an upward direction from the middle of the face to the sides (towards the ears).

- To help increase tone on the affected side of the face, use kneading movements with the fingertips.

- Light tapotement (tapping) and vibration movements may be used to help stimulate paralysed muscles.

- To help maintain tone, the face massage can be performed two to three times a day.

- The client may also be shown facial exercises:

  i To exercise the orbicularis oculi, ask the client alternately to close and open the eyes with and without mild resistance to the eyelids.

  ii To exercise the buccinator, ask the client to puff the cheeks out and in, and then try to whistle.

  iii To exercise the orbicularis oris, the mouth should be puckered.

  iv Saying the letters P, B, M and N helps to exercise the labials.

  v To exercise the frontalis muscle, ask the client to raise and lower the eyebrows.

- Electrotherapy (non-surgical face-lift machines or faradic) may be used to reduce the atrophy of the affected muscles.

Bronchitis

A chronic or acute inflammation of the bronchial tubes. Chronic bronchitis is common in smokers and may lead to emphysema, which is caused by damage to lung structure. Acute bronchitis can result from a recent cold or flu.

Cautions, Restrictions and Recommendations

- Clients with bronchitis may find Indian Head Massage more comfortable because of the fact that they are seated.

- Encourage the client to breathe slowly and deeply throughout the treatment.

- As sufferers of chronic bronchitis are prone to respiratory infection, therapists should avoid treating such clients if they have even the mildest form of acute chest infection.

Cerebral Palsy

A condition caused by damage to the central nervous system of the baby during pregnancy, delivery or soon after birth. The damage could be caused by bleeding, lack of oxygen, or other injuries to the brain.

The signs and symptoms of this condition depend on the area of the brain affected. Speech is impaired in most individuals and there may be difficulty in swallowing. There may or may not be mental retardation. Muscles may increase in tone to become spastic, making coordinated movements difficult. The muscles are hyperexcitable and even small movements, touch, stretch of muscle or emotional stress can increase the spasticity.

The posture is abnormal because of muscle spasticity and the gait is also affected. Some may have abnormal involuntary movements of the limbs that may be exaggerated on voluntarily performing a task. Weakness of muscles may also be associated with the condition, along with seizures. There may also be problems with hearing and vision.

Cautions, Restrictions and Recommendations

- Seek the support of the doctors, nurses, physiotherapist and the family before proceeding.

- Indian Head Massage can help to reduce stress, prevent contractures, improve the circulation to the skin and muscles that are unused and provide tremendous emotional support.

- Perform a shorter treatment (15 to 20 minutes) using mild to moderate pressure.

- Since any form of stress increases the symptoms, concentrate on relaxation as this will help to reduce muscular spasms and involuntary movements.

- Be aware that some clients may have reduced sensations and because of mental retardation may be unable to give adequate feedback regarding pressure and pain.

- Also be aware that the spasticity in an individual may change from day to day, with changes in posture, and is related to emotional stress.

Dandruff (pityriasis capitis)

An extremely common condition which presents with visible scaling from the surface of the scalp and is associated with the presence of the yeast pityrosporum ovale. It is the precursor of seborrhoeic eczema of the scalp, in which there is a degree of inflammation in addition to the greasy scaling.

Cautions, Restrictions and Recommendations

- Place a clean towel over the client's shoulders when proceeding to the scalp massage to prevent dead skin cells from the scalp falling on to their clothing.

- Regular scalp massage and use of oils help to remove dead skin cells and increase the circulation.

- Vitamin A is useful to improve a dry, scaly scalp.

Depression

This combines symptoms of lowered mood, loss of appetite, poor sleep, lack of concentration and interest, lack of sense of enjoyment, occasional constipation and loss of libido. On occasions there can be suicidal thinking, death wish or active suicide attempts.

Depression can be the result of chemical imbalance, usually related to serotonin and noradrenalin. There might be no medical cause for the depression, instead it might be linked to genetic predisposition, the result of physical illness, actual loss of a close relative, object, limb or loss of a relationship. A depressed person looks miserable, hunchbacked and downcast, and will usually avoid eye contact. The severity, as suggested above, can be variable but may become severe enough to become psychotic, manifested by hallucinations, delusions, paranoia or thought disorders.

Cautions, Restrictions and Recommendations

- A depressed client can present with physical ailments including backache, gastrointestinal symptoms (usually constipation) and headaches.

- Physical illness can present with depression and can include, for example, long-term illness, terminal illness, Parkinson's disease and arthritis.

- Therapists need to ensure that clients do not become emotionally dependent on them; they may need to be referred to another professional.

- If there is any indication of suicidal thinking at any time, the client should be referred to their GP.

- Indian Head Massage is thought to help increase levels of serotonin from the brain and may be effective in helping to lift depression.

Epilepsy

A neurological disorder that makes the individual susceptible to recurrent and temporary seizures. Epilepsy is a complex condition and classifications of types of epilepsy are not definitive.

Generalised

This may take the form of major or tonic–clonic seizures (formerly known as grand mal) in which at the onset the patient falls to the ground unconscious with their muscles in a state of spasm (tonic phase). This is then replaced by convulsive movements (the clonic phase) when the tongue may be bitten and urinary incontinence may occur. Movements gradually cease and the patient may rouse in a state of confusion, complaining of a headache, or may fall asleep.

Partial

This may be idiopathic or a symptom of structural damage to the brain. In one type of partial idiopathic epilepsy, often affecting children, seizures may take the form of absences (formerly known as petit mal), in which there are brief spells of unconsciousness lasting for a few seconds. The eyes stare blankly and there may be fluttering movements of the lids and momentary twitching of the fingers and mouth. This form of epilepsy seldom appears before the age of three or after adolescence. It often subsides spontaneously in adult life, but may be followed by the onset of generalised or partial epilepsy.

Focal

This is partial epilepsy caused by brain damage (either local or caused by a stroke). The nature of the seizure depends on the location of the damage in the brain. In a Jacksonian motor seizure, the convulsive movements may spread from the thumb to the hand, arm and face.

Psychomotor

This type of epilepsy is caused by dysfunction of the cortex of the temporal lobe of the brain. Symptoms may include hallucinations of smell, taste, sight and hearing. Throughout an attack the patient is in a state of clouded awareness and afterwards may have no recollection of the event.

Cautions, Restrictions and Recommendations

- Always refer to the client's GP regarding the type and nature of epilepsy.

- As epilepsy is a complex condition and Indian Head Massage involves stimulation of the brain, caution is advised.

- If the client is on controlled medication, the chances of a seizure are minimal; however, caution is advised because of the complexity of this condition.

- It has never been reported that holistic therapies have ever provoked the onset of epilepsy, although there is a theoretical risk to be considered in that deep relaxation or overstimulation could provoke an attack (although this has never been proven in practice).

Fibromyalgia

A chronic condition that produces musculosketetal pain. Predominant symptoms include widespread musculoskeletal pain, lethargy and fatigue. Other characteristic features include a non-refreshing sleep pattern in which the patient feels exhausted and more tired than later in the day, and interrupted sleep. Other recognised symptoms include early-morning stiffness, pins and needles sensation, unexplained headaches, poor concentration, memory loss, low mood, urinary frequency, abdominal pain and irritable bowel syndrome. Anxiety and depression are also common.

Cautions, Restrictions and Recommendations

- Avoid deep massage on localised tender areas (which include base of skull, cervical vertebrae C5–7, midpoint of the upper border of the trapezius, above the spine of the scapula).

- Caution is advised regarding stiffness.

- Relaxation is integral to reduce muscle spasm and feeling of stress.

Frozen Shoulder (adhesive capsulitis)

A chronic condition in which there is pain and stiffness and reduced mobility, or locking, of the shoulder joint. This may follow an injury, a stroke or myocardial infarction, or may develop because of incorrect lifting or a sudden movement.

Cautions, Restrictions and Recommendations

- If the condition is severe, refer the client to a physiotherapist.
- Avoid massaging the affected areas while there is acute inflammation.
- This condition can cause neck pain and pain at the base of the skull, which result in a headache.
- Be aware that the synovial capsule of the shoulder joint will be tender and surrounding muscles and tendons will also be affected.
- The client will benefit from gentle stretching exercises to help mobilise the shoulder joint.

Headache (tension)

This is the most common type of headache. It involves contraction and spasm of the neck and scalp muscles. The pain is produced by the pressure of the contracted muscle on the nerves and blood vessels in the area. The resultant blood flow increases the accumulation of waste products (such as lactic acid) in the area, which perpetuate the pain. The sufferer will usually complain of a dull, persistent ache and a feeling of tightness around the head, temple, forehead and occiput. Factors that may precipitate an attack include mental strain, noise, bright lights, alcohol consumption, menstruation and fatigue.

Cautions, Restrictions and Recommendations

- It is important to try to identify the precipitating cause of the headache.
- Indian Head Massage is usually very successful in helping to relieve this type of headache, particularly if it is stress-induced.
- Encourage the client to relax the shoulder and neck muscles with relaxation exercises before commencing the massage.
- Concentrate on relaxing areas that are less tense with effleurage (smoothing/stroking) and gentle kneading and then move on to muscles which are in spasm with frictions (it is likely that these will be the neck muscles, trapezius, levator scapula and the rhomboids).
- Massage of the scalp and face can be helpful (concentrating on the temporalis muscle, the masseters and the frontalis).
- Remember that clients may be taking painkillers and therefore may give inadequate feedback.

Kyphosis

A deformity of the spine that produces a rounded back. The condition presents with a rounded back and a flattened chest. There may be difficulty in breathing because of shortening of the pectoral muscles and the back muscles become weakened. In this condition the scapula tends to be pulled forward and the head is pushed forward.

Cautions, Restrictions and Recommendations

- A postural assessment is required in order to identify range of motion.
- Take care with the positioning of the client and if necessary offer supporting cushions/pillows.
- Concentrate on relaxing the muscles of the shoulders and neck.
- Gentle stretching exercises for the back and neck may help to improve posture.
- The aim of the treatment will be to relax and reduce pain in tense muscles.
- Deep diaphragmatic breathing should be encouraged to help mobilise the thorax.
- Avoid joint mobilisation if the condition is caused by changes in bone or connective tissue.

Migraine

Specific form of headache, usually unilateral (one side of the head), associated with nausea or vomiting and visual disturbances (usually scintillating light waves or zigzag patterns). Client may experience a visual aura before an attack actually happens. This is usually called a classical migraine. On occasions they cause painful, red and watery eyes, classified as ophthalmoplegic migraine.

Another form of migraine can cause one-sided paralysis and weakness of the face and body; this is called neuropathic migraine. Abdominal migraine can affect children, who present with recurring attacks of abdominal pain with or without nausea/vomiting. Migraine can be treated with simple analgesics or more specialised medication.

Cautions, Restrictions and Recommendations

- Avoid treatment during acute attacks and especially if the condition has not yet been diagnosed.
- Indian Head Massage is well known in helping migraine sufferers, as the relaxation and relief from stress and tension can help reduce frequency of attacks.
- Remember that women are likely to have more attacks during premenstrual periods, when they are taking the contraceptive pill, during the menopause or when starting HRT.
- Tension headaches can be a variant of migraine. Indian Head Massage is an ideal therapy in this event.

Myalgic encephalomyelitis (chronic fatigue syndrome)

A condition which is characterised by extreme disabling fatigue that has lasted for at least six months and is made worse by physical or mental exertion and is not resolved by bed rest. The symptom of fatigue is often accompanied by some of the following: muscle pain or weakness, poor coordination, joint pain, slight fever, sore throat, painful lymph nodes in the neck and armpits, depression, inability to concentrate and general malaise. It can happen in any age group, but recently children and adolescents have been noticed to have a higher incidence.

Cautions, Restrictions and Recommendations

- This is a condition which can benefit from Indian Head Massage, but avoid any claim which could be misinterpreted as curative.

- Relaxation can help the client to cope.

- Be aware of tenderness in the muscles and joints.

- Clients may require a lot of support and understanding.

Multiple Sclerosis

Disease of the central nervous system in which the myelin (fatty) sheath covering the nerve fibres is destroyed and various functions become impaired, including movement and sensations. Multiple sclerosis is characterised by relapses and remissions. It can present with blindness or reduced vision and can lead to severe disability within a short period. It can also cause incontinence, loss of balance, tremor and speech problems. Depression and mania can occur.

Cautions, Restrictions and Recommendations

- Be aware of loss of sensation.

- Be aware that massage and joint movement may trigger muscle spasm.

- Relaxation therapies and exercises may be helpful in decreasing tone in rigid muscles and preventing stiffness and contractures.

- Temperature extremes may make the symptoms worse.

- Treatments should be slow and gentle and of short duration, as clients may tire easily.

Psoriasis (of the scalp)

A chronic skin disease which presents as erythematous (red) scaly lesions on the scalp (other common areas affected include the knees, elbows, hands, nails and the sacral area). The client with psoriasis of the scalp may complain of a severe case of dandruff. However, unlike dandruff, scalp psoriasis can be easily felt as thick plaques occurring in patches. It may cause some hair thinning which tends to recover with successful treatment of this psoriasis.

Cautions, restrictions and recommendations

- See *dandruff* (pityriasis capitis) p. 94.

- Caution is advised regarding the application of oils – avoid oils which are too hot or too stimulating to the scalp (almond and coconut are good choices).

- Acute flare-up of psoriasis can cause painful and tender lesions of skin, and care is needed during massage.

- As psychological stress is a considerable cause of the exacerbation of psoriasis, Indian Head Massage can help clients to cope with their condition.

Seborrhoeic eczema (or dermatitis)

This condition presents with redness and diffuse scaling of the scalp (see *dandruff* p. 94) which may be mild or severe. Red scaly areas may also occur on the face, especially in the eyebrows and the nasolabial folds. A similar rash may occur behind the ears.

Cautions, Restrictions and Recommendations

See *dandruff* (p. 94) and *psoriasis* (p. 99).

Sinusitis

A condition involving inflammation of the paranasal sinuses. It is usually caused by a viral or bacterial infection or may be associated with a common cold or allergy. The congestion of the nose results in a blockage in the opening of the sinus into the nasal cavity and a build-up of pressure in the sinus.

The condition presents with nasal congestion followed by a mucous discharge from the nose. The pain is located to specific areas depending on the sinuses affected. If the frontal sinuses are affected, a major symptom is a headache over one or both eyes. If the maxillary sinuses are affected, one or both cheeks will hurt and it may feel as if there is toothache in the upper jaw.

Cautions, Restrictions and Recommendations

- Be aware of the site of inflammation where there will be pain and swelling.

- Pressures around the eyes and around the zygomatic bones can help to drain the sinuses and help relieve pain.

- Encourage the client to drink plenty of water after the treatment to increase elimination; encourage them to consider a cleansing diet.

Stroke

A blocking of blood flow to the brain by an embolus in a cerebral blood vessel. A stroke can result in a sudden attack of weakness affecting one side of the body, caused by the interruption of the flow of blood to the brain. A stroke can vary in severity, from a passing weakness or tingling in a limb to a profound paralysis and a coma if severe. Sometimes the term is used to describe cerebral haemorrhage when an artery or congenital cyst of blood vessels in the brain bursts, resulting in damage to the brain and causing similar signs to thrombus of cerebral vessels. Haemorrhage is usually associated with severe headaches and can cause neck stiffness.

Cautions, Restrictions and Recommendations

- Therapists will normally deal with clients who have recovered or are recovering from a stroke and Indian Head Massage can benefit and aid recovery.
- Be aware of muscle spasm and jerking movements in a paralysed limb.
- Neck massage is best avoided.

Temporomandibular Joint Tension (TMJ syndrome)

A collection of symptoms and signs produced by disorders of the temporomandibular joint. It is characterised by bilateral or unilateral muscle tenderness and reduced motion. It presents with a dull, aching pain around the joint, often radiating to the ear, face, neck or shoulder. The condition may start off as clicking sounds in the joint. There may be protrusion of the jaw or hypermobility and pain on opening the jaw. It slowly progresses to decreased mobility of the jaw, and locking of the jaw may occur.

Causes include chewing gum, biting nails, biting off large chunks of food, habitual protrusion of the jaw, tension in the muscles of the neck and back and clenching of the jaw. It may also be caused by injury and trauma to the joint or through a whiplash injury.

Cautions, Restrictions and Recommendations

- Be aware that the masseter, temporalis and pterygoid muscles may be in spasm and will be tender.
- The muscles of the neck, base of skull and shoulders should be massaged thoroughly to help reduce tension and spasms.
- The client needs to be educated on relaxing the muscles of the jaw. Ask the client to clench the jaw firmly and concentrate on the feeling of tightness in the jaw, then relax and let the jaw fall open.
- Clients may benefit from a posture assessment and breathing exercises.
- Clients should be encouraged to consult their dentist and a physiotherapist for specific treatment techniques.

Tinnitis

A condition where there is the sensation of sounds in the ears or head in the absence of an external sound source. The most common cause is ordinary age-related hair cell loss in the cochlear. Other causes include wax blocking the ear canal, damage to the ear drum, diseases of the inner ear such as Ménière's disease, and abnormalities of the auditory nerve.

Cautions, Restrictions and Recommendations

- Indian Head Massage has been known to be effective in clearing congestion in the head and may help relieve the symptoms.

- Concentrate on relaxing the neck muscle and work thoroughly above, in front of and behind the ears to increase lymph drainage.

- Be aware that some clients may experience dizziness and loss of balance upon rising.

Trigeminal Neuralgia

A painful condition caused by irritation of the 5th cranial nerve (the trigeminal nerve). The condition is characterised by excruciating intermittent pain confined to one or both sides of the face, along the distribution of the trigeminal nerve. The pain may be triggered by any touch or movement such as eating, chewing or swallowing. Exposure to hot or cold may also trigger an attack. Some cases of facial neuralgia are caused by a previous attack of shingles which has left a predisposition to life-long pain.

Cautions, Restrictions and Recommendations

- Obtain a detailed history of the signs and symptoms and refer the client to their GP before proceeding.

- The client may not allow you to touch the affected side of the face.

- If the client finds massage beneficial, use smoothing movements and light frictions over the skull. Then stroke gently from the middle of the face towards the temples, starting in the least sensitive area and moving gradually towards the more sensitive areas.

- Do not overwork the area as it may irritate the nerve and induce pain and discomfort.

- Treatment may be scheduled every other day initially.

Whiplash

A condition produced by damage to the muscles, ligaments, intervertebral discs or nerve tissues of the cervical region by sudden hyperextension and/or flexion of the neck. The most common cause is a road traffic accident when acceleration/deceleration causes sudden stretch of the tissue around the cervical spine. It may also occur as a result of hard impact sports. It can present with pain and limitation of neck movements, with muscle tenderness which can start hours to days after the accident and may take months to recover. This is usually affected by complicated physical, psychological and legal issues.

Cautions, Restrictions and Recommendations

- The condition may last for a few months or many years.

- Consider compensation as a reason for delayed healing and therefore avoid making any comments about reasons, prognosis or suitability of the therapy.

- Ascertain that the client is not seeking a cure; neither should the client receive any promise to be cured.

- Take care when massaging the neck and avoid manipulation or moving vigorously.

- Relaxation exercises can help.

- Holistic therapies such as Indian Head Massage may help clients to cope with the condition.

- Remember that clients with this condition would have seen many professionals and there may be legal issues you may want to avoid becoming involved with.

Self-Assessment Questions

1   Which of the following statements is correct?

    a   alopecia is a term used to describe temporary baldness with scaly patches

    b   alopecia is a term used to describe permanent baldness with scaly patches

    c   alopecia is a term used to describe temporary baldness without scaly patches

    d   alopecia is a term used to describe permanent baldness without scaly patches

2   Rheumatoid arthritis is

    a   a progressive disease affecting the rhomboids

    b   a chronic inflammation of peripheral joints

    c   a condition present only in elderly clients

    d   a condition also known as degenerative arthritis.

3   Bell's palsy is

    a   a disorder of the 11th cranial nerve resulting in temporary paralysis on one side of the face

    b   a disorder of the 7th cranial nerve resulting in temporary paralysis on one side of the face

    c   a disorder of the 11th cranial nerve resulting in permanent paralysis on one side of the face

    d   a disorder of the 7th cranial nerve resulting in permanent paralysis on one side of the face

4   Which of the following statements is correct?

    a   psychomotor epilepsy seizure depends on the location of the damage in the brain

    b   psychomotor epilepsy was formerly known as grand mal seizure

    c   psychomotor epilepsy is caused by dysfunction of the cortex of the temporal lobe of the brain

    d   psychomotor epilepsy was formerly known as petit mal seizure

5   For a client with multiple sclerosis

    a   treatments should be quick and firm and of short duration, as clients may tire easily

    b   treatments should be slow and gentle and of short duration, as clients may tire easily

    c   treatments should be quick and firm and of longer duration, to increase clients' stamina

    d   treatments should be slow and gentle and of longer duration, to increase clients' stamina

6   If a client is suffering with sinusitis

    a   avoid pressure around the eyes

    b   it may feel as if there is a toothache if the frontal sinuses are affected

    c   one or both cheeks will hurt if the maxillary sinuses are affected

    d   the congestion of the nose results in a blockage in the pharynx

7   A deformity of the spine that produces a rounded back is known as

    a   lordosis

    b   fibromyalgia

    c   osteoarthritis

    d   kyphosis

8   The condition pityriasis capitis is otherwise known as

    a   seborrheic dermatitis

    b   seborrheic eczema

    c   dandruff

    d   psoriasis

4 Consultation for Indian Head Massage

A client consultation involves professional communication between a client and a therapist and is a critical skill that helps establish a positive and trusting therapeutic relationship between both parties.

The time spent in establishing a professional relationship with the client will often result in client satisfaction and their continued patronage. Therapists therefore need to have effective communication skills which involve both talking and listening to clients in order to be able record and respond positively to the information elicited.

By end of this chapter you will be able to:

- Carry out a consultation for Indian Head Massage.

- Understand how contraindications and precautions may affect the proposed treatment.

- Liaise with other health care professionals.

- Formulate a treatment plan for Indian Head Massage.

Client Consultation Skills

As with all holistic therapy treatments, a consultation for Indian Head Massage involves one-to-one communication. During a consultation, a therapist's contact with the client involves talking, listening, non-verbal communication, as well as the recording of written information.

When carrying out a consultation, therapists need to adopt a warm, calm, open and understanding attitude towards the client, in order to facilitate a channel of positive communication. Clients presenting for treatment may be nervous or apprehensive about the treatment and it is therefore important for a therapist to adopt a sensitive, respectful and friendly attitude to the client at all times.

Although talking is an important part of a consultation, one of the most important skills a therapist can develop is in listening. Through effective listening, a therapist can customise the treatment with the aim of meeting the client's needs and expectations. It is important for therapists to realise that clients often communicate without the spoken word and non-verbal messages may be projected without the client's awareness. Therapists therefore need to be aware of what a client may be communicating in the tone of their words, gestures they may make, the posture they may present or by their facial expressions. With this in mind, therapists may realise that there may be a difference between what a client is expressing in words and what their body language may be indicating.

Consultation Environment

In order to facilitate a positive approach to a consultation, it is important to be aware of the environment in which it is undertaken. The environment for a consultation should ideally be private in order to respect the client's privacy and dignity in disclosing personal information. Attention to aspects such as lighting, smell, temperature and comfort of a consultation area can all help to aid client relaxation and decrease apprehension.

Client Education

Consultations provide an ideal opportunity for therapists to educate clients on what Indian Head Massage involves, its potential benefits along with the costs and time involved. Clients do not usually want to become passive recipients of the treatment and if they are to invest time and money in a therapy they need to be educated so that they become partners in their healing process.

Consultations also provide the client with the opportunity to ask questions about the treatment for reassurance and clarification. Based on the information and the education provided about the service, the client is then responsible for making a decision as to the treatment objectives. It is the therapist's responsibility to provide a treatment to suit their needs but to accurately inform them if their objectives and expectations are unrealistic. It is essential for therapists to stress to clients the importance of regular treatments to maintain long term benefits.

Clients may also be empowered to take charge of their own healing through client education of adjustments to lifestyle, posture and the correct use of ergonomics (the positioning of furniture at work).

Client Confidentiality

Client confidentiality is an important factor in a therapeutic relationship between a client and a therapist. Clients should be reassured that all information recorded will remain confidential and is stored securely, and that no information will be disclosed to a third party without the client's written consent. Maintaining client confidentiality will also help to establish a trusting professional relationship between a client and a therapist.

Written Documentation

Written documentation is essential in a consultation as it provides a systematic and continued record of the client's progress. Consultation documents should always be used as a guide to facilitate communication, and questions may need to be phrased in a certain way to maximise communication and receive qualitative information. For instance, upon asking a client about their stress levels, they may merely reply 'high'. In order to gain more information, a therapist may pose the question, 'In which part of the body do you feel stress most often?' or 'What factors are involved in your stress levels being high at the moment?'

It is important for therapists to realise that information received from the client is largely subjective in that it is from their viewpoint, and this information may differ from the evaluation of the therapist. Important information to be discussed during the consultation includes any factors which may affect the client's physical and emotional health such as medical history, diet, lifestyle, occupation, sleep patterns, exercise and relaxation, which may all contribute to an overall picture of the client from a holistic point of view.

Besides talking, listening and recording information on a client's records, client consultation involves other assessment skills such as:

- **Visual assessment** – This commences from the first point of contact with the client. Observations as to the client's mood, rate and depth of breathing, posture and gait may all help to contribute to the state of the client's physical and emotional health.

- **Manual assessment of the tissues** – the most effective form of communication a therapist can facilitate is in touch, and throughout the Indian Head Massage treatment the therapist can assess the tissues for tension, restrictions, temperature changes, and so on.

Contraindications and Cautions

Despite Indian Head Massage being an extremely safe and effective treatment, it is important for therapists to be aware of:

a Conditions that are totally contraindicated and for which treatment cannot be provided.

b Conditions that require referral to the client's GP, or another professional before treatment may be given.

c Conditions that present as localised contraindications; therefore treatment should be avoided in the affected area.

d Additional cautions which may affect the proposed treatment plan.

Knowledge of contraindications and precautions enables a therapist to work safely and effectively.

Conditions that are Totally Contraindicated to Indian Head Massage

These include:

- **fever/high temperature** – this is a contraindication due to the risk of spreading infection as a result of the increased circulation. During fever, the body temperature rises as a result of infection.

- **acute infectious diseases** (for example, colds, flu, measles, mumps, tuberculosis, chicken pox) – acute infectious diseases are contraindicated due to the fact they are highly contagious.

- **skin or scalp infections** – these should be avoided due to the risk of cross-infection. Some of the most common skin diseases that may be encountered on the head and neck include: herpes simplex (cold sores), impetigo, ringworm, scabies, conjunctivitis, folliculitis, pediculosis capitis (head lice) and tinea capitis (ringworm of the scalp). *See pages 26–30 for more detail on these and other skin and scalp disorders.*

- **recent haemorrhage** – haemorrhaging is excessive bleeding which may be either internal or external. Indian Head Massage should be avoided due to increasing the risk of blood spillage from blood vessels.

- **intoxication** – it is inadvisable to carry out treatment if a client is under the influence of alcohol, as the increase of blood flow to the head could make them feel dizzy and nauseous.

- **migraine** – it is inadvisable to carry out treatment if a client indicates the onset of an attack of migraine due to the fact they may become nauseous, dizzy, experience visual disturbances with severe headache and possible vomiting. In reality, clients experiencing an acute attack of migraine will usually be incapacitated from its effects and would be unable to receive treatment, let alone desire a treatment, at the time of the attack. *However, Indian Head Massage may help as a preventative treatment, particularly if the migraine is stress induced.*

- **recent head or neck injury** – in the case of a recent blow to the head with concussion, or an acute neck injury due to a recent accident, such as whiplash, it would be inadvisable to treat due to the risk of exacerbating the condition and increasing the inflammation and pain. However, if there is an old injury, massage may help to reduce scar tissue, decrease pain and increase mobility. Always obtain medical advice to ensure the client's condition is suitable for treatment.

Conditions that May Be Contraindicated to Indian Head Massage, but Require Medical Advice Before Deciding Whether Treatment is Advisable

- **severe circulatory disorders/heart conditions** – medical advice should always be sought before massaging a client with a severe heart condition or circulatory problem, as the increased circulation from the massage may overburden the heart and can increase the risk of a thrombus or embolus. *If medical advice indicates massage is advisable, it is recommended that a lighter massage is given, of a shorter duration initially.*

- **thrombosis/embolism** – always seek medical advice before massaging a client with a history of thrombosis or embolism, as there is a risk that the blood clot could become detached and be carried to another part of the body where it could obstruct the flow of blood to a vital organ. *If medical advice indicates massage is advisable, it is recommended that a lighter massage is given, of a shorter duration initially.*

- **high blood pressure** – clients with high blood pressure should have medical referral prior to massage, even in they are on prescribed medication, due to their susceptibility to form clots. Clients on anti-hypertensive medication may be prone to postural hypotension and may feel light headed and dizzy after treatment. Therapists are advised to carefully monitor a client's reaction and advise clients to get up slowly from the chair following treatment. *If medical advice indicates massage is advisable, techniques applied are generally soothing and relaxing.*

- **low blood pressure** – care should be taken with a client suffering from low blood pressure when sitting or standing up after massage due to the fact they may experience dizziness and could fall.

- **dysfunction of the nervous system** – clients with any dysfunction of the nervous system should be referred to their GP before treatment is given. A light relaxing massage may be indicated in the case of a client with cerebral palsy, multiple sclerosis or Parkinson's disease as massage may help to reduce spasms and involuntary movements and reduce rigidity and stiffness. *Always seek medical advice before offering treatment.*

- **epilepsy** – always refer to the client's GP regarding the type and nature of epilepsy the client may suffer from. Caution is advised due to the complexity of this condition and the risk that deep relaxation or overstimulation could provoke a convulsion (although this has never been proven in practice). *As some types of epilepsy may be triggered by smells, care should be taken with choice of oils or medium.*

- **diabetes** – this is a condition which requires medical advice, as some clients with diabetes may be prone to arteriosclerosis, high blood pressure and oedema. Pressure should be carefully monitored and administered carefully, due to any loss in sensory nerve function resulting in the client being unable to give accurate feedback regarding pressure. *If the client is receiving insulin by injection, care should be taken to avoid massage on recent injection sites. Clients should have their necessary medications with them when they attend for treatment, in the event of an emergency.*

- **cancer** – medical advice should always be sought before massaging a client with a cancerous condition. There is a risk of certain types of cancer spreading through the lymphatic system; massage is also thought to aid in the metasis of the cancer. It is unlikely that gentle massage can cause cancer to spread through the stimulation of lymph flow; however, it is important to always obtain advice from the consultant/medical team concerning the type of cancer and the extent of the disease. Once medical advice has been sought, massage may help in relaxing the body and supporting the immune system. It may also be used in palliative care (therapy that eases or reduces pain or other symptoms). *If massaging a cancer patient always avoid massage over areas of the body receiving radiation therapy, close to tumour sites and areas of skin cancer. It is usual to offer short light massage, which is beneficial in relaxing the client and supporting the immune system.*

- **recent operations** – depending on the nature of the operation and the area/s affected, it may be necessary to seek medical advice before proceeding with treatment. If a client has recently undergone surgery to the head and neck, Indian Head Massage should be avoided as it may interfere with the healing process. Medical advice is often necessary to establish when the area has completely recovered.

- **osteoporosis** – due to the fact that bones can break easily and vertebrae can collapse with this condition, it is advisable to seek medical advice before giving treatment. *If medical advice indicates treatment is advisable, care needs to be taken to ensure comfortable client positioning; avoid excessive joint movement and apply a lighter pressure.*

Conditions that Present as Localised Contraindications

- **skin disorders** – care should be taken as the condition may be worsened. Some skin conditions such as eczema, dermatitis and psoriasis should be treated as a localised contraindication as affected areas may be hypersensitive and the condition may be exacerbated by massage.

- **recent scar tissue** – massage should only be applied once the tissue is fully healed and can withstand pressure. Gentle frictions may be applied over healed scar tissue in order to help break down adhesions.

- **severe bruising, open cuts or abrasions** – these should be treated as localised contraindications, and if presented in the treatment areas they should be avoided.

- **undiagnosed lumps, bumps and swellings** – the client should be referred to their GP for a diagnosis. Massage may increase the susceptibility to damage in the area by virtue of pressure and motion.

Additional Cautions

- **allergies** – care should be taken to ensure that any oils or products used do not contain items to which the client may be allergic. Patch tests should be carried out to avoid adverse reactions.

- **asthma** – care should be taken to position the client comfortably during treatment, and to avoid using any massage mediums or substances a client may be allergic to.

- **medication** – certain medications may inhibit or distort the client's ability to give feedback regarding pressure, discomfort and pain. Always check with the client's GP if you are unsure as to type of medication and its effects.

- **pregnancy** – although pregnancy is not strictly a contraindication, unless there are serious complications, special care should be taken for a pregnant client to ensure that they are comfortable during the treatment. Therapists should be aware that some women may experience side effects as a result of the pregnancy, such as dizziness and high blood pressure. Pressure and duration of treatment may need to be adjusted according to the individual circumstances.

Total contraindications	Referral to GP/medical advice
■ High temperature or fever ■ Infectious/contagious diseases ■ Recent haemorrhage ■ Recent head or neck injury ■ Intoxication ■ Migraine	■ Recent surgery ■ Severe circulatory disorder/heart condition ■ Thrombosis/embolism ■ High/low blood pressure ■ Dysfunction of the nervous system ■ Epilepsy ■ Diabetes ■ Cancer ■ Undiagnosed lumps, bumps or swelling
Localised contraindications	**Special cautions**
■ Recent scar tissue ■ Bruising, open cuts or abrasions in treatment area	■ Allergies ■ Medication ■ Pregnancy

Liaising with other Health Care Professionals

As the benefits of Indian Head Massage become more widely known and validated, there are more opportunities opening up for therapists to work alongside other health care professionals. Therapists therefore need to be aware of professional and medical etiquette when liaising with other professionals.

Referral to a Health Care Professional

If a contraindication is established with a client at the time of consultation, treatment cannot usually proceed without reference to the client's GP. In this case, it is helpful to have a pre-prepared referral form on headed notepaper that may be taken by the client to their doctor, or may be posted with a stamped-addressed envelope.

When referring to a client's GP, it is important to note that a doctor's insurance will not cover them for giving permission or consent to holistic therapy treatments. It is therefore essential that therapists make it clear that they are seeking advice about the client's medical condition, in order to decide whether Indian Head Massage treatment is suitable, and that their proposed treatment is in accordance with medical advice.

In order to raise awareness of Indian Head Massage among doctors and other health care professionals, it is important for a therapist to include literature on Indian Head Massage concerning its methodology, benefits and effects.

Handling Referral Data from other Health Care Professionals

If a client has been referred to you by another health care professional, it is professional etiquette to reply with a status report on the client's progress. Report writing is an essential part of networking with other professionals, as it helps to raise awareness of the benefits of the treatment and its value in a client's physical and emotional well-being.

A status report should include the following information:

- a general introduction to the client and how he or she was referred

- a summary of the client's main presenting problems

- an evaluation of the therapist's findings

- the treatment used and explanation of the techniques involved

- the client's progress

- recommendations for future/continued treatment.

The most important factor in the consultation besides whether the client is medically suitable for treatment, is their expectations and objectives of the treatment.

Example of referral form

Therapist's Name
Clinic Address
Date

Doctor's Address
Surgery

Dear Dr _____

I am writing with regard to one of your patients _____ of

_____

who has requested **Indian Head Massage** treatment *(please see attached information on Indian Head Massage).*

Your patient has informed me that he/she suffers from _____.
(high blood pressure, etc)

Please can you advise me in your medical opinion if there is any reason why this patient should not receive an Indian Head Massage.

Thank you for your assistance in this matter

Therapist's name and signature

- -

Doctor's advice note
The proposed treatment of Indian Head Massage you suggest would be suitable/unsuitable for this patient.

_____

Doctor's name and signature

Setting Professional Boundaries

In order to have a healthy and professional relationship with clients there should be a balance between care and compassion for the client, and keeping a distance from any personal involvement. The setting of boundaries can provide the foundation upon which a therapist can build a professional relationship with a client. A therapeutic relationship should always involve distance between a therapist and a client, in order to make it safe for both parties.

There is always a risk of transference in a client-therapist relationship, in which a client begins to personalise the professional relationship and thus steps over the professional boundary. There is also risk of counter-transference when a therapist has difficulty in maintaining a professional distance from the client's problems and begins to step into a friend/counsellor role. If either of these situations occurs, it is important to realise how potentially damaging this can be for a client and for the therapist, and how it detracts from the healing process.

When to Refer a Client to Another Member of a Health Care Team

While Indian Head Massage can be very beneficial in relaxing a client and relieving minor stress-related conditions, it is important to realise that all treatments have their limitations.

If a client presents a condition that is beyond the scope of their treatment, such as a serious medical physical or psychological condition, it is essential that a therapist is able to recognise this and refer the client to the professional who can best help them. In this instance, it is useful for therapists to have resources available for clients to access such as information on:

- other complementary therapies
- counsellors or psychotherapists
- professional therapy organisations whom members of the public can contact for details of qualified members
- advice centres
- self help groups.

Displaying information offers the client the chance to choose for themselves a way of moving forward with their own situation. Holistic therapy treatments such as Indian Head Massage always tend to work best when there is a combined treatment strategy; this may involve a client receiving regular treatments, making lifestyle adjustments and attending for treatment with another health care professional.

An example of a consultation form that may be used for Indian Head Massage is shown opposite.

INDIAN HEAD MASSAGE CONSULTATION FORM

Client Note

The following information is required for your safety and to benefit your health. Whilst Indian head massage is a very safe treatment, there are certain contra-indications which may require special care. The following information will be treated in the strictest of confidence. It may however, be necessary for you to consult your GP before any treatment can be given.

Date of initial consultation: _____ Client ref. No. _____

Personal Details

Name: _____ Title: Mr / Mrs / Miss / Ms / Other _____

Address: _____

_____

Telephone Number – Daytime: _____ Evening: _____

Date of birth: _____ Occupation: _____

Marital status: _____ No of children (inc ages): _____

Medical Details

Name of Doctor : _____ Surgery: _____

Address: _____

Telephone Number : _____

Do you have/have you ever suffered with any of the following?

(Please give dates and details)   Dates and Details

Recent head or neck injury?	Y	N	_____
Cardiovascular condition?	Y	N	_____
Thrombosis or embolism?	Y	N	_____
High or low blood pressure?	Y	N	_____
Dysfunction of the nervous system?	Y	N	_____
Recent haemorrhage?	Y	N	_____
Cuts or abrasions in the treatment area?	Y	N	_____
Recent operation?	Y	N	_____
Diabetes?	Y	N	_____
Epilepsy?	Y	N	_____
Spastic conditions?	Y	N	_____
Migraine ?	Y	N	_____
Skin/scalp or hair disorder or infection?	Y	N	_____
Any recent scar tissue/bruises/ open cuts/large moles lumps/other swellings?	Y	N	_____
Any allergies?	Y	N	_____
Any medical condition (not mentioned above)?	Y	N	_____
Are you currently under the influence of drugs or alcohol?	Y	N	_____

►

Current medical treatment: _____
_____
_____

Current medication (list dosages):
_____
_____

GP referral required: Yes ( )   No ( )
Clearance form sent: Yes ( )   No ( ) Date : _____
Clearance form received :   Yes ( )   No ( ) Date : _____

General state of health

Do you smoke: Yes ( ) average per day _____ No ( )
Do you drink alcohol   Yes ( ) average consumption _____ daily / weekly   No ( )
How many glasses of water do you drink daily? _____
How would you describe your diet? _____
Stress levels :   High ( )   Medium ( )   Low ( )
Sleep pattern :   Good ( )   Average ( )   Poor ( )
Exercise undertaken / lifestyle: _____
_____
Do you follow a regular exercise program : Yes ( ) No ( )   Details : _____
_____
Do you have any hobbies / time set aside for relaxation (give details) : _____
_____
Reason for seeking treatment: _____
Have you had an Indian head massage treatment before: Yes ( )   No ( )
If yes please give brief details of previous treatments and succes : _____
_____
Are you currently having any other forms of alternative / complementary treatment? (please
give details) _____
_____

Client declaration

I declare that the information I have given is true and correct and that as far as I am aware, I can undertake
treatment without any adverse effects. I have been fully informed about contraindications and am therefore willing
to proceed. I understand that Indian Head Massage does not substitute medical treatment.

Client's signature : _____   **Date :** _____

Formulating a Treatment Plan for Indian Head Massage

Once the verbal and non-verbal information has been elicited from the client, the therapist is then in a position to suggest a treatment plan, or strategy, and obtain the client's agreement before proceeding.

A treatment plan for Indian Head Massage will include the following information:

- the date of the treatment

- feedback from any previous treatment, if applicable

- any updated information on the client's condition since the original consultation

- the treatment objectives

- client expectations

- any special considerations, such as specific areas to be worked on, special needs or requirements

- an outline of the proposed treatment to include areas for treatment, length and cost of treatment

- suggested treatment frequency (this may also be reviewed at the end of the treatment)

- skin and hair type (including any allergies)

- type of oils used (if applicable) and reasons for choice

- the client's agreement.

KEY NOTE

An important consideration in a client's treatment plan may be the time of day the treatment is undertaken. A client may require the treatment in the morning to gently awaken the nerves and prepare the body for a day's activities or may require the appointment later in the day to help remove the stresses of the day and promote sleep.

Treatments should be reviewed at regular intervals in order to monitor progress and elicit client satisfaction. By discussing a treatment plan regularly with a client, their individual needs can be taken into consideration and changes can be made, as required.

Example of a Treatment Plan for Indian Head Massage

Client's name: *Chris Parkin*   **Date of Treatment:** *19 September*

Proposed treatment: *Indian Head Massage treatment of all areas, concentrating on neck and shoulders due to tension. Client has recently had a head cold and has been experiencing sinus congestion.*

Time of treatment: *early evening appointment required – 6.30 p.m.*

Treatment timing: *30 minutes*

Client expectations
- *To feel calm and more relaxed.*
- *To improve sleep pattern.*
- *To reduce muscular tension in the neck and shoulders.*
- *To help relieve sinus congestion.*

Treatment objectives
- *General stress relief and relaxation.*
- *Concentrate on reduction of muscular tension in the neck and shoulder regions.*
- *Concentrate on relieving sinus congestion with pressure points to the face.*

Special client considerations
As the client's posture is poor due to occupational stress, consideration needs to be given to client comfort and client awareness (advice to be given on basic stretches to improve posture). Client's stress levels are high presently, so emphasis will be on relaxation and good breathing throughout.

Oils to be used
Coconut oil to be used for dry scalp condition.

Recommended treatment frequency
Because of client's high stress levels at present, it is recommended that treatment is commenced at weekly intervals for a month and then reviewed.

Self-Assessment Questions

1 Which of the following is the most essential skill needed for a therapist to carry out an effective consultation for Indian Head Massage?

  a talking

  b being friendly

  c showing empathy

  d listening

2 What action should be taken if, during a consultation, a client informs you that they have very high blood pressure?

  a offer a lighter treatment which is soothing and relaxing

  b proceed with a normal treatment but keep checking that the client doesn't feel dizzy

  c ask the client to seek advice from their GP to see if treatment is advisable

  d do not offer a treatment unless the client is taking medication

3 Which of the following conditions would indicate that Indian Head Massage treatment could not be offered?

  a recent scar tissue

  b low blood pressure

  c acute infectious disease

  d open cut or abrasion

4 Which of the following conditions would not require referral to a GP for advice before offering treatment?

  a thrombosis/embolism

  b dysfunction of the nervous system

  c recent head or neck injury

  d open cut or abrasion

5 Why is it important to avoid using the words 'permission' or 'consent' on a doctor's referral note?

  a it is unethical

  b the correct medical terminology must be used for insurance purposes

  c it is not professional etiquette

  d a doctor's insurance will not cover them for giving permission or consent to holistic therapy treatments

▶

6   An Indian Head Massage treatment plan should contain

a   treatment objectives

b   the client's agreement

c   the type of oils used

d   all of the above

5 Indian Head Massage Case Studies

As part of the development process for therapists studying to become professional practitioners of Indian Head Massage, it is necessary to carry out a number of case studies to explore the practical efficacy of the techniques and most importantly, to gain valuable practical experience of the skills learnt.

Carrying out several treatments on case studies encourages repetitive practice and can help to increase confidence levels through client feedback.

This chapter is devoted to providing general guidelines on how to approach case studies, along with three examples.

By the end of this chapter you will:

■ Know how to present an Indian Head Massage case study as part of an assessment for a professional qualification.

Indications for Treatment

There are many conditions which a client may present that may benefit from Indian Head Massage. Common conditions Indian Head Massage has been known to help with include:

■ tension headaches

■ eyestrain

■ muscular tension

■ emotional stress

■ anxiety and depression

■ insomnia and disturbed sleep patterns

■ sinusitis

■ poor hair condition.

What is a Case Study

A case study is a record of a series of treatments carried out on a client, which has been evaluated for effectiveness. Outlined below are some general guidelines on how to present case studies. When considering who to choose for your case studies, it is advisable to choose as wide a range of clients as possible in order to meet the requirements of a professional award and to prepare yourself for commercial practice.

The essential components of a case study are as follows.

Client Profile

This is a general introduction to the client and will include background information such as age range, occupation, lifestyle issues, sleep patterns, hobbies and interests along with their main presenting problems/any factors that may affect them in their daily life.

Consultation Form

Before any treatment commences, the client needs to be assessed in order that their individual considerations may be taken into account (health problems or special needs). A full consultation must be carried out and recorded, including personal, medical and lifestyle details, along with a declaration and the client's signature. See the example of an Indian Head Massage Consultation Form on pages 115–116.

Observations

This may include initial and ongoing observations from information elicited from the original consultation and subsequent treatments. Therapists need to be perceptive of non-verbal signs the client may exhibit, such as their posture, facial expressions, breathing rate. These are all factors which will not be evident from the recording paperwork. The noting of these factors will assist the reader or assessor to build a fuller picture of your case study, and will reflect the development of your perceptive skills.

Treatment Plan

Once the initial consultation has taken place a course of treatment may then be recommended. A treatment plan will typically include the following information:

- client's name
- date and time of treatment
- outline of proposed treatment and areas to concentrate on
- treatment timing
- cost
- client expectations
- treatment objectives
- special client considerations
- oils to be used
- recommended treatment frequency.

Record of treatments

It is important that a record is kept of all treatments carried out. This will typically include:

- an assessment of the client's physical condition (noting any areas of tension, physiological responses) as well as psychological responses and body language (client nervous or apprehensive)
- visual assessment of the client (noting posture, non-verbal signs)
- any known reactions, their effects and any advice given
- aftercare advice given
- homecare advice, along with any oils or products suggested for home use
- outcome and general evaluation of the treatment
- recommendations for future treatment and the suggested frequency.

Evaluation

Evaluation is an essential part of a case study, as it is only through feedback and evaluation that a therapist can gauge the effectiveness of the treatments given, and ultimately measure their own professional development.

Factors to consider in evaluating the treatment are:

- Was the course of treatments effective. If so, in what ways?
- What benefits, if any, were derived from the treatments?
- Were there any particular parts of the treatment the client liked or disliked?
- Were there any contra-actions?
- Is the client keen to continue with regular treatments?

Written Testimonial

Once the course of treatments has been completed, it is necessary for the purposes of assessment and authenticity to ask your case studies to complete a written testimonial, which is a handwritten letter to confirm that they have received a course of treatment on the dates concerned, and should outline any benefits they have noticed as a result.

Self-evaluation

It is also important for therapists to carry out their own self-evaluation, in order to assess their own development. By objectively analysing their own performance, therapists can perfect their skills and commit to continual improvement.

Examples of Case Studies

Case Study 1

Client Profile

Name: Jan

Age: 42 years

Occupation: mature student and homemaker

Jan is a mature student with two girls of 17 and 14 years of age. She is currently training to be a counsellor and is on work placement at a local doctor's surgery.

Her life is therefore very busy, looking after her two daughters, completing her studies and looking after their home. Despite her busy schedule, Jan does find some time to relax; she swims, goes for walks and loves reading.

Physically, Jan is fit and healthy with no medical conditions. However, she does sometimes feel stressed out due to the pressures of her studies and running a home. She finds her neck muscles are often tight, in particular the right trapezius muscle often aches, causing her a degree of discomfort.

Jan's energy and stress levels are average.

Treatment Objectives

Jan had never experienced Indian Head Massage before. The effects and benefits of the treatment were therefore explained to her.

After consultation, it was agreed with Jan that the treatment objectives were to:

- help relieve muscular tension in the shoulders and neck
- aid general relaxation and relief of tension
- help uplift Jan psychologically and aid stress relief.

Treatment Plan

It was agreed with Jan that a course of three treatments would be given over a period of two weeks; the first two were given in a week, and the third in the following week.

Coconut oil was to be used on the scalp as Jan's hair and scalp has a tendency to dryness.

Account of Treatments

Treatment 1

On commencement of the first treatment Jan indicated that she was very tired mentally, as she had just returned from her work placement.

The treatment uncovered a lot of tension in the neck and shoulder area. The neck and shoulders were very stiff. A lot of deep breathing was suggested throughout the treatment to help ease tension. By the time we reached the scalp massage Jan was almost asleep.

After the treatment Jan reported that at the start she was aware of all her thoughts and her mind was not still; however, at the end of the treatment she felt calm, extremely relaxed but at the same time energised.

Jan was advised to drink plenty of water following treatment, to rest, have a light meal and to avoid alcohol or caffeine consumption. She was also encouraged to leave the oil on for a few hours following treatment before shampooing.

Jan did not have any adverse reactions after the treatment and reported that she felt quite energetic the next day.

Treatment 2

The second treatment was given three days after the first. Jan had been at college all day and was tired, but less tension was noticeable. She relaxed from the beginning and fell asleep. At the conclusion of the treatment, she felt relaxed, calm and contented.

Jan did not report any adverse reactions after her second treatment and reported that she felt relaxed but energetic the next day.

Treatment 3

The third treatment was given a week later. During this treatment Jan commented on the overall improvement she was experiencing and how the muscular tension had decreased to the point where it no longer caused her discomfort. She reported she was also feeling more relaxed and energetic.

Outcomes and Recommendations

The course of three treatments have proved very beneficial to Jan. During and after each treatment, the improvements have been visibly noticeable. Jan has also commented enthusiastically on how much better she has felt.

Further treatments were recommended to maintain Jan's progress and condition and it was suggested that treatments were continued once fortnightly as a preventative measure against tension build-up.

Client Testimonial

'The experience of the head was quite different from anything I had experienced before. I was aware of my tension during the first treatment and found the shoulder and upper arm movements quite strange. However, the pressure was just right and by the second and third treatments I knew what to expect and was much more relaxed. In the second and third treatments I actually fell asleep – something I never realised I could do sitting upright in a chair!

'I think I slept better and definitely felt more invigorated in the days afterwards, and less tense.

'I really enjoyed and appreciated the experience and shall definitely be continuing with regular treatments.'

Case Study 2

Client Profile

Name: Pam

Age: 59 years

Occupation: retired librarian

Pam is a widow with two daughters and four grandchildren who she looks after on a regular basis. Although Pam is retired, she has quite an active social life playing tennis and swimming and she enjoys gardening.

Generally Pam is in good health and has no major illnesses, but sometimes suffers from sinusitis, headaches and disturbed sleep. She takes HRT and cholesterol tablets for which she has regular reviews with her GP.

During the consultation Pam revealed that she had manipulation on her left shoulder under anaesthetic two years ago. However, Pam's current condition did not prove to be contraindicated to treatment, although caution was observed when treating the shoulder and upper arm area. She did not present with any other conditions or considerations for treatment.

Generally Pam has low levels of stress and medium energy levels, but recently has been experiencing low energy levels. While the benefits were explained to her, Pam mentioned her dry scalp and thinning hair.

Treatment Objectives

After consultation, it was agreed that the treatment objectives were to:

- aid general relaxation
- improve congestion in the sinus area
- improve scalp and hair condition
- relieve muscular tension
- improve energy levels.

Treatment Plan

It was agreed with Pam to give a course of three treatments over a four-week period. The first and second treatments would be weekly and the third after a fortnight.

Account of Treatments

Treatment 1

Pam has never had any form of massage treatment before and was quite apprehensive. As a result she was unable to relax fully during her first treatment. She enjoyed the scalp massage and felt that the pressure points over the sinus area on the face helped to ease congestion. Pat commented that she felt relaxed at the conclusion of the treatment.

She felt calm and she experienced no adverse reactions the next day.

Treatment 2

During this treatment the muscles in Pam's neck and upper back felt very tight. She explained this was due to the fact she had been gardening during the day. Deep breathing was advised to help ease tension during the treatment. Pam was visibly more relaxed during this session and commented that her neck and upper back felt better.

Pam reported that she experienced a headache for a couple of days after the second treatment; this she felt was caused by congestion and the sinuses.

Treatment 3

The third treatment was given two weeks later. During the treatment Pam commented on how the pressure points over the sinus area helped and how the use of oil had helped with the dryness of the scalp and hair. Pam relaxed really well during this treatment and almost fell asleep.

Aftercare advice was given after each treatment: to drink plenty of water, rest, have a light meal and avoid consumption of alcohol and stimulants. Pam was also shown some simple massage techniques to use at home with oil for the long-term care of the hair and scalp condition.

Outcomes and Recommendations

The course of treatments has been successful for Pam. She felt relaxed after each treatment and indicated how they have helped with her sinusitis, sleep pattern and her hair and scalp condition. Pam also commented on how her energy levels have improved since treatments commenced.

Pam has requested that she continue with regular treatments for relaxation and body maintenance. Suggested frequency is once a fortnight.

Client Testimonial

'The course of Indian Head Massage I have received has been a beneficial and new experience for me. Having never received a massage, I was unsure of what to expect and felt quite nervous to start with. Everything was so well explained, and the pressure was perfect for me. Although I felt relaxed after the first treatment, I was able to relax more fully on the second and third knowing what to expect. I would very much like to continue with regular treatment, as this seems an ideal way to relax. It has certainly helped to improve my sinusitis and headaches, and after each treatment I found I slept more soundly and woke feeling more refreshed.'

Case Study 3

Client Profile

Name: Kelly

Age: 18 years

Occupation: student

Kelly is completing her A levels in Maths and the Sciences. She is fit and in good health, but suffers from hay fever for which she takes antihistamines.

Kelly has never experienced Indian Head Massage before; however, due to exam stress she was keen to try the treatment for stress relief and relaxation.

Treatment Objectives

After consultation, it was agreed with Kelly that the treatment objectives were to:

- help relieve muscular tension
- help relieve mental fatigue
- promote psychological uplift
- aid relaxation and stress relief.

Treatment Plan

It was agreed with Kelly that, due to her high stress levels at exam time, two treatments would be given in the first week and the third treatment given a week later.

Account of Treatment

Treatment 1

During the first treatment Kelly was unable to relax to start with; however, she began to relax with the neck massage and actually feel asleep during the scalp massage. A lot of tension was found in the neck and shoulder muscles. A little more time was devoted to treating the shoulder area and Kelly was advised to take plenty of deep breaths throughout the treatment to help ease tension.

Kelly was quite surprised how relaxed the treatment had made her feel and commented she could not believe she fell asleep sitting up. She felt calm, relaxed and energetic at the end of the first treatment.

She was advised to drink lots of water, to rest, eat a light meal following treatment and to avoid consumption of alcohol and stimulants.

Treatment 2

The second treatment was carried out after four days. Kelly reported that after the first treatment she felt relaxed and a bit tired the next day, but became more energetic as the day went on.

At the commencement of the second treatment, Kelly's neck and shoulders felt much looser. During the treatment she relaxed and fell asleep, but during the face massage she was awake and alert. After treatment, she was keen to go to an aerobics class, but was advised against it and told to rest in order that the energy could be utilised in the body for the healing process. The same aftercare advice was given as that in the first treatment.

Treatment 3

The third treatment was given a week later. Kelly reported that she had a slight headache the day after the second treatment, but also felt more calm and relaxed. She commented that she also felt dehydrated and felt better after drinking more water.

During the third treatment Kelly fell asleep soon after the treatment started but remained awake and energetic during the face massage.

Aftercare advice was specified as in the previous treatments.

The day following the third treatment, Kelly reported that she felt quite tired and lethargic in the morning. She also felt dehydrated but felt better after drinking more water. As the day progressed, she commented on how much more energetic she felt.

Outcomes and Recommendations

The series of treatments given have been successful for Kelly. She felt she was able to relax, unwind and relieve the mental fatigue she was feeling due to the pressure of her exams. After each treatment Kelly felt tired, lethargic and dehydrated due to toxins being released; however, after drinking more water Kelly felt much better – energetic, calm and relaxed.

Kelly is keen to continue treatments for relaxation; suggested frequency would ideally be once a fortnight.

Client Testimonial

'I thoroughly enjoyed my head massage sessions. I had never experienced a head massage before and found some of the sensations quite strange for the first time, yet at the same time they were very relaxing. While my back, shoulders and arms were being massaged I felt very lethargic and fell asleep every time these areas of my body were massaged. However, I found that when my neck, scalp and face were massaged I felt very energised and revitalised. The massage always left me feeling energetic and lively, yet calm and relaxed inside. During each massage I was aware that my body was relaxing, my heart rate slowed slightly and I fell asleep very easily as I became used to the movements. I also noticed that during the massage I was unaware of time passing as I was so relaxed.

'The days following the massages I sometimes felt quite tired and lethargic. I was also slightly dehydrated, but soon felt better when I increased my intake of water.

'I feel the head massage sessions have enabled me to relax and cope with my increased stress levels at this time and therefore I feel I have really benefited from the treatments. I would also like to continue with the treatments regularly to maintain the benefits.'

6 Indian Head Massage Techniques

In India massage has long been adopted as a daily practice in order to help maintain a healthy mind and body throughout the course of life. In the modern day of high stress levels in the western world, massage is a must for relaxing both mind and body, and recharging depleted energy levels. Indian Head Massage is uniquely different from other types of therapeutic massage practised in the West in that it is applied through the clothes to a client in a seated position and so there is no need for special or sophisticated equipment.

By the end of this chapter you will be able to:

- Understand the massage movements used in Indian Head Massage along with their effect.

- Prepare a treatment area for Indian Head Massage.

- Understand the properties and benefits of oils and herbs used in Indian Head Massage.

- Understand how to balance the chakras.

- Carry out a step-by-step Indian Head Massage treatment to the upper back and shoulders, upper arms, neck, scalp and face.

- Provide aftercare advice.

Massage Movements Used in Indian Head Massage

The massage techniques used in Indian Head Massage are simple but extremely effective. They consist of a combination of traditional Indian techniques and westernised techniques.

Effleurage

Effleurage is one of the principal techniques used in Indian Head Massage. It is a stroking or *smoothing* movement that signals the beginning and end of a massage. Effleurage is also used as a linking movement to facilitate the flow from one technique to another.

Effleurage is applied with the whole hand, fingers or the forearms. Pressure can be superficial or deep, depending on the effects to be achieved. Effleurage can be applied slowly and gently to produce a calming and soothing effect or applied more briskly to stimulate the circulation and energise and revitalise the person being massaged. In Indian Head Massage a combination of slow, gentle stroking and brisker energetic effleurage is used.

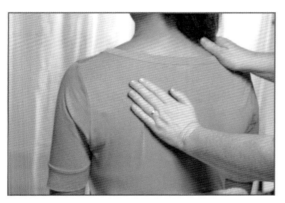

Fig 6.1 Effleurage/smoothing

Effects of effleurage

- dilates the capillaries and increases the circulation
- relaxes the client by soothing sensory nerve endings in the skin
- prepares the area for deeper strokes
- aids in moving waste out of congested areas
- soothes tired, achy muscles
- warms the tissues making them more extensible.

Petrissage

Petrissage movements are deeper movements using the whole hand, thumbs or fingers. There are many types of petrissage used in Indian Head Massage (for example, picking up, squeezing and releasing, rolling). Petrissage movements involve the skin and muscular tissue being moved from their position and squeezed with a firm pressure away from the underlying structure and then released.

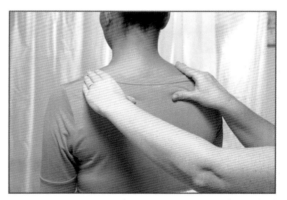

Fig 6.2 Petrissage

Effects of petrissage

- increases in the removal of waste products from the tissue and encourages fresh oxygen and nutrients to be delivered to the tissues
- stretches muscle tissue and fascia
- reduces adhesions and muscular spasms
- relaxes muscle tissue and reduces accumulated stress and tension from the muscles.

Tapotement

These techniques are performed with the fingers and are similar to percussion movements in Swedish massage. They involve a series of light, brisk, springy movements applied with both hands in rapid succession.

The main tapotement movements used in Indian Head Massage are as follows:

Hacking

This technique involves flicking the hands rhythmically up and down in quick succession using the ulnar borders of the hands.

Champi

This technique is also known as 'double hacking'. It is performed by holding the hands in a prayer position, and allowing them to relax so that the heels of the hands and the pads of the fingers and thumbs are gently touching. A series of light, rapid striking movements are then performed across areas such as the shoulders.

Tabla playing (tapping)

Tabla refers to a drum used in the classical and popular music of northern India. It is a light technique that uses the fingertips to tap on the head.

Effects of tapotement

- stimulates the nerve endings
- increases the circulation and local blood flow
- increases muscle tone through stimulation of muscle fibres
- wakens and refreshes the body.

When applied lightly, tapotement strokes are soothing and bring about relaxation and a release of tension and when applied more deeply they have a stimulating effect on the nerves and are refreshing.

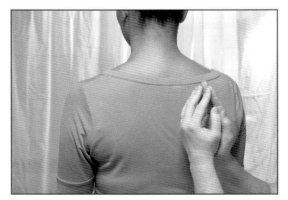

Fig 6.3 Champi/double hacking

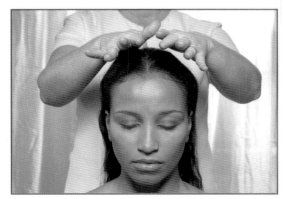

Fig 6.4 Tabla playing

Frictions

A strong feature of the Indian Head Massage is friction movements which are performed with the whole of the hand, the heel of the hand, the fingers or thumbs. They are deeper more penetrating movements that causes the skin to rub against the underlying structures.

Frictions are excellent for breaking down tension nodules that have accumulated due to stress and tension. Frictions are particularly useful in Indian Head Massage for working around the scapulae and on either side of the spine.

Effects of frictions

- dilate the capillaries and increase the circulation

- generate heat locally in the area massaged

- loosen stiffness and tension by relaxing muscles

- break down and help free adhered tissue in restricted areas.

Vibrations

These are fine shaking, trembling or oscillating movements that are applied with one or both hands, using either the whole palmar surface of the hand or the fingertips. A fine trembling movement may be achieved by moving the fingers up and down or side to side while maintaining contact with the skin.

Vibrations may be performed either in a static form or where the hands or fingertips travel over a point while still vibrating. Vibration movements may be fine, deep or vigorous depending on the effect required.

Effects of vibrations

- help relieve tension and aid relaxation, creating a sedative effect

- stimulate and clear nerve pathways, creating a refreshing effect

- stimulate muscle spindles, thereby creating minute muscle contractions

- help relieve pain.

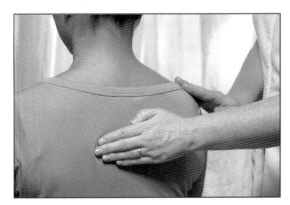

Fig 6.5 Frictions

Pressure Points

Pressure points are vital energy points similar to acupressure used in Chinese medicine. In Ayurveda it is said that the 'life force' is located in the head. By balancing the energy within these vital points, health at all levels within the body is promoted. The stimulation of pressure points in the head is said to stimulate the hypothalamus, pituitary and other areas of the brain to encourage healing to be relayed to various parts of the body.

Effects of pressure points

Pressure points are applied with the fingers and the thumbs and their effects are to:

- clear congestion in the nerve pathways
- relieve pressure and pain from tense muscles
- relieve sinus congestion
- encourage lymph drainage
- increase circulation locally to the area
- restore the energy balance to the body.

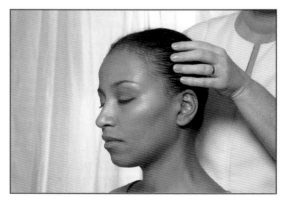

Fig 6.6 Pressure points

Marma points

Marma points are an integral part of Ayuveda and are the subtle pressure points, similar to points used in acupressure, that stimulate the life force or *pranic* flow. The marmas are anatomical places on the body, mostly composed of flesh and bones.

There are a total of 107 marmas in the body:

- 37 in the head and neck
- 12 in the front of the body
- 22 in the upper limbs
- 14 in the back of the body
- 22 in the lower limbs.

Marma points are naturally sensitive points, measured by finger widths known as *anguli*. The finger width is the finger of the person being treated and not the therapist's own finger. The location of marmas are given in this way because each person is made differently and has a different size and proportion. The location of marmas may vary from one to eight finger widths, and often relate to regions of the body and not a point.

In Indian Head Massage the marmas may be used to:

- treat the *pranas*
- treat a specific organ or system of the body
- treat a specific dosha imbalance.

Marma points relating to the head and neck

Marma point	Location	Helps with
1. Adhipati	at the crown of the head and the midline (11 finger widths above the eyebrows)	calming the mind, heightening perception, assisting with spinal alignment and mental clarity
2. Brahma randra	over the anterior fontanelle	insomnia, elevation of mood, easing headaches
3. Shiva andra	over posterior fontanelle	lowering of high blood pressure, relieving dizziness, improving the memory and sense of alertness
4. Vidhura	behind and slightly below the mastoid process (bony bump behind the ear lobe)	congestion in the ears, relief of tension in the jaw and facial muscles, mental tension and anxiety
5. Krikatika	either side of spine, where the neck meets the skull	releasing neck and shoulder tension, relaxing the body, improving posture
6. Simanta	bony joints at the top of the skull	whole body relaxation, aids sleep
7. Arshak	on top surface of the collar bone in the L made with the large neck muscles you feel as you turn the head from side to side	stimulates energy to the liver and spleen, aiding digestion, stabilising blood sugar levels
8. Manya	side of the neck, four finger widths below the ear lobe	improves circulation to the face, stimulates lymph drainage, helps ease a sore throat or upper chest congestion
9. Sira matrika	either side of the windpipe on the upper half of the neck	helps improve circulation and improves the voice
10. Nila	either side of the windpipe on the lower half of the neck	helps the voice and helps ease a sore throat
11. Kantha	in the middle of the neck at the level you feel your voice vibrate	healthy functioning of the thyroid gland and expression of inner feelings, helps regulate the mood

▶

Marma point	Location	Helps with
12. Kathanadi	behind the top of the sternum	helps sore throats and upper respiratory congestion
13. Hanu	in the middle of the chin	increases circulation to the face and helps your head connect with your heart feelings
14. Oshta	in the middle of the upper lip	mental clarity and improves sexual desire
15. Phana	either side of the nose, just above the flare of your nostrils	helps clear lung energy, clears the sinuses and helps to balance functioning of right and left sides of brain enabling us to feel more able to cope with stress
16. Gandu	either side of the nose, just above Phana	clears the sinuses and brightens the eyes
17. Apanga	in the corner of the eye, slightly on the inner surface of the bony orbit of the eye	relieves puffiness around the eyes and eye strain, clears the upper sinuses
18. Bhruh	either side of the very top of the nose where you can feel little bumps just above the eyes	eases eye strain and headaches
19. Avarta	in the middle (above) of each eyebrow	brings energy to the head, helps you feel more centred
20. Shankha	in the hollow of the temples	calms and nourishes the brain and the mind
21. Sthapani	just above the eyebrows, in the centre of the forehead (third eye area)	brings peace and harmony to the mind

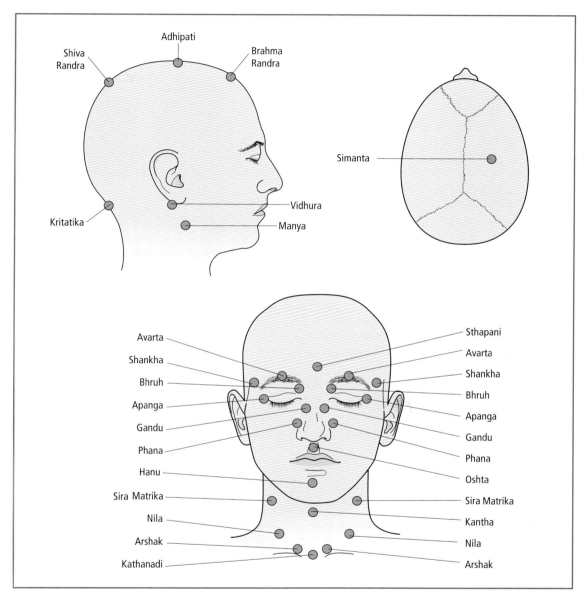

Fig 6.7 Marma points relating to the head and neck

Treatment methods of marma points

Marma points may be treated with pressure, circular massage, heat and with oils. Pressure is used on the marmas in the same way as any other form of pressure therapy. The marma is first found and located by the practitioner finding a hard, tender or sensitive point. Pressure is then increasingly applied with conscious breathing, in the knowledge that *prana* is going out from the fingers and into the client. When enough pressure has been applied, small counterclockwise massage movements may be used to break up the tension from the point.

In general, clockwise movements stimulate or energise a marma point and a counterclockwise movement dispels and liberates blocked or stagnant *prana*.

The key to using pressure therapy on a marma point is to go slowly and deeply and to work within the comfort zone of the client. It is essential to avoid pushing forcibly through a marma, as this can go against the internal harmony and interfere with the healing process.

Health and safety note

Although the treatment of marma points is part of traditional Ayurvedic massage, it is essential that practitioners undergo additional professional training and study in order to promote safe and effective use of them, as any injury to these subtle energy points may cause danger to life.

Compression

This is a form of petrissage in which the muscles are gently pressed against a surface such as the scalp, top of the shoulders or the upper arms, with the palms of both hands, and then slowly released.

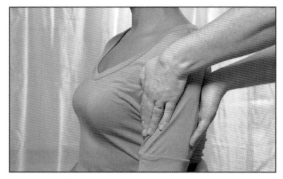

Fig 6.8 Compression

Effects of compression

In general the effects are to:

■ increase blood flow locally to the area being treated

■ help relieve tension in the muscles and alleviate pain, through gentle compression of the blood vessels and nerves.

Hair Tugging

This is a technique used in the scalp massage where the roots of the hair are lifted in-between the fingers of both hands and pulled upwards. Hair tugging stimulates hair growth by stimulating the nerves in the hair root.

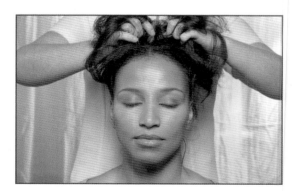

Fig 6.9 Hair tugging

Equipment and Materials for Indian Head Massage

The beauty of Indian Head Massage lies in its simplicity. It can be performed in an ordinary chair, without the need to purchase expensive equipment.

The type of chair best suited to Indian Head Massage treatments is one with a relatively low back and without an armrest.

An important factor for the therapist is the height of the chair; it is therefore preferable to use a chair with an adjustable height and backrest, so that the therapist's working position is comfortable.

It is also important for a therapist practising Indian Head Massage to have

- a variety of oils for optional use on the scalp

- a selection of small towels for draping across the shoulders/wrapping up the hair after the scalp oil massage, or for wrapping up the feet
- a dry hand cleanser (the type of hand cleanser most suited to a visiting therapist is a dry anti-bacterial cleanser which is easy and practical to use)
- a comb or brush to ensure the hair is unknotted and free from hair products prior to the massage
- a variety of clips to help secure the client's hair out of the way when massaging the upper back, neck and shoulders
- a small footstool/cushion (for the client to rest their feet if desired).

Hair Types

An important factor in deciding on the type of oil to use is identifying the client's hair type.

Hair type	Description
Dry	■ dry, flaky appearance ■ scalp may also be dry and flaky ■ may have a coarse appearance, lacking in shine
Oily	■ oily hair presents with a shiny appearance due to excess sebum ■ may look lank and lifeless
Fine	■ fine hair is smaller in diameter than medium or coarse hair ■ generally limper but shinier than coarse hair
Thick/dense	■ thick/dense hair is larger in diameter than thin or fine hair ■ may also be coarse
Chemically treated	■ hair may be weak and damaged ■ may be dry and brittle due to over processing
Coarse	■ coarse hair has a larger diameter and fewer hair follicles, which means the hair produces less oil, therefore it can tend to be dry

Oils Used in Indian Head Massage

The use of oil is optional when massaging the scalp. Oil that is applied to the head is absorbed into the roots of the hair which are connected with nerve fibres leading to the brain. Applying oil to the head helps to strengthen the hair, remove dryness, and by relaxing the muscles and nerves of the head, fatigue is eliminated leaving the recipient feeling refreshed and revitalised. Massaging the head increases the supply of oxygen and glucose to the brain and improves the circulation of spinal fluid around the brain and the spinal cord.

There are several oils which may be used for Indian Head Massage. Traditionally oils such as sesame, coconut, olive, mustard and almond have been used by Indian women as part of their grooming ritual to keep their hair in good condition.

Oil	Description	Properties	Hair/skin type	Additional notes
Almond	a popular oil full of nutrients, which makes an excellent hair conditioner	■ high in nutrients such as unsaturated fatty acids, protein, vitamins A, B, D and E ■ helps to soften, moisturise and protect the hair ■ has warming effects on the body and is therefore useful for stimulating hair growth, as well as helping to reduce muscular pain and tightness	suitable for all hair/skin types	**caution**: avoid this oil if your client has an allergy to nuts

Oil	Description	Properties	Hair/skin type	Additional notes
Coconut	this is a popular light oil for Indian Head Massage and is widely used in southern parts of India, especially in the spring	■ very moisturising and softening on the skin and the hair ■ also helps to relieve inflammation	■ dry, brittle and lifeless hair ■ dry, dehydrated skins	**caution**: take care with hypersensitive skin
Sesame	■ this is one of the most popular oils used in the western part of India ■ it is used as a base oil for all oils used in head massage and is very popular in Ayurveda	■ sesame seeds are high in minerals such as iron, calcium and phosphorus which help to strengthen, nourish and protect the hair ■ can also help to improve skin texture, reduce swellings and alleviate muscular pain	all skin types, especially dry skin and hair	it is particularly popular in India during the summer as it does provide some protection from the rays of the sun.
Olive	■ this oil is very popular in the western world ■ of viscous consistency with a strong smell, it is often mixed with another lighter oil such as almond	■ contains high levels of unsaturated fatty acids and has excellent moisturising properties ■ is soothing and penetrative ■ has stimulating properties which help to increase heat in the body and is therefore helpful in reducing swellings and alleviating muscular tightness and pain	all skin/hair types, especially dry skin and hair	

▶

Oil	Description	Properties	Hair/skin type	Additional notes
Mustard	■ this oil is often found in Indian grocery stores and is one of the most popular oils used in north-west India ■ especially used during the winter months because of the hot, warming sensation it creates ■ strong and pungent smell and, by increasing body heat, its effects are very warming ■ popular among wrestlers and bodybuilders in India	well known for its ability to break down congestion and swellings from tense muscles and to relieve pain	for dryness of the scalp, using mustard oil with a small amount of turmeric powder can prove very effective	**caution**: this oil may irritate the skin because of its stimulating nature

KEY NOTE

When the body is subjected to stress and illness, the skin and hair are often affected, resulting in dryness and sometimes loss of hair.

With tension the scalp becomes tight, restricting the flow of the nutrients which promote healthy hair growth.

Using oils on a regular basis can help to encourage healthy shiny hair, nourish the hair follicles, slow down hair loss and soften and moisturise the hair.

NB: *the oils used in Indian Head Massage are seasonal, with mustard and olive being a popular choice in the winter due to their warming effects and sesame and coconut being more popular in the summer months.*

In addition to the oils mentioned above there are other oils which are traditionally used in India for the treatment of hair. These oils are blended with eastern herbs and spices not readily available in the West. These may be imported and sold in traditional Indian supermarkets and health stores.

Hair oils

Name of oil	Properties/benefits
Amla	In combination with henna, this is an excellent hair tonic. It promotes the growth of healthy and lustrous hair and has a cooling and nourishing effect.
Brahmi	This is a unique combination of carefully selected exotic herbs blended with pure coconut oil. Brahmi oil is used medicinally in India as a tonic for the nervous system for those suffering from anxiety and emotional exhaustion. Brahmi oil helps the growth of long, lustrous hair and provides relief from dandruff and joint pain. It is also said to help improve the memory and dispel mental fatigue.
Bhringraj	This is a popular oil for daily head and scalp massage in India. As well as helping to promote hair growth, it is said to nourish brain cells, help encourage better sleep and relieve stress and tension.
Neem oil	This oil is native to India and has antiseptic, astringent and antibacterial properties. Early Sanskrit medical writings refer to the attributes of neem. It is particularly effective for relieving itching and irritation, on the scalp and the skin.
Pumpkin seed	This oil is extremely nourishing for dry and stressed hair, as pumpkin seeds are rich in vitamins A, E, C and K, unsaturated fatty acids and proteins.
Shikakai	This is an excellent hair rejuvenator and has astringent and antiseptic properties. Is said to help with eczema and dry scalp.

The Use of Essential Oils in Indian Head Massage

Traditionally essential oils such as sandalwood, jasmine and rosemary have long been used in India as part of Ayurvedic preparations. While the properties of essential oils can be extremely beneficial on the hair and the scalp, it is recommended that essential oils are not individually blended by a therapist practising Indian Head Massage unless they are qualified and insured for the practice of selecting and blending essential oils.

Many essential oils suppliers offer pre-blended preparations for sale which may be used in Indian Head Massage. However, caution is advised on safe proportions due to the fact that when carrying out Indian Head Massage you are close to the brain and the olfactory response, and the effects of essential oils may be enhanced.

Significant Points on the Head for Oil Application

There are three important points on the head according to the Ayurvedic tradition:

- The **first point** can be found by measuring eight finger widths above the eyebrows. This is where it is recommended that oil is poured on to the scalp initially and then distributed symmetrically down both sides of the head with the fingers.

- The **second point** is at the crown of the head on the midline: an important therapeutic point and it is where blood vessels, nerves and lymphatics meet. Oil is traditionally poured on to the crown and then evenly distributed down the sides of the scalp.

- The **third point** is at the base of the skull and is the point at which the neck meets the skull. Oil is traditionally poured on to this point, with the person's head inclined forwards and then mixed in either side and towards the ears.

Chakra Balancing and Indian Head Massage

Chakras

Everything that happens to us on an emotional level has an energetic impact on the subtle body, which in turn has an impact on the physical body. Chakras are non-physical energy centres located about an inch away from the physical body. The energy field of each chakra extends beyond the visible body of matter into the subtle body or aura.

It is important to remember that chakras do not have a physical form and any illustration of the chakras is merely a visual aid to the imagination and not a literal physical reality. Chakras are a way of describing the flow of subtle energy and are often said to be related to an endocrine gland, which the chakra is thought to influence.

With stress, the chakras can lose their ability to synchronise with each other and become unbalanced. If negative energy becomes stored in a chakra, it can accumulate and the function of the chakra becomes impaired. Ultimately, this can lead to the energy blocks where the chakras virtually ceases to function and creates an imbalance as other chakras attempt to compensate for the blocked centre, creating additional strain for the energy system.

The effects of an accumulation of negative energy in the chakras can manifest itself as an emotional or physical condition. Often we are only aware of a change in the physical body as our attention is drawn to a physical body in the form of pain or disease; this may not always be linked to being a symptom of a cause within the subtle body.

Chakras are the focal points for the energies of the subtle bodies and are the key to restoring balance. By placing hands along the axis of the chakras, energy can be aligned and harmony restored. By working with the subtle energy of the chakras, energy may be strengthened, decreased or balanced as needed by the body at the time of the treatment.

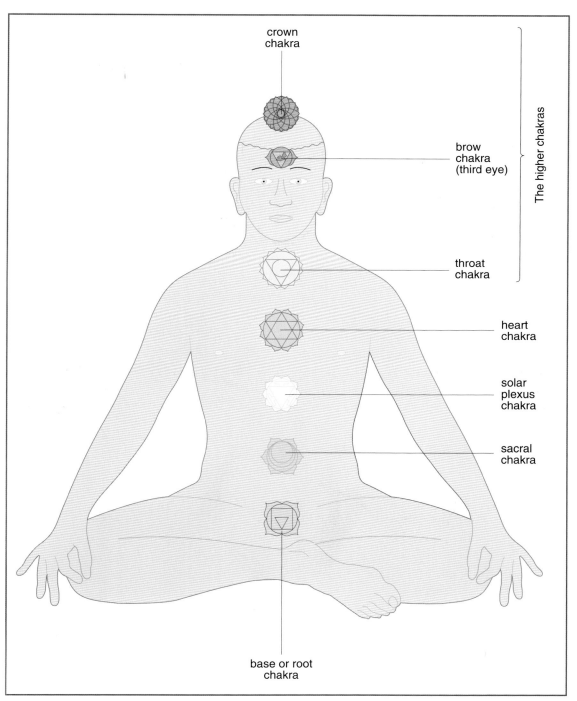

crown
chakra

brow
chakra
(third eye)

throat
chakra

The higher chakras

heart
chakra

solar
plexus
chakra

sacral
chakra

base or root
chakra

Fig 6.10 Seven major chakras

The Base or Root Chakra (Muladhara)

Location – at the base of the spine.

Relevance – it is the foundation chakra and is linked with nature and planet Earth. It is concerned with all issues of a physical nature: the body, the senses, sensuality, a person's sex, survival, aggression and self-defence. At a physical level, it is linked to the endocrine system through the adrenal glands. Its energies also affect the lower parts of the pelvis, the hips, legs and feet.

Imbalance – if this chakra is unbalanced it can make a person feel as if they are ungrounded and unfocused. They may feel weak, lack confidence and feel unable to achieve their goals

Colour association – the colour to visualise in balancing the base chakra is red.

The Sacral Chakra (Swadhistana)

Location – at the level of the sacrum between the naval and the base chakra.

Relevance – concerned with all issues of creativity and sexuality. At the physical level, it is linked to the testes in the male and the ovaries in the female. Its energies also affect the urinogenital organs, the uterus, the kidneys, the lower digestive organs and the lower back.

Imbalance – a person with an imbalance in this chakra may bury their emotions and be overly sensitive. An imbalance may also lead to sexual difficulties and energy blocks with creativity.

Colour association – the colour to visualise in balancing the sacral chakra is orange.

The Solar Plexus Chakra (Manipura)

Location – at approximately waist level.

Relevance – this chakra relates to our emotions, self-esteem and self-worth. Feelings such as fear, anxiety, insecurity, jealousy and anger are generated here. At a physical level, it is linked to the islets of Langerhans in the pancreas. Its energies also affect the solar and splenic nerve plexuses, the digestive system, the pancreas, liver, gall bladder, diaphragm and middle back.

Imbalance – people who are under a degree of stress will show imbalance in this chakra; shock and stress have a greater impact on this chakra than on the others. It is in the solar plexus chakra that negative energies relating to thoughts and feelings are processed. People with an imbalance in this chakra may feel depressed, insecure, lacking in confidence and may worry what other think.

Colour association – the colour to visualise in balancing the solar plexus chakra is yellow.

The Heart Chakra (Anahata)

Location – in the centre of the chest.

Relevance – this chakra is concerned with love and the heart. It deals with all issues concerned with love and affection. At a physical level it is linked to the thymus gland. Its energies also affect the cardiac and pulmonary nerve plexuses, the heart, lungs, bronchial tubes, chest, upper back and arms. It is also the point of connection between the upper and lower chakras.

Imbalance – if the energy does not flow freely between the solar plexus and the heart, or between the heart and the throat, it can lead to some form of imbalance due to the energy withdrawal into the body. A person with an imbalance in this chakra may feel sorry for themselves, be afraid of letting go, feel unworthy of love or feel terrified of rejection.

Colour association – the colour to visualise in balancing the heart chakra is green.

The Throat Chakra (Vishuddha)

Location – at the base of the neck.

Relevance – this chakra is concerned with communication and expression, it also deals with the issue of truth and true expression of the soul. At a physical level, it is linked to the thyroid and parathyroid glands. Its energies also affect the pharyngeal nerve plexus, the organs of the throat, the neck, nose, mouth, teeth and ears.

Imbalance – if this chakra is out of balance it may result in the inability to express our emotions; as a result of unexpressed feeling bottling up it can lead to frustration and tension. A person with an imbalance in this chakra may feel unable to relax.

Colour association – the colour to visualise in balancing the throat chakra is blue.

The Brow Chakra (Ajna)

Location – in the middle of the forehead over the third eye area.

Relevance – commonly known as the 'third eye', the brow chakra is the storehouse of memories and imagination and is associated with intellect, understanding and intuition. At a physical level, it is linked to the hypothalamus and pituitary gland. Its energies also affect the nerves of the head, brain, eyes and face.

Imbalance – if this chakra is not functioning correctly it can lead to headaches and nightmares. A person with an imbalance in this chakra may be oversensitive to the feelings of others, be afraid of success, be non-assertive and undisciplined.

Colour association – the colour to visualise in balancing the brow chakra is indigo.

The Crown Chakra (Sahasrara)

Location – on top of the head.

Relevance – this chakra is the centre of our spirituality and is concerned with thinking and decision making. At a physical level it is linked to the pineal gland. Its energies also affect the brain and the rest of the body.

Imbalance – an imbalance in this chakra may be reflected in those who are unwilling or afraid to open up to their own spiritual potential. An imbalance may also show as being unable to make decisions.

Colour association – the colour to visualise in balancing the crown chakra is violet.

KEY NOTE

An important part of Indian Head Massage treatment is the eastern tradition of balancing of the higher chakras (the throat chakra, the brow chakra (or third eye) and the crown chakra).

With stress and tension the chakras lose their ability to synchronise with one another and become unbalanced.

By placing the hands along the axis of the higher chakras, energy can be realigned and a sense of balance and harmony can be restored.

Keeping Chakras Healthy

Chakras are like the power stations of our body, bringing it to life, and keeping it healthy. Each chakra is associated with different parts of us and they need to spin totally in balance for us to feel good.

In a healthy, fully functioning person the chakras should all be close to the same size and spinning in the same direction. They should be fully functional, clean and translucent and with no blockages. When they malfunction, unwanted physical and emotional problems may result.

The chakras absorb energy that comes from our thoughts, feelings and outside environment and feed this to our body. Our body is affected by the quality of the energy that passes through the chakras. For instance, if we have negative feelings, we will be filtering negative energy through our chakras and into our body. Over time this can make our body ill. Our chakras also absorb energy from the environment. Other people's negative emotions or a room full of clutter will produce an unhealthy energy which we absorb.

Chakra balancing

We cannot avoid coming into contact with negative energy or feeling down sometimes, but we can help to change our feelings from negative to positive and to protect ourselves from harmful energy in the environment. Keeping our chakras in tip-top condition is the key, in other words keeping them spinning in balance.

Chakra balancing is a bit like spring-cleaning the chakras and fine-tuning them. No one is immune; it is therefore important to balance and cleanse the chakras regularly. This is particularly important for therapists, as they are exposed to a considerable amount of emotional energy from their clients, and in order to help their clients effectively their chakras need to be in balance to facilitate the right healing energies.

The technique of balancing or clearing your chakras is based on meditation, and is a relaxation and energy technique recognized for its rejuvenating and healing power. We know that chakras are non-physical centres, therefore you need a non-physical method to stimulate them. This is achieved by focusing your awareness in the area of a chakra and using your mind to manipulate it. You need a localized, mental opening effect in a chakra to stimulate it with your imaginary hands. By moving your point of awareness to the site of a chakra and causing a mental opening effect with your hands, you are directly stimulating the chakra.

There are many different methods of chakra balancing; it is a question of finding one which is effective for you.

Some people use coloured crystals, as the energy vibrations of colours aids balancing; some use essential oils for their healing vibrations. Visualisation is powerful, as thought is energy. Affirmations made while chakra balancing create positive feelings. There are many specific exercises associated with each chakra and different books give suggestions for different exercises; find one that you feel intuitively attracted to, and go with that (see resources for suggested further reading and see also the chakra balancing exercise detailed below).

Whichever methods are used or combined, chakra balancing offers very positive results, improving your health and making you feel good about yourself.

Chakra Balancing Exercise

Firstly, it is important to do some relaxation and breathing exercises, meditate, or do whatever you usually do to get centred. This method will only work effectively if you are in a peaceful and centred state.

Once centred start to visualize your chakras. Don't worry if you feel you can't see them perfectly in your mind. As you do this regularly seeing them will become clearer and clearer.

Start with the 1st charka (the root chakra). Visualize it in your mind. Use the colour (red) and see it as an orb. Look at it closely in your mind. Does it look clean and spotless, or do you see any spots?

If you feel you can't see it, then imagine whether it has spots or not. Your imagination is the key to everything spiritual and it is highly accurate in telling you what is there.

Now imagine a golden beam of light shining on your 1st chakra, removing any impurities or blockages and opening the chakra up to positive energy. Now try to feel the light shining on your chakra. It may be difficult at first to perceive it, but with practice you will soon feel a tingling sensation where your chakra is.

This golden beam is the light of universal energy, the power that flows through everything and gives it life. Allow your intuition to tell you when the light has done the job and burned away the dark spots and blockages. In most cases under a minute is all the time that is necessary. With practice it will become more obvious.

Now work you way up the chakras, going through the same procedure and concentrating on each one individually; to the 2nd chakra (sacral), visualizing the colour orange, followed by the 3rd chakra (solar plexus) visualizing the colour yellow, to the 4th chakra (heart) visualizing the colour green, to the 5th chakra (throat) visualizing the colour blue, to the 6th chakra (third eye) visualizing the colour indigo, working your way up to the 7th chakra, visualizing the colour violet. This whole procedure should take less than 10 minutes.

Once you have purified your crown chakra then look at all seven chakras at once in your mind's eye, as a stack. Perceive whether they are all the same size or whether there are a few larger or smaller ones. Concentrate your energy to help balance them all to the same size and get all of the vortexes spinning in the same direction. Hold the image in your mind and 'imagine' them shifting to the same size and the vortexes spinning in the same direction.

KEY NOTE
The base, or root chakra, is the master chakra and is the most important one to activate. This chakra is the doorway for the Kundalini energy. Unless this is opened sufficiently, the energy cannot flow into the other chakras.

Chakra sensations

The sensations you will feel in your chakras can vary from a gentle warmth, a localized pressure, or bubbling, a localized dizziness, a tingling, a gentle pulsing, to a heavier throbbing, or a combination of some or all of the above. The heavier the thrumming, the more active the chakra. If you place your hand on a chakra, when it is active, you will actually feel the flesh pulsing.

You may, however, feel a slight internal contracting, a feeling that is not muscular, while you are stimulating your chakras. These are the glands and nerve ganglia linked to the chakras contracting in response to the stimulation. This internal contracting is normal.

NB: *You may feel a stronger sensation in some chakras and little or none in others. Concentrate on the lowest ones with the least sensation. This will help balance the energy flow in the chakra systems.*

Preparation for an Indian Head Massage Treatment

Client Preparation

- Check client is a suitable candidate for treatment by carrying out a consultation.

- Formulate the client's individual treatment plan.

- Seat client comfortably in a chair, ensuring that their legs are uncrossed and feet are placed on the ground. It is usually more comfortable and relaxing for the client to remove their shoes before treatment. Comfort may be assisted further by the use of a cushion, pillow or stool for clients to rest their feet on, and a comforting therapeutic touch is to wrap the feet in a warm towel.

- Drape a towel over the back of the chair and have a clean towel ready for placing over the shoulders for the scalp massage.

- Ask the client to remove any obtrusive jewellery such as necklaces, earrings and noserings, and to remove glasses.

- Ask the client to brush their hair to remove any residue of hairspray, gel and mousse, and to remove face make-up.

- If the client's hair is long, it should be tied up with a suitable hair clip.

Therapist Preparation

- Present a smart and professional appearance.

- Tie hair back off the face.

- Remove all obtrusive jewellery and wristwatch.

- Ensure chair is at a suitable height for you and your client.

- Prepare oil for the scalp massage, if required (approximately 2–5 ml depending on the length of the hair and the condition of the scalp). The client may prefer the oil to be warmed before application to the scalp. If this is desired, place the oil container in a bowl of warm water before treatment.

KEY NOTE

Breathing techniques

It is important for therapists to be aware of their own breathing during an Indian Head Massage treatment, and realise that correct breathing can help to increase the effectiveness of the treatment.

Correct breathing helps the therapist and the client to relax and regain their natural balance, whilst helping the therapist to maintain concentration and provide the right energy needed for a positive treatment outcome.

Hygiene Precautions

- Cleanse hands before and after treatment.

- Check client for any infectious conditions.

- Avoid carrying out treatment if you have any infection which may be transmitted.

- Cover any open cuts or abrasions with a waterproof plaster.

- Pour oil into a separate container for individual client use and dispose of residual oil.

Correct Body Mechanics

Body mechanics involves using correct posture in order to apply Indian Head Massage techniques with the maximum efficiency and with the minimal trauma to the therapist. Initially, therapists often find it difficult adjusting from massaging a client on a couch to massaging a client who is seated in a chair. It is therefore essential that correct adjustments are made to body mechanics in order to increase the effectiveness of the massage, help prevent repetitive strain injuries, decrease fatigue and increase comfort for the therapist.

Guidelines for correct body mechanics:

- Check the chair height: a chair at the correct height will enable a therapist to use body weight effectively to develop pressure.

- Wear low heeled shoes with good support.

- Keep the back straight by tilting the pelvis forwards.

- Use body weight effectively, by lunging in order to create pressure needed.

- Keep the shoulders and upper back relaxed (avoiding raising shoulders to ears).

- Keep feet firmly placed on the ground.
- Bend knees slightly and keep knees soft, taking care to avoid locking them straight.
- Keep wrists as straight as possible.
- Avoid joint hyperextension.
- Keep the body in correct alignment by maintaining head erect over neck and shoulders.
- Keep head-forward posture to a minimum and avoid spending too much time looking down.
- Take breaks between clients to stretch the neck, shake out the arms and relax.
- Vary the massage techniques used and vary hand and foot placements.
- Have regular treatments in order to keep your body working at an optimum level.

Adaptations to an Indian Head Massage Treatment

Indian Head Massage, like any other massage techniques, should always be adapted and varied to suit the differences in the physical characteristics of clients, such as their body size, muscle tone, age and hair type. Therapists are likely to encounter many clients that may require a degree of adaptation due to their physical and health-related situations.

KEY NOTE

The best approach to massage is to see every client's situation as a different challenge and view their individual needs as part of the treatment plan. When adapting a massage it is not the massage movements themselves that change, the difference is in the way in which the therapist modifies or adjusts the pressure, speed, duration and frequency of the massage.

A Pregnant Client

It is advisable to avoid carrying out Indian Head Massage in the first trimester until the pregnancy is established. The first trimester can be an unsettling time and some clients may experience nausea and sickness.

Once past the first trimester and provided the pregnancy has no complications, Indian Head Massage can often be a popular choice due to the fact that pregnant clients can sit comfortably in a chair for treatment, and no special positioning is required.

Care should be taken when massaging a pregnant client due to the fact that some clients may experience a feeling of dizziness, Care should also be taken, and if necessary, GP referral sought, for those clients who experience high blood pressure during their pregnancy.

A Disabled Client

The first consideration for the therapist is to establish the nature of the disability, and if necessary research the condition beforehand to be prepared. It is important for a therapist to tactfully enquire about the limitations of the condition and not to assume anything; just because a client is disabled it is does not mean they are paralysed.

If a client is in a wheelchair, then due to the portability of Indian Head Massage they may be treated quite easily while sitting in the wheelchair. If the client is in a wheelchair it is advisable for the therapist to sit or kneel when carrying out the consultation in order that they may talk to the client at eye level. It is essential to take care not to appear patronising to disabled clients and you should not discriminate against them because of their disability.

An Elderly Client

There are several considerations to be borne in mind with an elderly client.

- Take care to ensure the client is warm enough throughout the treatment.

- Many elderly people experience a sudden drop in blood pressure, so if you are helping the client up, do it gently and carefully to avoid the risk of loss of balance and falls.

- Avoid deep massage due to decreased reaction time, possible insensitivity to pain and thinning of skin and blood vessels.

- There may be loss of hearing and vision.

- There will be a decrease in muscle tone, bones will not be as strong and flexible, and joints may be worn.

- Skin may appear pale, wrinkled, thinner, looser and more fragile.

- The circulation may not be as efficient, especially if the client is inactive.

It is best to make the treatment sessions shorter as the client may tire easily, to take care when applying pressure and avoid extreme joint mobilisation due to loss of bone integrity.

A Large-framed Client

Clients with a large frame may find Indian Head Massage more comfortable due to positioning and the fact that no undressing is required.

Pressure should be applied carefully to areas with dense areas of adipose tissue in order to avoid tissue damage and client discomfort. It may be tempting for the massage therapist to consider that areas of fatty tissue are insensitive and apply too firm a pressure. Adipose tissue is in fact highly vascular, making it very susceptible to bruising and damage. General pointers are to consider pressure and monitor client feedback and use body mechanics correctly.

The therapist may also need to adjust the chair height to suit the size of the client.

A Small-framed Client

Care needs to be taken with a thin client to avoid deep massage or pressure over bony areas, which may cause discomfort. Stimulating techniques such as hacking should be avoided over unprotected areas, and pressure applied should be carefully monitored in line with client feedback. It is important for the therapist to avoid assuming that because the client is thin they require a light massage.

Male Clients

In general terms the male body presents more muscle bulk than the female body and therefore an adaptation of technique is often required. Male clients will generally require a firmer pressure and the therapist should take care to apply the correct body mechanics and posture in order to be able to carry out the techniques effectively and to the client's satisfaction.

Adaptations for Clients with Long/Thick Hair

When carrying out an Indian Head Massage on a client with long or thick hair, the first consideration is that generally more oil will be needed, and in some cases it may be necessary to section off the hair for the oil application. When establishing contact with the head/scalp it is best to slide the fingers from the hair root upwards above the ears. When dealing with thick hair, which has a tendency to be coarse, it is best to use a softening and moisturising oil such as coconut.

Adaptations for Clients Without Hair

Clients without hair will require a slightly different approach when massaging the scalp. Any techniques involving manipulation or tugging of the hair will obviously be omitted. However it is still important to work over the scalp, as regardless of whether the client has hair or not, the scalp muscles are still liable to develop tension due to their attachments.

Indian Head Massage Techniques

An Indian Head Massage treatment typically consists of massage to the upper back and shoulders, upper arms, neck, scalp and face. Treatment is traditionally applied through the clothes with the use of oil being optional on the scalp.

Due to the fact that Indian Head Massage has been taught within families for generations and has now also been westernised, it should be noted that techniques may vary in their content and application.

The Shoulders

The shoulders are the place where most people hold a considerable amount of tension. When the body is in a state of tension the shoulders are lifted towards the ears and often remain this way, causing the muscles to go into spasm. This restricts the blood flow to the head, neck and shoulders and causes the neck and shoulders to become stiff and inflexible. Sitting with hunched shoulders can reduce chest capacity and thus impair breathing.

> **KEY NOTE**
> Indian Head Massage can help to counterbalance the effects of stress, as by relaxing the shoulders they will drop and allow the energy to flow more freely to the area, encouraging deeper and easier breathing and improved joint flexibility.

Upper Back and Shoulder Massage

1 Starting Position with hands over the top of the client's shoulders

Therapist's stance
Standing behind the client in a relaxed posture.

Technique
- Commence by holding your hands lightly on your client's shoulders.
- Ask your client to take three deep breaths, with the emphasis on breathing in and out slowly and deeply.

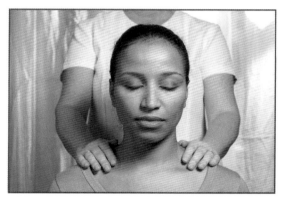

Fig 6.11 Starting position

> **KEY NOTE**
> This helps both the client and therapist relax and prepare themselves for treatment.

2 Holding Position over the top of the head

Therapist's stance
Standing behind the client in a relaxed posture.

Technique
- Hold your hands lightly on either side of the head for about a minute, waiting for a feeling of relaxation and calm.
- You are now ready to commence the massage.

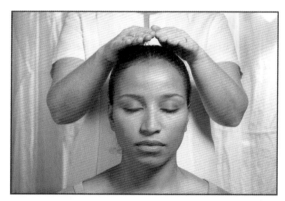

Fig 6.12 Holding position

> **KEY NOTE**
> The holding position helps to create a feeling of stillness and calm before commencing the massage.

3 Effleurage/Smoothing across the shoulders and upper back

Therapist's stance
Standing behind the client in a walk standing position. The walk standing posture is used to lunge forward and increase the pressure and effectiveness of the techniques.

Technique
- Use one hand to support one side of the upper back.

- Use the palmar surface of the other hand to stroke up either side of the spine, across the top of the shoulder and around the lateral border of the scapula to return to the starting position.

- The stroke upwards should be deeper than the stroke downwards.

- Repeat three times one side and then repeat the other side, gradually increasing in pressure with each stroke.

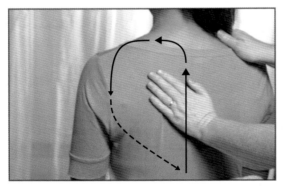

Fig 6.13 Effleurage/smoothing

> **KEY NOTE**
> Effleurage/smoothing is the first communication across the shoulders and enables the therapists to establish contact and feel for any areas of tension.

4 Petrissage/Thumb Sweeping across the shoulders

Therapist's stance
Standing behind the client in a walk standing position. Therapist uses walk standing posture to lunge forward and increase the pressure and effectiveness of the techniques.

Technique
- With fingers resting on the top of the client's shoulders, reach down the upper back with your thumbs and place them as far as they can go either side of the spine, across the lower border of the trapezius muscle.

- Now draw the thumbs up and across the trapezius muscle fanning out towards the little finger.

- Repeat three times, gradually increasing in pressure.

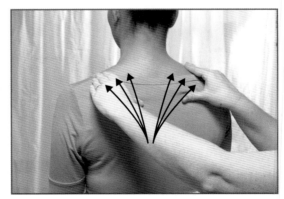

Fig 6.14 Petrissage/thumb sweeping

- Now draw the thumbs up towards the middle finger and repeat three times.

- Then draw the thumbs up towards the index finger and repeat three times.

KEY NOTE
Petrissage/thumb sweeping is a deeper technique that helps to unlock tension and free fibrous adhesions from the trapezius muscle.

5 Frictions with the Heel of the Hand rubbing around the scapulae

Therapist's stance
Standing to the side so that you are facing your client's shoulder from the side.

Technique
- Support one side of the back with one hand.

- Use the *heel* of your other hand to rub lightly and briskly (in a side to side motion) across the top of the scapula, in-between the scapula and below the scapula in the characteristic 'C' shape.

- Repeat three times each side.

KEY NOTE
Frictions help create a considerable amount of heat in the tissues which helps to break down fibrous adhesions and restrictions around the scapulae.

6 Frictions with the Finger rubbing around the scapulae

Therapist's stance
Standing to the side so that you are facing the clients shoulder from the side.

Technique
- Support one side of the back with one hand.

- Join the fingers of the other hand and place fingertips so that they face away from the spine.

- Rub vigorously backwards and forwards across the top of the scapula, in-between and below the scapulae in the characteristic 'C' shape.

- Repeat three times each side.

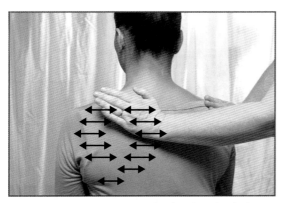

Fig 6.15 Frictions with the heel of the hand

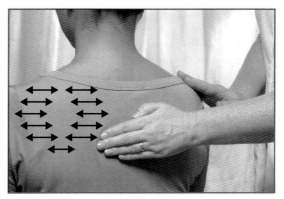

Fig 6.16 Frictions with the fingers

KEY NOTE
This technique is similar to the previous technique in helping to free restrictions and tension from around the scapulae.

7 Effleurage/Smoothing (as Step 3)

8 Pressures with the knuckles either side of the spine

Therapist's Stance
Standing behind the client in a walk standing position.

Technique
- Place the middle knuckles of the forefinger *and* middle finger on either side of the spine at the top of the shoulders.
- Ask the client to take a deep breath in and *as they breathe out* apply pressure inwards and then slowly release back towards you.
- Continue working down either side of the spine, approximately an inch at a time until you reach the mid spine.

- Light sweep back up to the top of the shoulders. Repeat twice.

KEY NOTE
Pressures stimulate the nerve endings either side of the spine, releasing blockages in the nerves and easing tension.

9 Thumb Pushes over the shoulders

Therapist's Stance
Standing behind the client in a walk standing position.

Technique
- Place the palms of the hands around the cap of the shoulder (deltoid muscle) with thumbs resting above shoulder blades.
- Starting from the outer edge of the shoulder, use the pads of the thumbs to push in one long sweep from the trapezius muscle (back of the shoulders) over to the pectoralis major muscle (front of the chest).

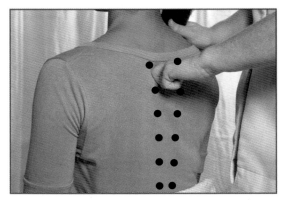

Fig 6.17 Pressures with the knuckles

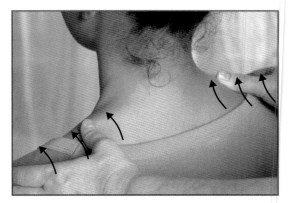

Fig 6.18 Thumb pushes over the shoulders

- Slowly release and then move further in towards the neck and repeat.

- Repeat the movement until the whole of the top of the shoulders has been covered.

KEY NOTE

The thumb pushing technique loosens tension in the muscles across the top of the shoulders by squeezing the toxins from the muscle and mobilising the tissues.

10 Finger Pulls across the top of the shoulders

Therapist's Stance
Standing behind the client in a walk standing position

Technique
- Place both hands over the top of the shoulders, with the thumbs anchored across the back and the fingers in front of the shoulders.

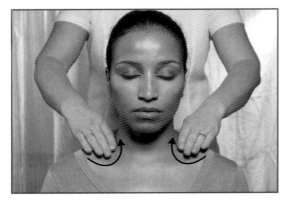

Fig 6.19 Finger pulls

- Draw the muscles in-between your fingers and thumbs and lift upwards and back towards you.

- Repeat several times until the whole of the top of the shoulder has been thoroughly covered.

KEY NOTE

The finger pulls technique helps to squeeze the toxins from the muscle fibres and encourages fresh oxygen and nutrients into the muscles. It also helps to soften and loosen the muscles , thereby easing tension.

11 Squeezing and Releasing across the top of the shoulders

Therapist's Stance
Standing behind the client in a walk standing position.

Technique
- Place palms of both hands on the top of the shoulders with the heel of the hand lying on the trapezius muscle and fingers resting on the front of the shoulder.

- Lift and squeeze the muscles in an upwards motion, heel of the hands and fingers clasping them tightly in the palm of the hands.

- Squeeze using medium pressure and hold for a few seconds before releasing.

- Move further in towards the neck and repeat until the area across the top of the shoulders has been covered.

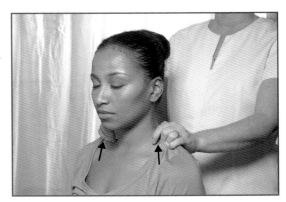

Fig 6.20 Squeezing and releasing across the top of the shoulders

KEY NOTE

The squeeze and release technique helps to squeeze and release toxins from the muscles, as well as softening and loosening tight muscle fibres.

12 Heel Pushes across the tops of the shoulders

Therapist's Stance
Standing behind the client in a walk standing position.

Technique
■ Place palms of both hands on the top of the shoulders with the heel of the hand lying on the trapezius muscle and fingers resting on the front of the shoulder.

■ Lift up and squeeze the muscles in an upwards motion and then roll the hands forwards across to the front of the shoulders, slowly releasing the muscle from your hands as you go.

■ Repeat several times until the whole of the top of the shoulders has been covered.

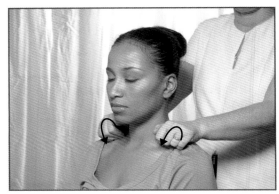

Fig 6.21 Heel pushes

KEY NOTE

The heel pushes technique helps to mobilise and loosen the muscles across the top of the shoulders, encouraging the client to release tension.

13 Smoothing with the forearms

Therapist's Stance
Standing behind the client in a walk standing position.

Technique
- Place the inside of the forearms across the top of your client's shoulders and gently apply pressure downwards.
- Glide the forearms across the top of the shoulders, rotating them as you proceed to the outer edge of the shoulder and down the upper arms to just above the elbow.
- Release and then brush the forearms back up the arms and on to the top of the shoulders
- Repeat three times.

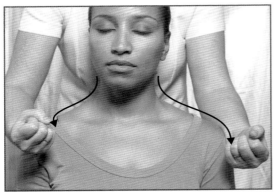

Fig 6.22 Smoothing with the forearms

KEY NOTE
The smoothing with the forearms technique stretches and releases the muscles across the top of the shoulders and helps to encourage the drainage of toxins from the tissues. It also encourages the shoulders to release tension.

14 Chopping across the shoulders and upper back

Therapist's Stance
Behind the client, kneeling down or standing up with the knees bent, depending on preference and client height.

Technique
- Place the palms of both hands across the upper back, with fingers together and fingertips pointing upwards.
- Perform light brisk chopping movements by quickly moving the index fingers of both hands together, picking up and squeezing the tissue between the index fingers of both hands before releasing them.
- Work across the whole of the upper back and shoulders.

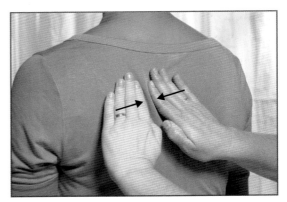

Fig 6.23 Chopping

KEY NOTE
The chopping technique helps to loosen the muscles across the upper back and shoulders and stimulates the blood circulation and nerve endings, giving a refreshing feeling.

15 Champi/Double Hacking across the shoulders and upper back.

Therapist's Stance
Standing behind the client in a walk standing position.

Technique
- Hold your hands in a praying position, leaving the heels of the hands and the fingertips loosely in contact.
- Relax the hands and wrists.
- Using the tips of both fingers joined like a cage, lightly strike the surface and then spring off again.
- Start on one side of the spine of the upper back, around the shoulders and then back down again.
- Repeat the other side.

NB: Take care to ensure that hacking is NOT performed directly over the spine.

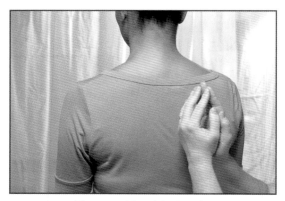

Fig 6.24 Champi/double hacking

KEY NOTE
Champi or double hacking stimulates the nerve endings and blood circulation, giving a refreshing and revitalising feeling.

16 Squeezing and Releasing across the tops of the shoulders (as Step 11)

17 Effleurage/Smoothing (as Step 3)

18 Holding Position over the tops of the shoulders (as Step 1)

Upper Arms

The upper arms are important for upper body movement and when the shoulders are tense they tighten and restrict movement. When in a state of tension, the upper arms tend to hug the chest, either at the sides or in front, while the elbows bend up.

> **KEY NOTE**
> Indian Head Massage can help to reduce tension and tightness in the upper arm muscles to help improve flexibility of the arms and shoulders.

1 Squeezing and Releasing to the upper arms

Therapist's Stance
To the side of the client, standing behind the upper arms.

Technique
- Stand to one side of your client, behind the upper arm.
- Place the palms of both hands (one above the other) around the upper arm (thumbs resting towards the back of the upper arm and fingertips resting towards the front).

- Starting at the top, gently squeeze and release the upper arm muscles by pressing the fingers towards the thumbs, and then slowly releasing.
- Continue working down the upper arm towards the elbow.
- Stroke lightly back up to the top of the upper arm and repeat three times.
- Then lightly brush across the top of the client's shoulders to repeat the movement on the client's other arm.

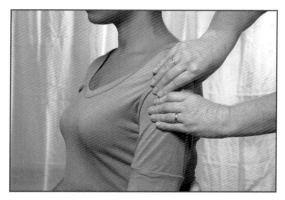

Fig 6.25 Squeezing and releasing to the upper arms

> **KEY NOTE**
> The squeezing and releasing technique helps loosen tension in the upper arms.

2 Compression of the upper arms

Therapist's Stance
To the side of the client, standing behind the upper arms.

Technique
- Stand to face your client's upper arm.

- With fingers facing towards the floor, place one palm on the front of the upper arm and one on the back.

- Starting from the top of the upper arms, use the palms of both hands to compress towards one another gently, squeezing the muscles of the upper arms.

- Slowly release and then continue working down the upper arm until you reach the elbow.

- Brush lightly back up to the top and repeat two times.

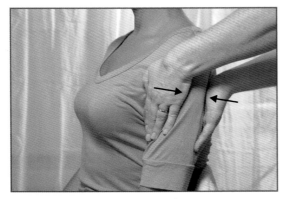

Fig 6.26 Compression of upper arms

KEY NOTE
The compression technique helps to encourage lymphatic drainage by squeezing toxins from the tissues of the upper arms.

3 Heel Rolls embracing the upper arms

Therapist's Stance
Behind the client in a walk standing position.

Technique
- Place your hands facing forwards on top of the deltoid muscles, heels of the hands behind.

- Roll the heels of your hands over the muscles of the upper arm until they reach your fingertips.

- Repeat at the middle of the upper arm and just above elbow.

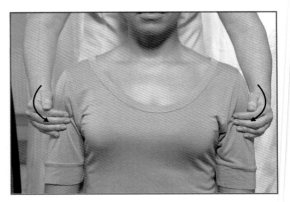

Fig 6.27 Heel rolls

KEY NOTE
The heel rolls technique helps relax and loosen the muscles of the upper arms and top of the shoulder (Biceps, Triceps and Deltoid muscles)

4 Squeezing and Kneading down the upper arms

Therapist's Stance
Behind the client in a walk standing position.

Technique
- Cup the hands around the cap of the shoulder, thumbs pointing forwards and fingertips behind.

- Draw your hands from under the back of the client's upper arm and squeeze up and round towards the front of the upper arms.

- Repeat this movement down to the elbows and then sweep back up to the cap of the shoulder and repeat.

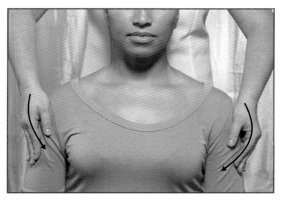

Fig 6.28 Squeezing and kneading down the upper arms

KEY NOTE
The squeezing and kneading technique mobilises the muscles of the upper arm and helps release tension.

5 Shoulder Mobilisation

Therapist's Stance
Standing to one side of the client, facing the shoulder and upper arm.

Technique
- Place one hand on the top of the client's shoulder and one hand under the elbow, supporting your client's hand in the crook of your elbow.

- Gently mobilise the shoulder in a clockwise and anticlockwise direction taking the shoulder through its full range of movement.

- Repeat on the other side.

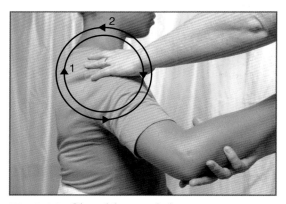

Fig 6.29 Shoulder mobilisation

KEY NOTE
The shoulder mobilisation technique encourages joint mobility and helps release tension and restrictions in the shoulder joint.

6 Squeezing and Kneading to the forearms

Therapist's Stance
Standing to one side of the client, facing the shoulder and upper arm.

Technique
- Support the weight of the client's forearm with one hand and with the other hand gently use a squeeze and release action down the forearm to just above the wrist.
- Repeat three times.

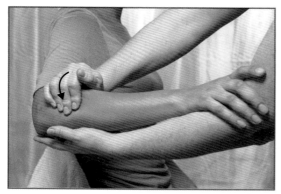

Fig 6.30 Squeeze and knead forearms

KEY NOTE

The squeezing and kneading technique mobilises the muscles of the lower arm and helps release tension.

7 Squeezing and Kneading to the fingers

Therapist's Stance
Standing to one side of the client, facing the shoulder and upper arm.

Technique
- Support the client's wrist from underneath with one hand.
- Take each finger between your thumb and fingers and use the squeeze and release technique from the bottom of the finger to the tips, ending on the thumb. End with a gentle traction to each digit.

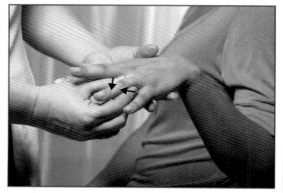

Fig 6.31 Squeeze and knead fingers

KEY NOTE

The squeezing and kneading technique to the fingers helps mobilise the fingers and helps release tension from the hand.

8 Circular Pressure Massage to the pressure point between the thumb and index finger

Therapist's Stance
Standing to one side of the client, facing the shoulder and upper arm.

Technique
- While supporting the client's wrist from underneath with one hand, use the thumb and the index finger to apply gentle circular pressure massage to the area on the top of the hand, between the thumb and finger.

- Apply the circular pressure massage in a clockwise direction, followed by an anticlockwise direction, to slowly release any stagnant energy.

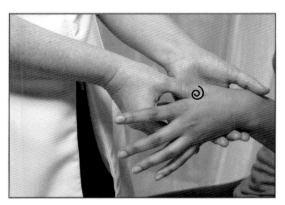

Fig 6.32 Circular pressure massage between thumb and index finger

KEY NOTE
Applying pressure to the pressure point between the thumb and index finger can help relieve tension and headaches.

9 Circular Pressure Massage to the pressure point in the centre of the palm

Therapist's Stance
Standing to one side of the client, facing the shoulder and upper arm.

Technique
- Turn the client's hand over to reveal the palm.

- Use the thumb to apply circular pressure massage, as above, to the centre of the palm.

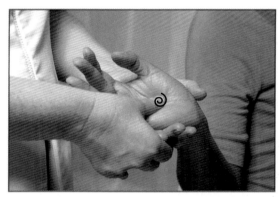

Fig 6.33 Circular pressure massage on palm

KEY NOTE
Applying circular massage to the centre of the palm helps calm and relax the client as you are working on the solar plexus (palm charka).

10 Shoulder Lift

Therapist's Stance
Standing behind the client and bending the knees.

Technique

- Ask your client to place their hands on their lap.

- Place your hands under their elbows and ask the client to take in a long, deep breath.

- As they breathe in pull the shoulders up and outwards.

- On the client's out breath release the shoulders back down.

- Repeat twice.

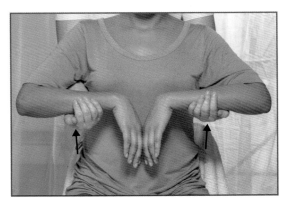

Fig 6.34 Shoulder lift

> **KEY NOTE**
> The shoulder lift technique symbolises letting tension go and helps the clients to drop their shoulders and release the tension.

11 Effleurage/Smoothing with the Forearms down the upper arms

Therapist's Stance
Standing behind the client in a walk standing position.

Technique

- Using the inside of the forearms apply gentle pressure on both sides across the top of the shoulders.

- Glide the forearms across the top of the shoulders, rotating them as you proceed to the outer edge of the shoulder and down the upper arms to just above the elbow.

- Release and then brush the forearms back up the arms.

- Repeat three times.

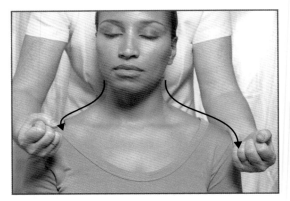

Fig 6.35 Effleurage/smoothing with forearms

The Neck

When the body is balanced, the neck is designed to allow the head to move in a variety of directions. When the body is out of balance and under stress, the head tends to come forwards and the chin juts out. This then throws the body out of alignment as the neck muscles tense and take the weight of the head. The neck muscles are then in a permanent state of contraction and can cause the neck to become stiff and tight. The tension then reduces mobility of the neck and shoulders.

KEY NOTE

Working on the neck with Indian Head Massage helps to open up the energy flow from the spine to the whole head and can help to reduce tension and improve posture by realigning the muscles, thereby increasing mobility and allowing the head to move more freely.

Health and safety note

During the neck massage it is important to fully support the client's head to avoid neck strain.

Neck Massage

1 Rocking the head backwards and forwards

Therapist's Stance
Standing to the side of the client.

Technique
- Place one hand on the forehead and one hand at the back of the neck.

- Ask your client to drop the head slightly forwards so you can support its weight.

- Gently rock the head forwards and backwards, taking care to avoid hyperextending the neck.

- If the neck appears tight, ask the client to breathe deeply three times to relax, after which the head should move more freely and with less resistance.

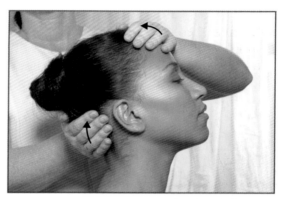

Fig 6.36 Rocking the head backwards and forwards

KEY NOTE

Gently rocking the head back and forth helps the therapist to assess how much tension there is in the neck and can help the client to relax the neck muscles.

2 Squeeze and Release the muscles at the back of the neck

Therapist's Stance
Standing to the side of the client.

Technique
- Place one hand on the client's forehead.
- Ask your client to tip their head back slightly.
- Spread your thumbs and fingers of the other hand on either side of the base of the neck (forming a V shape).
- Using firm contact with the skin, slide your hand in to squeeze and lift the muscles of the back of the neck and then release by pulling the hand backwards.
- Start from the bottom of the neck and gradually work upwards until you reach the base of the skull.

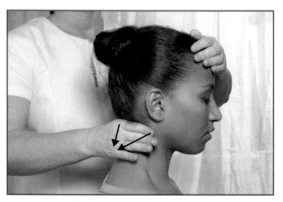

Fig 6.37 Squeeze and release muscles at back of neck

KEY NOTE
The squeeze and release technique helps release tension that builds up in the back of the neck and the skull.

3 Finger Frictions to the top of the shoulders and up the side of the neck

Therapist's Stance
Standing behind the client to one side.

Technique
- Tilt the client's head gently to one side.
- Support your client's head by using your forearm to cup around the side of their head so that it rests comfortably into your forearm.
- Perform frictions using the pads of the fingers in a side-to-side motion across the top of the shoulder and up the side of the neck to behind the ear.
- Repeat three times.
- Repeat techniques to the other side of the neck.

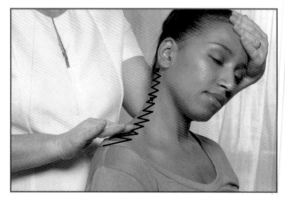

Fig 6.38 Finger frictions to shoulders

KEY NOTE
This technique helps increase the blood and lymph supply to the neck. It also builds up heat in the muscles from the frictions and helps to relieve tightness in the muscles at the side of the neck.

4 Thumb Pushes to the side of the neck

Therapist's Stance
Standing behind the client to one side.

Technique
- Retain the same support for the client's head as in technique 3.
- Use the thumb to push deeply into the muscles of the neck by pushing forwards horizontally across from the back of the neck to the side of the neck just below the ears.
- Repeat to the other side of the neck.

NB: *Caution is necessary during this technique in order to avoid applying pressure to the carotid arteries at the side of the neck and to respiratory structures such as the trachea at the front of the neck.*

5 Squeezing and Releasing at the side of the neck

Therapist's Stance
Standing behind the client to one side.

Technique
- Still retain the same support for the head as in technique 4.
- Form a V shape between the thumb and the forefinger (thumb is anchored at the back).
- Squeeze and release the muscles at the side of the neck by lifting the tissue and pulling the forefinger back towards the thumb.
- Start from the side of the neck and work from the bottom upwards to up behind the ears.
- Repeat to the other side of the neck.

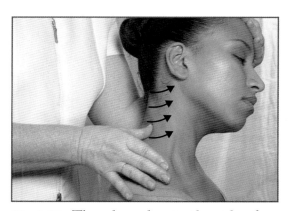

Fig 6.39 Thumb pushes to the side of the neck

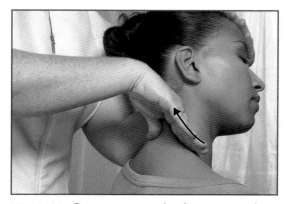

Fig 6.40 Squeezing and releasing at the side of the neck

KEY NOTE
The thumb pushes technique helps to break down fibrous adhesions that restrict movements of the head and neck.

KEY NOTE
The squeeze and release technique to the side of the neck helps to squeeze the toxins from the muscles and encourages lymph drainage to the neck.

6 Finger Frictions to the base of the skull

Therapist's Stance
Standing to one side of the client.

Technique
- Support the client's forehead with one hand.

- Use your other hand to perform frictions up and down the back of the neck with the pads of the fingers.

- Work from the base of the neck to the base of the skull.

- Repeat until the back of the neck and skull has been covered.

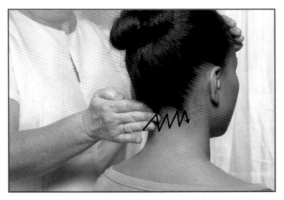

Fig 6.41 Finger frictions to base of skull

KEY NOTE
The finger frictions technique helps encourage heat to release tight congested muscles at the back of the neck and the base of the skull, where tension builds up.

7 Heel of the Hand Frictions to the base of the skull

Therapist's Stance
Standing to one side of the client.

Technique
- Retaining the supporting hand on the forehead, use the heel of the other hand to apply friction at the base of the skull.

- Mould the heel of the hand to the base of the skull and use a side-to-side motion to friction briskly across the base of the skull.

- Repeat until the whole area of the base of the skull has been covered.

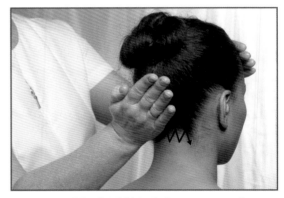

Fig 6.42 Heel of hand frictions to base of skull

KEY NOTE
The heel of the hand frictions technique helps to encourage the release of toxins from tight congested muscles at the base of the skull.

8 Effleurage/Smoothing to the back of the neck

Therapist's Stance
Standing to one side of the client.

Technique
- Still retaining the supporting hand across the forehead, use the other hand to smooth the base of the skull and neck in a circular motion.
- Repeat several times.

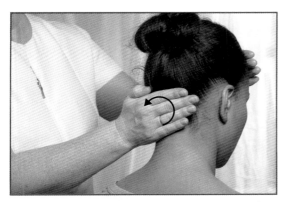

Fig 6.43 Effleurage/smoothing to back of neck

KEY NOTE

Effleurage/smoothing technique helps relax and soothe the neck muscles.

9 Pressure Points at the base of the skull

Therapist's Stance
Standing to one side of the client.

Technique
- Maintain the supporting hand across the front of the head.
- Use the tip of the middle finger to gently press into the pressure point in the centre of the base of the skull for a few seconds, while at the same time gently rocking the head backwards.
- Pause for a second and then move the head forwards to release.
- Then using the thumb and the middle finger, press on the points approximately one inch either side of the central point and rock the head gently backwards.
- Pause and then move the head forwards to release.

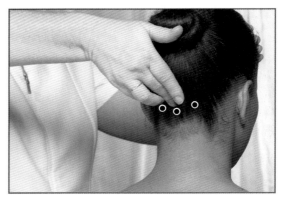

Fig 6.44 Pressure points at base of skull

KEY NOTE

The pressure points technique helps to relieve pressure from congested nerves and muscles relating to the head and neck.

10 Gentle Stretching to the side of the neck

Therapist's Stance
Standing behind the client to one side.

Technique
- Tilt your client's head gently to one side.

- Support your client's head by using your forearm to cup around the side of their head, so that it rests comfortably into the forearm.

- Place your other forearm on top of the client's shoulder.

- Ask your client to take a deep breath in and as they breathe out gently press down on the top of the shoulder and hold for a few seconds before sweeping down and over the top of the upper arm.

- Repeat twice.

- Then repeat the technique on the other side of the neck.

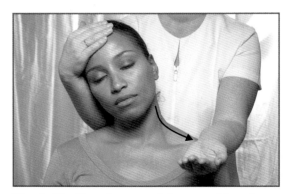

Fig 6.45 Gentle stretching to side of neck

KEY NOTE
This technique creates a gentle stretch up the side of the neck.

11 Smoothing with the Whole Hand at the base of the skull (as in Step 8)

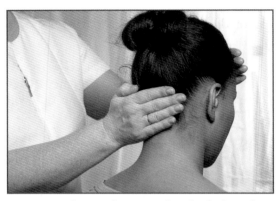

Fig 6.46 Smoothing with whole hand

The Scalp

The scalp muscles tighten when under stress restricting the blood flow leading to headaches, eyestrain and neck and shoulder tension.

> **KEY NOTE**
>
> Indian Head Massage helps to counter-balance stress in the head by improving the circulation and the condition of the hair. Regular head massage also helps to relax the muscles and nerve fibres of the scalp, thereby relieving tension and fatigue.

Scalp Massage

1 Rubbing to the side of the scalp, around the ears

Therapist's Stance
Standing behind the client.

Technique
- Support one side of the head with one hand.
- Use the fleshy part of the palm of the other hand to carry out a light rubbing movement with side-to-side motion, across the temporalis muscle above, in front of and behind the ears.

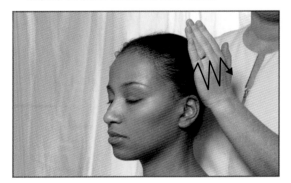

Fig 6.47 Rubbing to side of scalp, around the ears

- Work backwards and forwards three times.
- Repeat to other side.

> **KEY NOTE**
>
> The rubbing technique helps to lightly increase the circulation of blood to the scalp.

2 Frictions to the side of the scalp, around the ears

Therapist's Stance
Standing behind the client.

Technique
- Support one side of the head with one hand.
- Use the pad of the fingers of the other hand to perform frictions briskly to the same area as the previous technique (in front of, above and behind the ears).
- Repeat on the other side of the scalp.

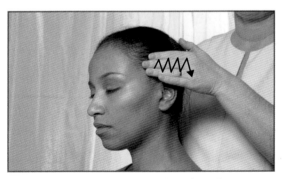

Fig 6.48 Frictions to side of scalp

> **KEY NOTE**
>
> The frictions technique helps to loosen tension from the temporalis muscle that can cause headaches.

3 Rubbing to the whole of the scalp

Therapist's Stance
Standing behind the client.

Technique
- Support one side of the client's head with one hand.
- Use the soft fleshy part of other hand to carry out a rubbing motion using a broad zigzag motion from side to side.
- Work over one side of the head from front to back and then repeat on the other side.

4 Frictions with the whole of the hand

Therapist's Stance
Standing behind the client.

Technique
- Support one side of your client's head.
- Apply firm pressure using the whole hand in a side-to-side zigzag motion, moving the scalp up and down.
- Work over one side of the scalp from the front of the scalp to the back.
- Repeat to the other side.

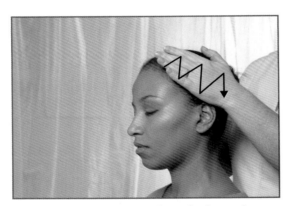

Fig 6.49 Rubbing to the whole scalp

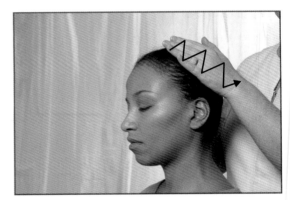

Fig 6.50 Frictions with whole hand

KEY NOTE
The rubbing technique helps to loosen up tight scalp muscles and encourages blood and lymph supply to the scalp.

KEY NOTE
The frictions technique increases the circulation to the scalp and loosens tight scalp muscles.

5 Ruffling through the hair

Therapist Stance
Standing behind the client.

Technique
- Support one side of the client's head with one hand.
- Separate the fingers of the other hand and use the tips of the fingers to perform a light wave-like movement from side-to-side through the hair.
- Work from the front of the scalp towards the back.
- Repeat three times.

6 Hair Tugging

Therapist's Stance
Standing behind the client.

Technique
- Draw the fingers of both hands through the client's hair, from root to tip, in an upwards direction.
- Release the hair from your fingers, repeating several times.
- Then gather the hair between your fingers and give the hair a tug to stimulate its growth.

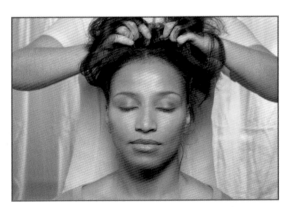

Fig 6.51 Ruffling through hair   **Fig 6.52** Hair tugging

KEY NOTE
This ruffling technique has a very soothing and soporific effect on the nerves if performed slowly and is more stimulating and invigorating if performed more vigorously.

KEY NOTE
The hair tugging technique helps to stimulate the circulation to the scalp and helps bring fresh blood and lymph to the surface.

7 Effleurage/Smoothing through the hair

Therapist's Stance
Standing behind the client.

Technique
- With alternate hands, stroke through the hair using the fingertips.
- Work repetitively from the front of the scalp towards the back several times.
- If your client requires more stimulation to the scalp, use the nails of both hands to comb through the hair from front to back.

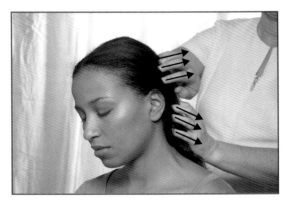

Fig 6.53 Effleurage/smoothing through hair

KEY NOTE
The effleurage/smoothing technique has a very calming and soothing effect on the client.

8 Tabla Playing over the scalp

Therapist's Stance
Standing behind the client.

Technique
- Use the fingertips of both hands to perform a light drumming over the head.
- Work from the front of the head towards the back.

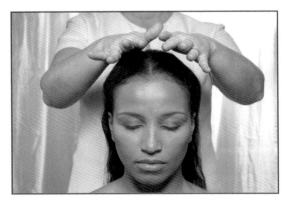

Fig 6.54 Tabla playing

KEY NOTE
The tabla playing technique is very stimulating and energising to the scalp.

9 Pressure Points over the scalp

Therapist's Stance
Standing behind the client.

Technique
- Support one side of the client's head.
- With the other hand, use the tips of all the fingers and the thumb to perform pressures (with a pumping action) across the scalp, at approximately one inch intervals.
- Work from the hairline towards back of head.
- Use the fingers and thumb to press in slowly for a couple of seconds and then release.
- Work across from one side of the head to the other, changing the supporting hand when you reach the centre of the scalp.

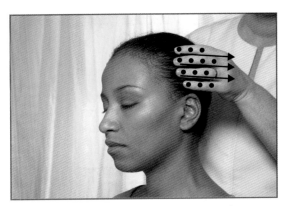

Fig 6.55 Pressure points over scalp

KEY NOTE
The pressure point technique over the scalp helps to release blockages from the nerves relating to the head and neck and has a stimulating effect on the head.

10 Squeeze and Release the scalp muscles

Therapist's Stance
Standing behind the client.

Technique
- Place your fingers on top of client's head with the heels of the hands placed behind the ears.
- Using the heels of the hand, squeeze inwards with medium pressure.
- Hold and then lift and release upwards.
- Repeat the movement with the heels of hands above the ears.
- Repeat the movement with the hands placed in front of the ears.

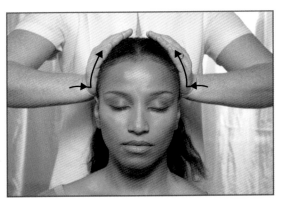

Fig 6.56 Squeeze and release the scalp muscles

KEY NOTE
The squeeze and release technique to the scalp muscles helps to relieve

11 Circular Frictions using the heel of the hands across the temples

Therapist's Stance
Standing behind the client.

Technique
- Support client's head against you.
- Use the heels of both hands to make circular movements against the temples.
- Lift upwards and back towards you.
- Repeat several times.

12 Compression to the head

Therapist's Stance
Standing to the side of the client.

Technique
- Place one hand round front of head and one round the back.
- Squeeze inwards with the palms of the hands and then release.
- Repeat three times.

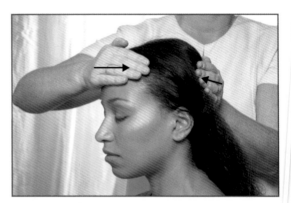

Fig 6.58 Compression to head

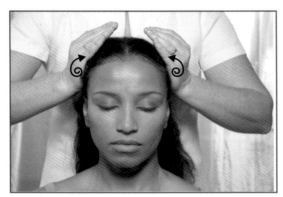

Fig 6.57 Circular frictions using the heel of the hands across the temples

KEY NOTE
This technique is very effective at helping to release tension headaches.

KEY NOTE
Applying circular frictions to the temples is also very effective at helping to relieve tension headaches and eyestrain.

13 Effleurage/Smoothing through the hair (as in Step 7)

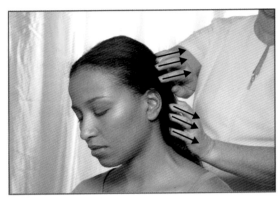

Fig 6.59 Effluerage/smoothing through hair

The Face

The face is an area of the body that cannot help but show tension. When feeling tense the jaw tends to clamps tight, teeth grind together and the lips tighten.

> **KEY NOTE**
>
> Indian Head Massage can help to relax the facial muscles and melt away tension, leaving the client feeling calm and refreshed.

Before commencing the face massage, you may wish to use a dry hand cleanser to cleanse your hands of any oil or sebum that may be left on the hands from the scalp massage.

For the face massage, the client's head needs to be tilted back slightly to rest against the therapist's upper thorax. Ensure that the client's neck is comfortable and offer a neck support or cushion.

1 Effleurage/Smoothing across the face

Therapist's Stance
Standing behind the client.

Technique
- Start with the fingers across the chin.
- Use the fingers of both hands to smooth the face with gentle flowing movements in an upwards direction.
- Work across the chin and jaw, then across cheeks and across the forehead.
- Repeat three times.

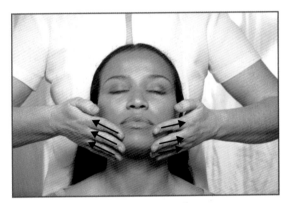

Fig 6.60 Effleurage/smoothing across face

> **KEY NOTE**
>
> The effleurage/smoothing technique helps to relax and soothe tired facial muscles.

2 Pressure Points across the forehead, around the eye sockets and cheekbones

Therapist's Stance
Standing behind the client.

Technique
- Support the client's head with one hand.
- Use the pads of the forefinger and middle finger of the other hand to press the following pressure points in pairs at the midline of the forehead:

  Pair 1: half an inch above the bridge of the nose

  Pair 2: halfway up the forehead

  Pair 3: at the hairline.

- Then move both fingers outwards approximately half an inch and repeat.
- Then press points on the ridge of bone all round the eyes – outwards along the top and inwards along the bottom.
- Now move to points on either side of the nose and across the curve of the cheekbones and drain sinuses by curving forefingers under the cheekbones and holding for a few seconds.

KEY NOTE
Using this pressure point technique on the face helps to relieve sinus congestion and encourage lymphatic drainage from the head.

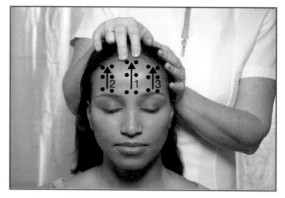
Fig 6.61 Pressure points across forehead

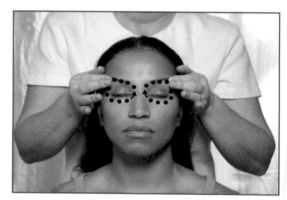
Fig 6.62 Pressure points around eyesockets

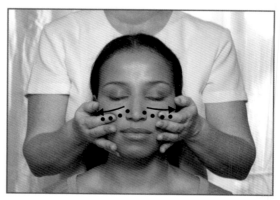
Fig 6.63 Pressure points on cheekbones

3 Circular Temple Frictions with the tips of the fingers

Therapist's Stance
Standing behind the client.

Technique
- Support the client's head against you.
- Use the pads of the fingers to perform circular frictions to the temples.
- Work slowly and deeply over the area several times.

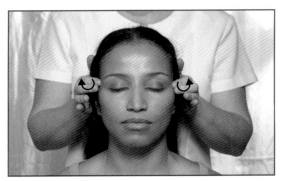

Fig 6.64 Circular temple frictions with the tips of the fingers

KEY NOTE
This technique helps to relieve tension in facial muscles, relieves headaches and eyestrain and helps relax the eyes.

4 Squeezing and Twiddling the ear lobes

Therapist's Stance
Standing behind client.

Technique
- Place your fingers behind the client's earlobes and the thumbs in front.
- Squeeze the earlobes between thumb and forefinger.
- Hold for a few seconds and then slowly release.
- Then twiddle the ears by rolling the thumb and the forefinger across the earlobe in a brisk manner.
- Repeat several times.

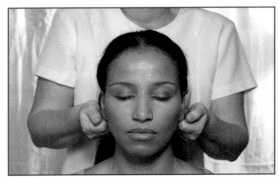

Fig 6.65 Squeeze and twiddle ear lobes

KEY NOTE
The squeezing and twiddling technique applied to the ears stimulates the nerve endings to the whole of the body and creates an energising feeling.

5 Effleurage/Smoothing (as in Step 1)

6 Relaxing the facial muscles

Therapist's Stance
Standing behind the client.

Technique

- Gently place both of your hands so that they cover the lower part of the jaw and cheeks.

- Relax the hands and keep them still and relaxed for a few seconds.

- Gradually move the hands up the face, stopping to place the hands so that the tips of the middle fingers meet at the bridge of the nose.

- Continue up the face stopping to place the hands so that they cover the eyes.

- Continue up the face to finally place hands over the top of the forehead.

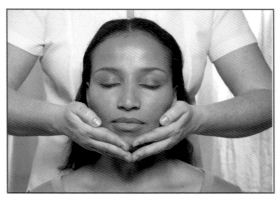

Fig 6.67 Relaxing facial muscles

KEY NOTE
This technique relaxes the facial muscles and the eyes, and creates a feeling of stillness and calm.

7 Higher Chakra Balancing

Therapist's Stance
Standing to the side of the client.

Technique

- Place one hand lightly over the crown chakra (top of the client's head) and cup the other hand over the throat chakra (without touching throat).

- Hold your hands there for a short while, breathing deeply and slowly to concentrate.

- Retaining the hand over the crown chakra, move the other hand up to place lightly over the third eye and hold there for a few moments.

- Then place both hands over the crown.

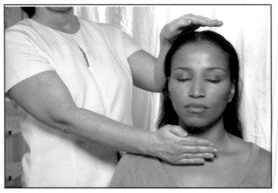

Fig 6.68 Higher chakra balancing

KEY NOTE
Chakra balancing helps to realign the client's energy and is very soothing and calming, helping to bring about a sense of peace and harmony.

8 Squeeze and Release to the back of the neck

Therapist's Stance
Standing to the side of the client.

Technique
- Place one hand over the third eye area of the client's forehead.
- Spread the thumbs and fingers of your other hand on either side of the base of the neck (forming a V shape) and gently squeeze and release the muscles at the back of the neck.

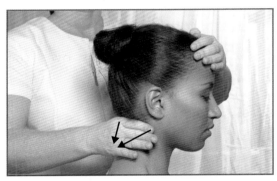

Fig 6.69 Squeeze and release back of neck

9 Effleurage/Smoothing across the upper back

> **KEY NOTE**
> The use of effleurage/smoothing at the end of the massage helps to get the client grounded and brings them back from a deep state of relaxation.

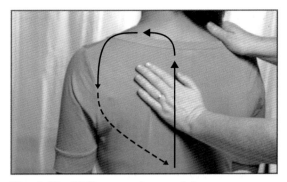

Fig 6.70 Effleurage/smoothing across upper back

10 Slowly Leave the Client's Aura
After squeezing the top of the shoulders take a step back from the client's aura and gently shake your hands.

Wash your hands.

Full Routine Quick Reference Guide

Upper Back and Shoulder Massage

1 **Starting Position** with hands over the top of the client's shoulders

2 **Holding Position** over the top of the head

3 **Effleurage/Smoothing** across the shoulders and upper back

4 **Petrissage/Thumb** Sweeping across the shoulders

5 Frictions with the Heel of the Hand rubbing around the scapulae

6 Frictions with the Finger rubbing around the scapulae

7 Effleurage/Smoothing (repeated as in 3)

8 Pressures with the knuckles either side of the spine

9 Thumb Pushes over the shoulders

10 Finger Pulls across the top of the shoulders

11 Squeezing and Release across the top of the shoulders

12 Heel Pushes across the tops of the shoulders

13 Smoothing with the forearms

14 Chopping across the shoulders and upper back

15 Champi/Double Hacking across the shoulders and upper back

16 Squeezing and Releasing across the tops of the shoulders (repeated as in 11)

17 Effleurage/Smoothing (repeated as in 3)

18 Holding Position over the tops of the shoulders (repeated as in 1)

Upper Arms

1 Squeezing and Releasing the upper arms

2 Compression of the upper arms

3 Heel Rolls embracing the upper arms

4 Squeezing and Kneading down the upper arms

5 Shoulder Mobilisation

6 Squeezing and Kneading to the forearms

7 Squeezing and Kneading to the fingers

8 Circular Pressure Massage to the pressure point between the thumb and index finger

9 Circular Pressure Massage to the pressure point in the centre of the palm

10 Shoulder Lift

11 Effleurage/Smoothing with the Forearms down the upper arms

The Neck

1 Rocking the head backwards and forwards

2 Squeezing and Releasing the muscles at the back of the neck

3 Finger Frictions to the top of the shoulders and up the side of the neck

4 Thumb Pushes to the side of the neck

5 Squeezing and Releasing at the side of the neck

6 Finger Frictions to the base of the skull

7 Heel of the Hand Frictions to the base of the skull

8 Effleurage/Smoothing to the back of the neck

9 **Pressure Points** at the base of the skull

10 **Gentle Stretching** to the side of the neck

11 **Smoothing with the Whole Hand** at the base of the skull (repeated as in 8)

The Scalp

1 **Rubbing** to the side of the scalp, around the ears

2 **Frictions** to the side of the scalp, around the ears

3 **Rubbing** to the whole of the scalp

4 **Frictions** with the whole of the hand

5 **Ruffling** through the hair

6 **Hair Tugging**

7 **Effleurage/Smoothing** through the hair

8 **Tabla Playing** over the scalp

9 **Pressure Points** over the scalp

10 **Squeeze and Release** the scalp muscles

11 **Circular Frictions Using the Heel of the Hands** across the temples

12 **Compression** to the head

13 **Effleurage/Smoothing** through the hair (repeated as in 7)

The Face

1 **Effleurage/Smoothing** across the face

2 **Pressure Points** across the forehead, around the eye sockets and cheekbones

3 **Circular Temple Frictions** with the tips of the fingers

4 **Squeezing and Twiddling** the ear lobes

5 **Effleurage/Smoothing** (repeated as in 1)

6 **Relaxing** the facial muscles

7 **Higher Chakra Balancing**

8 **Squeeze and Release** to the back of the neck

9 **Effleurage/Smoothing** across the upper back

10 **Slowly Leave the Client's Aura**

Aftercare advice

Clients will often feel deeply relaxed following treatment. It is therefore important that clients have a suitable rest period and are offered a glass of water before rising. If oils has been used on the scalp, then clients should be encouraged to leave the oil on for a few hours after treatment before shampooing.

When washing their hair after oil application, clients should be advised not to wet their hair first but to apply shampoo to the scalp before the water in order to help to emulsify the oil.

As part of a client's homecare programme, therapists may wish to teach clients simple self-massage techniques with oils, particularly if the client requires an improvement to their hair condition.

In order to aid the healing process and to get the maximum benefit from their treatments, clients are advised to:

- increase intake of water following treatment to assist the body's detoxification process

- have a suitable rest period after the treatment

- avoid eating a heavy meal after the treatment; try to keep the diet light while the body is using its energy for healing

- avoid smoking

- cut down on the consumption of stimulants such as tea, coffee, alcohol and drugs

- take time out to relax and practise stress-relieving techniques such as yoga or meditation, if appropriate

- participate in regular manageable exercise

- practise the correct breathing techniques to create a feeling of calm

- use oils and simple head massage techniques at home for long-term haircare.

Reactions to Indian Head Massage

A client's reaction to Indian Head Massage may vary according to their physical and emotional condition. If the body has been under a considerable amount of stress, it is not unusual for there to be some kind of reaction as the body adjusts itself back to balance. This is often referred to as a 'healing crisis'. Clients should be made aware of the fact that some of these reactions may occur and be reassured that if they do occur, they will only be temporary.

Discussed below are some of the healing reactions that may occur following an Indian Head Massage treatment:

- a feeling of tiredness and lethargy due to the release of toxins

- a feeling of dizziness or nausea

- an aching and soreness in the muscles due to the release of toxins and the nerve fibres responding to the massage

- a heightened emotional state – depression, weepiness or laughter

- increased urination

- increased secretions of mucous from the nose and mouth

- cold-like symptoms

- a disturbed sleep pattern (restlessness).

Many clients report the following positive reactions following an Indian Head Massage:

- relief from stress and muscular tension

- an increased feeling of awareness; clients often experience a feeling of calm, peace and tranquillity due to the rebalancing of the chakras

- improved sleep pattern (deep and restful)

- a feeling of alertness and clarity in mental thought

- increased energy levels

- elevation of mood

- pain relief

- increased joint mobility.

Important information to be recorded after the treatment includes:

- an assessment of the client's physical condition (noting any areas of tension, physiological responses) as well as psychological responses

- visual assessment of the client (noting posture, non-verbal signs)

- any known reactions, their effects and any advice given

- aftercare advice

- homecare advice, along with any oils or products suggested for home use

- outcome and general evaluation of the treatment

- recommendations for future treatment and the suggested frequency.

Frequency of Treatment

In India, head massage is often part of a daily schedule. In the western world, as part of a stress management programme, Indian Head Massage should ideally be carried out once or even twice a week for maximum benefit. It is advisable to offer clients a course of treatments (between four and six initially) and to recommend the client takes the treatments close together initially.

Frequency of treatment may vary due to a client's resources, namely time and money, and clients should be encouraged to attend for treatments as frequently as their schedule and financial resources will allow.

Benefits of Regular Indian Head Massage Treatments

In order to maximise the benefits of Indian Head Massage, it is important for clients to receive regular treatment.

Benefits of regular treatment include:

- improvement in hair condition

- reduction in stress levels

- increased energy levels

- a general sense of well-being

- improved sleep patterns

- improvement in circulation.

Self-Assessment Questions

1 Which of the following statements is *false* in relation to Indian Head Massage techniques?

a   effleurage is a stroking or smoothing movement that signals the beginning and end of the massage

b   petrissage movements are deeper, using the whole hand, thumb or fingers

c   tapotement movements are heavy and applied with both hands in a slow motion

d   friction movements are a strong feature of Indian Head Massage, and are performed with the whole of the hand, heel of the hand, the fingers or thumbs

2 Friction movements are used in Indian Head Massage to

a   prepare the area for deeper strokes

b   stimulate and clear nerve pathways

c   break down tension nodules caused by stress and tension

d   restore energy balance to the body

3 A form of tapotement used in Indian Head Massage called 'double hacking' is also known traditionally as

a   tabla playing

b   tapping

c   cupping

d   champi

4 Which of the following is *not* considered to be a form of petrissage?

a   picking up

b   squeezing and releasing

c   smoothing

d   rolling

5 Which of the following statements is *false*?

a   marma points are naturally sensitive points measured by finger widths

b   marma points are subtle pressure points that stimulate the life force

c   in Indian Head Massage the marmas may be used to treat a client's internal illness

d   the marmas are anatomical places on the body, mostly composed of flesh and bones

6 How many marma points are located in the head and neck area?

   a   107

   b   27

   c   37

   d   57

7 The marma point located on the top of the head/crown in known as the

   a   apanga marma point

   b   adhipati marma point

   c   avarta marma point

   d   none of the above

8 Which of the following oils would not be suitable for a client with dry skin and hair?

   a   sesame

   b   mustard

   c   olive

   d   coconut

9 In Indian Head Massage the idea of working on the higher chakras is to

   a   enable the client to breathe more easily

   b   de-stress the client

   c   restore a sense of balance and harmony to the client's energy

   d   to open up a client's spiritual potential

10 The colour associated with the crown chakra is

   a   indigo

   b   violet

   c   blue

   d   red

11 The throat chakra is associated with

   a   creativity and sexuality

   b   emotions and self-worth

   c   communication and expression

   d   memories and imagination

▶

12 Which of the following may be considered a contra-action to Indian Head Massage?

a   improved sleep pattern

b   feeling of alertness

c   headache and nausea

d   increased energy levels

7 Stress Management

Stress is a common feature of modern life and is therefore something everyone experiences. Nobody is born knowing how to handle stress and, as there is no immunity from it, the best way to protect the body from the harmful effects of stress is to learn how to manage it.

Stress undermines the state of physical and emotional well-being; learning how to manage stress effectively can therefore help to maintain good health and vitality. It is now acknowledged that many medical conditions are stress-related and therefore more importance is being placed on being able to handle stress in order to improve health.

The increasing pressures of modern life have influenced the growth in popularity of holistic therapies such as Indian Head Massage, as the stress relief and relaxation provided by these treatments can be a major factor in helping clients to manage their own stress.

By the end of this chapter, you will be able to relate the following to your work in Indian Head Massage:

- Definition of stress.
- Different types of stress and how they affect the body.
- Recognising stress.
- Strategies to help clients to take control of and manage their own stress.

- Indian Head Massage as a counterbalance to stress.

By the very nature of their work, holistic therapists are exposed to a considerable amount of emotional energy when dealing with clients. It is therefore important for them to be able to use stress management techniques in order to help both their clients and themselves.

Indian Head Massage can be a very effective treatment in counterbalancing some of the negative effects of stress. However, for long-term stress relief, clients often need to consider many other factors in their life. This chapter considers the basic tools of stress management, from identifying the symptoms and causes to employing strategies for coping with stress.

Definition of Stress

There is no conclusive definition of 'stress'. It is a difficult term to define, as stress means different things to different people. However, it can be said that stress is the adaptive response to the demands or pressures placed upon an individual, and can involve any interference that disturbs a person's emotional and physical well-being. The stress becomes unacceptable when the pressures are beyond the control of the individual, and the results of the stress can then be harmful to others. Stress is therefore the imbalance between the demands of everyday life and the ability to cope with them.

Stress can be positive in that it can act as a stimulus and increase levels of alertness, but it can also be negative when too much stress affects the ability to function effectively. It is the depth and number of stressors at any time that causes stress to become beyond control, which then requires the body to make adjustments to re-establish a normal balance.

Types of Stress

Survival Stress

This type of stress is when the body reacts to meet the demands of a physically or emotionally threatening situation. The reaction is mediated by the release of adrenaline and produces the so-called 'fight or flight' reaction.

This type of stress is positive in that it enables the body and mind to react quickly and effectively. It is only when the effects of adrenaline are long-term that it can lead to negative stress.

Internally Generated Stress

This type of stress is often caused by the view of or reaction to a situation, rather than the situation itself. Anxiety and worry can lead to negative thought processes and often lead to a feeling that circumstances are out of control.

There is a relationship between personality and stress, in particular with anxious and obsessional personalities. What may be stressful for one person may be enjoyable and exciting for another.

Work/lifestyle-related Stress

Many stresses that are experienced may relate to work or lifestyle. In this context, stress may come from some of the following:

- having too much or too little work
- time pressures and deadlines
- demands of a job with limited resources
- insufficient working or living space
- disorganised working conditions
- limited time, to the detriment of leisure and family life
- pollution
- financial problems
- relationship problems
- ill health
- family situations such as a birth, death, marriage or divorce.

Negative Stress

This type of stress is caused by the inability to manage long-term stress.

How to Recognise Stress

Recognising stress can be very difficult. It is important to realise that as stress levels increase, the ability to recognise stress usually decreases. Stress can manifest itself in different ways, and symptoms may be presented in a number of different ways. These are discussed below.

Short-term Physical Stress Signals

These are symptoms of survival stress as the body adapts to situations that are perceived as a threat. Effects of short-term physical stress include an increased heart beat, rapid breathing, increased sweating, tense muscles, dry mouth, frequency of urination and feeling of nausea.

While the effects of short-term physical stress may help you survive in a threatening situation, negative stress can result when the adrenaline is not put to this use. The effects of excess adrenaline can lead to anxiety, frustration, negative thinking, reduction in self-confidence, distraction, and may cause difficult situations to be seen as a threat rather than a challenge.

Long-term Stress Signals

Common complaints relating to long-term stress are back pain, headaches, aches and pains, excessive tiredness, digestive problems, frequent colds, skin eruptions and exacerbation of asthma. Stress and pressure can also lead to the following:

Internal stress signals

When the body is subjected to long-term stress, the mind becomes unable to think clearly and rationally about situations and problems. This can lead to feelings of anxiety, worry, confusion, feeling out of control or overwhelmed, restlessness, frustration, irritability, hostility, impatience and helplessness, and also lead to depression and mood changes.

People who suffer from long-term stress may generally feel more lethargic, find difficulty sleeping, change their eating habits, rely more on medication, drink and smoke more frequently and have a reduced sex drive.

Behavioural stress signals

When people are under pressure this can be exhibited in some of the following ways: talking too fast, twitching and fiddling, being irritable, defensive, aggressive, irritated, critical and overreacting emotionally to situations. They may also find that they start becoming more forgetful, make more mistakes, are unable to concentrate, are unrealistic in their judgement and become unreasonably negative. Pressure may cause some people to neglect their personal appearance and have increasing amounts of time absent from work.

If the body is subjected to excessive short-term stress, it may lead to ineffective performance which should be treated as a warning sign; stress management strategies can be adopted to avoid the problem in the future. The effects of long-term stress, however, can be much more severe as it can lead to extreme fatigue, exhaustion, burn-out or even breakdown.

Summary of Signs and Symptoms of Stress

Behavioural changes

People who suffer from stress may:

- be argumentative
- be less friendly
- become withdrawn
- avoid friends and relatives
- lose creativity
- work longer and harder and achieve less
- be reluctant to do their own job properly
- procrastinate.

Change of feelings

People who experience stress may:

- lose their sense of humour
- have a sense of being a failure
- lack self-esteem and have a cynical and bitter attitude
- experience irritability with conflict at home and work
- feel apathetic.

Change of thinking

Stress can cause people to:

- be rigid in their thinking, with resistance to change
- be suspicious
- have poor concentration
- feel like leaving a job or relationship.

Physical

People who are stressed may:

- feel tired all the time
- experience sleep problems (usually poor sleep)
- be increasingly absent from work because of prolonged minor illnesses
- have aches and pains
- suffer backache
- experience headaches and migraine
- have indigestion
- hyperventilate
- have palpitations.

Mental health

The effects of stress can cause feelings of:

- anxiety
- depression
- fear of rejection.

Cognitive distortion

Individuals suffering from stress may view themselves in a distorted way:

- **Jumping to conclusions**: even in the absence of proof, stressed individuals may jump to conclusions. They may assume that other people see them in a certain way, or they may anticipate that things will turn out badly and act as if their predictions are facts.
- **All or none**: this is the feeling that, if you fail in one way, you see yourself as a total failure. There is then the tendency to over-generalise and see this single failure as a proof of your life's failure.

■ **Mental filter**: this is when people pick out negative events and dwell on them to the exclusion of everything else. Eventually, the positive aspects of life become rejected and ignored.

The Effects of Stress on the Body

When the body is placed under physical or psychological stress, it increases the production of certain hormones such as cortisol and adrenaline. These hormones produce marked changes in the heart rate, blood pressure levels, metabolism and physical activity. While this physical action can help a person to function more effectively when under pressure for short periods of time, it can also be extremely damaging and debilitating in the long term.

Dr Hans Selye called the body's response to stress the 'general adaptation syndrome' which he suggested be divided into three stages.

The first stage is the **alarm** stage, which is the body's initial reaction to the perceived stressor. This involves the so-called 'fight or flight' syndrome which involves the sympathetic nervous system and the release of the hormones adrenaline and cortisol.

The effects on the body are to effect an alert response, and include:

■ increased heart rate

■ increased ventilation rate

■ increased diversion of blood to the muscles and brain

■ increase in perspiration

■ increased release of glucose from the liver

■ inhibited digestion.

The alarm stage allows the body to cope and respond and when the threat is over the body returns to a state of balance through repair and rest (parasympathetic system). However, problems can start to occur when the restoration of balance does not happen because the body is not allowed to rest sufficiently, or due to perceived or real encounters with repeated stressful situations. Repeated alarm reactions can lead to symptoms such as breathlessness, a dry mouth, aching, a clenched jaw or fists, dizziness, palpitations and sweating.

The second stage is known as the **resistance** stage which, through the secretion of the circulating hormones, allows the body to continue fighting long after the effects of the alarm reaction have dissipated. This eventually leads to symptoms of disease as the body's energy resources are drained without adequate recuperation and repair. Symptoms associated with the resistance stage include colds and flu, anxiety and depression, high blood pressure, chest pains, tiredness, insomnia, indigestion, headaches and migraine.

The third stage is the **exhaustion** stage which takes place if the stress response continues without relief and can result in organs becoming more and more compromised until the adaptation becomes degenerative.

KEY NOTE

Increased cortisol secretion in stressful situations reduces the body's immune response and the anti-inflammatory effect of cortisol can slow down healing too.

Areas of the body most vulnerable to stress

When the body is moving or stationary, a combination of muscle tension and relaxation exists in order to maintain posture. If a good balance is not achieved then the body suffers excessive muscle tension, which can cause pain and fatigue. If muscles are held tightly in a state of contraction, circulation is impeded which results in a build-up of the products of fatigue. This can then result in muscular spasms, aches and pains.

When under stress, the entire body becomes tense and posture changes. Hours spent sitting and working at a desk can cause tension to accumulate in the upper body, particularly around the neck and shoulders. Large amounts of time spent in front of the computer screen can result in eyestrain where the eyes and surrounding muscles become tired.

Being tense and in a permanent state of alert can be uncomfortable and has the ability to throw the body out of balance. Tension uses up energy, but the energy is unproductive. Muscle tension can also affect our ability to function well as it makes our thought processes less efficient.

KEY NOTE

Tension can also have a debilitating effect on the immune system, predisposing people to colds and other diseases because when we are in a constant state of alert, healing and tissue repair are inhibited. The key to stress relief is therefore relaxation as healing can only take place when the body is at rest.

Shoulders

The shoulders are the place where most people hold a considerable amount of tension. When the body is in a state of tension the shoulders are lifted toward the ears and often remain this way, causing the muscles to go into spasm. This restricts the blood flow to the head, neck and shoulders and causes the neck and shoulders to become stiff and inflexible. Sitting with hunched shoulders can reduce chest capacity and thus impair breathing.

KEY NOTE

Indian Head Massage can help to counterbalance the effects of stress by relaxing the shoulders; they will then drop and allow the energy to flow more freely to the area, encouraging deeper and easier breathing and improved joint flexibility.

Upper arms

The upper arms are important for upper body movement; when the shoulders are tense they tighten and restrict movement. When in a state of tension, the upper arms tend to hug the chest either at the sides or in front, while the elbows bend up.

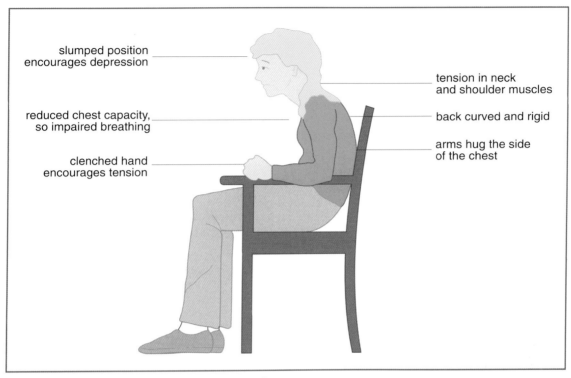

slumped position encourages depression

reduced chest capacity, so impaired breathing

clenched hand encourages tension

tension in neck and shoulder muscles

back curved and rigid

arms hug the side of the chest

Fig 7.1 Postural changes due to muscular tension

KEY NOTE

Indian Head Massage can help reduce tension and tightness in the upper arm muscles to help improve flexibility of the arms and shoulders.

Neck

When the body is balanced the neck is designed to allow the head to move in a variety of directions. When the body is out of balance and under stress, the head tends to come forwards and the chin juts out. This then throws the body out of alignment as the neck muscles tense and take the weight of the head.

The neck muscles are then in a permanent state of contraction and can cause the neck to become stiff and tight. This tension then reduces mobility of the neck and shoulders.

KEY NOTE

Working on the neck with Indian Head Massage helps to open up the energy flow from the spine to the whole head and can help to reduce tension and improve posture by re-aligning the muscles, thereby increasing mobility and allowing the head to move more freely.

Head

The face is an area of the body that cannot help but show tension; the jaw clamps tight, teeth grind together and the lips tighten. The scalp and temporal muscles tighten when under stress, restricting the blood flow and leading to headaches, eyestrain and neck and shoulder tension.

> **KEY NOTE**
>
> Indian Head Massage helps to counterbalance stress in the head by improving the circulation and relaxing the muscles and nerve fibres, thereby relieving tension.

When the body is in balance it facilitates relaxation and a positive mental outlook, which are critical to successful stress management. If the shoulders and chest are free of tension the ribs are free to allow deep relaxed breathing; if the head and neck are well-balanced they can support the shoulders and take pressure from the neck muscles.

The body is ideally equipped to deal with many different types of stressors; however, the ability to deal with stress can be inhibited by a heavy load of unresolved stress, which contributes to the development of disease and pain.

Stress-related Disorders

Stress is considered to be a contributory factor in many conditions. Listed below are areas susceptible to stress-related diseases:

- **skin** – as the skin is often a manifestation of what is felt inside, skin disorders such as eczema and psoriasis are often exacerbated by stress. Allergies may also be triggered by stress

- **hair** – some forms of hair loss are linked to stress

- **heart** – high blood pressure and conditions such as angina may be exacerbated by stress. If the blood supply to the heart is restricted by arteriosclerosis and the person's life is very stressful, a heart attack can result

- **lungs** – symptoms of asthma often worsen when the body is subjected to high levels of emotional stress

- **muscles** – muscle tension is often the result of stress

- **brain** – anxiety and depression may be triggered by stress

- **reproductive** – the reproductive hormones are reduced at times of stress; this is evidenced by stress-related problems such as infertility and menstrual disorders

- **digestion** – conditions that may be aggravated by stress include ulcers and irritable bowel syndrome.

Adaptation to Stress

Fortunately, the body has the capacity to cope with stress as the purpose of all the body's systems is to maintain a constant internal environment through homeostasis.

However, there are several factors that may affect the body's ability to deal with stress, including the following:

■ **genetics** – the effects of stress on the body can be determined by genetic make-up and can dictate how well different organs respond and adapt to stressful situations

■ **physiological reserve** – the body's response to stress depends on the ability to increase or decrease function according to its needs. If the ability of an organ to respond is diminished, it is difficult for the body to maintain homeostasis; even with small demands, imbalance and disease may ensue

■ **age** – with age the ability to adapt is diminished and while a young, healthy individual may respond and adapt to stress easily, an elderly client may find the situation considerably more stressful

■ **health status** – clients who are mentally and physically fit are able to adapt to stress placed on them more easily than others who are not

■ **nutrition** – deficiencies or excesses of nutrition can impair one's ability to adapt to stressful situations

■ **sleep** – irregular sleep patterns and wakefulness can reduce immunity as well as physical and psychological functions. Sleep is important for restoring energy and if sleep is inadequate, it can impair the body's ability to deal with stress

■ **psychological factors** – psychological conditions such as anxiety and depression can make a person more susceptible to stress.

Managing Stress

In order to be able to work towards preventing stress, it is important to be able to identify its causes. Part of the problem with stress is its familiarity; as people become used to living with stress they may be unaware of how it is affecting them or those around them.

Mental attitude is a critical factor in dealing with stress, along with finding ways of reducing the effects of stress. Focusing on the ownership of the sources of the stress and not on the feelings they generate is the first step to counterbalancing it. Stress management can be approached in several different ways and a client's stress management programme may typically consist of experiencing a range of holistic therapies, the use of relaxation and stress reduction techniques, as well as implementing lifestyle changes.

Holistic therapists can help clients to recognise their own stress by advising on ways in which they can combat it and start to manage their own stress positively. Stress management has to take into account the recognition of an individual's vulnerability to stress and their ability to be aware of possible sources of stress and identify signs and symptoms of stress. What is most important is helping clients to learn how to manage stress and be able to identify the factors that contribute to it and so be able to control it.

Optimum Stress Levels

Stress levels vary, like any other human characteristic, and what may seem challenging and exciting to one person may seem stressful and threatening to another. The most positive approach to successful stress management is finding an optimum stress level in which the body can be sufficiently stimulated to perform well, while not becoming overstressed and unhappy.

KEY NOTE

It is important that each individual is able to monitor their own stress levels. Some people may operate most effectively at a low level of stress, while this may leave another person feeling bored or unmotivated. Alternatively, someone who performs only moderately at low level may find they excel at a high level when they are under more pressure.

The most effective way of finding an optimum level of stress is to keep a stress diary for a short period of time in order to identify what is causing the stress and whether it is being controlled effectively. The type of information that could be recorded in a stress diary is the stressful event and time, how stressful the event was (on a scale of 1 to 10), what made the event stressful and how the situation was handled. This can be the key to identifying whether it was the cause that was tackled or the symptom.

When analysing a stress diary, it should be possible to extract the following information:

- the level of stress that is optimum for an individual

- the main sources of unpleasant or negative stress and whether the strategies for managing them are effective or not.

Managing Stress Effectively

Once there is an understanding or recognition as to what is causing the stress and the level under which an individual can work effectively, the next stage is to work out how to manage the stress. An action plan for managing stress may include:

- controlling or eliminating the problems that are causing the stress

- using stress-reduction techniques

- making lifestyle changes

- taking a holiday or break more often

- social and family support

- time management
- hobbies and leisure time
- being prepared to ask for help
- looking back at action taken and evaluating the effects.

Stress Reduction Techniques

When choosing methods for stress reduction, different strategies may be required for different people and different circumstances.

The main objective in managing stress is to help the client to improve the quality of their lives and their resistance to stress by employing certain techniques, as well as making certain lifestyle changes. It is important to realise that as people react differently to stress, different techniques or combinations of techniques may be required for each individual. Stress can only be eliminated if the root causes are recognised and resolved. However, there are ways in which the unpleasant effects of stress may be reduced.

Relaxation Techniques

Physical relaxation is something which often appears easy but in reality is a skill that needs to be learned and practised. By teaching clients physical relaxation techniques you can help them to take responsibility for their stress reactions and reduce the distress of many conditions.

Tensing muscles and holding breath when tense becomes habitual; the key to relaxation is training the body to feel tension and recognise when breathing reflects tension. The body's reaction to stress involves breathing and muscle tension: the parts over which a person can gain control. The aim of relaxation is to control breathing and muscle tension in order to calm the mind and body.

Through learning physical relaxation, a person can learn to slow down their breathing, breathe deeply and relax their muscles. As the relaxation response starts to happen, other responses change automatically and as the breathing calms down and the muscles relax, the heart rate simultaneously slows down. With relaxation, the key is in gaining control over breathing and muscles: the rest will happen automatically as the body responds positively to being in a state of relaxation.

Relaxation can help to:

- maintain emotional and physical health
- aid restful sleep
- reduce the harmful effects of stress
- relieve muscular tension
- promote optimum oxygen levels for the body
- aid the body to recover and repair.

Breathing

Deep breathing is a very effective method of relaxation and works well combined with other relaxation techniques such as relaxation imagery, meditation and progressive muscular relaxation.

On inhaling, the intercostal muscles, abdominal muscles and the diaphragm contract in order to increase the volume of the thoracic cavity which causes air to pass into the lungs. While the breath is held, all these muscles remain tensed. When they relax, the volume of the thoracic cavity decreases as the muscles return to their original relaxed position. Comfortable, healthy breathing brings air down into the depth of the lungs and the body is able to relax as the breath is let out. When the body is still tense, breathing becomes fast and the muscles in the upper part of the chest take over to cause panting.

The experience of any physical or emotional stress will affect breathing. At times of stress, breathing becomes shallow and irregular, resulting in the brain being deprived of sufficient oxygen. This leads to a feeling of dizziness, inability to concentrate, and agitation. Learning how to breathe deeply helps to fill the body with positive energy and clears the mind. It can also help to prevent a person from getting stressed, or can help them gain control more quickly when they are feeling stressed.

Most people use only half of their lung capacity and breathe with their chest and not their diaphragm. Below are two breathing exercises which may be taught to clients for self-help. It is important for clients to practise breathing exercises regularly, in order that they may be prepared to use them the next time they feel anxious and stressed.

Breathing exercises for successful stress control

Breathing exercise 1

1 Sit in a comfortable position and loosen tight clothing.

2 Place one hand on the chest and the other across the stomach.

3 Inhale deeply through the nose to fill the upper chest cavity and down to the lower part of the lungs, as if breathing into the stomach for a count of 6.

4 Exhale slowly to a count of 12, allowing the air to escape from the top of your lungs first before the lower part deflates.

5 Repeat this exercise 6–8 times.

Breathing exercise 2

1 Apply the first two fingers of the right hand to the side of the right nostril and press gently to close it.

2 Breathe in slowly through the left nostril and hold for a count of 3.

3 Transfer the first two fingers to the left nostril to close it.

4 Breathe out slowly through the right nostril on a count of 3. Breathe in through the right nostril and hold for a count of 3 and while holding transfer the fingers to the right nostril and breathe out.

5 Repeat the exercise 6 times.

KEY NOTE

After completing breathing exercises, clients should be advised to wait a few moments before getting up, in order to avoid dizziness.

Correct breathing is something which really needs to be practised often until it feels natural and it may then be utilised as a counterbalance to stress. Breathing properly enables the body to relax and regain its natural balance, whilst calming the mind. If a client has difficulty breathing correctly, it may be advisable for them to attend classes which involve structured breathing, such as yoga.

The effects of poor breathing on the body can be damaging in that it:

- weakens the nervous system
- encourages muscle tension
- starves the body of nutrients
- blocks the circulation
- weakens the immune system
- disturbs digestion.

Progressive Muscular Relaxation

This is a physical technique designed to relax the body when it is tense. It may be applied to any group of muscles in the body, depending on whether one area is tense or whether it is the whole body.

PMR is achieved by tensing a group of muscles so that they are as tightly contracted as possible. The muscles are then held in a state of tension for a few seconds and relaxed. This should result in a feeling of deep relaxation in the muscles.

For maximum effect, this exercise should be combined with breathing exercises and imagery (such as the image of stress leaving the body).

Relaxation exercise

1 Find a place where you can feel comfortable.

2 Close your eyes and pull your feet towards you as far as you can, hold them for a count of 5 and let them relax. Let them drop as if you are a puppet on a string and the string had broken.

3 Curl your toes as if you were holding a pencil, hold them for a count of 5 and then relax.

4 Tighten and tense the calf muscles, count to 5 and then relax.

5 Tighten and tense the thighs, press them tightly together, count to 5 and then relax, allowing them to fall apart.

6 Tighten the abdominal muscles, pulling in the muscles, count to 5 and then relax.

7 Tighten the muscles in the hips and the buttocks, count to 5 and then relax.

8 Arch the back and tense the back muscles, count to 5 and then relax.

9 Tense the shoulders by raising them to the ears, count to 5 and then drop them.

10 Lift your arms up with the hands outstretched as if you were reaching for something. Hold for a slow count of 5 and then let the arms drop down.

11 Tense the muscles in the forehead, count to 5 and then relax.

12 Tense the muscles around the eyes tightly, count to 5 and then relax.

13 Tense the muscles in the jaw and cheeks (as if gritting your teeth), hold for 5 and then relax.

14 By now you should feel relaxed and heavy, as if you are sinking into the floor or chair.

15 Check that all body parts are free from tension and if there are any areas left with tension, hold that part tense again before relaxing.

16 When you're ready, get up gradually, taking your time.

NB *This exercise will be easier to do if the instructions are on CD or tape, preferably spoken by a person with a slow, calm and relaxing voice.*

Imagery and Visualisation

Imagery techniques can be useful in recreating a retreat from stress and pressure, by imagining a place or event that was happy and restful, and calling upon it to help manage a stressful period.

Imagery and visualisation are often more effective and real if combined with sounds, smell, taste and warmth. It is important to realise that visualisation is a very individual skill. Clients should be encouraged to call upon a happy experience and to gear their visualisation towards that image. Imagery and visualisation can often be enhanced by a relaxation tape, which may be played while the client is receiving treatment and can be purchased for home use.

Meditation

This is a very effective way of relaxing, as the idea is to focus your thoughts on relaxing for a period of time, leaving the mind and body to recover from the problems and worries that have caused the stress. Meditation can help to reduce stress by slowing down breathing, helping muscular relaxation, reducing blood pressure, and encouraging clear thinking by focusing and concentrating the mind. The key to meditation is to quieten the mind and focus completely on one thing.

With meditation, it is important for the body to be relaxed and in a comfortable position.

Meditation is a very personal experience and can involve a person sitting or lying quietly and focusing the mind, or it can be taught in a class situation. Therapists may also facilitate meditation by using positive mental imagery and visualisation, in order to help clients focus their minds and lift themselves into a state of passive awareness in order to relax.

Relaxing at Work

When a person spends hours sitting at a desk, driving or in meetings, tension can accumulate in the areas of the body most vulnerable to stress, such as the head, neck and shoulders. Using a simple relaxation routine while at work can help to release tension, reduce stress and renew the body's energy to carry on working effectively.

Start by loosening any tight clothing (collar, tie, scarf) and removing your shoes.

5-minute stress reliever

Sit comfortably with your back supported against the back of the chair, your feet firmly on the ground and your hands and arms open and relaxed and supported by armrests.

1 With a deep breath in, raise the shoulders towards the ears and hold them raised for a few seconds (be aware of the tension that may be accumulating in the shoulders); now take a long slow breath out and drop the shoulders down. Repeat this exercise several times.

2 Now lift your right shoulder and slowly pop it backwards several times, ensuring that the arms are kept loose and relaxed. Repeat the exercise with the left shoulder. Now pop both shoulders together. Repeat several times.

3 Place your left hand on your right shoulder and squeeze gently and then release. Repeat the exercise down the right arm to the elbow. Repeat several times. Now place your right hand on your left shoulder and repeat the exercise.

4 Place your hands over your shoulders. As you exhale, let your head fall backwards and slowly draw your fingers over the clavicles (collar bones). Repeat several times.

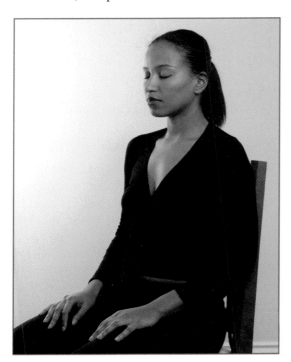

Fig 7.2 Meditation

5 Place your hands over the top of your head and pull your head gently downwards, feeling the slight stretch in the back of the neck. Hold this position for several seconds and then repeat.

6 Place the fingers of both hands at the base of your skull; apply slow circular pressures from the base of the skull and behind the ears, gradually working down the neck. Repeat several times.

7 Exhale and turn the head to the right side. Hold there for a few seconds and use the right hand to massage the right side of the neck from behind the eye down to the clavicle (collar bone). Repeat the exercise on the other side of the neck.

8 Now close your eyes and relax the muscles in your face. Be aware of your eye muscles, your jaw and your forehead. Place the fingers of both hands on each side of the temples and slowly massage in a circular motion, repeating several times.

9 Place the fingertips of both hands in the centre of the forehead and perform slow circular movements with both hands, working out towards the temples. Repeat several times.

10 Finish by cupping your hands over your eyes and holding for several seconds. This helps to release tension and tightness left in the face.

Clients can be encouraged to practise these exercises at least once a day during a break, and they may use individual exercises whenever they start to feel tense, to avoid stress building up.

Stress management is something which needs to be assessed in a holistic way, and will undoubtedly involve many other factors which are outlined below.

Welcoming Change

It is important to realise that in implementing a stress management programme, there will be an element of change, and success will often depend on the adaptation to change. Changes in circumstances and lifestyle can be stressful; however, it is often the anticipation of the change that is more stressful than the change itself.

Attitude to Stress

Attitude is a fundamental factor in stress management. A negative attitude can cause stress by alienating and irritating other people, whereas a positive attitude can help to draw the positive elements out of a situation and can make life more pleasurable and stress more manageable.

When the body is under stress, it is very easy to lose perspective; relatively minor problems can be perceived as threatening and intimidating. When faced with a seemingly overwhelming problem it may help to view the problem in a different way, for instance as a challenge or seeing what may be learned from it, whatever the outcome. It is important to be able to view mistakes as learning experiences, and realise that if something has been learned from an experience, then it has a positive value. Learning how to change the response to stress can help to transform it from a negative to a positive experience.

It may help to talk to someone who has had similar problems, or write the problem down in order to help put it into perspective. It is often helpful to break the problem down in order that it may be reduced to a smaller, more manageable size.

Positive Thinking/Cognitive Therapy

Negative thoughts can cause stress as they can damage confidence and harm effective performance by stifling rational thoughts. Common negative thoughts are feelings of inadequacy, self-criticism, dwelling on past mistakes and worrying about how you appear to others.

Awareness of negative thoughts can be the first step to counterbalancing stress. It is important to write negative thoughts down and review them rationally, deciding whether they are based on reality. It is useful to counter negative thoughts with positive affirmations in order to change a negative thought into a positive one, such as 'I can do this'.

Stress from the Environment

Disorganised living and working conditions can be a major source of stress. A well-organised and pleasant environment can usually make a large contribution to reducing stress and increasing productivity. Stress may be reduced in the environment by improving air quality, lighting, decoration, untidiness and noise levels. Natural light can lift moods and help prevent eyestrain. Creating order out of disorder can help clear a space mentally and physically to regain a state of calm.

When working in an office, it is advisable to consider the ergonomics of furniture as a potential source of stress. If you are working at a computer station, chairs should be checked for comfort and height and the keyboard and monitor comfortably positioned and at the right height. Taking a short break from computer/desk work every hour or so can help prevent tension and eyestrain from building up.

Health and Nutrition

Eating an unbalanced diet can cause stress to the body by depriving it of essential nutrients. Eating a well-balanced diet can help to eliminate chemical stress that may be caused by consumption of too much caffeine, too much alcohol, smoking, and food with high levels of sugar and salt.

Drinking more water may help to increase energy levels and the resistance to stress, by clearing the toxins from the bloodstream. Eating sensible well-balanced meals can help to calm or energise the mind and body and counteract the effects of stress. The best defence against negative stress is a healthy and nutritious diet.

Implementing the following guidelines with diet and nutrition can help towards successful stress control:

- taking time out to eat properly (avoid working lunches)

- eat slowly and chew food well to aid digestion

- rest for a few minutes after eating

- eat fresh food to provide the body with essential vitamins and minerals

- avoid eating late at night to allow the body time to digest food properly

- avoid overeating, as it will decrease energy levels

- avoid eating if you are feeling angry, agitated or upset (practise relaxation techniques before eating).

A healthy diet to help beat stress will consist of:

- eating food rich in vitamins such as citrus fruits and dark green leafy vegetables

- eating foods rich in vitamin A and folic acid

- cutting back on alcohol, caffeine, refined sugars, salt and saturated fats

- eating iron-rich foods such as dried beans, peas and leafy green vegetables

- eating foods high in zinc and magnesium (seafood, wholegrains and dried beans)

- eating balanced amounts of protein, fat and carbohydrates to help provide the body with energy to be able to cope with stress

- eating plenty of whole, unprocessed foods (wholegrain bread and cereals, dried beans and peas, fresh fruit and vegetables, low-fat milk)

- drinking at least two pints of water a day.

Exercise

Taking frequent exercise is one way of reducing stress, as it helps to improve your health, relaxes tense muscles, relaxes the mind and helps induce sleep. Exercise can help to accelerate the flow of blood through the brain, helping the brain to function more clearly, and will remove waste products that have built up as a result of intensive mental energy. Exercise also releases chemicals called endorphins into the blood stream that give a feeling of well-being.

When considering incorporating exercise into a stress management programme, thought should be given to the type of exercise and its suitability to the individual, as if it is difficult or unenjoyable it may cause stress and may not be continued long enough to produce long-term benefits.

Taking Time Out

A successful way of reducing long-term stress is to take up a hobby where there is little or no pressure for performance. Long-term stress can also be reduced by taking time out for undirected activities such as reading a book, taking a walk, having a long bath, listening to music. It is important to take regular holidays or breaks in order to refresh mind and body and recharge energy levels. Taking a break can also help put problems into perspective.

Managing Relationships (Home and Work)

Stress can be caused by relationships with other people and although it is not possible to change a person's personality, a change of attitude will often determine the amount of stress experienced from the situation.

A useful technique to employ when dealing with other people is to try to understand the way they think and why they feel the way they do. Unfortunately, it is human nature that people will often attempt to exploit a relationship at the expense of another person. In this case, it is important to project the right approach – by being positive and pleasant but assertive.

When dealing with a difficult, annoying or frustrating person, it is always a good policy to stay calm and neutral (take deep breaths) in order to be able to think more clearly and react more rationally. It is also important to be able to respect other people's opinions and to accept that some people or situations may not change.

Indian Head Massage as an Antidote to Stress

Holistic therapies such as Indian Head Massage can help clients to manage their stress, as they provide a period of time away from everyday stresses in order to relax and regain a sense of physical and emotional balance. A combination of relaxation and a holistic therapy programme can relieve tension and stress and allow the body energies to flow more freely. When the body reaches a state of relaxation, tense muscles start to unknot, blood pressure starts to lower, breathing becomes more regular and deeper, and the mind drifts into a state of passive awareness.

Indian Head Massage is particularly effective as an antidote to stress as it relaxes and revitalises the mind and body, and can help with anxiety, tension and many stress-related conditions.

Other professional help

Although holistic therapies can provide a positive counterbalance to the negative effects of stress, it is important that a client does not become dependent on a therapist for any advice or service, other than that which is associated with the chosen treatment. Clients may need to consult another professional; for instance, if they are deeply depressed they may need to be referred to their GP or to a counsellor.

KEY NOTE
It is unhealthy for a client to become reliant on a holistic therapist for their problems and see them as the one to provide a solution to their stress. The key to successful stress management is for clients to be able to recognise their own stress and for the therapist to help guide them in managing it.

NB: *Therapists should always take care to ensure that they remain objective with clients at all times and realise that by not taking responsibility for the client's problems they are in fact helping them to help themselves.*

Time Management

By employing time management skills effectively, time can be utilised in the most productive and effective way. Time management can help to reduce stress by increasing productivity, therefore allowing more time to relax outside work activities.

The important factor in time management is to concentrate on results and not on activity. This can be achieved by:

- assessing the value of your time and how it may be used most effectively
- focusing on priorities, while deciding which tasks can be delegated and which may be dropped

- managing and avoiding distractions
- finishing work that has been started and working systematically
- learning when to say no and avoiding feeling guilty for doing so
- avoiding being someone else's time problem and reducing commitments
- having a planner for the weeks of the year, including a plan for holidays and leisure.

This can help to reduce the effects of long-term stress by helping to put things back into perspective, giving a feeling of control and direction and freeing more quality time for relaxation and enjoyment of life outside work.

Evaluating stress from experience

In a stress management programme, it is important to look back and reassess in order to plan for the future. Planning ahead can help you to manage stress more effectively, rather than waiting for the distress signals. It is always useful to look back on a stressful situation, in order to assess whether it was dealt with successfully and to decide what could be repeated or what needs to be changed.

Stress Management in the Workplace

Stress is a significant factor, costing billions of pounds a year, as it is thought that 60 per cent of absenteeism in the workplace is caused by stress-related disorders.

Over the last century, ever-increasing technological changes have led to a faster pace of life and to people being required to perform the job descriptions that may previously have been assigned to several people.

Stress occurs when the body is required to perform beyond its normal range of capabilities and the net results of this can be harmful to both individuals and organisations. It is also important to realise that stress can be a motivator and that people need a certain amount of pressure in order to stimulate them into action. Positive stress is the type of stress that gives the body a kick-start when needed. It is a known fact that people with too much time on their hands and not enough stimulus suffer from symptoms of stress, just as do those with too much work and too little time.

Companies are starting to realise that their staff members are more productive when they are able to deal with stress creatively and any factors that can help to reduce the damaging effects of stress can make the workforce happier and increase productivity.

Part of an action plan for stress management at work may include the following:

- Learn to recognise the warning signals of stress and act on them in order to start taking control of stress responses.

- Enlist the support of colleagues and do not be afraid to talk about stressful situations in order to relieve some of the feeling of pressure.

- Take regular breaks away from the desk or workspace and get some fresh air (even if it means opening a window or door).

- Pay attention to the ergonomics of office furniture and try to keep your workspace uncluttered.

- Eat healthily and regularly.

- Eat slowly and digest food properly.

- Learn to delegate and use time management skills – making lists and prioritising.

- Keep a stress diary, noting the days when high stress levels are experienced and learn from this to help counterbalance the negative effects in the future.

- Set realistic goals to avoid the stress of failing to meet an unrealistic deadline.

- Concentrate on one task at a time.

- Pause after completing one task before starting another.

- Plan activities for days off.

- Try to view problems as challenges and as opportunities.

- Think positively – negative thought processes can be disabling and very destructive.

- Learn to see the funny side of stressful situations.

- Look after yourself.

- Use relaxation techniques regularly.

Indian Head Massage as a Counterbalance to Stress in the Workplace

Many companies and individuals are now aware of the costs negative stress can have on their company and their staff. Staff illness can lead to reduced productivity and increased pressure being placed on other individuals, leading to low morale and high staff turnover. Frequent complaints of work-related stress include the following:

'My neck and shoulders ache constantly from using the phone all day'

'I frequently suffer from headaches at work and feel under pressure all the time to meet tight deadlines'

'I never have time for a lunch hour as there is always too much work and not enough time to complete it in'

'I feel stressed-out and tired before I even start work and am too exhausted to enjoy a social life'

Comments like those above sound all too familiar to those suffering from the negative effects of stress at work, who could benefit from stress reduction techniques.

Some organisations have occupational health advisors who look after the welfare of their staff and are interested in ways in which staff stress levels may be managed effectively. Indian Head Massage is well suited to the work environment due to its portable nature. An area of the workplace (preferably private) can be assigned for the treatment, which is performed in an ordinary chair and is short enough in duration to be slotted into a break or lunch hour. It is also advantageous in that the client does not have to undress.

The benefits of Indian Head Massage to organisations and individuals are that it helps to:

- increase staff morale by alleviating depression and anxiety
- relieve stress and muscular tension
- relieve headaches, neck and backache
- relieve eyestrain
- relieve mental and physical strain
- improve concentration levels, memory and mental alertness
- increase energy levels to improve productivity.

Self-Assessment Questions

1 Which of the following statements is *false*?

   a   stress is the imbalance between the demands of everyday life and the ability to cope

   b   too much stress can affect a person's ability to function effectively

   c   stress is caused by external pressures, such as work

   d   stress can involve any interference that disturbs a person's emotional and physical well being

2 Which of the following is a symptom of short-term stress?

   a   rapid breathing

   b   digestive problems

   c   excessive tiredness

   d   mood changes

3 Which hormone increases in production when the body is under stress?

   a   thyroxine

   b   adrenaline

   c   oestrogen

   d   oxytocin

4   Which of the following factors may affect the body's capacity to deal with stress effectively?

   a   age

   b   psychological factors

   c   physiological reserve

   d   all of the above

5   Which of the following effects on the body are associated with the alarm stage of stress, as defined by Dr Hans Selye?

   a   increased heart and ventilation rate

   b   colds and flu

   c   high blood pressure

   d   anxiety and depression

6   Which of the following is a symptom of long-term stress?

   a   dry mouth

   b   headaches

   c   nausea

   d   increased sweating

8 Health, Safety, Security and Employment Standards

In order to be fully competent in their working role, a therapist is required to support and maintain workplace standards and codes of practice. This role covers following health, safety and security procedures when providing services to the general public and safeguarding their own safety and that of their colleagues and clients.

The success of a therapist lies not only in their ability to perform their own job roles effectively but to be able to contribute to the overall efficiency and operation of a business, upon which their livelihood ultimately depends.

By the end of this chapter you will be able to understand and apply the following knowledge to your workplace practice:

- Workplace standards and industry codes of practice.
- Hygienic precautions required for the professional practice of Indian Head Massage.

- Health, Safety and Security procedures in the workplace.
- Professional codes of practice in the workplace.
- Supporting and maintaining efficient workplace services and operations.
- The implications of relevant legislation in relation to Indian Head Massage.

Workplace Standards and Industry Code of Practice

A therapist carrying our the professional practice of Indian Head Massage needs to understand that their work activities and responsibilities must comply with the individual establishment rules in which they are working.

Establishment rules lay down a benchmark of standards required by the workplace and are set according to the requirements of the individual business. They will include codes of professional dress, conduct and specific responsibilities. Below is an example of an establishment's rules.

Establishment Rules

It is each therapist's responsibility to ensure the following procedures and regulations are observed and adhered to during salon operational periods. These duties are required in line with establishment rules, health and safety policies, local bye-laws and awarding body guidelines.

Professional appearance

Workwear All therapists must wear professional workwear for **ALL** practical sessions in the Salon, in order to present a professional image of the establishment and to maintain hygiene.

Footwear This should be low-heeled, comfortable, clean, enclosed at the toes and of smart and professional appearance.

Hair This should be clean, neatly styled and secured away from the face. It is important to tie long hair back for hygienic and practical reasons.

Jewellery and accessories Hands and arms should be bare of jewellery, other than a wedding band. All other jewellery must be unobtrusive.

Hands These should be kept as soft as possible and protected from harsh chemicals. Nails must be kept **short** and **without nail enamel**. Hands must be cleansed immediately before and after physical contact with the client.

Personal hygiene Due to the close nature of therapy treatments, close attention should be paid to maintaining personal hygiene to avoid offending a client by having bad breath and body odour. Attention is also drawn to the need to avoid strong-smelling foods, smoking and the wearing of highly scented products when in close contact with clients.

Professional conduct

Reasonable and professional behaviour must be demonstrated by the therapist at all times, and workplace practices adhered to, including being punctual and fully ready for work, as required.

Therapists should adopt a professional attitude to clients, colleagues and staff at all times. This will include adherence to establishment rules and workplace policies in order to promote a continuity of professional service within the workplace.

All therapists need to observe the salon's Code of Ethics at all times.

Health and safety

All therapists are reminded of the importance of health and safety and hygiene precautions, and these must be observed at all times in accordance with the specific treatment/s provided.

Damages, breakages and accidents

All incidents, including damages, breakages or accidents must be reported to the Salon Manager. All accidents must be recorded in the accident book.

Liaising with colleagues

All therapists are to contribute to the efficiency of the salon's operation by assisting colleagues and informing them of any changes in procedures (client running late/client arriving early/client cancelled, etc.)

Security

Windows and doors

Please ensure that all windows and doors are secured at the end of each session.

Personal belongings

The salon is unable to accept liability for loss or damage to personal possessions while on the premises. Therapists must therefore be vigilant over their own property, as well as that of clients, and keep handbags and other items of value in a safe place.

Records

In order to maintain confidentiality, it is essential that client records and other confidential papers are secured and locked away when unattended.

In the event of any problems or breaches of security, report to the Salon Manager.

Dealing with clients

Greeting clients

Clients visiting the salon are to be attended to promptly and efficiently in a professional manner at all times. Therapists are responsible for greeting their own clients promptly at Reception, carrying out the treatment in a professional manner and booking the client's next appointment.

Processing client payments

It is each therapist's responsibility to ensure that the correct fee is taken for the treatment provided. The treatment and payment made must be recorded on the record of payments sheet so that a reconciliation may be made at the end of the session.

Record-keeping

It is essential that a central record is kept of all salon treatments and that client confidentiality is observed at all times. It is each therapist's responsibility to ensure that all records are completed fully at the conclusion of the treatment and are updated accordingly.

Cost-effectiveness

It is each therapist's responsibility to ensure that cost-effective use of all resources is maintained. Due to the volume of products used in the clinic, please ensure that you split couch roll and only use the designated amount of products/towels, etc. for each treatment, in order to avoid wastage.

NB: *Attention is also drawn to the requirement of carrying out treatments in a commercially acceptable time.*

Maintaining salon resources

Work areas

All therapists are responsible for the preparation of their work area prior to the client's arrival, and for tidying up and leaving the work area ready for re-use

Equipment/resource cupboards

All items, which are designated for storage in specific cupboards, should be placed in the relevant cupboard on the shelves clearly marked for that item. The cupboard should always be kept clean and tidy, as should the items placed within.

Shortages of stock

All breakages, spillages, damages or shortages in salon stock are to be reported immediately to the Salon Manager for action.

Laundry

All dirty linen should be folded neatly into a dirty linen bag, ready for laundering.

Bins

All bins and waste must be emptied at the end of each session.

Final check

At the end of your working day please ensure that:

- All waste has been removed and disposed of.
- Client records have been updated and filed away.
- Your work area is tidy and ready for reuse.
- All electrical appliances have been switched off.
- The salon has been left secure (windows and doors locked).

Maintaining a Hygienic Working Environment

A therapist is responsible for applying the appropriate hygiene procedures at all times to

- ensure compliance with legislative and workplace requirements
- prevent cross-infection and contamination
- promote client confidence.

Hygiene Precautions

- A smart and hygienic appearance should be presented at all times (including attention to personal hygiene).
- All equipment should be disinfected regularly.

- Rubbish should be disposed of regularly, in a sealed bin.
- Open cuts or abrasions should be covered with a waterproof plaster.
- All jewellery should be removed from the client and the therapist before treatment (with the exception of a wedding band).
- All materials and consumables used should be clean and hygienic, ensuring all tops are secured tightly after use.
- Therapists hands should be washed with an antibacterial soap/hand cleanser before and after each client.

Health and Safety

Health and safety procedures are of paramount importance in the workplace. The law demands that every place of employment is a healthy, and above all safe, place to work, not only for employees but also for their clients and other visitors who may enter the workplace.

Failure to comply with legislation may have serious consequences such as:

- claims from injured staff or clients
- loss of trade through bad publicity
- closure of the business.

Health and Safety Legislation

Health and Safety at Work Act 1974

The Health and Safety at Work Act provides a comprehensive legal framework to promote and encourage high standards of health and safety in the workplace. The Health and Safety at Work Act covers a range of legislation relating to health and safety. Both the employer and employee have responsibilities under the Act.

The responsibilities of the employer

- To safeguard as far as possible the health, safety and welfare of themselves, their employees, contractors' employees and members of the public.
- To ensure all equipment meets health and safety standards.
- To have safety equipment checked regularly.
- To ensure the environment is free from toxic fumes.
- To ensure that all staff are aware of safety procedures by providing safety information and training.
- To ensure safe systems of work.

The responsibilities of the employee

- To adhere to the workplace rules and regulations concerning safety.
- To follow safe working practices and attending training as required.
- To take reasonable care to avoid injury to themselves and others.
- To cooperate with others in all matters relating to health and safety.
- To not interfere or wilfully misuse anything provided to protect their health and safety.

The Health and Safety Executive (HSE) have produced a guide to the laws on health and safety and it is a requirement that an employer displays a copy of this poster in the workplace.

What health and safety law requires

The basis of British health and safety law is the **Health and Safety at Work Act 1974**. The Act sets out the general duties which employers have towards employees and members of the public, and employees have to themselves and to each other.

These duties are qualified in the Act by the principle of 'so far as is reasonably practicable'. In other words, the degree of risk in a particular job or workplace needs to be balanced against the time, trouble, cost and physical difficulty of taking measures to avoid or reduce the risk. What the law requires here is what good management and common sense would lead employers to do anyway: that is, to look at what the risks are and take sensible measures to tackle them.

Besides the Health and Safety at Work Act itself, the following apply across the full range of workplaces:

Legislation	Requirements
Management of Health and Safety at Work Regulations 1999	require employers to carry out risk assessments, make arrangements to implement necessary measures, appoint competent people and arrange for appropriate information and training
Workplace (Health, Safety and Welfare) Regulations 1992	cover a wide range of basic health, safety and welfare issues such as ventilation, heating, lighting, workstations, seating and welfare facilities
Health and Safety (Display Screen Equipment) Regulations 1992	set out requirements for work with Visual Display Units (VDUs)
Personal Protective Equipment at Work Regulations 1992 (PPE)	require employers to provide appropriate protective clothing and equipment for their employees
Provision and Use of Work Equipment Regulations 1998 (PUWER)	require that equipment provided for use at work, including machinery, is safe
Manual Handling Operations Regulations 1992	cover the moving of objects by hand or bodily force
Health and Safety (First Aid) Regulations 1981	cover requirements for first aid
Health and Safety Information for Employees Regulations 1989	require employers to display a poster telling employees what they need to know about health and safety
Employers' Liability (Compulsory Insurance) Regulations 1998	require employers to take out insurance against accidents and ill health to their employees

Legislation	Requirements
Reporting of Injuries, Diseases and Dangerous Occurrences Regulations 1995 (RIDDOR)	require employers to notify certain occupational injuries, diseases and dangerous events
Noise at Work Regulations 1989	require employers to take action to protect employees from hearing damage
Electricity at Work Regulations 1989	require people in control of electrical systems to ensure they are safe to use and maintained in a safe condition
Control of Substances Hazardous to Health Regulations 2002 (COSHH)	requires employers to assess the risks from hazardous substances and take appropriate precautions. In addition, specific regulations cover particular areas, for example asbestos and lead
Gas Safety (Installation and Use) Regulations 1998	cover safe installation, maintenance and use of gas systems and appliances in domestic and commercial premises

Management of Health and Safety at Work Regulations 1999 (the Management Regulations)

These regulations generally make more explicit what employers are required to do to manage health and safety under the Health and Safety at Work Act. Like the Act, they apply to every work activity.

Put simply, the regulations primary concerns are:

- Avoiding risks.

- Evaluating the risks which cannot be avoided.

- Combating the risks at source.

- Adapting the work to the individual, especially with regard to the design of workplaces, the choice of work equipment and the choice of working and production methods, with a view to alleviating monotonous work and work at a predetermined work-rate and to reducing the effect of these ways of working on employees' health.

- Adapting to technical progress.

- Replacing the dangerous by the non-dangerous or the less dangerous.

- Developing a coherent overall prevention policy which covers technology, organisation of work, working conditions, social relationships and the influence of factors relating to the working environment.

- Giving collective protective measures priority over individual protective measures.

- Giving appropriate instructions to employees.

The regulations require employers to carry out a **risk assessment**. Employers with five or more employees need to record the significant findings of the risk assessment. Risk assessment should be straightforward in a simple workplace such as a typical office. It should only be complicated if it deals with serious hazards such as those on a nuclear power station, a chemical plant, laboratory or an oil rig.

How to undertake a risk assessment

Step 1: Identify the hazards

Step 2: Decide who might be harmed and how

Step 3: Evaluate the risks and decide on precautions

Step 4: Record your findings and implement them

Step 5: Review your assessment and update if necessary

The process does not need to be complicated. In many organisations, the risks are well-known and the necessary control measures are easy to apply. Remember, communication is important; all staff should be aware of the procedures put in place.

If you run a small organisation and you are confident you understand what's involved, you can do the assessment yourself. You don't have to be a health and safety expert.

If you work in a larger organisation, you could ask a health and safety advisor to help you. If you are not confident, get help from someone who is competent. In all cases, you should make sure that you involve your staff or their representatives in the process.

They will have useful information about how the work is done that will make your assessment of the risk more thorough and effective. But remember, you are responsible for seeing that the assessment is carried out properly.

When thinking about your risk assessment, remember:

- A **hazard** is anything that may cause harm, such as chemicals, electricity, working from ladders, an open drawer, etc.

- The **risk** is the chance, high or low, that somebody could be harmed by these and other hazards, together with an indication of how serious the harm could be.

Besides carrying out a risk assessment, employers also need to:

- make arrangements for implementing the health and safety measures identified as necessary by the risk assessment

- appoint competent people (often themselves or company colleagues) to help them to implement the arrangements

- set up emergency procedures

- provide clear information and training to employees

- work together with other employers sharing the same workplace.

Other regulations require action in response to particular hazards, or in industries where hazards are particularly high.

If there are more than five employees a written Health and Safety Policy is required.

Manual Handling Operations Regulations 1992

This legislation covers musculoskeletal disorders primarily caused by manual handling and lifting, repetitive strain disorders and unsuitable posture causing back pain.

The regulations cover minimising the risks of lifting and handling large or heavy objects and require certain measures to be taken, such as correct lifting techniques, to avoid musculoskeletal damage.

Cash handling

Under the Health and Safety at Work Act, failure to provide a safe system of cash handling could lead to prosecution of the employer. Employers must therefore ensure compliance with this legislation and avoid sending an individual to the bank in a way that exposes the employee to risk.

Health and Safety (First Aid) Regulations 1981

Under the Health and Safety (First Aid) Regulations 1981, workplaces must have first aid provision. The form it should take will depend on various factors including the nature and degree of hazards at work, what medical services are available and the number of employees.

The HSE booklet *COP 42 First Aid at Work* (ISBN 0 11 885536 0) contains an Approved Code of Practice and guidance notes to help employers meet their obligations. The number of first-aiders needed in the workplace depends primarily on the degree of hazards. If the workplace is considered to be low-hazard (such as a holistic therapy clinic) there should be at least one first-aider

for every 50 employees. If there are fewer than 50 employees, there should always be an appointed person present when people are at work if no trained first-aider is available.

First-aiders must undertake training and obtain qualifications approved by the HSE. At present, first aid certificates are valid for three years. Refresher courses should be started before a certificate expires, otherwise a full course will need to be taken.

First-aid kits

First-aid kits should only contain items that a first-aider has been trained to use. They should always be adequately stocked and should *not* contain medication of any kind. A general purpose first-aid kit will contain the following items: bandages, plasters, wound dressings, antiseptic cream, quick sling, eye pads, scissors, safety pins and vinyl gloves.

First-aiders should record all cases they treat. Each record should include at least the name of the patient, date, place, time and circumstances of the accident and details of the injury and treatment given.

Personal Protective Equipment at Work Regulations 1992 (PPE)

This legislation requires an employer to:

- provide suitable protective clothing and equipment for all employees to ensure safety in the workplace
- ensure staff are adequately trained in the use of chemicals and equipment
- ensure that equipment is suitable for its purpose and is kept in a good state of repair.

Control of Substances Hazardous to Health Regulations 2002 (COSHH)

Regulations under this legislation require employers to regulate employees' exposure to hazardous substances, which may cause ill health or injury in the workplace, and involves risk assessment.

For the risk assessment, an itemised list of all the substances used in the workplace or sold to clients that may be hazardous to health must be made. Attention is drawn to any substances which may cause irritation; cause allergic reactions, burn the skin, or give off fumes.

Instructions for handling and disposing of all hazardous substances must be made available to all staff and training provided, if required.

Manufacturers will usually supply information relating to their products and therapists should be able to recognise hazard warning symbols on labels and packaging.

Gas Safety (Installation and Use) Regulations 1998

This legislation relates to the use and maintenance of gas appliances. All work carried out on gas appliances must be undertaken by installers who are registered under the CORGI scheme. The Rights of Entry Regulations 1996 gives Gas and HSE inspectors the right

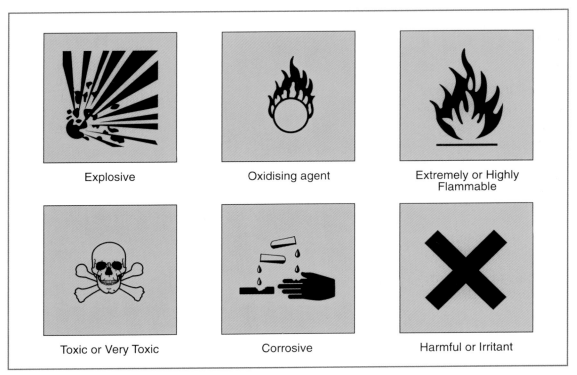

Fig 8.1 Hazard Symbols

to enter premises and order the disconnection of dangerous appliances. (HSE inspectors will not normally be CORGI registered and cannot personally undertake any work on a gas appliance, including disconnection).

Electricity at Work Regulations 1989

Regulations under this legislation are concerned with safety in connection with the use of electricity. It is recommended that electrical equipment be checked regularly (at least once a year) by a competent person, such as a qualified electrician, to verify correct fusing, no loose or frayed wires, proper insulation, no earth leakage, and so on.

All checks should be listed in a record book, stating the results of the tests and the recommendations and action taken in the case of defects. In the event of legal action, a record book may serve as important evidence.

Reporting of Injuries, Diseases and Dangerous Occurrences Regulations 1995 (RIDDOR)

This legislation requires that all accidents occuring in the workplace, however minor, *must* be entered into an accident register. This is a requirement of the Health and Safety at Work Act.

An accident report form should detail the following information:

- details of the injured person (age, sex, occupation and contact details)
- date and time of the accident
- place where the accident occurred
- a brief description of the accident

- the nature of the injury
- the action taken
- signatures of all parties concerned (preferable).

The regulations under this legislation also require that if anyone is seriously injured or dies in connection with an accident in the workplace, or if anyone is off work for more than three days as a result of an accident at work, or if a specified occupational disease is certified by a doctor, then the employer must send a report to the Local Authority Environmental Health Department within seven days.

Local authority bye-laws

Larger local authority areas in the UK may impose their own legislation under which therapy establishments are licensed. Their position is not uniform and therefore practising therapists should obtain advice from the local Environmental Health Officer.

Fire Precautions (Workplace) Regulations 1997

This legislation is for compliance with fire regulations and procedures in the workplace.

The Act requires that:

- all premises have fire-fighting equipment that is in good working order
- the equipment is readily available and is suitable for all types of fire
- all staff are familiar with the establishments evacuation procedures and the use of fire-fighting equipment

- fire escapes are kept free from obstruction and clearly signposted

- smoke alarms are fitted

- fire doors are fitted to help control the spread of fire.

It is a legal requirement for an employer to apply for a fire certificate if the business employs twenty or more staff. It is important for all establishments to have set procedures in the event of a fire and that all staff are aware of it.

Fire-fighting and fire detection

Where necessary (whether due to the features of a workplace, the activity carried on there, any hazard present or any other relevant circumstances) the safety of employees should be safeguarded in case of fire by taking certain measures.

- A workplace shall, to the extent that is appropriate, be equipped with appropriate fire-fighting equipment and with fire detectors and alarms.

- Any non-automatic fire-fighting equipment shall be easily accessible, simple to use and indicated by signs.

- Measures for fire-fighting in the workplace shall be taken, adapted to the nature of the activities if necessary, and also take into account persons other than employees who may be present.

- Employees shall be nominated to implement those measures, ensuring that the number of such employees, their training and the equipment available to them are adequate, taking into account the size and the specific hazards of the workplace concerned.

- Arrangements will be made for any necessary contacts with external emergency services, particularly with regards to rescue work and fire-fighting.

Fire extinguishers

There are different fire extinguishers designed to deal with different types of fire. Since 1997, all fire extinguishers must be coloured red, but they have different symbols and colour codes to show what type of fire they should be used for. Any old extinguishers that are not coloured red will be replaced when they become unserviceable.

Water extinguishers are usually colour-coded red and will have the Class A fire symbol on them. Other types of extinguishers fall into different categories, either:

- the entire body of the extinguisher is coloured in the type colour

- predominately red with a 5 per cent second colour to indicate the contents of the extinguisher

- predominately red with a bold coloured block in the relevant colour stating its type.

The main types of fire extinguishers are given on page 228.

Fire extinguisher colour-coding	Contents	Type of fire
Red	water	paper, wood, fabrics and textiles (*not* on burning liquids, electrical or flammable metal fires)
Black	carbon dioxide (CO_2)	electrical fires, grease, oils, paint, flammable liquids (*not* on flammable metal fires)
Blue	dry powder	Electrical fires, oils, alcohols, solvents, paint, flammable liquids and gases (*not* on flammable metal fires)
Cream	foam	flammable liquids, paper, wood, fabrics and textiles (*not* on electrical or flammable metal fires)
Canary yellow	wet chemical	cooking oil and fat (*not* on electrical or flammable metal fires)

Fire extinguishers are coded in order to allow quick and easy identification and to avoid the risk of using the wrong type and putting yourself and others in danger.

If you are in any doubt about the type of fire extinguisher to use in the workplace, it is advisable to contact your local Fire Safety Department for advice.

Emergency routes and exits

In order to safeguard the safety of employees in case of fire, routes to emergency exits from a workplace and the exits themselves shall be kept clear at all times. Specific safety requirements relating to emergency routes and exits have been laid down and must be complied with.

- Emergency routes and exits shall lead as directly as possible to a place of safety.
- In the event of danger, it must be possible for employees to evacuate the workplace quickly and as safely as possible.

- The number, distribution and dimensions of emergency routes and exits shall be adequate having regard to the use, equipment and dimensions of the workplace and the maximum number of persons that may be present there at any one time.
- Emergency doors shall open in the direction of escape.
- Sliding or revolving doors shall not be used for exits specifically intended as emergency exits.
- Emergency doors shall not be locked or fastened so that they cannot be easily and immediately opened by any person who may require to use them in an emergency.
- Emergency routes and exits must be indicated by signs.
- Emergency routes and exits requiring illumination shall be provided with emergency lighting of adequate intensity in the case of failure of their normal lighting.

Maintenance

The workplace and any equipment and devices shall be subject to a suitable system of maintenance and be maintained in an efficient state, in efficient working order and in good repair.

Environmental Protection Act 1990

This Act legislates for the improved control of pollution arising from certain industrial operations and other processes such as:

- waste on land
- the collection and disposal of waste
- offensive trades or businesses
- the extension of the Clean Air Acts to prescribed gases
- litter control
- radioactive substances
- genetically modified organisms
- potentially hazardous substances.

Special waste and non-controlled waste

If any kind of controlled waste is, or may be, so dangerous or difficult to treat, keep or dispose of that special provision is required, it is imperative to adhere to waste regulation authorities' rulings.

Waste other than controlled waste

If a person deposits waste that is not controlled waste (or if that person knowingly causes or permits the waste to be deposited), they are guilty of an offence and liable to be punished accordingly. This also applies if the waste is special waste and a waste management licence is not in force.

Dealing with Spillages, Breakages and Waste in the Workplace

Spillages

Wipe up spillages immediately and warn staff and clientele. If the area is still wet display a sign indicating the potential hazard.

Breakages

Clear up the pieces immediately. Wrap up sharp items such as glass before placing them into the waste container.

Waste

Use a covered bin for waste and empty it daily.

Safety and Security in the Workplace

The proprietor of a salon or clinic is required by law to ensure adequate security of their business premises. Therapists also require knowledge of security issues and measures in connection with premises, people and their belongings. Staff should also know the business requirements for the security of stock, equipment, money and records.

The following steps may be taken to ensure maximum security. This is important not only for peace of mind but also for insurance requirements.

Security recommendations include:

- fitting locks and bolts on doors and windows
- installing a burglar alarm
- fitting security lights
- ensuring there is a minimum number of key holders
- leaving a light on at night, preferably at the front of the premises
- ensuring all windows and doors are checked by the last person to leave the premises.

Money

- Have a safe for short-term storage of money and valuables.
- Always keep the till locked with a minimum number of key holders.
- Never leave money in the till overnight.

Stock

A good stock control system is needed in order to monitor the use of consumables and retail products and this should be documented in a stock control book.

Recommendations for safeguarding stock include:

- always keeping supplies in a locked cupboard
- issuing keys to a limited number of authorised staff only
- have a locked cabinet for display purposes or use 'dummy stock' to prevent shoplifting.

Records

In order to maintain confidentiality, it is essential that client records and other confidential papers are secured and locked away when unattended.

Personal Belongings

It is not possible for therapists to take responsibility for a client's personal belongings when they attend for treatments. Make clients aware of this by displaying a disclaimer sign in the reception area.

When clients are removing jewellery, it is important that valuable items are placed in a safe place for the duration of the treatment. In order to minimise risks, it is advisable to recommend that clients keep a minimum amount of money and valuables on them.

Staff should be vigilant over their own property as well as that of clients and keep handbags and other items of value in a safe place.

Health and Safety of the Client

Therapists need to have knowledge of health and safety in relation to the client, which includes risk assessment, contraindications and contra-actions. A therapist needs to fully understand that a contraindication may mean a client being adversely affected by the treatment, or that the treatment could be ineffective, and an adapted or shortened treatment might be possible.

NB: *Therapists must understand that diagnosis of a medical condition is the role of the medical profession, therefore suggestions should never be made to a client about a condition. It is the responsibility of the client to ask for medical advice concerning a contraindication.*

Any condition that does not appear to be normal should be brought to the attention of the client and medical consultation advised before treatment is given.

Contra-actions (adverse reactions) to treatment must be explained and avoided where possible. In the event of a contra-action, the corrective action to be taken must be understood, and the therapist must know how to advise the client. It is also important to ensure that contra-actions are recorded.

Consumer Protection Act 1987

This Act provides the consumer with protection when buying goods or services. It ensure that products are safe for use on the client during the treatment or are safe to be sold as a retail product. In the past, those injured had to prove a manufacturer negligent before they could successfully sue for damages. The Consumer Protection Act removed the need to prove negligence. The Act provides the same rights to anyone injured by a defective product, whether the product was sold to them or not.

The Act also covers giving misleading price indications about goods, services or facilities. The term price indication also includes price comparisons. The term 'misleading' includes any wrongful indications about conditions attached to a price, about what you expect to happen to a price in the future and what you say in price comparisons. It is essential to understand the implications of this legislation, including the promotion of special offers, as an offence could result in legal proceedings.

Sale and Supply of Goods Act 1994

As consumers of products and services, clients do have rights under this legislation. This legislation identifies the contract of sale, which takes place between the retailer (the clinic/salon) and the consumer (the client). This Act amends the previous Act (Sale of Goods Act 1979), which was the first of the modern consumer laws and covers rights including the goods being accurately described without misleading the consumer.

The Sale and Supply of Goods Act 1994 is associated with the Supply of Goods and Services Act 1982, the Unfair Contract Terms Act 1977 and the Supply of Goods (Implied Terms) Act 1973. These Acts cover consumer rights including goods being of satisfactory quality, the conditions under which goods may be returned after purchase and whether goods are fit for their intended purpose.

Trade Descriptions Act 1968 (amended 1988)

This Act prohibits the use of false descriptions or the selling or offering for sale of goods that have been described falsely. This Act covers advertisements such as oral descriptions or display cards and applies to quality and quantity as well as fitness for purpose and price.

It is important to understand this legislation, especially where the description is given by another person and repeated. Thus, to repeat a manufacturer's claim is to be equally liable.

Local Government (Miscellaneous Provisions) Act 1982

Part 8 of this Act provides local authorities with powers of registration of persons practising acupuncture, tattooing, electrical epilation and ear piercing, among other things. This applies to those operating from permanent premises or with home-visiting practices.

The primary concern of this legislation is within hygiene practices and may include qualifications. The precise bye-laws may vary between local authorities, as does the licence and inspection system involved. In areas where this is required, only those who are registered are allowed to practise, both from permanent premises and by home visiting. Operators working under medical control (as in a hospital) are specifically excluded from registration.

Employers' Liability (Compulsory Insurance) Act 1969

This legislation requires the employer to take out and maintain an approved insurance policy with authorised insurers against liability for bodily injury or disease sustained by their employees in the course of their employment. A certificate of Employers' Liability insurance must be displayed at each place of business for the information of the employees. Local authorities are specifically excluded from this Act.

Performing Rights Act (under Copyright Designs and Patents Act 1988)

If a therapist is using relaxation music when carrying out treatments in the workplace it may be necessary to obtain a licence from Phonographic Performance Ltd (PPL), or the Performing Rights Society (PRS), which is a organisation that collects licence payments as royalties on behalf of performers and record companies whose music is protected under the Copyright Designs and Patents Act 1998.

Any use of music in treatment premises or waiting rooms, or music played on a switchboard holding system, is termed a public performance. The PPL and PRS have the backing of the Copyright Designs and Patents Act 1988 and can take legal action against those who seek to avoid paying its licence fees. However, it should be noted that a lot of music comes from composers who are not members of the above organisations. In such cases the music is 'copyright free' and no fee is due to PPL or PRS. Therapists are advised to check the position with the supplier of the music.

Data Protection Act 1998

This legislation protects clients' personal information being stored on a computer. If client records are stored on computer, the establishment must be registered under this Act. The Data Protection Act operates to ensure that the information stored is only used for the purposes for which it was given. Therefore none of the information may be given to any outsider without the client's permission.

Clients can seek compensation through the Courts for any infringement of their rights established by giving information in the first instance for a specific purpose.

Businesses should therefore ensure that they:

- only hold information which is relevant

- allow individuals access to the information held on them

- prevent unauthorised access to the information.

Cosmetic Products (Safety) Regulations 2003

This legislation implements EEC regulations regarding the description of cosmetic products, their labelling, composition and marketing.

It is concerned with the supply of any cosmetic product, which is liable to cause damage to human health when it is applied under:

a normal conditions of use; or

b conditions of use which are reasonably foreseeable taking into account all the circumstances, including the cosmetic product's presentation, labelling, any instructions for its use and disposal and any other information or indication provided by the manufacturer, his agent or the person who supplies the cosmetic product on the first occasion that it is supplied in the Community.

Marking

Cosmetic products must be supplied in packaging which bears (in lettering which is visible, indelible and easily legible):

- a list of its cosmetic ingredients (preceded by the word 'ingredients')

- the weight or volume

- the name or trade name of the product

- the address or registered office of the manufacturer of the product

- a 'Best Before' date (if the shelf life is less than 30 months)

- any particular precautions to be observed in use and any special precautionary information on a cosmetic product for professional use, in particular in hairdressing

- a means of identifying the batch in which the product was manufactured

- the function of the product, unless this is clear from its presentation.

Professional Codes of Practice

The role of a professional representative therapy body is in defining limitations on procedures and practices for public protection. A professional therapist is bound by the rules of a professional representative therapy body (such as the Federation of Holistic Therapists) and its Code of Ethics, which exists to ensure that social, ethical and moral standards exist in a professional's day-to-day work.

Codes of ethics are rules of conduct binding on those who join a professional body. Infringement of these codes are taken very seriously by professional bodies and can result in penalties, including expulsion from membership. A code of ethics also exists to determine the demarcation lines that enable a non-medical therapist to exist harmoniously in the industry with medical and medical-auxiliary practitioners. Therapists must, therefore, not practise beyond the scope of their profession.

Code of Ethics

Professional codes of ethics are standards of acceptable professional behaviour by which a person or business conducts their business. Each professional association has its own code of ethics, to which they require their members to adhere. The following guidelines reflect, in general terms, a code of ethics expected from a professional therapist.

Therapists must:

- not treat any person who is suffering from a medical condition; in the event of a client presenting a medical condition they should be referred to their GP

- conduct themselves in a professional manner and be courteous and respectful to a client at all times

- always bear in mind that their primary concern should be for the client and that they should practise their skills to the best of their ability at all times

- have respect for the religious, spiritual, social or political views of the clients, irrespective of creed, race, colour or sex

- never abuse the relationship between themselves and a client

- act in a cooperative manner with other health care professionals and refer cases, which are out of the sphere of the therapy field in which they practise

- explain the treatment and discuss any fees involved with the client before any treatment commences

- keep accurate, up-to-date records of treatments carried out on a client and the results, which should include client's confidential details, a medical history, dates and details of treatment, and any advice given

- never disclose client information without the prior written permission of the client, except when required to do so by law

- never claim to cure

- never diagnose a medical condition

- never give unqualified advice

- keep their personal and professional lives separate

- ensure that any advertising represents their business in the most professional manner

- ensure that their working premises comply with all current health, safety and hygiene legislation

- be adequately insured to practise the therapy in which they are qualified

- become a member of a professional association which sets high standards for the industry

- continue their own professional development.

Anti-Discrimination Practices

Anti-discrimination practices involve therapists ensuring equal treatment of all those with whom they come into contact. It is each therapist's responsibility to examine their procedures and practices to ensure that they are not discriminatory, and that cultural differences are fully respected when dealing with clients and colleagues.

A therapist needs to understand the nature and diversity of communities. There are sub-groups of different economic, cultural or other divisions co-existing within any geographical location. Knowledge of the different communities within the larger community as a whole is necessary in order to ensure that the provision of services encompasses the needs of these different groups. This may involve communication with other professionals (medical and non-medical) within the community. The forging of relationships that foster mutual respect and raise awareness will encourage integration of the therapist's chosen therapy within the community.

Therapists should understand that through making professional contact with all parts of the community, they can improve knowledge of and raise awareness of the benefits of their therapy.

Anti-Discrimination Legislation

Discrimination occurs if an individual is treated less favourably than another on the grounds of race or sex.

The Sex Discrimination Act 1975 (SDA) and the Race Relations Act 1976 (RRA)

These Acts provide that it is unlawful to discriminate on grounds of sex, marital status or race (defined as including colour, race, nationality or ethnic national origins).

Both sex and race discrimination legislation specifically state that it is unlawful to discriminate against people in the following situations:

a recruitment (including job advertisements, interviews, refusal to offer employment)

b promotion

c transfer

d training

e benefits or facilities

f dismissal.

Protection for the Therapist and the Client

When in professional practice, therapists may be in contact with various members of the community including the elderly, infirm, those unable to give consent, special needs clients and clients of the opposite gender to the therapist.

Specific attention is drawn to the law regarding the protection of minors (a person below the legal age of consent). Therapists need to be aware that a minor should not be examined or treated unless a parent or guardian is present, or has given written permission for examination and a chaperone is present.

Specific precautions also exist in relation to those individuals in specific categories (elderly, infirm, those unable to give consent, special needs clients). In the treatments of these client groups, attention is drawn to the need for a companion or appropriate adult (such as a carer) to be present to offer protection for the individual and the therapist. Any special precaution should be considered and requested before any treatment is undertaken.

A competent therapist needs to be sensitive to apparent signs of abuse, which could be in the form of physical, verbal, mental (bullying or discrimination), sexual, neglect or self-harming. However, it is imperative that under no circumstances must the therapist make comments or judgements, as this is outside their professional sphere. Therapists must understand that their role is in adopting a supportive but professional attitude at all times, but at no time must they become directly involved.

Therapists need to be aware that the client may exhibit non-verbal signs indicating anxiety, or concern and these should be observed and responded to appropriately.

Any signs of prior abuse should be noted by the therapist and treated confidentially within the law. Therapists need to be aware of any signs of inappropriate behaviour (which may include an action or statement from a minor not appropriate to their age, signs of being bullied, withdrawn or introverted behaviour, or may be in the form of bullying and discrimination). Therapists have a duty to report any abnormal statement, event or observation to a senior person in the establishment, and request advice if in any doubt as to how to proceed.

Providing a Safe Working Environment

Therapists need to be aware of special precautions to ensure that clients do not feel vulnerable or at risk at any time. The working environment in which the therapist practises must allow clients to feel comfortable and at ease at all times. Treatment processes should be not be invasive and all procedures must be explained to the client beforehand to ensure their consent is given for treatment to proceed.

Special precautions that therapists need to be aware of include having someone else nearby, working in an easily accessible working area and checking clients' details before offering treatment. As far as therapists are concerned, for personal protection they may refuse to treat anyone they have concerns about.

A therapist must exhibit professional conduct at all times to allay fears of any inappropriate behaviour. In addition, therapists may themselves be subject to unwanted attention and therefore must know how to avoid giving misleading signals.

Legislation for the Protection of Minors

Children Act 1989

The Children Act is an important piece of legislation concerning children and the way they are treated. The Children Act gives children the right to be consulted, listened to, protected and given the chance to voice their feelings and opinions. Most importantly, the Act recognises that children should be treated with respect and as individuals.

The key points of the Children Act are as follows:

- children's welfare in both private and public sectors is made a priority
- recognition that children are best brought up within their families, wherever possible
- aims to prevent unwarranted interference in family life
- requires local authorities to provide services for children and families in need
- promotes partnership between children, parents and local authorities
- improves the way that Courts deal with children and families
- gives a right of appeal against court decisions
- protects the rights of parents with children being looked after by local authorities
- aims to ensure children looked after by local authorities are provided with a good standard of care.

Protection of Children Act 1999

This Act requires a list to be kept of persons considered unsuitable to work with children. It also makes provisions to extend the powers of the Education Reform Act 1988. It is also designed to enable the protection afforded to children to be extended to persons suffering from mental impairment.

NB: The Criminal Records Bureau may be consulted by employers with reference to employees who have access to minors.

Youth Justice and Criminal Evidence Act 1999

This Act makes provision for the referral of offenders under 18 to youth offender panels. It includes the giving of evidence or information for the purposes of criminal proceedings and makes pre-consolidation amendments relating to youth justice.

Crime and Disorder Act 1998

This Act includes provisions for preventing crime and disorder, including certain racially aggravated offences. It also includes abolishment of the death penalty for treason and piracy. It makes further provision for dealing with offenders and also with respect to remands and committals for trial, and the release and recall of prisoners.

Sex Offenders Act 1997

This Act primarily requires persons who have committed certain sexual offences to report to the police and provide information in relation to the offences.

NB: *Any person convicted of a sexual crime will be placed on the Sex Offenders Register.*

Care Standards Act 2000

This Act establishes a National Care Standards Commission. It covers the registration and regulation of children's homes, independent hospitals, independent clinics, care homes, residential family centres, independent medical agencies, domiciliary care agencies, fostering agencies, nursing agencies and voluntary adoption agencies. It also covers the regulation and inspection of local authority fostering and adoption services.

The Act establishes a General Social Care Council and a Care Council for Wales and covers the registration, regulation and training of social care workers. Within the UK it establishes a Children's Commissioner for Wales, in order to make provision for the registration, regulation and training of those providing child-minding or daycare. It also makes provision for the protection of children and vulnerable adults and covers the law about children who are being looked after in schools and colleges.

Children (Leaving Care) Act 2000

This Act covers provisions for children and young persons who are being, or have been, looked after by a local authority.

Human Rights Act 1998

This Act gives effect to the rights and freedoms guaranteed under the European Convention on Human Rights (ECHR).

AUTHOR'S NOTE

While the acts and legislation provided in this book are current at the time of writing, legislation is constantly changing and being amended regularly. Good sources of information on the most current legislation and act amendments can be found at www.opsi.gov.uk

Maintaining Operations and Services

The role of a therapist in the context of the workplace is not merely in the provision of treatments, but in monitoring and maintaining the operations to meet the requirements of both the establishment and the client. Therapists are concerned with helping the business run smoothly and efficiently, with the ultimate aim of clients who are satisfied with the service provided and the result of repeat business. Therapists are expected to understand what is required to support workplace efficiency, within their given area of responsibility.

There are several important factors to be taken into account when working as a therapist, in order to monitor and maintain the standard of service offered to clients. It is not only important to be able to perform a skill competently, but also to be able to apply it in a commercially acceptable way.

In the workplace, therapists have a responsibility to their manager or supervisor, to their clients and to their colleagues.

The Responsibilities of a Therapist to a Supervisor

These are to ensure that they:

- adhere to the establishments rules

- understand and adhere to legislation applying to the provision of services

- report any hazard or potential danger observed in the workplace

- have a sincere commitment to providing a high standard of work to enhance the reputation and image of the establishment

- carry out work practices with honesty and integrity

- complete records fully and accurately

- work on their own initiative to make the best use of time at work

- carry out their work to a high standard to ensure client satisfaction and repeat business

- create a good working relationship with other colleagues to contribute to a good working environment

- avoid wastage of resources

- make recommendations for improvement in workplace practices, where appropriate

- understand how their job role contributes to the success of the business.

The Responsibilities of a Therapist to a Client

These are to:

- treat clients with dignity and respect

- respond to clients requests politely and efficiently

- accurately inform them of the services provided by the establishment

- provide treatment only when there is a reasonable expectation that it will be advantageous to the client

- take appropriate measures to protect the client's right to privacy and confidentiality

- provide a high standard of service to ensure client satisfaction and the fostering of repeat business

- make recommendations for future treatments that would benefit the client

- make recommendations for homecare products that may benefit their condition.

The Responsibilities of a Therapist to their Colleagues

These are to:

- create a good working environment by being friendly, helpful and approachable

- share responsibilities fairly to create a good team spirit

- ensure good communication channels, pass on messages promptly and record messages accurately

- inform others of any changes in establishment procedure.

Maintaining Effective Relationships with Colleagues

A successful business depends on a good image and reputation, but also depends on the way in which staff work together as a team to maintain the image and professionalism of the establishment. Working with colleagues as a team helps ensure smooth operations and promotes a pleasant working environment and a friendly atmosphere.

Working as a team involves:

- building a good rapport with each other

- understanding each other's responsibilities

- working efficiently within your own job responsibilities

- responding to each other's requests politely and cooperatively

- providing support and assistance when required

- working together for the needs of the business.

Communication is essential when working with others in a team. Regular meetings can help to maintain effective working relationships.

Meetings provide an opportunity to:

- identify and resolve problems in the workplace

- avoid misunderstandings and a breakdown in communication

- contribute and exchange ideas on how workplace practices may be enhanced

- identify training needs

- maintain good working relationships.

Communication Skills

Whether small or large, a successful business relies on good communication to promote good understanding and efficient working relationships. Communication skills are extremely important when there are several colleagues working together, and if communication breaks down it can have a dramatic effect on the service given and the overall efficiency and image of the establishment. It is therefore important for a therapist to be able to communicate effectively with clients, colleagues and other visitors who may visit or telephone the establishment.

Communication skills may be used to:

- identify clients needs

- inform clients about a service

- inform clients and colleagues of changes in procedures and problems arising

- maintain workplace records

- pass on recommendations for improving employment standards.

Communication skills involve verbal communication, listening, non-verbal communication and written communication.

Verbal communication

This involves sending and receiving information and is a cooperative effort between two parties. In order to facilitate effective verbal communication it is important to pause periodically, in order to verify that the message received was the message intended. In this way, alterations and corrections to the conversation may be made. The objective of verbal communication to be heard and also understood. For clarity, it is important to choose words which convey intent clearly, concisely and tactfully.

Listening

Although it is important to use effective verbal communication, it is equally important to have good listening skills in order to develop optimal client-therapist/client-colleague relationships. Effective listening involves understanding and evaluating the person's needs, and includes paying attention to the tone and emotion in which the message is delivered. The objective of listening is focusing on understanding the message heard through interpreting all the clues given.

Good listening may be enhanced by maintaining eye contact, nodding, using verbal phrases or facial expressions to encourage the speaker to continue. It is important for therapists to clarify information received from clients or colleagues, in order to ensure the message has been understood correctly.

Non-verbal communication

This involves messages transmitted other than by the spoken word and may be exhibited by posture, gestures and facial expressions. Non-verbal communication often projects more information about how a person is feeling and their emotions. It is helpful to be aware of body language as this may convey more meaning than the spoken word.

Written communication

An efficient working environment providing services to clients relies on accurate, legible record-keeping, which is kept up to date. These records may either be computer-generated or handwritten.

Written communication may involve the recording of messages to colleagues to ensure continuity of service, or the completion of client records in the workplace to ensure therapeutic continuity. Client records should be complete, accurate and legible at the time of the treatment and stored securely and confidentially.

It is very important that all messages are recorded accurately to ensure continuity of operation and services. Written communication should be clear, dated and timed, with information as to the action required. It should also be left in a place where the person it is intended for will notice it.

Responding to Clients' Requests

Requests for information may come from a telephone enquiry, a personal caller to the workplace or may be in the form of a written request. As clients are at the centre of every business, it is essential for therapists to respond to their requests promptly, accurately and enthusiastically. It is important to assume a friendly and approachable manner and use phrases such as 'How may I help you?'

It is also important to provide accurate information on treatments such as:

- the benefits of the services
- the cost (of individual and courses of treatment)
- the treatment duration
- any pre-treatment advice
- how often the client should attend for maximum benefit.

Providing as much useful information at the time of request will increase the chances of the client booking an appointment and even if the client does not book immediately, it will certainly give them a good impression of the professionalism of the establishment.

The best source of information is the professional herself (the therapist), however, when this is not possible it is important to consider that leaflets and brochures may also help to sell treatments to clients. The information contained within leaflets and brochures should therefore be educational and informative to increase client awareness of the treatment, as well as being attractive enough to stimulate interest.

Quality Assurance

Every business, however small, should have a quality assurance policy in order to ensure their services and operation are conducted in a systematic way. Quality assurance policies help to monitor the quality and standard of the service provided and are useful in analysing whether the client's needs are met efficiently, effectively and consistently.

Effective ways of monitoring quality assurance include:

- examining your own workplace practice and how it relates to client needs and the needs of the business
- ensuring that you don't become complacent and continue updating your skills and knowledge
- distributing client satisfaction questionnaires
- introducing a client suggestions box
- implementing changes based on recommendations from clients and staff.

Encouraging communication with clients on a regular basis can help to monitor the quality assurance policy of the establishment.

Cost-effectiveness

Efficient work practice requires a therapist to perform a skill to the required standard of the establishment and the industry, and in a time, which is considered to be commercially acceptable.

Cost-effectiveness in terms of the workplace means maintaining treatment times and minimising waste, in order to avoid loss of revenue for the establishment. Therapists need to be aware that by adhering to their appointment times and avoiding wastage they are in fact helping to preserve the business's precious resources and thereby helping to maintain their security of employment.

Self-Assessment Questions

1   Why is it important to understand national and local legislation?

    a   because it is part of the Health and Safety Act

    b   so that you do not inadvertently break the law

    c   to make sure you are offering the correct treatments

    d   it will help the business to operate more efficiently

2   COSHH stands for

    a   Control of Special Health Hazards

    b   Control of Substances Hazardous to Health

    c   Control of Severe Hazards to Health

    d   Control of Substances and Health Hazards

3   RIDDOR stands for

    a   Reporting of Incidents, Diseases and Dangerous Occurrences

    b   Reporting of Injuries, Damages and Dangerous Occurrences

    c   Reporting of Injuries, Diseases and Dangerous Occupations

    d   Reporting of Injuries, Diseases and Dangerous Occurrences

4   The Health and Safety at Work Act provides a comprehensive legal framework to

    a   promote and encourage high standards of health and safety in the workplace

    b   promote standards of responsibility in the workplace

    c   encourage employers to be more responsible

    d   encourage employees to be more responsible

5   Why is it important to wear professional clothing when carrying out therapy treatments?

    a   because it is a requirement of the Workplace (Health, Safety And Welfare) Regulations 1992 Act

    b   in order to maintain a professional image and maintain hygiene

    c   so that clients think you are a professional

    d   in order to maintain personal hygiene

6 Good communication skills are essential in order to develop optimal client-therapist/client-colleague relationships. Effective communication involves which important skill?

   a   talking loudly so that the client can hear you

   b   maintaining eye contact at all times

   c   listening

   d   verbal communication

7 What are the legislative regulations which require employers to carry out risk assessment in the workplace?

   a   The Employers' Liability Act

   b   The Consumer Protection Act

   c   The Fire Precautions (Workplace) Regulations 1997

   d   The Management of Health and Safety at Work Regulations 1999

8 What is a workplace risk assessment?

   a   checking if the workplace is at risk

   b   a means of identifying hazards and potential problems

   c   a procedure to check risks associated with staff

   d   a procedure to check risks associated with clients

9 State the Act that is concerned with all electrical equipment being checked regularly.

   a   COSHH

   b   RIDDOR

   c   Electricity at Work Regulations

   d   Employers' Liability Act

10 State the Act that is concerned with the reporting of accidents

   a   COSHH

   b   RIDDOR

   c   Electricity at work regulations

   d   Employers' Liability Act

11 State the Act that is concerned with regulating exposure to hazardous substances

   a   COSHH

   b   RIDDOR

   c   Electricity at Work regulations

   d   Employers' Liability Act

12 By law, what insurance certificate must be displayed in a place of work?

    a   public liability

    b   employers' liability

    c   professional indemnity

    d   personal injury indemnity

13 In the event of a problem in the workplace, who would you report to?

    a   the Health and Safety Executive

    b   a colleague

    c   a friend

    d   your manager

14 The hazard symbol that shows a skull and crossbones is used to indicate items which are

    a   highly flammable

    b   corrosive

    c   explosive

    d   toxic

15 State which of the following is *not* the correct colour coding and use for a fire extinguisher

    a   water: red marking, used on paper fires

    b   carbon dioxide: black marking, used on electrical fires

    c   foam: green marking, used on electrical fires

    d   dry powder: blue marking, used on electrical fires

16 What does The Fire Precautions (Workplace) Regulations 1997 enforce?

    a   fire doors are fitted to help stop the spread of fire

    b   fire escapes are kept free from obstruction and clearly indicated

    c   smoke alarms are clearly indicated

    d   all premises have some fire-fighting equipment

17 What is the first consideration in the event of a fire in the workplace?

    a   collect your client's belongings and make sure your client is safe

    b   try to put the fire out with a fire axe

    c   check that no one is trapped

    d   raise the alarm and exit the premises

▶

18 Who is responsible for the client's personal belongings in the workplace?

   a   the salon

   b   the owner

   c   the therapist

   d   the client

19 Why is it important to understand cultural differences when dealing with colleagues, customers and other visitors to the workplace?

   a   in order to ensure equal treatment of all those with whom you come into contact

   b   because it is part of the Care Standards Act

   c   because it will be helpful if visiting other countries

   d   to make sure that you use the correct products when providing treatments

20 Why must you take care to avoid discrimination in your practices and procedures at all times?

   a   to ensure that all treatments keep to the same timings

   b   because it will increase business

   c   because it is the law and good business practice

   d   in order to protect the client

21 Why is confidentiality important?

   a   to protect the client and comply with the Data Protection Act

   b   to protect the client and comply with the Consumer Protection Act

   c   to protect the client and comply with the Children Act

   d   in case information is needed by other professionals

9 Promotion and Marketing

Marketing is the means by which you tell potential clients what you have to offer and how it will benefit them. In order to be successful in business, it is not enough for therapists to have excellent skills in the therapy they practise; they also need to get to grips with the important skill of marketing. Holistic therapists need to consider the marketing of services such as Indian Head Massage carefully, as it is a specialist market and the marketing must therefore be selective.

By the end of this chapter, you will be able to:

- Understand the fundamental issues of marketing and promotion.

- Design a marketing plan for business success in Indian Head Massage.

Marketing in the holistic therapy industry is educational and is about raising awareness of who you are and what you do. It is important for therapists to consider that marketing is about matching their service to clients' needs and therefore the focus is not so much on selling but on identifying needs. The key to successful marketing is to view every aspect of your marketing through the clients' eyes and match their needs and desires to your products and services.

Marketing involves finding out:

- who your potential clients are

- what their needs are

- how much they would be prepared to pay for the service

- where they are and how to reach them

- how often they would visit.

Researching Clients

It is essential to use market research to assess the needs of the market. Knowing and understanding who your potential clients are is crucial to devising a marketing plan and deciding who to target in advertising and promotion. Market research enables you to identify potential clients, discover what influences them and find out how to reach them. Knowing the market then enables you to refine the message you wish to send to potential clients. There are very few services that will appeal to everyone; there is always a sector of the market that is going to be more inclined to buy. Therefore you need to find out who makes up this sector and focus the attention of your marketing on them.

When building client profiles, it is helpful to consider the following factors:

- age
- gender
- income
- interests
- location.

Gathering Client Information

As clients are at the centre of every business, it is vital to find out about them and what they want. Carrying out marketing surveys using questionnaires is an effective way of gathering information. A great deal of thought needs to be given to the design of a marketing questionnaire, in order to give both quantitative and qualitative results.

When designing marketing questionnaires, it is important to keep questions short, simple and to the point in order to get an exact answer. If questions are structured it is simpler and quicker for the respondent to reply. Another important consideration is the type of questions to ask. Closed questions require only yes/no/don't know responses, while open questions are such that the respondent has to answer in their own way.

When designing questionnaires it is also important to remember to avoid prejudging the participant's response: in other words, do not assume that you know what they are going to say. Neither should you leave them with no alternative but to agree with you.

In order to get the best results from your marketing questionnaire, bear in mind the following:

- Keep it simple, attractive, interesting and relevant.

- Include a short introduction to the questionnaire in order to stimulate the respondent's enthusiasm and motivation to complete it.

- Offer an incentive to complete the questionnaire (such as a free prize or entry into a free prize draw).

- Make it known to the respondents that there is a deadline for reply to the questionnaire.

You may wish to carry out a pilot survey on a group of individuals (friends, family, colleagues); however, check that the individuals concerned are among the right category of potential clients, otherwise this may prove to be a fruitless exercise.

There is an example of a market research questionnaire for Indian Head Massage at the end of the chapter (page 262).

Client surveys are useful tools in market research in that by gaining the client's input they:

- demonstrate your desire to offer the best possible service
- help you to fulfil the client's needs
- direct you towards potential sales triggers

- guide you towards potential strengths and weaknesses.

If sending out market research questionnaires, always make the response easy for the client by providing a stamped addressed envelope.

As Indian Head Massage involves a personal and specialised service, it tends to appeal to certain segments of the market. By selecting a target market it enables you to modify your advertising and promotional activities to appeal to a specific group.

Consider the type of clientele you want to attract or, if you have an existing clientele, examine who is already using your services and what they have in common.

When targeting client markets it is wise to have more than one sector, the number being dependent on your preference, expertise and the size of your practice.

In order to make marketing more effective, it is helpful to create a niche market by addressing the needs of a specific group of people. Your name then becomes linked with providing a particular service for a particular target group.

Assessing Marketing Needs

Marketing needs will be dependent on the following factors:

- your target market
- the size of your practice

- the amount of money you can afford
- the amount of time you can devote.

If you are a therapist starting out in business and do not have a large clientele, more time and energy can be devoted to making contacts and giving talks and presentations to help get your name and what you do known. The activities involving client education and awareness will be low-cost but time-consuming.

If you are an established business, you may have the financial budget to concentrate on other marketing methods such as targeted advertising or mailshots to announce the introduction of a new service such as Indian Head Massage into the business. An important factor to consider in marketing is that it takes time and money to become known in business.

Compiling a marketing plan

Once you have established where the market for Indian Head Massage is and how extensive it is, the next stage is to put all the findings together in the form of objectives – this will form a marketing plan. A marketing plan will form the basis of how you intend to promote the service to generate clients. Before compiling a marketing plan, it is essential to carry out a SWOT analysis in order to self-assess your Strengths, Weaknesses, Opportunities and Threats, in order to be realistic in your plan.

Strengths

These may include:

- specialism
- location of the business
- pricing
- the opening hours
- personality
- customer service
- flexibility.

> **KEY NOTE**
>
> A marketing plan should also include your **unique selling point** (USP) which is what makes your business and service different.

Weaknesses

Possible weaknesses may be:

- lack of experience
- opening hours
- location
- range of skills offered.

Opportunities

These could include:

- expansion into other sectors of the market, for example, the workplace.

Threats

Potential threats may include:

- local competition.

Getting the Balance Right in Marketing

Successful marketing usually involves a mix of different methods and the chemistry or 'mix' has to be right for the individual business.

Marketing can be divided into four factors and each of these will influence how you develop your marketing plan. Marketing can be seen as a balancing act and if adjustments are made to one or more of the four factors, then a compensating adjustment has to be made among the other factors in order for the approach to be balanced.

Product/service

This includes the features and benefits of the product/service being offered, including the quality of service. For marketing to be effective, it is important to create a demand. With products and services, it is also important to consider the image of the business being projected by the service itself, the marketing material and the staff.

Price

This is the cost of the service to the client. When setting prices for services it is vital to consider the following:

- charge enough to cover your overheads, meet your expenses and make a profit
- charge what clients are prepared to pay
- be in line with your competitors.

Place

This is where you are located in relation to your clients. Careful consideration needs to be given to the location and opening hours of the business to ensure that the service is available to potential clients.

Location is an important factor in business; it affects the distribution of services. Because of the portable nature of Indian Head Massage, therapists should consider the many locations or settings in which the therapy may be practised (for example, in the workplace, in hairdressing salons and hospitals as well as beauty spas and clinics).

Promotion

The objective of promotion is to become known and to create a desire in potential clients to use your services. The promotion of services such as Indian Head Massage is largely educational in nature and is the means by which potential clients learn who you are, what you do and how your services will benefit them.

In the holistic therapy industry it is important for therapists to realise that they are marketing themselves as well as their treatments. Marketing is the art of promoting yourself and the services you offer in order to attract clients. There are many marketing strategies that can be used to sell the services you intend to offer. However, one of the most important attributes for a holistic therapist is to have self-confidence, a positive attitude and belief in themselves and their abilities. As the holistic therapy business is a personal service, it is essential that therapists feel confident enough to sell their services and products to potential clients.

In order to be able to sell a service or product effectively, it is important for a therapist to:

- know the services well enough and have enough experience to be able to sell their benefits to potential clients
- be aware of the services of competitors and have identified their strengths and weaknesses
- be able to sell solutions
- identify with the potential client's needs and personalise the sale.

Personality Selling

The concept of personality selling is very important in business. Some clients may decide whether to have a treatment based on factual information. In this case the benefits of the treatment need to be stressed in a very factual and analytical way. Other clients may need to have a picture created for them, enhanced by imaginative therapeutic words to stimulate their interest.

KEY NOTE

Some therapists may feel uncomfortable with the idea of selling and may need to attend sales training in order to enhance this very important skill.

No amount of advertising can make up for the personal touch and with Indian Head Massage it is best to consider the direct and more personal approach first and turn personal skills to your advantage. By creating a positive environment for treatment provision, therapists can sell through one of the most powerful senses – the therapeutic touch. When planning advertising and promotion, it is essential to use a mix of methods in order to reach different target markets and to help evaluate the overall effectiveness of the activities.

The Direct Approach to Marketing and Promotion

Personal Recommendation/ Word of Mouth

This is the most valuable form of advertising for personal treatments like Indian Head Massage. Once a therapist has established a reputation for excellent customer service and quality skills, a satisfied client will automatically recommend the service to another potential client. It is important for therapists to tell as many people as possible about Indian Head Massage and communicate their enthusiasm. Positive enthusiasm is infectious and even if the person you are speaking to does not need the information, they may pass it on to someone who does. The power of the spoken word is very effective in the marketing of services.

Talks and Demonstrations

Talks and demonstrations are an effective way of presenting the service to a targeted group and they usually work best when presented together.

Talks should be informative and educational in nature (they should tell potential clients how Indian Head Massage will benefit them) and the demonstration should show the target audience the effects and help to break down barriers or preconceptions they may hold about the therapy.

It is useful to identify the needs of the target audience prior to the presentation, as this gives the therapist the advantage of being able to personalise the session. Talks and demonstrations are best limited to a maximum of 30–40 minutes, with time left to answer questions and to distribute business cards and literature.

The focus of the talk should be about identifying with and providing solutions to the client's needs.

A useful checklist when preparing for talks is to:

- find out as much as possible about the target group before the talk
- confirm the number of people that will be attending
- check out the venue and its suitability
- plan out the talk with a basic outline format
- have a plentiful supply of literature to hand out
- prepare a list of possible questions you may be asked
- take some relaxation music to help create a relaxing ambience
- aim to involve the audience in the session (encourage questions or volunteer models for demonstrations)
- take your appointment book with you!

Exhibitions

Exhibitions are an effective way to communicate with lots of potential clients in one place. They are a useful way of distributing brochures and leaflets and persuading new clients to watch a demonstration of a new service and sample it. When exhibiting at a show it is important to ensure that it is the right type of show for the image of the business. It is also important to speak to people who have attended the show to gain feedback from them.

In order to project the right image at an exhibition it is important to ensure that:

- the stand looks attractive, neat and tidy
- the stand is accessible and situated to your best advantage
- staff manning the stand look warm and welcoming, and are approachable and easy to talk to
- there is space for people to browse without feeling intimidated.

It is also important, if possible, to take the names and telephone numbers of those who visited the stand so you may contact them after the exhibition.

Building a Referral Network

This is one of the most successful and inexpensive ways of creating new business. Current satisfied clients are one of the most effective means of advertising.

Referrals can be encouraged by:

- offering existing clients incentives to introduce new clients to use your service
- establishing links with other professionals by making yourself and what you do known to them.

Public Relations

This is a way for therapists to get their name in the public eye without actually paying for advertising.

There is a variety of ways in which it can be done.

1 Offering a free talk and demonstration to a particular client group in the community is an ideal way of marketing Indian Head Massage and helping to get your name and reputation established.

Public interest in holistic therapies is increasing all the time and there are many groups that meet regularly who may be keen to hear from you (a list of contact names, addresses and phone numbers may be obtained from your local library).

See Talks and Demonstrations, page 252.

2 Send information or news concerning your business to editors of newspapers or magazines in the form of a news article. Every day, editors and journalists are looking for stories and information to fill their newspapers or magazines.

An important consideration when sending information to journalists is to send only information that is truly of interest to the community and their readers.

3 Donating your time, money or products to a local worthwhile charity. There are many charitable organisations who rely on donations each year in order to survive. An event linked to funding or sponsoring a charity would be a newsworthy article, as well as helping to meet the needs of the community.

4 Getting a regular or one-off slot on local radio (see radio, page 259).

5 Compiling a press release which may be sent to local and national newspapers and magazines.
When compiling a press release the following guidelines may help to increase your chance of publication:

- think of an original, interesting, thought-provoking or even humorous headline

- avoid trying to sell your service

- it should be newsworthy and of interest to the journalists and their readers

- address the information directly to a named editor or journalist, preferably one with whom you have already established contact

- ensure that it is laid out clearly (preferably double-line spacing) and is no longer than two pages

- always include a contact name, address and telephone number.

> **KEY NOTE**
> Editorials in newspapers and magazines are seen to be credible and true as readers place a considerable amount of trust in the objectivity of journalists. It is therefore worth getting to know editors and journalists and being persistent, as the articles they write tend to hold a lot of weight with readers.

Indirect Approach to Marketing and Promotion

There are several other methods of advertising or marketing which may be used in order to reach the potential clients you cannot reach in person, and these include:

- newspaper advertising

- specialist magazines

- national directories

- mailshots

- leaflets and promotional material

- the Internet

- local radio

- cross-merchandising promotional literature.

Advertising strategies usually involve a mix of different media and should be scheduled over a period of time for maximum effect. Isolated advertisements rarely sustain enough interest.

Advertising is about getting your message across. Important considerations when considering an advertisement are:

- what do you want to say to potential clients?

- who is your target audience?

- how will you communicate to them what you want to say?

It is essential to follow the tried and tested **AIDA** formula when considering your publicity:

A – attracting *attention*: this can be created by an appropriate heading that attracts attention.

I – generating *interest*: this can be created by stating what is on offer.

D – creating *desire*: this can be created by stating why what you have to offer is needed and getting potential clients to believe in the benefits.

A – motivating *action*: this can be created by offering the reader an incentive (special offer).

Good advertisements are usually targeted to the right audience, are accurate and not misleading, catchy, concise and memorable. Effective adverts must have a good headline (select a major benefit for this) to have immediate impact. A good headline will:

- attract the reader's attention

- compel the person to read further

- improve response

- express the most important benefits.

A good advert should be easy to read and be written to:

- touch people's emotions

- be informative

- promote the service

- raise awareness

- motivate the reader to act.

When designing adverts, ask yourself what adverts you responded to and why.

KEY NOTE

Words that tend to sell in adverts include: You, New, Results, Health, Free, Complimentary, Benefits, Now, Yes.

Local Papers

There are two types of advertisements in newspapers and these are display advertisements and business classified. Display advertising is more expensive and could appear anywhere in the paper, unless you have paid to have a particular space such as the front or back page, or the television page (any of which could prove very expensive).

It is always a gamble when relying on display advertising as it may be largely dependent on the following:

- the day of the week the paper is printed

- the time of the year

- the page the advert appears on

- the layout of the advert in relation to the other advertisers.

An important point to consider with display advertising is that people buy papers for many reasons other than to read adverts (reading news, announcements and events, crosswords, horoscopes). It is therefore important to consider how your advert is going to grab their attention, bearing in mind that newspapers have a short lifespan, and also bearing in mind the AIDA principle.

It is also useful to consider that the person reading the news and features may come across your display advert and may not be thinking about a massage until he or she sees your advert, or they may not be ready to have a massage for some while. In fact it may take many exposures to your advert before this person feels you are sufficiently familiar to give you a try. It is important therefore that adverts are repeated regularly in the same way, in order to create familiarity. It can also help to have a picture of yourself in the advert, as it will be more eye-catching and will help the potential client to feel they know you.

It is important to remember when writing adverts that you are speaking directly to your potential clients and the reader will be initially attracted by your headline message, rather than the name of your business. It is often helpful to give the reader a reason to reply now, such as a deadline on a special offer, as this motivates action.

When you have designed an advert, it is often helpful to ask friends and colleagues to cast an eye over the design and the wording for critical review; often by looking with a fresh pair of eyes they can add constructive comments.

Display advertising is usually more effective when it is combined with some editorial. Often papers run special features on health-related matters and it may be more appropriate to consider a display advert within a feature as it draws the reader's attention to a more focused subject. Classified advertising is more cost-effective than display advertising as it is more targeted to the service to be provided. The disadvantage with classified advertising is that there may not always be an appropriate section for holistic therapists and advertisements will need to be placed frequently in order to make it effective.

Specialist Magazines

These are usually targeted to a specific audience and those related to health are normally of interest to a holistic therapist. The main drawback with them is that they are not local but national and will depend on the readership and the location of the therapist as to whether the advertising will be effective.

KEY NOTE

Check the readership profile before committing to advertising in magazines and check circulation radius and readership numbers.

Promotional Material

When writing and designing promotional material the key to success is to write it as if you know the client personally. Choose words carefully so they strike a chord with the client. Remember that many clients reading promotional material may not know they are looking for your service until they see it.

It is also important when developing marketing material to ensure that it reflects the image you wish to portray and that it appeals to the target market.

Promotional materials such as leaflets, brochures and posters are the means by which clients will decide whether to contact you for an appointment. Promotional material must be attractive enough to make clients read it and wording should be positive, direct and above all personal. Brochures and posters with a question and answer format can help clients to overcome their reservations and visual aids can help to attract attention.

It is also important to use positive language and turn a negative statement (such as a client's problem) into a positive one (how your treatment is going to help them). Including testimonials from satisfied clients (with their permission) can also help to build credibility and break down barriers.

Mailshots

Mailshots can be a worthwhile exercise but require a degree of planning and forethought. It is far more effective to target a specific group when designing a mailshot, as the main theme has to address the needs of all the recipients.

You may choose to target self-help groups with a common need of relaxation or to write to the Occupational Health Adviser at local companies, offering to give free talks and demonstrations as part of their stress management programme.

The letter should be sent on headed notepaper and be brief and concise. The focus should be on the recipient's needs, although it is helpful to send background information on yourself, as well as information on Indian Head Massage.

Mailshots usually have a success or response rate of around 2 per cent, although this may be enhanced to 5 per cent by follow-up phone calls.

> **KEY NOTE**
>
> When writing to companies it is worth offering the incentive of corporate membership as a promotion to motivate more clients to use your service. Each employee may be issued with a corporate membership card which entitles them to a certain percentage discount.

When sending a mailshot it is important to consider the day it is mailed out as this could have a significant effect on the result. If sending a mailshot to clients' homes, aim to send it to arrive on a Friday or Saturday, ready for the weekend, when they may have more time to consider what you are offering. If sending mailshots to companies, aim to send the information to arrive on a Tuesday or Wednesday and not on a Friday or Monday.

Getting Corporate Clients

Indian Head Massage is ideally suited to the workplace because of its unique selling points:

- it is portable in nature
- it is quick
- it provides a solution to the client's problems

- it is a personal service
- there is no need for the client to undress
- no special resources are required.

If your objective is to secure contracts with corporate clients, first consider which companies (both large and small) are within your catchment area and the profile of the staff members.

When approaching corporate clients, it is important to create a corporate image for yourself, even if you are not part of a large organisation. The first point of contact should be by letter directly to the person within the organisation who is responsible for the health and welfare of staff (this may be an Occupational Health Adviser, Staff Nurse, Health and Safety Officer, or Managing Director). The letter should be sent on quality headed notepaper; the main theme of the letter should focus on the workplace benefits of Indian Head Massage and how it can benefit the staff and the organisation (see Chapter 7, Stress Management). When approaching corporate clients it is advisable to avoid 'flowery' therapy language and be specific and accurate in terms of the outcome (the benefits). Offer to come in and give a free talk and demonstration with no obligation. Once the letter has been sent, keep a record of it and follow it up with a phone call approximately seven to ten days afterwards.

Remember that businesses, whether large or small, receive a lot of paperwork through the post. Do not assume that the reason you have not heard from them is that they are not interested. They may simply not have had the time to read your letter.

Publications and Directories

Advertising in national publications and directories such as Yellow Pages can be an effective way of advertising as entries are classified by therapy type. It is also a long-term form of advertising and can prove to be cost-effective as many are annual publications.

Therapists should also consider their geographical location; if they are situated between two counties, it may be advisable to take an advert in more than one directory.

If there are several therapists advertising under the same category then it is important to consider your USP (unique selling point) and stress this in order to make your entry stand out from the competitors.

Internet

Some therapists are now taking advantage of the Internet as a means of advertising their treatments. An attractively designed web page, including a treatment menu and a photograph of the therapist, can be factors that may enhance the chances of contact from any interested parties. It can also help to give a therapist a more corporate image, which is especially important if it is this sector of the market you are interested in pursuing.

Some feel that the Internet is a little impersonal but others who are constantly using it feel it is a very effective means of communication.

It is certainly worth considering this as a potential source of enquiries and contact, but remember that not everyone will have access to the Internet and many may prefer the more traditional means of contact.

Radio

Radio is an excellent form of media in raising awareness of treatments such as Indian Head Massage. Consider contacting your local radio station with a view to having either a regular or one-off spot on the radio to promote Indian Head Massage. It is important when approching the station to make the proposal interesting and one which will interest their listeners. It is important to respond to local trends or issues (for instance lifestyle or reducing stress) when presenting information on the radio, as it has to be topical and of value to listeners. Assessing growth trends within the industry will help you to assess the opportunities afforded to you.

When preparing to talk on the radio it is important to find out as much as possible about the programme you will be appearing on, the profile of the listeners and most importantly the style of the radio presenter. Some presenters prefer to work to a script and will run through a list of questions before the programme; others prefer to work unscripted and make the presentation more spontaneous.

KEY NOTE
Local radio stations often look for gifts that can be given to listeners in exchange for on-air promotions. Donating your services is an easy and effective way of getting your name out on the airwaves without buying advertising time.

Cross-Merchandising Promotional Literature

Consider other local businesses that cater for clientele similar to yours (for example, hairdressers, osteopaths, and so on) and who may be in a position to influence clients to try Indian Head Massage. Exchange promotional literature and brochures with them and this will allow each party additional exposure to the type of clients they wish to attract. When approaching other local businesses with a view to cross-merchandising, it is important to establish a friendly, approachable and cooperative working relationship, as this will enhance the success of the promotion on both sides.

Encouraging Client Retention

The first goal of marketing is to encourage potential clients to try out your services; the next goal is to encourage them to come back again. There are several ways of fostering repeat business:

- Create an understanding of the benefits of the treatments you provide to clients by encouraging them to book regular treatments.

- Award loyalty bonuses and reward schemes (such as ones offered by major supermarket chains).

- Stay in touch with your clients and informing them of special offers and any new treatments you may have added to your treatment menu (and how these can benefit them).

- Invite clients to attend talks and events you may be holding.

Maximising Marketing Opportunities

Because of the widespread appeal of Indian Head Massage it is well suited to clinics, salons and spas, as well as other associated trades such as hairdressers, osteopaths, chiropractors and health clinics. Consider all places where people attend regularly for reasons of health, beauty and relaxation.

A local hairdresser's may be interested in adding Indian Head Massage to their treatment menu to give a different marketing angle to their customer service. Osteopaths and chiropractors may be interested in Indian Head Massage for clients with soft-tissue problems of the head, neck and shoulders. A GPs surgery may be interested in helping clients with stress, anxiety and depression or people with musculoskeletal problems.

If you have a local regional airport nearby, they may be interested in a business proposal to offer treatments to tired business executives in need of stress relief. A local school may benefit from a regular visit to help teachers and students to manage their stress levels.

If you use your imagination, there is a multitude of different opportunities and reasons for marketing Indian Head Massage.

Selling of associated products

As providing treatments is a labour-intensive service, consider selling complementary products for clients' home use. Clients are more likely to buy products such as scalp oils and relaxation tapes at the time of their treatment. It is therefore advisable to have a display of items available for purchase at reception or wherever the client is likely to pay. Clients are also more likely to buy from their therapist, with whom they have a trusting relationship.

Creative marketing opportunities

Other creative marketing opportunities could be to offer gift certificates linked to promotions at specific times of the year such as Christmas, Valentine's Day, birthdays, Mother's Day or Father's Day. Specially packaged courses of treatment often attract interest as they are designed specifically to address the needs of the recipient.

Male clients

An area that is often left unexploited is the male market. Marketing treatments such as Indian Head Massage can require a different strategy from selling to female clients. Men often respond more to factual and benefit-related words rather than the more aesthetic language women tend to respond to. Think of male-dominated markets and how that target may be reached. Local sports clubs and associations may be a good start; also men's barbers, health clubs.

An important consideration when marketing to male clients is whether the environment you are practising in is male-friendly (it will be difficult to attract male clients into a salon that looks too pretty and feminine). Some men are also conscious of their body image; it may therefore be more prudent to schedule specific times for male clients to attend.

Defining Marketing Objectives

Once you have put together the right mix of marketing methods, the next stage is to define your marketing objectives. Marketing objectives are closely linked to overall business objectives and will define what you want to achieve from your marketing and how you intend to meet the objectives.

Example of Marketing Objectives for a Therapist Practising Indian Head Massage

Objectives

Short term

To introduce Indian Head Massage to existing clientele.

Medium term

To expand the existing client base to secure new clients.

Long term

To introduce Indian Head Massage into the workplace.

Strategy

1 Send a newsletter to all existing clients advising them of the benefits of Indian Head Massage and how it can help them. Include a voucher with a special introductory offer.

2 Contact the editor of a local newspaper to offer an article on Indian Head Massage that is going to be of interest to readers, and a free demonstration.

3 Write to 20 local companies with a short but informative introductory letter. Offer a corporate discount. Follow up with a phone call in 7 to 10 days with a view to securing a meeting to offer a free talk and demonstration.

Monitoring marketing methods

It is important to regularly monitor the response to marketing methods, so you can assess which methods are working to help you meet your business objectives. It is essential to constantly monitor, review and adapt your strategies in order to ensure continued business success. Marketing methods may change with a difference in trend or may simply become out-dated.

A simple and effective way of monitoring the response to your marketing methods is to ask each new client how they heard of you and keep a record of this, in order to review it in line with your business objectives. Provided you know how much a particular method cost and how many clients were generated from it, you are then in a position to analyse which methods are cost-effective. Once you establish a clientele you can then build up information such as how often they attend for treatments, how much they spend and what marketing methods they respond to.

For marketing to have the desired effects it should be:

- **sufficient** – it has to be done regularly, even when you are busy

- **efficient** – it has to be cost-effective to be worthwhile

- **effective** – it has to work and get results.

How to Encourage Repeat Business

Maintaining excellent customer service is the key to encouraging repeat business.

It is important to make it easy for clients to come to you by:

- making client needs a priority
- concentrating all your actions and efforts for the business with the client in mind
- treating every client like a new client and avoiding complacency
- delivering an excellent service
- building an open relationship with clients by encouraging feedback.

Keeping Ahead of Business

Many businesses fail to realise their potential because they don't continually market themselves. An important factor to consider is that many clients may have to see your advert or marketing material many times before responding.

Many therapists fail to be consistent in marketing methods, believing they already have enough clients. Even if the appointment book is full, it is important to keep on marketing to raise client awareness and maintain your professional image, as you never know when you are going to lose current clients because of various circumstances (for example, client's personal or financial circumstances, client moving out of the area, and so on).

INDIAN HEAD MASSAGE QUESTIONNAIRE

Indian Head Massage is a traditional massage treatment originating in India. It involves the application of massage technique to the upper back and shoulders, upper arms, neck, face and scalp. The treatment is applied through the clothes, with the recipient remaining seated in a chair.

Indian Head Massage has many benefits, including helping to relieve muscular tension, relieving headaches and reducing stress levels.

This questionnaire is designed to establish current levels of awareness and interest in Indian Head Massage.

1 Have you heard of Indian Head Massage before?   Yes/No

2 If yes, when did you hear about it?

_____

_____

3 Do you experience any of the following on a regular basis?

high stress levels? ☐   muscular tension in the back, neck or shoulders? ☐

headaches? ☐   eyestrain? ☐   anxiety? ☐   depression? ☐

poor concentration levels? ☐

4 What measures do you take (if any) to help with any of the above?

_____

_____

5 Would you be interested in trying a treatment?   Yes/No

6 Would you like further information on Indian Head Massage and its benefits?   Yes/No

Thank you for your time and cooperation in completing this form. If you would like further information or would like to book a complimentary introductory treatment, please give your details below.

Name _____

Address _____

Telephone Number Work: _____   Home: _____

ACTIVITY

Design a Marketing Plan for Indian Head Massage based on the following outline:

1 Description of the service to be offered (i.e. Indian Head Massage)

Include your unique selling points (USPs) and a full description of the service and how it can benefit clients

2 Objectives of the marketing campaign

This could be to increase your client market, or to raise awareness of Indian Head Massage, etc.

3 A profile of your intended client market

This is who you want to target and why you think they will pay for the service. Include as much information as possible, based on what you have discovered about your potential clients (market questionnaires, interviews etc.). Also include information on competitors, if applicable, as this will help you to identify how much your potential clients are currently spending on a similar service.

4 Where you intend to offer the service (location)

Because of its portability, consider the different locations in which Indian Head Massage treatment may be offered

5 Details of your SWOT analysis

(strengths, weaknesses, opportunities, threats)

6 Intended marketing strategies

Consider how you intend to advertise the service, what media you will use and how often you will advertise.

Consider all the direct and indirect forms of marketing and promotions that will help your business succeed.

Design a promotional leaflet for Indian Head Massage.

Remember to allocate a budget for marketing activities and to plan the activities out over a period of time for maximum effect.

FAQs

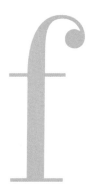

Can Indian Head Massage be carried out daily as it is in India?
Indian Head Massage is generally carried out daily in Indian families as it is part of family life. Treatment is short and is mainly restricted to the head only. Indian Head Massage has developed in the western world into a more comprehensive treatment, which if carried out daily may prove too stimulating and provoke adverse reactions. It is therefore best to leave 48 hours between treatments to allow the body to rest and respond to any reactions.

When massaging the scalp I find the oil application difficult. Do you have any advice?
Firstly it is best to use a bottle with a slow drip cap to ensure that only a small amount of oil is released at a time. If you are massaging a client with thick or long hair it is best to section the hair off with clips by parting down the centre and then dividing the scalp into quarter sections to ensure even coverage of the oil to be absorbed into the scalp and hair follicles.

If a client has curly hair, what is the best way of carrying out the hair tugging without causing the client discomfort/getting your fingers stuck in the hair?
Firstly ensure the hair is free from hair products such as mousse, hairspray or gel. When carrying out the hair tugging on curly hair, ensure that you tug the hair from the root only, by clasping the hair between the fingers but keeping them *fixed at the root* as you tug. If you attempt to draw the fingers upwards and through the hair (as is usual with this technique), your fingers will invariably get stuck and will be likely to cause discomfort.

With clients with little or no hair do I simply miss the scalp massage out?
No, you can still carry out the scalp massage, omitting techniques such as the hair tugging, because despite the fact your client may have little or no hair they will still benefit from the relaxation of the muscle fibres of the scalp.

Where is the best place to buy authentic Indian oils for Indian Head Massage?
The best place to buy authentic Indian oils is from a local Indian supermarket, or from an Ayurvedic supplier (see resource section on pages 267–270).

What is the best way to promote Indian Head Massage?

The best way to promote Indian Head Massage is simply to demonstrate it in as many locations as possible; the more public the place the better (such as exhibitions and shows). Take advantage of the fact that Indian Head Massage is portable and demonstrate an aspect of the treatment where clients look most relaxed (massaging the scalp).

When I was carrying out Indian Head Massage on one of my clients recently, she started to experience a feeling of faintness when I started to massage the head. Why is this, and what action should be taken in the event of this happening during a treatment?

This can be a common reaction to Indian Head Massage due to the increased blood supply to the head. Some clients may feel dizzy due to stress, tiredness, or their blood sugar levels or blood pressure may have dropped during the treatment. Always monitor and discuss your client's reactions during treatments, and if they start to feel faint it is best to stop the treatment and ensure their continued comfort by offering them a glass of water and advising that they get some fresh air, if appropriate.

I have a client who suffers from osteoarthritis in the neck who wants to try Indian Head Massage. Is it possible to carry out a treatment on this client?

It may be possible to carry out an adapted form of treatment, but this depends on the severity of the client's condition. In cases where pain and discomfort are severe it is best for a client to seek medical advice.

Care must be taken to ensure there is no excessive movement of the neck joint during treatment to avoid pain, discomfort and potential joint damage. In most cases gentle massage can help to ease pain and gently increase mobility. Care should also be taken to position the client according to individual comfort and offer additional supports for the neck.

Remember that if the client's condition is *acutely* inflamed at the time of the treatment, massage would be best avoided as the increased circulation arising from the massage may exacerbate the symptoms.

Resources

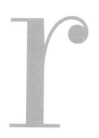

For professional training courses, training DVDs and posters

Helen McGuinness
Health and Beauty Training
International

www.helenmcguinness.com

For a selection of authentic Indian massage and hair oils contact

Maharishi Ayur-Veda Products
Beacon House
Willow Walk
Skelmersdale
Lancs
WN8 6UR

01695 51015

www.maharishi-european-sidhaland.org.uk

For an extensive range of therapy books and DVDs

Willen Limited
Three Crowns Yard
High Street
Market Harborough
Leicestershire
LE16 7AF

01858 410233

www.willenbooks.co.uk

DVDs

Indian Head Massage DVD
Helen McGuinness

Synopsis

A demonstration of a professional Indian Head Massage which covers the area around the upper back, neck, scalp, shoulders, arms and face. This DVD is suitable for those studying for a professional qualification as well as a reference for qualified professionals.

Also includes: Contraindications, Contra-actions, Aftercare.

Further reading

Aldred, Elaine Mary
A Guide to Starting Your Own Complementary Therapy Practice: A Manual for the Complementary Healthcare Profession
Churchill Livingstone (2006)
ISBN-10: 0443103097
ISBN-13: 978-0443103094

Brennan, Dr Donn
Live Better: Ayurveda Remedies and Inspirations for Well-being
Duncan Baird Publishers (2006)
ISBN-10: 1844832910
ISBN-13: 978-1844832910

Cash, Mel and Wadmore, Anne
The Pocket Atlas of the Moving Body
Ebury Press (1999)
ISBN-10: 0091865123
ISBN-13: 978-0091865122

Davis, Martha, Eshelman, Elizabeth Robbins and McKay, Matthew
The Relaxation and Stress Reduction Workbook, 5th edition
New Harbinger Publications Inc. (2000)
ISBN-10: 1572242140
ISBN-13: 978-1572242142

Duncan, Mary, Cahill, Finbar and Heighway, Penny
Health and Safety at Work Essentials: The One-stop Guide for Anyone Responsible for Health and Safety Issues in the Workplace, 5th edition
Lawpack Publishing Ltd (2006)
ISBN-10: 1905261241
ISBN-13: 978-1905261246

Edwards, Douglas
Getting Business to Come to You: Complete Do-it-yourself Guide to Attracting All the Business You Can Handle
Jeremy P. Tarcher (1998)
ISBN-10: 087477845X
ISBN-13: 978-0874778458

Frawley, David, Ranade, Subhash and Lele, Avinash
Ayurveda and Marma Therapy: Energy Points in Yogic Healing
Lotus Press (2004)
ISBN-10: 0940985594
ISBN-13: 978-0940985599

Gardner, Joy
Vibrational Healing Through the Chakras
Celestial Arts, Ten Speed Press (2006)
ISBN-10: 1580911668
ISBN-13: 978-1580911665

Gardner-Gordon, Joy
Pocket Guide to the Chakras
Pilgrims Publishing (2002)
ISBN-10: 8173032211
ISBN-13: 978-8173032219

Goodheart, Herbert P.
Photoguide to Common Skin Disorders: Diagnosis and Management, 2nd edition
Lippincott Williams and Wilkins (2003)
ISBN-10: 0781737419
ISBN-13: 978-0781737418

Hayden, C.J.
Get Clients Now! A 28-day Marketing Program for Professionals and Consultants
Amacom (1999)
ISBN-10: 0814479928
ISBN-13: 978-0814479926

Jenkins, Gail, Kemnitz, Christopher and Tortora, Gerard J.
Anatomy and Physiology: From Science to Life
John Wiley and Sons Inc., Book and CD-Rom edition (2006)
ISBN-10: 0471613185
ISBN-13: 978-0471613183

Johari, Harish
Ayurvedic Massage: Traditional Indian Techniques for Balancing Body and Mind
Healing Arts Press, Inner Traditions, Bear and Company (1996)
ISBN-10: 0892814896
ISBN-13: 978-0892814893

Johari, Harish
Chakras – Energy Centers of Transformation, Revised and Enlarged Edition
Destiny Books, Inner Traditions, Bear and Company (2000)
ISBN-10: 0892817607
ISBN-13: 978-0892817603

Kingsley, Philip
The Hair Bible, New Edition
Aurum Press Ltd (2003)
ISBN-10: 1854109065
ISBN-13: 978-1854109064

McGuinness, Helen
Anatomy and Physiology: Therapy Basics, 3rd edition
Hodder Arnold H&S (2006)
ISBN-10: 0340908084
ISBN-13: 978-0340908082

McGuinness, Helen
Facials and Skin Care in Essence (In Essence Series)
Hodder Arnold (2007)
ISBN-10: 0340926937
ISBN-13: 978-0340926932

McGuinness, Helen
Holistic Therapies: An Introductory Guide
Hodder Arnold (2000)
ISBN-10: 0340772964
ISBN-13: 978-0340772966

Mehta, Narendra
Thorsons First Directions: Indian Head Massage
HarperCollins (2001)
ISBN-10: 0007123566
ISBN-13: 978-0007123568

Mehta, Narendra and Mehta, Kundan
The Face Lift Massage: Rejuvenate Your Skin and Reduce Fine Lines and Wrinkles
HarperCollins (2004)
ISBN-10: 000715741X
ISBN-13: 978-0007157419

Mitchell, Tim and Kennedy, Cameron
Common Skin Disorders: Your Questions Answered
Churchill Livingstone (2006)
ISBN-10: 0443074631
ISBN-13: 978-0443074639

Premkumar, Kalyani
Pathology A to Z: A Handbook for Massage Therapists, 2nd edition
Lippincott Williams and Wilkins (2002)
ISBN-10: 0781740983
ISBN-13: 978-0781740982

Rickman, Cheryl D. and Roddick, Dame Anita
The Small Business Start-up Workbook: A Step-by-step Guide to Starting the Business You've Dreamed of
How To Books Ltd (2005)
ISBN-10: 1845280385
ISBN-13: 978-1845280383

Tortora, Gerard J.
Principles of Anatomy and Physiology, 11th edition
John Wiley and Sons Inc. (2005)
ISBN-10: 0471718718
ISBN-13: 978-0471718710

Turkington, Carol and Dover, Jeffrey S.
The Encyclopedia of Skin and Skin Disorders, 3rd edition
Facts on File Inc. (2006)
ISBN-10: 0816064032
ISBN-13: 978-0816064038

Werner, Ruth
A Massage Therapist's Guide to Pathology 3rd edition
Lippincott Williams and Wilkins (2005)
ISBN-10: 0781754895
ISBN-13: 978-0781754897

Williams, Sara
Lloyds TSB Small Business Guide, New edition
Vitesse Media plc (2003)
ISBN-10: 0954562127
ISBN-13: 978-0954562120

Glossary

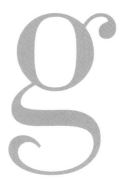

abducens nerve a mixed nerve that innervates only the lateral rectus muscle of the eye

abduction movement of a limb away from the midline

accessory nerve innervates muscles in the neck and upper back, as well as muscles of the palate, pharynx and larynx

acne vulgaris a common inflammatory disorder of the sebaceous glands which leads to the overproduction of sebum

adduction movement of a limb towards the midline

adipose tissue type of tissue containing fat cells, found in the subcutaneous layer of skin

adrenaline hormone secreted by the medulla of the adrenal glands; prepares the body for 'fright, fight or flight' response

Ajna the brow chakra located in the middle of the forehead, over the 'third eye' area

albinism a condition in which there is an inherited absence of pigmentation in the skin, hair and eyes

allergic reaction a disorder in which the body becomes hypersensitive to a particular allergen and produces histamine in the skin as part of the body's defence

alopecia term used to describe temporary baldness or severe hair loss which may follow illness, shock, or a period of extreme stress

Anahata the heart chakra located in the centre of the chest

angina pain in the left side of the chest and usually radiating to the left arm, caused by insufficient blood reaching the heart muscle

ankylosing spondylitis a systemic joint disease

anxiety a psychological illness that can vary from a mild form to panic attacks and severe phobias

arthritis: osteoarthritis a joint disease involving varying degrees of joint pain, stiffness, limitation of movement, joint instability and deformity

arthritis: rheumatoid chronic inflammation of peripheral joints, resulting in pain, stiffness and potential damage to joints

asthma shortness of breath and difficulty in breathing caused by spasm or swelling of the bronchial tubes

autonomic nervous system part of the nervous system that controls the automatic activities of smooth and cardiac muscle, and the activities of glands

ayurveda world's oldest Indian healing system ('the science of life and longevity')

basal cell layer (stratum germinativum) deepest and innermost of the five layers of epidermis

Bell's palsy a disorder of the 7th cranial nerve (facial nerve) that results in paralysis on one side of the face

biceps a muscle on the anterior of the upper arm

boil an inflamed nodule forming a pocket of bacteria around the base of a hair follicle, or a break in the skin

brachialis a muscle attaching to the distal half of the anterior surface of the humerus at one end and the ulna at the other

brachioradialis an anterior muscle of the forearm, connecting the humerus to the radius

brain stem the enlarged extension upwards within the skull of the spinal cord, consisting of the medulla oblongata, the pons and the mid-brain

bronchi two short tubes which carry air into each lung

bronchiole a subdivision of the bronchial tree

bronchitis a chronic or acute inflammation of the bronchial tubes

buccinator the main muscle of the cheek, attached to both the upper and lower jaw

cardiac muscle special type of involuntary muscle found only in the heart

carotid artery either of the two main arteries of the neck whose branches supply the head and neck

carpals eight small bones forming the wrist

central nervous system (CNS) part of the nervous system consisting of the brain and spinal cord

cerebellum cauliflower-shaped structure located at the posterior of the cranium, below the cerebrum

cerebral palsy a condition caused by damage to a baby's central nervous system during pregnancy, delivery or soon after birth

cerebrum largest portion of the brain and makes up the front and top part of the brain

cervical nodes lymph nodes located within the neck

cervical plexuses spinal nerves supplying the skin and muscles of the head, neck, and upper region of the shoulders

cervical vertebrae seven vertebrae of the neck

chakras non-physical energy centres located about an inch away from the physical body

chloasma a pigmentation disorder which presents with irregular areas of increased pigmentation, usually on the face

clavicle bone forming anterior of shoulder girdle

clear layer (stratum lucidum) epidermal layer below the most superficial layer

coccygeal plexus supplies the skin in the area of the coccyx and the muscles of the pelvic floor

coccygeal vertebrae (coccyx) four fused vertebrae at the base of spine forming the tail bone

collagen protein in the dermis which gives the skin its strength and resilience

comedone a collection of sebum, keratinised cells and wastes which accumulate in the entrance of a hair follicle

compression a form of petrissage in which the muscles are gently pressed against a surface

conjunctivitis a bacterial infection following irritation of the conjunctiva of the eye

contact dermatitis red, dry and inflamed skin caused by a primary irritant

corrugator a muscle located on the inner edge of the eyebrow

cranial nerves set of 12 pairs of nerves originating from the brain

cuticle outer layer of hair

deltoid thick triangular muscle that caps the top of the humerus and shoulder

depression a psychological condition which combines symptoms of lowered mood, loss of appetite, poor sleep, lack of concentration and interest

dermal papilla elevation at the base of the hair bulb; contains a rich blood supply

dermis deeper layer of the skin found below the epidermis

desquamation the shedding of dead skin cells from the horny layer (stratum corneum)

diabetes a metabolic disorder. Diabetes mellitus, in which sugars are not oxidised to produce enough energy due to lack of the pancreatic hormone insulin, is the most common form. Diabetes insipidus, in which a person produces large quantities of dilute urine and is constantly thirsty, is a less common form of diabetes.

diaphragm dome-shaped muscle of respiration that separates the thorax from the abdomen

dosha subtle life-giving force

eccrine gland simple coiled tubular sweat gland that opens directly on to the surface of the skin

effleurage a stroking, or smoothing movement that signals the beginning and end of a massage

embolism obstruction or closure of a vessel by an embolus

embolus substance such as a blood clot that is carried by the blood and obstructs a blood vessel

epidermis outermost, superficial layer of the skin

epilepsy a neurological disorder that makes the individual susceptible to recurrent and temporary seizures

erector pili muscle small smooth muscle attached at an angle to the base of a hair follicle

erector spinae a long postural muscle in three bands either side of spine, attaching to the spine, ribcage and head

erythema reddening of the skin due to the dilation of blood capillaries just below the epidermis

ethmoid skull bone forming part of the wall of the orbit, the roof of the nasal cavity and part of the nasal septum

extensor carpi radialis a muscle extending along the radial side of the posterior of the forearm

extensor carpi ulnaris a muscle extending along the ulnar side of the posterior of the forearm

extensor digitorum a muscle extending along the lateral side of the posterior of the forearm

facial nerve a mixed nerve that conducts impulses to and from several areas in the face and neck

fibromyalgia a chronic condition that produces musculosketetal pain

flexor carpi digitorum an anterior muscle of the forearm extending from the medial end of the humerus, the anterior of the ulna and radius to the anterior surfaces of the second to fifth fingers

flexor carpi radialis a muscle of the forearm extending along the radial side of the anterior of forearm

flexor carpi ulnaris an anterior muscle of the forearm extending along the ulnar side of the anterior of the forearm

folliculitis a bacterial infection which occurs in the hair follicles of the skin

frictions deeper massage movements causing the skin to rub against the underlying structures

frontal skull bone forming the forehead

frontalis muscle that extends over the front of the skull and the width of the forehead

frozen shoulder (adhesive capsulitis) a chronic condition in which there is pain and stiffness and reduced mobility, or locking, of the shoulder joint

glossopharyngeal nerve a mixed nerve that innervates structures in the mouth and throat

granular layer (stratum granulosum) layer of epidermis linking the living cells of the epidermis (basal and prickle cell layers) to the dead cells above

haemorrhage loss of blood from the circulatory system; bleeding

hair bulb the enlarged part at the base of the hair root

hair root part found below the surface of the skin

hair shaft part of the hair which lies above the surface of the skin

hair tugging a technique used in the scalp massage where the roots of the hair are lifted and pulled upwards in order to stimulate hair growth

herpes simplex (cold sores) a viral infection normally found on the face and around the lips

herpes zoster (shingles) painful infection along the sensory nerves by the virus that causes chicken pox

high blood pressure when the resting blood pressure is above normal (consistently exceeding 160 mmHg systolic and 95 mmHg diastolic)

homeostasis process by which the body maintains a stable internal environment for its cells and tissues

horny layer (stratum corneum) most superficial, outer layer of the skin consisting of dead, flattened, keratinised cells

humerus long bone of the upper arm

hypothenar eminence a projection of soft tissue located on the ulnar side of the palm of the hand; consists of three muscles: abductor digiti minimi manus, flexor digiti minimi manus and opponens digiti minimi

impetigo a superficial contagious inflammatory disease caused by streptococcal and staphylococcal bacteria

infraspinatus a muscle that attaches to the middle two-thirds of the scapula, below the spine of the scapula at one end and the top of the humerus at the other

intercostal muscles muscles that occupy the spaces between the ribs and are responsible for controlling some of the movements of the ribs

jugular vein major vein draining blood from the head and neck (divides into internal and external branches)

kapha one of the three doshas; said to be responsible for growth

keratin tough fibrous protein found in the epidermis, the hair and the nails

keratinisation process that cells undergo when they change from living cells with a nucleus to dead, horny cells without a nucleus

kyphosis an abnormally increased outward curvature of the thoracic spine

lacrimal bones smallest of the facial bones, and are located close to the medial part of the orbital cavity

larynx (voice box) short passage connecting the pharynx to the trachea

levator labii superiorus a muscle located towards the inner cheek beside the nose, extending from the upper jaw to the skin of the corners of the mouth and the upper lip

levator scapula a strap-like muscle that runs almost vertically through the neck, connecting the cervical vertebrae to the scapula

low blood pressure when the blood pressure is below normal (consistently 99 mmHg or less systolic and less than 59 mmHg diastolic)

lymph transparent, colourless, watery liquid, derived from tissue fluid

lymphatic capillaries minute blind-end tubes that commence in the tissue spaces of the body

lymphatic node oval or bean-shaped structure that filters lymph

lymphatic vessels tubes similar in structure to veins, with thin collapsible walls and valves; responsible for transporting lymph

malignant melanoma a deeply pigmented mole which is life-threatening if it is not recognised and treated promptly

mandible only moveable bone of the skull forming the lower jaw

Manipura the solar plexus chakra, located at approximately waist level

marma points subtle pressure points that stimulate the life force or pranic flow

masseter a thick muscle in the cheek extending from the zygomatic arch to the outer corner of the mandible

mastication the process of chewing food

mastoid nodes lymph nodes located behind the ear; they drain lymph from the skin of the ear and the temporal region of the scalp

matrix (hair) area of mitotic activity of the hair cells located at the lower part of the hair bulb

maxilla largest bone of the face and forming the upper jaw

mentalis a muscle radiating from the lower lip over the centre of the chin

metacarpals five long bones in the palm of the hand

migraine specific form of headache, usually unilateral (one side of the head), associated with nausea or vomiting

milia pearly, white, hard nodules under the skin

Muladhara the base or root chakra, located at the base of the spine, concerned with issues of a physical nature

multiple sclerosis disease of the central nervous system in which the myelin sheath is destroyed and various functions become impaired

muscle tone state of partial contraction of a muscle

nasal bone small facial bone forming bridge of nose

nasalis a muscle located at the sides of the nose

occipital bone skull bone forming the back of the skull

occipital nodes lymph nodes located at the base of the skull

occipitalis a muscle found at the back of the head, attached to the occipital bone and the skin of the scalp

oculomotor nerve a mixed nerve that innervates the internal and external muscles of the eye and a muscle of the upper eyelid

oedema an abnormal swelling of body tissues due to an accumulation of fluid

orbicularis oculi a circular muscle that surrounds the eye

orbicularis oris a circular muscle that surrounds the mouth

osteoporosis brittle bones due to ageing and the lack of the hormone oestrogen, which affects the ability to deposit calcium in the matrix of bone

palatine L-shaped bones which form the anterior part of the roof of the mouth

papillary layer most superficial layer of the dermis, situated above the reticular layer

parasympathetic nervous system one of the two divisions of the autonomic nervous system; creates the conditions needed for rest and sleep

parietal bones bones forming the upper sides of the skull and the back of the roof of the skull

parotid nodes lymph nodes located at the angle of the jaw; they drain lymph from the nose, eyelids and ear

pectoralis major a thick fan-shaped muscle covering the anterior surface of the upper chest

pectoralis minor a thin muscle that lies beneath the pectoralis major

pediculosis (lice) a contagious parasitic infection, commonly known as 'lice'; the lice live off blood sucked from the skin

petrissage deeper massage movements using the whole hand, thumbs or fingers (picking up, squeezing and releasing, rolling, etc.)

pharynx (the throat) serves as an air and food passage

pitta one of the three doshas, which is said to be responsible for the process of transformation or metabolism

pityriasis capitis (dandruff) a scaly, flaking scalp condition

platysma a superficial neck muscle that extends from the chest up either side of the neck to the chin

prana the vital force (pra = before, ana = breath)

pressure points vital energy points similar to acupressure used in Chinese medicine

prickle cell layer (stratum spinosum) binding and transitional layer between the stratum granulosum (granular layer) and the stratum germinativum (basal cell layer)

procerus a muscle located in-between the eyebrows

progressive muscular relaxation a physical technique designed to relax the body when it is tense

psoriasis chronic inflammatory skin condition

radius long bone of the forearm (on thumb side of forearm)

reticular fibres fibres found in the reticular layer of dermis which help to maintain the skin's tone, strength and elasticity

reticular layer deepest layer of the dermis, situated below the papillary layer

rhomboids either of the two muscles situated in the upper part of the back, between the thoracic vertebrae and the scapula

ringworm a fungal infection of the skin

risorius a triangular-shaped muscle that lies horizontally on the cheek, joining at the corners of the mouth

rodent ulcer a malignant tumour, starts off as a slow-growing pearly nodule, often at the site of a previous skin injury

rosacea a chronic inflammatory disease of the face, making the skin appear abnormally red

Sahasrara the crown chakra located on top of the head, concerned with thinking and decision making

scapula bone forming posterior of shoulder girdle

scar a mark left on the skin after a wound has healed

sebaceous cyst a round, nodular lesion with a smooth shiny surface, which develops from a sebaceous gland

sebaceous gland small sac-like pouches found all over the body (except for the soles of the feet and the palms of the hands) producing an oily substance called sebum

seborrhoea an excessive secretion of sebum by the sebaceous glands

seborrhoeic dermatitis a mild to chronic inflammatory disease of hairy areas that are well supplied with sebaceous glands. Common sites are the scalp, face, axilla and the groin.

serratus anterior a broad curved muscle located on the side of the chest/ribcage below the axilla

sinusitis a condition involving inflammation of the paranasal sinuses

skeletal/voluntary muscle attached to the skeleton, this type of muscle tissue is striped in appearance and is responsible for the movement of bones

smooth/involuntary muscle this type of muscle tissue is found in the walls of hollow organs such as the stomach, intestines, bladder, uterus and in blood vessels

sphenoid skull bone located in front of the temporal bone

squamous cell carcinoma a malignant tumour which arises from the prickle cell layer of the epidermis

sternomastoid long muscle that lies obliquely across each side of the neck

stress any factor which affects physical or emotional health

stroke the blocking of blood flow to the brain by an embolus in a cerebral blood vessel

stye acute inflammation of a gland at the base of an eyelash, caused by bacterial infection

subcutaneous layer thick layer of connective and adipose tissue found below the dermis

submandibular nodes lymph nodes located beneath the jaw; they drain lymph from the chin, lips, nose, cheeks and tongue

superficial cervical nodes lymph nodes located at the side of the neck, they drain lymph from the lower part of the ear and the cheek region

supraspinatus muscle located in the depression above the spine of the scapula

Swadhistana the sacral chakra located at the level of the sacrum, between the navel and the base chakra

tapotement a series of light, brisk, springy movements applied with both hands in rapid succession (hacking, double hacking, tapping)

telangiecstasis the term for dilated capillaries, where there is persistent vasodilation

temporal bone forms the sides of the skull below the parietal bones and above and around the ears

temporalis a fan-shaped muscle situated on the side of the skull above and in front of the ear

temporomandibular joint tension (TMJ syndrome) a collection of symptoms and signs produced by disorders of the temporomandibular joint (the hinge joint between the mandible of the jaw and the temporal bone of the skull)

teres major a muscle that attaches to the bottom lateral edge of the scapula at one end and the back of the humerus (just below the shoulder joint) at the other

teres minor a muscle that attaches to the lateral edge of the scapula, above teres major at one end, and into the top of the posterior of the humerus at the other

thenar eminence a mound of soft tissue located on the radial side of the palm of the hand

thoracic cavity group of body parts (sternum, ribs and thoracic vertebrae) which protect the heart and lungs

thrombosis the formation of a thrombus in an unbroken blood vessel

thrombus a clot of coagulated blood that remains at its site of formation

tinea capitis a fungal infection of the scalp (a type of ringworm)

tinnitis condition where there is the sensation of sounds in the ears in the absence of an external sound source

trachea the windpipe that passes down into the thorax and connects the larynx with the bronchi

trapezius a large triangular-shaped muscle in the upper back

triangularis a triangular-shaped muscle, located below the corners of the mouth

triceps a muscle on the posterior of the upper arm

trigeminal nerve a mixed nerve (containing motor and sensory nerves)

trigeminal neuralgia a painful condition caused by irritation of the 5th cranial nerve (the trigeminal nerve)

tumour an abnormal growth of tissue, which may be benign or malignant

turbinate bone layers of bone located either side of the outer walls of the nasal cavities

ulcer a slow-healing open sore in the skin, extending to all its layers

ulna long bone of the forearm (on little finger side of forearm)

urticaria (also known as 'hives') an itchy rash resulting from the release of histamine by mast cells

vacuole empty space within the cytoplasm containing waste materials or secretions formed by the cytoplasm

vagus nerve a cranial nerve with branches to numerous organs in the thorax and abdomen as well as the neck

vata one of the three doshas, which is said to govern the principle of movement and relates to the nervous system and the body's energy centre

vesicles small sac-like blister

vibrations fine shaking, trembling or oscillating movements that are applied with one or both hands

Vishuddha the throat chakra, located at the the base of the neck

vitiligo areas of the skin lacking pigmentation

vomer single bone at the back of the nasal septum

wart a benign growth on the skin caused by the human papilloma virus

weal a raised area of skin which contains fluid and is white in the centre with a red edge

whiplash condition produced by damage to the muscles, ligaments, intervertebral discs or nerve tissues of the cervical region by sudden hyperextension and/or flexion of the neck

zygomatic major and minor muscles lying in the cheek area, extending from the zygomatic bone to the angle of the mouth

zygomatic bone facial bone forming the cheeks

Index

abdominal muscles 82
abducens nerve 77
abuse 236
accessory nerve 77
accidents 218, 226
acid mantle 17
acne vulgaris 25
actin 44, 45, 46
adrenaline 194, 195, 197
advertising see promotion and marketing
aftercare advice 187–8
age 33, 35, 201
AIDA 255
air element 2, 3
alarm stage 197
albinism 30
alcohol intake 33, 108
all-or-nothing thinking 196
allergens 24, 92
allergic reactions 24, 34, 111
almond oil 140
alopecia 89
alveoli 80
amla oil 143
anaphylactic shock 24
anatomy and physiology 16–87
  blood 61–3
  circulatory system 64–6
  lymphatic system 67–72
  muscular system 43–61
  nervous system 72–9
  respiration 80–2
  skeleton 35–43
  skin 16–34
angina 89
anguli 134
ankylosing spondylitis 90
anti-discrimination practices 235
anxiety 90
aorta 64, 65
apocrine glands 23
arm(s)
  bones 40–1
  massage techniques for 163–8, 186
  muscles 53–7
  tension in the 198
arteries 62–6
arterioles 20, 62
arthritis 91, 266
assessments 107, 123
association (mixed) neurones 72, 74
asthma 92, 111, 200
athlete's foot (tinea pedis) 29
atlas 36
attitudes 208

auras 185
autonomic nervous system 77–9
availability of IHM 11
axis 36
Ayur-Veda 2
Ayurveda 1–8
  definition 1–2
  doshas 2, 3–4, 5–8
  five elements 2–3
  perspective 3–4
  prana 4
  pressure points 134
  principals of 2
  sub-doshas 4, 5–7

back
  massage techniques for the 155–63, 185–6
  muscles 51–3
  see also spine
bacterial infections 26–7
balance 2, 5, 7–8, 13, 148–50, 169, 200
baldness 89, 154, 265
barbers 9
basal cell layer (stratum germinativum) 19
basilar artery 66
Bell's palsy 92–3
benefits of IHM 10, 11–13, 23, 189
bhringraj oil 143
biceps 53, 54
bins 219
birthmarks 24, 31
blackheads 24
blisters 25
blood 61–3
blood clotting 62
blood pressure 109
blood supply 20–1
blood vessels 62–3
body language 241
body mechanics 151–2
boils 26
bone 35–43
boundaries 114
brachial plexus 76
brachiocephalic trunk 65
brachioradialis 54, 55, 56
Brahmi oil 143
brain 13, 73–5, 200, 210
brain stem 75
breakages 218, 229
breathing
  anatomy and physiology of 80–2
  techniques 151, 203–5
brochures 253

bronchioles 80
bronchitis 93
bruises 110
buccinator 48, 50, 92, 93

cancer 31, 110
capillaries 21, 25, 63
carbon dioxide 61, 63, 64, 80
Care Standards Act 2000 238
carotid artery 65
carpals 40
cartilage 35
case studies 121–9
  components 122–3
  examples 124–9
cautions, regarding IHM practice 88–104, 107–11
cell division 19, 20
cell regeneration 20
cellular wastes 61
central nervous system 73–7
cerebellum 74
cerebral haemorrhage 100
cerebral palsy 93–4
cerebrum 74
cervical plexus 75
chairs 139
chakras 144–50
  balancing 148–50, 184
  sensations 150
  types of 145–7
champi 9, 132, 162
charity work 254
chest muscles 58–9
children 236, 237–8
Children Act 1989 237
Children (Leaving Care) Act 2000 238
chiropractors 260
chloasma 30
chopping technique 161
chronic fatigue syndrome 98–9
CIBTAC (Confederation of International Beauty Therapy and Cosmetology) 11
circular pressure technique 167
circulation boosters 12, 13, 23, 66
circulatory disorders 109
circulatory system 64–6, 67–8
City and Guilds 11
clavicle 39
clear layer (stratum lucidum) 19
client profiles 122
client requests 241–2
coccygeal plexus 76
coccyx 36, 38

coconut oil   141
codes of ethics   233–5
codes of practice   216–19, 224, 233–4
cognitive therapy   208
cold sores (herpes simplex)   27
collagen   20
comedones   24
communication skills   105–6, 218, 240–1
compression   138, 164, 180
confidentiality   106
conjunctivitis   26
consciousness   2–3
consultations   105–20
    communication skills   105–6
    confidentiality   106
    consultation forms   115–16, 122
    contraindications   107–11
    environment   106
    GP referrals   109–13
    record keeping   107
    treatment plans   117–18, 122
Consumer Protection Act 1987   231
contra-actions (adverse
        reactions)   188, 230, 231, 266
contraindications   107–11, 230–1
    localised   107, 110, 111
    requiring medical
        advice   107, 109–10, 111
    special cautions   107, 111
    total   107, 108, 111
Control of Substances Hazardous
        to Health Regulations 2002
        (COSHH)   222, 225
CORGI   225–6
corporate market   11, 257–8, 260–1
corrugator   48, 49
cortisol   79, 197, 198
cosmetic products   233, 260
Cosmetic Products (Safety)
        Regulations 2003   233
cost-effectiveness   218, 242
counter-transference   114
cranial nerves   76–7, 92, 102
cranium   41
Crime and Disorder Act 1998   237
Criminal Records Bureau   237
cross-merchandising   259
cuts   110
cysts   24, 26

damages   218, 229
dandruff (pityriasis capitis)   32, 94
Data Protection Act 1998   232–3
deeper reticular layer   20
deltoid   53, 54
demonstrations   252, 253, 258, 266
dependence   211
depression   94–5, 211
dermal papillae   20
dermatitis
    contact   31
    seborrhoeic   32, 94, 100
dermis   18, 20–1
desquamation   20
diabetes   109–10
diagnosis, dangers of making   231
diaphragm   81, 82, 203–4
digestive disorders   200
directories   258

disabled clients   152–3
doshas   2, 3–4, 5–8, 140
dryness   5

ear lobes   183
earth element   2, 3
eccrine glands   17, 22–3
eczema   32
education, client   106, 241–2
effects of IHM   11–13
effleurage
    for the body   156, 158, 161, 168
    definition   130–1
    effects of   131
    with the forearms   161
    for the head and
        neck   173–4, 178, 181, 184–5
    whole hand   174
elastic fibres   20
elderly clients   153, 235–6
Electricity at Work Regulations
        1989   222, 226
electrotherapy   93
embolism   109
emergency routes/exits   228
emphysema   93
Employers' Liability (Compulsory
        Insurance) Act 1969   232
employment standards   216–19
endocrine glands   74
endomysium   44
endorphins   13, 210
energy flow/balance   13, 144, 150
    see also prana
Environmental Protection Act 1990   229
environmental stress   208–9, 213
epidermis   18, 19–20
epilepsy   95–6, 109
epiphysis   35
equipment   139–44
erector pili muscle   22
erector spinae   51, 52
ergonomics   209, 213
erythema   24
establishment rules   216–19
ethics, codes of   233–5
ethmoid bone   42
etiquette   218
evaluations   123
excretion   17
exhalation   80–2
exhaustion   197
exhibitions   253
extensors   56–7
eye muscles   13

face
    bones of the   42
    exercises for the   93
    massage techniques for the 181–5, 187
facial nerve   77, 92
fasciculi   44
fat   17, 21, 153
fatigue   198
fever   108
fibroblasts   20
fibromyalgia   96–7
'fight or flight' reaction   194, 197
finger frictions   157–8, 170, 172, 183

finger massage   166–7, 159
finger pulls   159
fire (element)   2, 3
fire extinguishers   227–8
fire hazards   226–8
Fire Precautions (Workplace)
        Regulations 1997   226–8
first aid   224
fissures   24
five elements   2–3
flexors   54, 55, 56
folliculitis   26–7
footwear   217
foramen magnum   42
frequency of treatments   189, 265
frictions
    circular   180, 183
    definition   133
    effects of   133
    with the fingers   157–8, 170, 172, 183
    with the heel of the hand 157, 172, 180
    technique   157–8, 170, 172, 175–6,
                                         180, 183
frontal bone   41
frontalis muscle   47, 48, 93
fungal infections   28–9

Gas Safety (Installation and Use)
        Regulations 1998   222, 225–6
general adaptation syndrome   197
genetics   201
glossopharyngeal nerve   77
GPs   211, 260
    referrals   88, 109–13
granular layer (stratum granulosum)   19
growth plate   35

hacking   132, 162
haemoglobin   61, 63
haemorrhage   100, 108
hair   21–2
    colour   22
    condition   23
    curly   265
    growth   22, 23, 34
    lifespan   22
    long/thick   154, 265
    and oils   142
    structure   21–2
    therapist's   217
    types of   139
hair follicle   22
hair loss   89, 200
    see also baldness
hair tugging   138, 177, 265
hairdressers   11, 260
hand(s)
    bones of the   40–1
    massage for   166–7
    muscles of the   57
    therapist's   217
hazards   223, 225
head
    blood flow to the   65–6
    injury   108
    lymphatic drainage   71–2
    muscles of the   47–50
    tension in the   200
head lice   29

headache   97, 98, 108
healing crisis   188
health and safety   216–18, 220–9, 230–6
Health and Safety at Work
     Act 1974   220, 221, 224
Health and Safety Executive
     (HSE)   220, 224
   inspectors   225–6
Health and Safety (First Aid)
     Regulations 1981   221, 224
heart   64
heart beat   45–6
heart conditions   89, 109, 200
heel pushes   160
heel rolls   164
herpes   27, 28
Hippocratic medicine   8
histamine   20, 24
history of IHM   1–9
hives (urticaria)   32
holding position   155
holistic therapies   11, 201–2, 211
hormones   33, 34, 61
horny layer (stratum corneum)   19–20
Human Rights Act 1998   238
humerus   40
hygiene   151, 217, 219–20
hyperhidrosis   26
hypertrophic disorders   31
hypoglossal nerve   77
hypothalamus   74
hypothenar eminence   57

imagery   206
imbalance   2, 5–8, 144, 146–7, 169
immune system   198
impetigo   27
indications, for IHM treatment   121
infections   26–9, 108
infestations   29–30
inflammation   12, 31–2
information provision   241–2, 106
infraspinatus   51, 53
inhalation   80, 81, 82, 203–4
insulin therapy   110
insurance   232
intercalated discs   45
intercostal muscles   81–2, 203–4
Internet advertising   258–9
intoxication   108
ITEC (International Beauty Therapy
     Education Council)   11

jaw bone   42
jewellery   217, 220, 230
jugular vein   66
jumping to conclusions   196

kapha   2, 3, 4, 7–8
keloid scars   24, 25
keratin   21, 22
keratinisation   19, 20
kneading technique   165, 166
Kundalini energy   150
kyphosis   60, 90, 97–8

lacrimal bones   42
large-framed clients   153

laundry   219
leaflets   253
lesions   24
levator labii superiorus   48, 50
levator scapula   51, 52
lice (pediculosis)   29
lifting   224
listening skills   105–6, 241
liver spots (lentigo)   30
local authority bye-laws   226
Local Government (Miscellaneous
     Provisions) Act 1982   232
lordosis   60
loyalty bonuses   259
lumbar plexus   76
lumps, undiagnosed   111
lungs   80, 81–2, 200
lymph   67, 68
lymphatic drainage   12, 68, 71–2
lymphatic system   21, 67–72
lymphocytes   62, 67, 70

macrophages   70
macules   24
magazines   253, 254, 256
mailshots   257
maintenance   229
male clients   154, 260
malignant melanoma   31
Management of Health and Safety at
     Work Regulations 1999   221, 222–3
mandible   42
Manual Handling Operations
     Regulations 1992   221, 224
marketing see promotion and marketing
marma points   134–8
masseter muscle   48, 50
mast cells   20
maxillae   42
medication   33, 34, 111
meditation   206
medulla oblongata   75
melanin   19, 22
melanocytes   17, 19, 22
melatonin   74
menopause   33, 34
menstruation   33, 34
mental filters   196
mentalis muscle   48, 50
metacarpals   41
mid-brain   75
migraine   98, 108
milia   24
minerals   34
minors   236, 237–8
mitosis   19, 20
moles   24
motor neurones   72, 74
multiple sclerosis   99
muscular relaxation   12
muscular spasticity   94
muscular system   43–61
   arms/hands   53–7
   back and shoulders   51–3
   cardiac muscle   44, 45–6
   chest area   58–9, 81–2
   functions   43–4
   head/scalp/neck   47–50

muscle tissue   44–7
muscle tone   47
   and posture   59–61
   skeletal/voluntary muscle   43–5
   smooth/involuntary muscle   44, 46
muscular tension   59, 73, 198–200
music   232, 260
mustard oil   142
myalgic encephalomyelitis   98–9
myelin   99
myofibrils   44
myosin   44, 45, 46

naevi   24, 31
nasal bones   42
nasalis muscle   48, 49
National Care Standards Commission 238
National Occupational Standards   11
neck
   blood flow   65–6
   cervical vertebrae   36, 37, 39
   injury/conditions   102–3, 108, 266
   lymphatic drainage   71–2
   massage techniques
      for the   169–74, 186–7
   muscles   48–50
   tension in the   199
neem oil   143
negative thoughts   208
nerve cells (neurones)   72
nerves   21, 75–7
nervous system   72–9
   disorders of the   109
neuralgia   102
newspapers   253, 254, 255–6, 261
nutrients   61
nutrition   33, 34, 61, 89, 201, 209

observations   122
occipital bone   41, 42
occipitalis muscle   47, 48
oculomotor nerve   76
oils   9, 139–44
   aftercare advice   187–8
   allergic reactions to   111
   application   144, 154, 265
   essential   143
   preparation   151
   and skin conditions   89, 99
   suppliers   265
   types of   140–3
   washing out the hair   187
olfactory nerve   76
olive oil   141, 142
optic nerve   76
orbicularis oculi   48, 49, 93
ossification   35
osteoarthritis   91, 266
osteoblasts   35
osteopaths   260
osteoporosis   110
oxygen   61–4, 80

pain   75, 198
palatine bones   42
palliative care   110
papules   24
parasympathetic nervous
     system   12, 77, 78, 79

parietal bones 41
payment 218, 224, 230
pectorals 58, 82
Performing Rights Act (under Copyright
        Designs and Patents Act 1988) 232
Performing Rights Society (PRS) 232
perimysium 44
peripheral nervous system 73, 75–6
personal appearance 217
personal belongings 218, 230
personal hygiene 217
Personal Protective Equipment at Work
        Regulations 1992 (PPE) 221, 224
personality 194, 251–2
petrissage 131, 156–7
    see also compression
phagocytes 20, 62
phalanges 41
Phonographic Performance Ltd 232
physical exercise 33, 210
physiology see anatomy and physiology
pineal gland 74
pitta 2–4, 6–8, 140
pituitary gland 74
plasma 61, 67
platysma muscle 48, 49
plexus 75–6
pollution 229
pons 75
portwine stain 31
positive thinking 208
posture 59–61, 151–2, 198–9
prana 4, 134, 138
pregnancy 9, 33–4, 111, 152
preparation for treatment 150–4
press releases 254
pressure points 134–8
    effects of 134
    marma points 134–8
    massage techniques
        for 158, 173, 179, 182
pricing 250
prickle cell layer (stratum spinosum) 19
procerus muscle 48, 49
products 233, 250, 260
professional conduct 217
progressive muscular relaxation 205–6
promotion and marketing 247–64, 266
    direct 252–4
    indirect 254–60
    keeping ahead with 262
    market research 247–9, 263
    needs 249
    objectives 261
    and personality selling 251–2
    plans 249–51, 261, 264
    and referral networks 253–4
    and repeat business 262
    and target markets 249
promotional material 256–7, 259, 261
promotions 260
pronation 40
Protection of Children Act 1999 237
protective legislation 235–8
psoriasis 32, 99–100
puberty 33
public relations 253–4
publications 258

pulmonary circulation 62, 64
pumpkin seed oil 143
pustules 25

quality assurance 242
questionnaires 248–9, 263

Race Relations Act 1976 (RRA) 235
radio advertising 259
radius 40
record keeping 107, 123, 189, 218, 230,
        232–4, 241
red blood cells (erythrocytes) 61
referral networks 253–4
referrals 88, 109–10, 111, 112–14
relationships 210
relaxation techniques 203–8
repeat business 259, 262
Reporting of Injuries, Diseases and
        Dangerous Occurrences
        Regulations 1995 (RIDDOR) 222, 226
reproductive disorders 200
reputation 252
resistance stage 197
respiration 13, 80–2
responsibilities, professional 238–42
retention of clients 259, 262
reticular fibres 20
rhomboids 51, 52
ribs 38, 39
ringworm 28–9
risk assessment 222, 223, 225
risorius muscle 48, 50
rocking the neck technique 169
rodent ulcers 31
rosacea 26
rubbing technique 176
ruffling technique 177

sacral plexus 76
sacrum 36, 38
Sale and Supply of Goods Act 1994 231
salon resources 219
scabies 30
scalp
    circulation boosters 13
    conditions 29, 94, 99–100, 108
    massage techniques
        for the 175–81, 187, 265
    muscles 47–8
scapula 39
scars 24, 25, 110
scoliosis 60–1
sebaceous cysts 26
sebaceous glands 17, 23, 25–6
seborrhoea 26
sebum 13, 17, 23
security 216, 218, 229–30
sedentary lifestyle 198
seizures 95–6
self-evaluation 123
Selye, Hans 197
semipermeable membranes 63
sensation 17
senses 2
sensory neurones 72, 74
sensory pathways 75
serotonin 79, 95

serratus anterior 58, 59, 82
service maintenance 238–42
services 250
sesame oil 141
Sex Discrimination Act 1975 (SDA) 235
Sex Offenders Act 1997 237
shikakai oil 143
shingles (herpes zoster) 28
shoulder lift 168
shoulder(s)
    bones 39
    frozen (adhesive capsulitis) 96–7
    massage techniques for 154–63, 185–6
    mobilization 165
    muscles 51–3
    tension in the 198
    see also back and shoulder muscles
sinoatrial node 45–6
sinuses 42–3
sinusitis 100
skeleton 35–43
    bone development 35
    bone structure 35
    bone types 35–6
    shoulder bones 39
    skull 41–3
    thoracic cavity 38–9
    upper limb bones 40–1
    vertebrae 36–8
skin 16–34
    appendages 21–3
    circulation boosters 23
    condition of 23
    factors affecting the 33
    functions of the 16–17
    structure 18–21
    terminology 24–5
    types of 6
skin cancer 31
skin conditions/disorders 24–32, 110, 200
skin pigmentation disorders 30
skin tags 25
skull 41–3
sleep 33, 201
small clients 153
smoking 33
space (ether) 2, 3
sphenoid bone 41, 42
spider naevi 31
spillages 229
spinal cord 75
spinal nerves 75
spine
    disorders of the 60–1, 90, 97–8, 110
    vertebrae 36–8
squamous cell carcinoma 31
squeezing technique 159–60, 163, 165–6,
        170–1, 179, 183, 185
starting position 155
sternomastoid muscle 48, 49, 82
sternum 38
stock 219, 230
strawberry marks 31
streptococci 27
stress 59, 193–201
    adaptations to 201
    attitude to 208
    definition 193–4

stress (continued)
effects of 195–200
optimum levels 202
recognition 195–7, 213
and the skin 33
types of 194
stress diaries 202, 213
stress hormones 79, 194–5, 197–8
stress management 10, 193, 201–14
5-minute stress reliever 206–7
action plan 202–3
experience in 212
IHM's role in 211, 213–14
and nutrition 202, 209
and physical exercise 210
and relationships 210
relaxation techniques for 203–8
and time management 211–12
and time out 210, 213
in the workplace 194, 206–7, 212–14
stress-related disorders 200
stretching 174
stroke 100–1
styes 27
sub-doshas 4, 5–7
subclavian artery 65
subcutaneous layer 18, 21
suicidal thoughts 95
superficial papillary layer 20
supination 40
supraspinatus 51, 52
surgery 110
surveys 248–9
survival stress 194, 195
sweat glands 17, 22–3, 26
sweating, excessive 26
SWOT analysis 250–1
sycosis barbae 27
sympathetic nervous system 12, 77–9
systemic circulation 64

tabla playing 132, 178
talks 252, 253, 259
tapotement 132
see also champi; hacking; tabla playing
techniques 130–92
adaptations 152–4
for the arms 163–8, 186
and the chakras 144–50
equipment for 139–44

for the face 181–5, 187
massage movements 130–8
for the neck 169–74, 186–7
preparation for 150–4
quick guide to 185–7
for the scalp 175–81, 187, 265
for the shoulders 154–63, 185–6
telangiecstasis 25
temperature regulation 17, 62
temporal bones 41
temporalis muscle 47, 48
temporomandibular joint tension
(TMJ) 101
teres major/minor 51, 53
thalamus 74
thenar eminence 57
thoracic cavity 38–9, 81–2
thoracic duct 71
thrombocytes (platelets) 61, 62
thrombosis 109
thumb pushes 158–9, 171
thumb sweeping 156–7
thyroid problems 34
time of day, treatment 117
time management 211–12, 242
time out 210, 213
tinea 28–9
tinnitis 101–2
tissue fluid 67
towels 139
Trade Description Act 1968 231–2
transference 114
trapezius 51, 52, 156, 158, 160
treatment plans 117–18, 122
example 124, 126, 128
triangularis muscle 50
triceps 54
trigeminal nerve 77, 102
trochlear nerve 76
tumours 25
turbinate bones 42

ulcers 25, 31
ulna 40
ultraviolet (UV) radiation 17
uniforms 217, 224

vagus nerve 77
vasoconstriction 17
vasodilatation 13, 17, 24

vata 2–5, 8, 140
vayus 4, 5–6
veins 62–3, 66
ventricles 64
venules 21, 63
verrucae 28
vertebrae 36–8
cervical 36, 37, 39
lumbar 36, 37, 38
thoracic 36, 37
vertebral artery 65–6
vertebral vein 66
vesicles 25
vestibulocochlear nerve 77
vibrations 133
viral infections 27–8
visualisation 149, 206
vitamins 17, 33–4
vitiligo 30
vomer 42
VTCT (Vocational Training Charitable
Trust) 11

warts 25, 28
waste 229, 242
water element 2, 3
water intake 33
weals 25, 32
wheelchair-bound clients 153
whiplash 102–3
white blood cells
(leucocytes) 20, 61, 62, 70
whiteheads 24
word of mouth 252
work colleagues 239–40, 241
workplace 209, 213, 219
IHM in the 11, 257–8, 260–1
stress management
in the 194, 206–7, 212–14
wrist 40
written communication 241
written testimonials 123, 125, 127, 129

yin and yang 8
Youth Justice and Criminal Evidence
Act 1999 237

zygomatic bone 42
zygomatic muscle 48, 50

Electrical and Electronic Principles and Technology

To Sue

Electrical and Electronic Principles and Technology

Fourth edition

John Bird, BSc (Hons), CEng, CSci, CMath, MIEE, FIIE, FIET, FIMA, FCollT

ELSEVIER

AMSTERDAM • BOSTON • HEIDELBERG • LONDON • NEW YORK • OXFORD
PARIS • SAN DIEGO • SAN FRANCISCO • SINGAPORE • SYDNEY • TOKYO
Newnes is an imprint of Elsevier

Newnes

Newnes is an imprint of Elsevier
The Boulevard, Langford Lane, Kidlington, Oxford OX5 1GB, UK
30 Corporate Drive, Suite 400, Burlington, MA 01803, USA

First edition 2000 previously published as *Electrical Principles and Technology for Engineering*
Reprinted 2001
Second edition 2003
Reprinted 2004, 2005, 2006
Third edition 2007
Fourth edition 2010
Reprinted 2011

British Library Cataloguing-in-Publication Data
A catalogue record for this book is available from the British Library.

Library of Congress Cataloging-in-Publication Data
A catalogue record for this book is available from the Library of Congress.

ISBN: 978-0-08-089056-2

For information on all Newnes publications
visit our Web site at *www.elsevierdirect.com*

Typeset by: diacriTech, India

Printed and bound in China
11 12 13 14   10 9 8 7 6 5 4 3 2

Contents

Preface   ix

| Section 1 | Basic Electrical and Electronic Engineering Principles | 1 |

1   Units associated with basic electrical quantities   3
    1.1   SI units   3
    1.2   Charge   4
    1.3   Force   4
    1.4   Work   4
    1.5   Power   4
    1.6   Electrical potential and e.m.f.   5
    1.7   Resistance and conductance   5
    1.8   Electrical power and energy   6
    1.9   Summary of terms, units and their symbols   7

2   An introduction to electric circuits   9
    2.1   Electrical/electronic system block diagrams   9
    2.2   Standard symbols for electrical components   10
    2.3   Electric current and quantity of electricity   11
    2.4   Potential difference and resistance   11
    2.5   Basic electrical measuring instruments   12
    2.6   Linear and non-linear devices   12
    2.7   Ohm's law   13
    2.8   Multiples and sub-multiples   13
    2.9   Conductors and insulators   15
    2.10   Electrical power and energy   15
    2.11   Main effects of electric current   17
    2.12   Fuses   18
    2.13   Insulation and the dangers of constant high current flow   18

3   Resistance variation   21
    3.1   Resistor construction   21
    3.2   Resistance and resistivity   21
    3.3   Temperature coefficient of resistance   24
    3.4   Resistor colour coding and ohmic values   26

4   Batteries and alternative sources of energy   30
    4.1   Introduction to batteries   30
    4.2   Some chemical effects of electricity   31
    4.3   The simple cell   31

    4.4   Corrosion   32
    4.5   E.m.f. and internal resistance of a cell   32
    4.6   Primary cells   35
    4.7   Secondary cells   36
    4.8   Cell capacity   38
    4.9   Safe disposal of batteries   38
    4.10   Fuel cells   38
    4.11   Alternative and renewable energy sources   39

| Revision Test 1 | 42 |

5   Series and parallel networks   43
    5.1   Series circuits   43
    5.2   Potential divider   44
    5.3   Parallel networks   46
    5.4   Current division   49
    5.5   Loading effect   53
    5.6   Potentiometers and rheostats   53
    5.7   Relative and absolute voltages   56
    5.8   Earth potential and short circuits   57
    5.9   Wiring lamps in series and in parallel   57

6   Capacitors and capacitance   61
    6.1   Introduction to capacitors   61
    6.2   Electrostatic field   62
    6.3   Electric field strength   62
    6.4   Capacitance   63
    6.5   Capacitors   63
    6.6   Electric flux density   64
    6.7   Permittivity   64
    6.8   The parallel plate capacitor   66
    6.9   Capacitors connected in parallel and series   67
    6.10   Dielectric strength   72
    6.11   Energy stored in capacitors   72
    6.12   Practical types of capacitor   73
    6.13   Discharging capacitors   75

7   Magnetic circuits   77
    7.1   Introduction to magnetism and magnetic circuits   77
    7.2   Magnetic fields   78
    7.3   Magnetic flux and flux density   78
    7.4   Magnetomotive force and magnetic field strength   79
    7.5   Permeability and B–H curves   80

7.6	Reluctance	83
7.7	Composite series magnetic circuits	83
7.8	Comparison between electrical and magnetic quantities	87
7.9	Hysteresis and hysteresis loss	87

Revision Test 2   **90**

8 Electromagnetism   **91**
8.1	Magnetic field due to an electric current	91
8.2	Electromagnets	93
8.3	Force on a current-carrying conductor	94
8.4	Principle of operation of a simple d.c. motor	97
8.5	Principle of operation of a moving-coil instrument	98
8.6	Force on a charge	99

9 Electromagnetic induction   **101**
9.1	Introduction to electromagnetic induction	101
9.2	Laws of electromagnetic induction	102
9.3	Rotation of a loop in a magnetic field	105
9.4	Inductance	106
9.5	Inductors	107
9.6	Energy stored	108
9.7	Inductance of a coil	108
9.8	Mutual inductance	110

10 Electrical measuring instruments and measurements   **114**
10.1	Introduction	115
10.2	Analogue instruments	115
10.3	Moving-iron instrument	115
10.4	The moving-coil rectifier instrument	116
10.5	Comparison of moving-coil, moving-iron and moving-coil rectifier instruments	116
10.6	Shunts and multipliers	116
10.7	Electronic instruments	118
10.8	The ohmmeter	119
10.9	Multimeters	119
10.10	Wattmeters	119
10.11	Instrument 'loading' effect	119
10.12	The oscilloscope	121
10.13	Virtual test and measuring instruments	126
10.14	Virtual digital storage oscilloscopes	127
10.15	Waveform harmonics	130
10.16	Logarithmic ratios	131
10.17	Null method of measurement	134
10.18	Wheatstone bridge	134
10.19	D.C. potentiometer	135
10.20	A.C. bridges	136
10.21	Q-meter	137
10.22	Measurement errors	138

11 Semiconductor diodes   **143**
11.1	Types of material	143
11.2	Semiconductor materials	144
11.3	Conduction in semiconductor materials	145
11.4	The p-n junction	146
11.5	Forward and reverse bias	147
11.6	Semiconductor diodes	150
11.7	Characteristics and maximum ratings	151
11.8	Rectification	151
11.9	Zener diodes	151
11.10	Silicon controlled rectifiers	152
11.11	Light emitting diodes	153
11.12	Varactor diodes	153
11.13	Schottky diodes	153

12 Transistors   **157**
12.1	Transistor classification	157
12.2	Bipolar junction transistors (BJT)	158
12.3	Transistor action	158
12.4	Leakage current	159
12.5	Bias and current flow	160
12.6	Transistor operating configurations	161
12.7	Bipolar transistor characteristics	161
12.8	Transistor parameters	162
12.9	Current gain	164
12.10	Typical BJT characteristics and maximum ratings	164
12.11	Field effect transistors	166
12.12	Field effect transistor characteristics	166
12.13	Typical FET characteristics and maximum ratings	168
12.14	Transistor amplifiers	168
12.15	Load lines	171

Revision Test 3   **178**

Formulae for basic electrical and electronic principles   **179**

Section 2   Further Electrical and Electronic Principles   **181**

13 D.C. circuit theory   **183**
13.1	Introduction	183
13.2	Kirchhoff's laws	183
13.3	The superposition theorem	187
13.4	General d.c. circuit theory	190
13.5	Thévenin's theorem	192
13.6	Constant-current source	197
13.7	Norton's theorem	197

13.8   Thévenin and Norton equivalent networks   200
13.9   Maximum power transfer theorem   204

14 Alternating voltages and currents   209
14.1   Introduction   209
14.2   The a.c. generator   209
14.3   Waveforms   210
14.4   A.C. values   211
14.5   Electrical safety – insulation and fuses   215
14.6   The equation of a sinusoidal waveform   215
14.7   Combination of waveforms   218
14.8   Rectification   221
14.9   Smoothing of the rectified output
         waveform   222

Revision Test 4   225

15 Single-phase series a.c. circuits   226
15.1   Purely resistive a.c. circuit   226
15.2   Purely inductive a.c. circuit   226
15.3   Purely capacitive a.c. circuit   227
15.4 R–L series a.c. circuit   229
15.5 R–C series a.c. circuit   232
15.6 R–L–C series a.c. circuit   234
15.7   Series resonance   238
15.8   Q-factor   239
15.9   Bandwidth and selectivity   241
15.10 Power in a.c. circuits   241
15.11 Power triangle and power factor   242

16 Single-phase parallel a.c. circuits   247
16.1   Introduction   247
16.2 R–L parallel a.c. circuit   247
16.3 R–C parallel a.c. circuit   248
16.4 L–C parallel circuit   250
16.5 LR–C parallel a.c. circuit   251
16.6   Parallel resonance and Q-factor   254
16.7   Power factor improvement   258

17 Filter networks   266
17.1   Introduction   266
17.2   Two-port networks and characteristic
         impedance   266
17.3   Low-pass filters   267
17.4   High-pass filters   270
17.5   Band-pass filters   274
17.6   Band-stop filters   275

18 D.C. transients   278
18.1   Introduction   278
18.2   Charging a capacitor   278
18.3   Time constant for a C–R circuit   279
18.4   Transient curves for a C–R circuit   280
18.5   Discharging a capacitor   283
18.6   Camera flash   286

18.7   Current growth in an L–R circuit   286
18.8   Time constant for an L–R circuit   287
18.9   Transient curves for an L–R circuit   287
18.10 Current decay in an L–R circuit   288
18.11 Switching inductive circuits   291
18.12 The effects of time constant on a
         rectangular waveform   291

19 Operational amplifiers   295
19.1   Introduction to operational amplifiers   295
19.2   Some op amp parameters   297
19.3   Op amp inverting amplifier   298
19.4   Op amp non-inverting amplifier   300
19.5   Op amp voltage-follower   301
19.6   Op amp summing amplifier   302
19.7   Op amp voltage comparator   303
19.8   Op amp integrator   303
19.9   Op amp differential amplifier   304
19.10 Digital to analogue (D/A) conversion   306
19.11 Analogue to digital (A/D) conversion   307

Revision Test 5   311

**Formulae for further electrical and electronic
principles   312**

Section 3   Electrical Power Technology   315

20 Three-phase systems   317
20.1   Introduction   317
20.2   Three-phase supply   317
20.3   Star connection   318
20.4   Delta connection   321
20.5   Power in three-phase systems   323
20.6   Measurement of power in three-phase
         systems   325
20.7   Comparison of star and delta connections   330
20.8   Advantages of three-phase systems   330

21 Transformers   333
21.1   Introduction   333
21.2   Transformer principle of operation   334
21.3   Transformer no-load phasor diagram   336
21.4   E.m.f. equation of a transformer   337
21.5   Transformer on-load phasor diagram   339
21.6   Transformer construction   341
21.7   Equivalent circuit of a transformer   341
21.8   Regulation of a transformer   343
21.9   Transformer losses and efficiency   344
21.10 Resistance matching   347
21.11 Auto transformers   349
21.12 Isolating transformers   351
21.13 Three-phase transformers   351

21.14 Current transformers   352
21.15 Voltage transformers   354

Revision Test 6   **357**

22 D.C. machines   358
22.1   Introduction   358
22.2   The action of a commutator   358
22.3   D.C. machine construction   359
22.4   Shunt, series and compound windings   360
22.5   E.m.f. generated in an armature winding 360
22.6   D.C. generators   362
22.7   Types of d.c. generator and their
       characteristics   362
22.8   D.C. machine losses   366
22.9   Efficiency of a d.c. generator   367
22.10 D.C. motors   368
22.11 Torque of a d.c. motor   368
22.12 Types of d.c. motor and their
       characteristics   370
22.13 The efficiency of a d.c. motor   374
22.14 D.C. motor starter   376
22.15 Speed control of d.c. motors   377
22.16 Motor cooling   379

23 Three-phase induction motors   383
23.1   Introduction   383
23.2   Production of a rotating magnetic field 384
23.3   Synchronous speed   385
23.4   Construction of a three-phase induction
       motor   386
23.5   Principle of operation of a three-phase
       induction motor   387
23.6   Slip   387
23.7   Rotor e.m.f. and frequency   388
23.8   Rotor impedance and current   389
23.9   Rotor copper loss   390

23.10 Induction motor losses and efficiency   390
23.11 Torque equation for an induction motor 392
23.12 Induction motor torque-speed
       characteristics   395
23.13 Starting methods for induction motors   396
23.14 Advantages of squirrel-cage
       induction motors   396
23.15 Advantages of wound rotor
       induction motors   397
23.16 Double cage induction motor   397
23.17 Uses of three-phase induction motors   398

Revision Test 7   **401**

Formulae for electrical power technology   **402**

Section 4   Laboratory Experiments   **403**

24 Some practical laboratory experiments   405
24.1   Ohm's law   406
24.2   Series-parallel d.c. circuit   407
24.3   Superposition theorem   408
24.4   Thévenin's theorem   410
24.5   Use of a CRO to measure voltage,
       frequency and phase   412
24.6   Use of a CRO with a bridge rectifier
       circuit   413
24.7   Measurement of the inductance of a coil 414
24.8   Series a.c. circuit and resonance   415
24.9   Parallel a.c. circuit and resonance   417
24.10 Charging and discharging a capacitor   419

Answers to multiple-choice questions   **420**

Index   423

Preface

'Electrical and Electronic Principles and Technology 4th Edition' introduces the principles which describe the operation of d.c. and a.c. circuits, covering both steady and transient states, and applies these principles to filter networks, operational amplifiers, three-phase supplies, transformers, d.c. machines and three-phase induction motors.

In this edition, new material has been added on resistor construction, the loading effect of instruments, potentiometers and rheostats, earth potential and short circuits, and electrical safety with insulation and fuses. In addition, a new chapter detailing some **10 practical laboratory experiments** has been included. (These may be downloaded and edited by tutors to suit local availability of equipment and components).

This fourth edition of the textbook provides coverage of the following latest syllabuses:

(i)   **'Electrical and Electronic Principles'** (BTEC National Certificate and National Diploma, Unit 5) – see Chapters 1–10, 11(part), 13 (part), 14, 15 (part), 18(part), 21(part), 22(part).

(ii) **'Further Electrical Principles'** (BTEC National Certificate and National Diploma, Unit 67) – see Chapters 13, 15–18, 20, 22, 23.

(iii) Parts of the following BTEC National syllabuses: Electrical Applications, Three Phase Systems, Principles and Applications of Electronic Devices and Circuits, Aircraft Electrical Machines, and Telecommunications Principles.

(iv) Electrical part of 'Applied Electrical and Mechanical Science for Technicians' (BTEC First Certificate).

(v)   Various parts of City & Guilds Technician Certificate/Diploma in Electrical and Electronic Principles/Telecommunication Systems, such as Electrical Engineering Principles, Power, and Science and Electronics.

(vi) 'Electrical and Electronic Principles' (EAL Advanced Diploma in Engineering and Technology).

(vii) Any introductory/Access/Foundation course involving Electrical and Electronic Engineering Principles.

The **text** is set out in four main sections:

Section 1, comprising Chapters 1 to 12, involves essential **Basic Electrical and Electronic Engineering Principles**, with chapters on electrical units and quantities, introduction to electric circuits, resistance variation, batteries and alternative sources of energy, series and parallel networks, capacitors and capacitance, magnetic circuits, electromagnetism, electromagnetic induction, electrical measuring instruments and measurements, semiconductors diodes and transistors.

Section 2, comprising Chapters 13 to 19, involves **Further Electrical and Electronic Principles,** with chapters on d.c. circuit theorems, alternating voltages and currents, single-phase series and parallel networks, filter networks, d.c. transients and operational amplifiers.

Section 3, comprising Chapters 20 to 23, involves **Electrical Power Technology**, with chapters on three-phase systems, transformers, d.c. machines and three-phase induction motors.

Section 4, comprising Chapter 24, detailing **10 practical laboratory experiments**.

Each topic considered in the text is presented in a way that assumes in the reader little previous knowledge of that topic. Theory is introduced in each chapter by a reasonably brief outline of essential information, definitions, formulae, procedures, etc. The theory is kept to a minimum, for problem solving is extensively used to establish and exemplify the theory. It is intended that readers will gain real understanding through seeing problems solved and then through solving similar problems themselves.

To aid tutors/lecturers/instructors, the following **free Internet downloads** are available with this edition (see page x for access details):

(i)   a **sample of solutions** (some 410) of the 540 further problems contained in the book.

(ii)   an **Instructors guide** detailing full worked solutions for the **Revision Tests**.

(iii) **10 practical laboratory experiments**, which may be edited.

(iv)   **Suggested lesson plans for BTEC units 5 and 67**, together with **Practise Examination questions (with solution)** for revision purposes.

(v)   a **PowerPoint presentation of all 538 illustrations** contained in the text.

'Electrical and Electronic Principles and Technology 4th Edition' contains **410 worked problems**, together with **341 multi-choice questions** (with answers at the back of the book). Also included are over **455 short answer questions**, the answers for which can be determined from the preceding material in that particular chapter, and some **540 further questions**, arranged in **146 Exercises**, all with answers, in brackets, immediately following each question; the Exercises appear at regular intervals - every 3 or 4 pages - throughout the text. **538 line diagrams** further enhance the understanding of the theory. All of the problems - multi-choice, short answer and further questions - mirror practical situations found in electrical and electronic engineering.

At regular intervals throughout the text are seven **Revision Tests** to check understanding. For example, Revision Test 1 covers material contained in Chapters 1 to 4, Revision Test 2 covers the material contained in Chapters 5 to 7, and so on. These Revision Tests do not have answers given since it is envisaged that lecturers/instructors could set the Tests for students to attempt as part of their course structure. Lecturers/instructors may obtain a free Internet download of full solutions of the Revision Tests in an **Instructor's Manual** – see next column.

A list of relevant **formulae** are included at the end of each of the three sections of the book.

'Learning by Example' is at the heart of 'Electrical and Electronic Principles and Technology 4th Edition'.

JOHN BIRD
Royal Naval School of Marine Engineering,
HMS Sultan,
formerly University of Portsmouth
and Highbury College, Portsmouth

Free web downloads

A suite of five sets of support material is available to tutors/lecturers/instructors - only from Elsevier's textbook website.

To access material, please go to *http://www.booksite.elsevier.com/newnes/bird*, find the correct title, and click on to whichever of the following resource materials you need.

(i) Solutions manual

Within the text there are some 540 further problems arranged within 146 Exercises. A sample of about 410 worked solutions has been prepared for lecturers.

(ii) Instructor's manual

This manual provides full worked solutions and mark scheme for all 7 Revision Tests in this book.

(iii) Laboratory Experiments

In Chapter 24, 10 practical laboratory experiments are included. It maybe that tutors will want to edit these experiments to suit their own equipment/component availability. These have been made available on the website.

(iv) Lesson Plans and revision material

Typical 30-week lesson plans for 'Electrical and Electronic Principles', Unit 5, and 'Further Electrical Principles', Unit 67 are included, together with two practise examinations question papers (with solutions) for each of the modules.

(v) Illustrations

Lecturers can download electronic files for all 538 illustrations in this fourth edition.

Section 1

Basic Electrical and Electronic Engineering Principles

Chapter 1

Units associated with basic electrical quantities

At the end of this chapter you should be able to:

- state the basic SI units
- recognize derived SI units
- understand prefixes denoting multiplication and division
- state the units of charge, force, work and power and perform simple calculations involving these units
- state the units of electrical potential, e.m.f., resistance, conductance, power and energy and perform simple calculations involving these units

1.1 SI units

The system of units used in engineering and science is the Système Internationale d'Unités (International system of units), usually abbreviated to SI units, and is based on the metric system. This was introduced in 1960 and is now adopted by the majority of countries as the official system of measurement.

The basic units in the SI system are listed below with their symbols:

Quantity	Unit
length	metre, m
mass	kilogram, kg
time	second, s
electric current	ampere, A
thermodynamic temperature	kelvin, K
luminous intensity	candela, cd
amount of substance	mole, mol

Derived SI units use combinations of basic units and there are many of them. Two examples are:

Velocity – metres per second (m/s)

Acceleration – metres per second squared (m/s^2)

SI units may be made larger or smaller by using prefixes which denote multiplication or division by a particular amount. The six most common multiples, with their meaning, are listed below:

Prefix	Name	Meaning
M	mega	multiply by $1\,000\,000$ (i.e. $\times 10^6$)
k	kilo	multiply by 1000 (i.e. $\times 10^3$)
m	milli	divide by 1000 (i.e. $\times 10^{-3}$)
μ	micro	divide by $1\,000\,000$ (i.e. $\times 10^{-6}$)
n	nano	divide by $1\,000\,000\,000$ (i.e. $\times 10^{-9}$)
p	pico	divide by $1\,000\,000\,000\,000$ (i.e. $\times 10^{-12}$)

DOI: 10.1016/B978-0-08-089056-2.00001-2

1.2 Charge

The **unit of charge** is the coulomb (C) where one coulomb is one ampere second (1 coulomb $= 6.24 \times 10^{18}$ electrons). The coulomb is defined as the quantity of electricity which flows past a given point in an electric circuit when a current of one ampere is maintained for one second. Thus,

$$\text{charge, in coulombs} \quad Q = It$$

where I is the current in amperes and t is the time in seconds.

Problem 1. If a current of 5 A flows for 2 minutes, find the quantity of electricity transferred.

Quantity of electricity $Q = It$ coulombs

$$I = 5\,\text{A}, t = 2 \times 60 = 120\,\text{s}$$

Hence $Q = 5 \times 120 = \mathbf{600\,C}$

1.3 Force

The **unit of force** is the **newton (N)** where one newton is one kilogram metre per second squared. The newton is defined as the force which, when applied to a mass of one kilogram, gives it an acceleration of one metre per second squared. Thus,

$$\text{force, in newtons} \quad F = ma$$

where m is the mass in kilograms and a is the acceleration in metres per second squared. Gravitational force, or weight, is mg, where $g = 9.81\,\text{m/s}^2$.

Problem 2. A mass of 5000 g is accelerated at $2\,\text{m/s}^2$ by a force. Determine the force needed.

Force = mass × acceleration

$$= 5\,\text{kg} \times 2\,\text{m/s}^2 = 10\,\text{kg m/s}^2 = \mathbf{10\,N}.$$

Problem 3. Find the force acting vertically downwards on a mass of 200 g attached to a wire.

Mass $= 200\,\text{g} = 0.2\,\text{kg}$ and acceleration due to gravity, $g = 9.81\,\text{m/s}^2$

$$\left. \begin{array}{l} \text{Force acting} \\ \text{downwards} \end{array} \right\} = \text{weight}$$

$$= \text{mass} \times \text{acceleration}$$

$$= 0.2\,\text{kg} \times 9.81\,\text{m/s}^2$$

$$= \mathbf{1.962\,N}$$

1.4 Work

The **unit of work or energy** is the **joule (J)** where one joule is one newton metre. The joule is defined as the work done or energy transferred when a force of one newton is exerted through a distance of one metre in the direction of the force. Thus

$$\text{work done on a body, in joules,} \quad W = Fs$$

where F is the force in newtons and s is the distance in metres moved by the body in the direction of the force. Energy is the capacity for doing work.

1.5 Power

The **unit of power** is the watt (W) where one watt is one joule per second. Power is defined as the rate of doing work or transferring energy. Thus,

$$\text{power, in watts,} \quad P = \frac{W}{t}$$

where W is the work done or energy transferred, in joules, and t is the time, in seconds. Thus,

$$\text{energy, in joules,} \quad W = Pt$$

Problem 4. A portable machine requires a force of 200 N to move it. How much work is done if the machine is moved 20 m and what average power is utilized if the movement takes 25 s?

Work done = force × distance

$$= 200\,\text{N} \times 20\,\text{m}$$

$$= \mathbf{4\,000\,Nm\ or\ 4\,kJ}$$

$$\text{Power} = \frac{\text{work done}}{\text{time taken}}$$

$$= \frac{4000\,\text{J}}{25\,\text{s}} = \mathbf{160\,J/s} = \mathbf{160\,W}$$

Problem 5. A mass of 1000 kg is raised through a height of 10 m in 20 s. What is (a) the work done and (b) the power developed?

(a) Work done = force × distance

and force = mass × acceleration

Hence,

$$\text{work done} = (1000\,\text{kg} \times 9.81\,\text{m/s}^2) \times (10\,\text{m})$$

$$= 98\,100\,\text{Nm}$$

$$= \textbf{98.1 kNm or 98.1 kJ}$$

(b) $\text{Power} = \dfrac{\text{work done}}{\text{time taken}} = \dfrac{98100\,\text{J}}{20\,\text{s}}$

$$= 4905\,\text{J/s} = \textbf{4905 W or 4.905 kW}$$

Now try the following exercise

Exercise 1   Further problems on charge, force, work and power

(Take $g = 9.81\,\text{m/s}^2$ where appropriate)

1. What quantity of electricity is carried by 6.24×10^{21} electrons?   [1000 C]

2. In what time would a current of 1 A transfer a charge of 30 C?   [30 s]

3. A current of 3 A flows for 5 minutes. What charge is transferred?   [900 C]

4. How long must a current of 0.1 A flow so as to transfer a charge of 30 C? [5 minutes]

5. What force is required to give a mass of 20 kg an acceleration of 30 m/s²? [600 N]

6. Find the accelerating force when a car having a mass of 1.7 Mg increases its speed with a constant acceleration of 3 m/s².   [5.1 kN]

7. A force of 40 N accelerates a mass at 5 m/s². Determine the mass.   [8 kg]

8. Determine the force acting downwards on a mass of 1500 g suspended on a string.   [14.72 N]

9. A force of 4 N moves an object 200 cm in the direction of the force. What amount of work is done?   [8 J]

10. A force of 2.5 kN is required to lift a load. How much work is done if the load is lifted through 500 cm?   [12.5 kJ]

11. An electromagnet exerts a force of 12 N and moves a soft iron armature through a distance of 1.5 cm in 40 ms. Find the power consumed.   [4.5 W]

12. A mass of 500 kg is raised to a height of 6 m in 30 s. Find (a) the work done and (b) the power developed.
[(a) 29.43 kNm (b) 981 W]

13. Rewrite the following as indicated:
(a) 1000 pF = ... nF
(b) 0.02 μF = ... pF
(c) 5000 kHz = ... MHz
(d) 47 kΩ = ... MΩ
(e) 0.32 mA = ...μA
[(a) 1 nF (b) 20000 pF (c) 5 MHz
(d) 0.047 MΩ (e) 320 μA]

1.6   Electrical potential and e.m.f.

The **unit of electric potential** is the volt (V), where one volt is one joule per coulomb. One volt is defined as the difference in potential between two points in a conductor which, when carrying a current of one ampere, dissipates a power of one watt, i.e.

$$\text{volts} = \frac{\text{watts}}{\text{amperes}} = \frac{\text{joules/second}}{\text{amperes}}$$

$$= \frac{\text{joules}}{\text{ampere seconds}} = \frac{\text{joules}}{\text{coulombs}}$$

A change in electric potential between two points in an electric circuit is called a **potential difference**. The **electromotive force (e.m.f.)** provided by a source of energy such as a battery or a generator is measured in volts.

1.7   Resistance and conductance

The **unit of electric resistance** is the **ohm**(Ω), where one ohm is one volt per ampere. It is defined as the resistance between two points in a conductor when a constant electric potential of one volt applied at the two points produces a current flow of one ampere in the conductor. Thus,

$$\text{resistance, in ohms}\quad R = \frac{V}{I}$$

where V is the potential difference across the two points, in volts, and I is the current flowing between the two points, in amperes.

The reciprocal of resistance is called **conductance** and is measured in siemens (S). Thus

$$\text{conductance, in siemens } G = \frac{1}{R}$$

where R is the resistance in ohms.

Problem 6. Find the conductance of a conductor of resistance: (a) $10\,\Omega$ (b) $5\,k\Omega$ (c) $100\,m\Omega$.

(a) Conductance $G = \dfrac{1}{R} = \dfrac{1}{10}$ siemen $= \mathbf{0.1\,S}$

(b) $G = \dfrac{1}{R} = \dfrac{1}{5 \times 10^3}\,S = 0.2 \times 10^{-3}\,S = \mathbf{0.2\,mS}$

(c) $G = \dfrac{1}{R} = \dfrac{1}{100 \times 10^{-3}}\,S = \dfrac{10^3}{100}\,S = \mathbf{10\,S}$

1.8 Electrical power and energy

When a direct current of I amperes is flowing in an electric circuit and the voltage across the circuit is V volts, then

$$\text{power, in watts } P = VI$$

$$\text{Electrical energy} = \text{Power} \times \text{time}$$

$$= VIt \text{ joules}$$

Although the unit of energy is the joule, when dealing with large amounts of energy, the unit used is the **kilowatt hour (kWh)** where

$$1\,kWh = 1000 \text{ watt hour}$$
$$= 1000 \times 3600 \text{ watt seconds or joules}$$
$$= 3\,600\,000\,J$$

Problem 7. A source e.m.f. of 5 V supplies a current of 3 A for 10 minutes. How much energy is provided in this time?

Energy $=$ power $\times$ time, and power $=$ voltage $\times$ current. Hence

$$\textbf{Energy} = VIt = 5 \times 3 \times (10 \times 60)$$
$$= 9000 \text{ Ws or J} = \mathbf{9\,kJ}$$

Problem 8. An electric heater consumes 1.8 MJ when connected to a 250 V supply for 30 minutes. Find the power rating of the heater and the current taken from the supply.

$$\text{Power} = \frac{\text{energy}}{\text{time}} = \frac{1.8 \times 10^6\,J}{30 \times 60\,s}$$
$$= 1000\,J/s = 1000\,W$$

i.e. **power rating of heater $= 1\,kW$**

$$\text{Power } P = VI, \text{ thus } I = \frac{P}{V} = \frac{1000}{250} = 4\,A$$

Hence the current taken from the supply is 4 A.

Now try the following exercise

Exercise 2 Further problems on e.m.f., resistance, conductance, power and energy

1. Find the conductance of a resistor of resistance (a) $10\,\Omega$ (b) $2\,k\Omega$ (c) $2\,m\Omega$ [(a) 0.1 S (b) 0.5 mS (c) 500 S]

2. A conductor has a conductance of $50\,\mu S$. What is its resistance? [$20\,k\Omega$]

3. An e.m.f. of 250 V is connected across a resistance and the current flowing through the resistance is 4 A. What is the power developed? [1 kW]

4. 450 J of energy are converted into heat in 1 minute. What power is dissipated? [7.5 W]

5. A current of 10 A flows through a conductor and 10 W is dissipated. What p.d. exists across the ends of the conductor? [1 V]

6. A battery of e.m.f. 12 V supplies a current of 5 A for 2 minutes. How much energy is supplied in this time? [7.2 kJ]

7. A d.c. electric motor consumes 36 MJ when connected to a 250 V supply for 1 hour. Find the power rating of the motor and the current taken from the supply. [10 kW, 40 A]

1.9 Summary of terms, units and their symbols

Quantity	Quantity Symbol	Unit	Unit Symbol
Length	l	metre	m
Mass	m	kilogram	kg
Time	t	second	s
Velocity	v	metres per second	m/s or m s^{-1}
Acceleration	a	metres per second squared	m/s^2 or m s^{-2}
Force	F	newton	N
Electrical charge or quantity	Q	coulomb	C
Electric current	I	ampere	A
Resistance	R	ohm	Ω
Conductance	G	siemen	S
Electromotive force	E	volt	V
Potential difference	V	volt	V
Work	W	joule	J
Energy	E (or W)	joule	J
Power	P	watt	W

Now try the following exercises

Exercise 3 **Short answer questions on units associated with basic electrical quantities**

1. What does 'SI units' mean?

2. Complete the following:
   Force = ... × ......

3. What do you understand by the term 'potential difference'?

4. Define electric current in terms of charge and time

5. Name the units used to measure:
   (a) the quantity of electricity
   (b) resistance
   (c) conductance

6. Define the coulomb

7. Define electrical energy and state its unit

8. Define electrical power and state its unit

9. What is electromotive force?

10. Write down a formula for calculating the power in a d.c. circuit

11. Write down the symbols for the following quantities:
    (a) electric charge   (b) work
    (c) e.m.f.   (d) p.d.

12. State which units the following abbreviations refer to:
    (a) A   (b) C   (c) J   (d) N   (e) m

Exercise 4 **Multi-choice questions on units associated with basic electrical quantities (Answers on page 420)**

1. A resistance of $50\,\text{k}\Omega$ has a conductance of:
   (a) $20\,\text{S}$ (b) $0.02\,\text{S}$
   (c) $0.02\,\text{mS}$ (d) $20\,\text{kS}$

2. Which of the following statements is incorrect?
   (a) $1\,\text{N} = 1\,\text{kg m/s}^2$ (b) $1\,\text{V} = 1\,\text{J/C}$
   (c) $30\,\text{mA} = 0.03\,\text{A}$ (d) $1\,\text{J} = 1\,\text{N/m}$

3. The power dissipated by a resistor of $10\,\Omega$ when a current of $2\,\text{A}$ passes through it is:
   (a) $0.4\,\text{W}$ (b) $20\,\text{W}$ (c) $40\,\text{W}$ (d) $200\,\text{W}$

4. A mass of $1200\,\text{g}$ is accelerated at $200\,\text{cm/s}^2$ by a force. The value of the force required is:
   (a) $2.4\,\text{N}$ (b) $2,400\,\text{N}$
   (c) $240\,\text{kN}$ (d) $0.24\,\text{N}$

5. A charge of 240 C is transferred in 2 minutes. The current flowing is:
   (a) 120 A (b) 480 A (c) 2 A (d) 8 A

6. A current of 2 A flows for 10 h through a 100 Ω resistor. The energy consumed by the resistor is:
   (a) 0.5 kWh   (b) 4 kWh
   (c) 2 kWh   (d) 0.02 kWh

7. The unit of quantity of electricity is the:
   (a) volt   (b) coulomb
   (c) ohm   (d) joule

8. Electromotive force is provided by:
   (a) resistances
   (b) a conducting path
   (c) an electric current
   (d) an electrical supply source

9. The coulomb is a unit of:
   (a) power
   (b) voltage
   (c) energy
   (d) quantity of electricity

10. In order that work may be done:
    (a) a supply of energy is required
    (b) the circuit must have a switch
    (c) coal must be burnt
    (d) two wires are necessary

11. The ohm is the unit of:
    (a) charge   (b) resistance
    (c) power   (d) current

12. The unit of current is the:
    (a) volt   (b) coulomb
    (c) joule   (d) ampere

Chapter 2

An introduction to electric circuits

At the end of this chapter you should be able to:

- appreciate that engineering systems may be represented by block diagrams
- recognize common electrical circuit diagram symbols
- understand that electric current is the rate of movement of charge and is measured in amperes
- appreciate that the unit of charge is the coulomb
- calculate charge or quantity of electricity Q from $Q = It$
- understand that a potential difference between two points in a circuit is required for current to flow
- appreciate that the unit of p.d. is the volt
- understand that resistance opposes current flow and is measured in ohms
- appreciate what an ammeter, a voltmeter, an ohmmeter, a multimeter, an oscilloscope, a wattmeter, a bridge megger, a tachometer and stroboscope measure
- distinguish between linear and non-linear devices
- state Ohm's law as $V = IR$ or $I = V/R$ or $R = V/I$
- use Ohm's law in calculations, including multiples and sub-multiples of units
- describe a conductor and an insulator, giving examples of each
- appreciate that electrical power P is given by $P = VI = I^2 R = V^2/R$ watts
- calculate electrical power
- define electrical energy and state its unit
- calculate electrical energy
- state the three main effects of an electric current, giving practical examples of each
- explain the importance of fuses in electrical circuits
- appreciate the dangers of constant high current flow with insulation materials

2.1 Electrical/electronic system block diagrams

An electrical/electronic **system** is a group of components connected together to perform a desired function.

Figure 2.1 shows a simple public address system, where a microphone is used to collect acoustic energy in the form of sound pressure waves and converts this to electrical energy in the form of small voltages and currents; the signal from the microphone is then amplified by means of an electronic circuit containing

DOI: 10.1016/B978-0-08-089056-2.00002-4

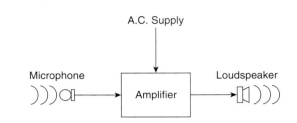

Figure 2.1

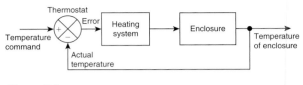

Figure 2.3

transistors/integrated circuits before it is applied to the loudspeaker.

A **sub-system** is a part of a system which performs an identified function within the whole system; the amplifier in Fig. 2.1 is an example of a sub-system.

A **component** or **element** is usually the simplest part of a system which has a specific and well-defined function – for example, the microphone in Fig. 2.1.

The illustration in Fig. 2.1 is called a block diagram and electrical/electronic systems, which can often be quite complicated, can be better understood when broken down in this way. It is not always necessary to know precisely what is inside each sub-system in order to know how the whole system functions.

As another example of an engineering system, Fig. 2.2 illustrates a temperature control system containing a heat source (such as a gas boiler), a fuel controller (such as an electrical solenoid valve), a thermostat and a source of electrical energy. The system of Fig. 2.2 can be shown in block diagram form as in Fig. 2.3; the thermostat compares the actual room temperature with the desired temperature and switches the heating on or off.

There are many types of engineering systems. A **communications system** is an example, where a local area network could comprise a file server, coaxial cable, network adapters, several computers and a laser printer; an **electromechanical system** is another example, where a car electrical system could comprise a battery, a starter motor, an ignition coil, a contact breaker and a distributor. All such systems as these may be represented by block diagrams.

2.2 Standard symbols for electrical components

Symbols are used for components in electrical circuit diagrams and some of the more common ones are shown in Fig. 2.4.

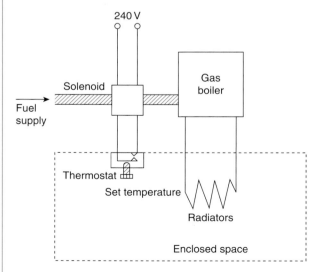

Figure 2.2

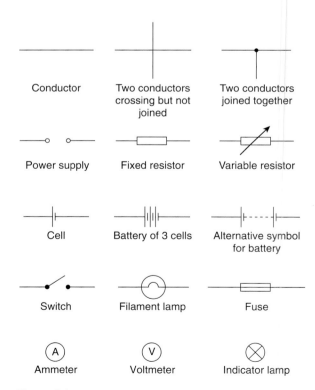

Figure 2.4

2.3 Electric current and quantity of electricity

All **atoms** consist of **protons, neutrons** and **electrons**. The protons, which have positive electrical charges, and the neutrons, which have no electrical charge, are contained within the **nucleus**. Removed from the nucleus are minute negatively charged particles called electrons. Atoms of different materials differ from one another by having different numbers of protons, neutrons and electrons. An equal number of protons and electrons exist within an atom and it is said to be electrically balanced, as the positive and negative charges cancel each other out. When there are more than two electrons in an atom the electrons are arranged into **shells** at various distances from the nucleus.

All atoms are bound together by powerful forces of attraction existing between the nucleus and its electrons. Electrons in the outer shell of an atom, however, are attracted to their nucleus less powerfully than are electrons whose shells are nearer the nucleus.

It is possible for an atom to lose an electron; the atom, which is now called an **ion**, is not now electrically balanced, but is positively charged and is thus able to attract an electron to itself from another atom. Electrons that move from one atom to another are called free electrons and such random motion can continue indefinitely. However, if an electric pressure or **voltage** is applied across any material there is a tendency for electrons to move in a particular direction. This movement of free electrons, known as **drift**, constitutes an electric current flow. **Thus current is the rate of movement of charge**. **Conductors** are materials that contain electrons that are loosely connected to the nucleus and can easily move through the material from one atom to another. **Insulators** are materials whose electrons are held firmly to their nucleus.

The unit used to measure the **quantity of electrical charge Q** is called the **coulomb C** (where 1 coulomb $= 6.24 \times 10^{18}$ electrons)

If the drift of electrons in a conductor takes place at the rate of one coulomb per second the resulting current is said to be a current of one ampere.

Thus   1 ampere = 1 coulomb per second or
$$1\,A = 1\,C/s$$
Hence   1 coulomb = 1 ampere second or
$$1\,C = 1\,As$$

Generally, if I is the current in amperes and t the time in seconds during which the current flows, then $I \times t$ represents the quantity of electrical charge in coulombs,

i.e. quantity of electrical charge transferred,

$$Q = I \times t \text{ coulombs}$$

Problem 1. What current must flow if 0.24 coulombs is to be transferred in 15 ms?

Since the quantity of electricity, $Q = It$, then

$$I = \frac{Q}{t} = \frac{0.24}{15 \times 10^{-3}} = \frac{0.24 \times 10^3}{15}$$
$$= \frac{240}{15} = \mathbf{16\,A}$$

Problem 2. If a current of 10 A flows for four minutes, find the quantity of electricity transferred.

Quantity of electricity, $Q = It$ coulombs. $I = 10\,A$ and $t = 4 \times 60 = 240$ s. Hence

$$Q = 10 \times 240 = \mathbf{2400\,C}$$

Now try the following exercise

Exercise 5   Further problems on charge

1. In what time would a current of 10 A transfer a charge of 50 C?   [5 s]

2. A current of 6 A flows for 10 minutes. What charge is transferred?   [3600 C]

3. How long must a current of 100 mA flow so as to transfer a charge of 80 C?
                    [13 min 20 s]

2.4 Potential difference and resistance

For a continuous current to flow between two points in a circuit a **potential difference (p.d.)** or **voltage**, V, is required between them; a complete conducting path is necessary to and from the source of electrical energy. The unit of p.d. is the **volt, V**.

Figure 2.5 shows a cell connected across a filament lamp. Current flow, by convention, is considered as flowing from the positive terminal of the cell, around the circuit to the negative terminal.

The flow of electric current is subject to friction. This friction, or opposition, is called **resistance R** and is the

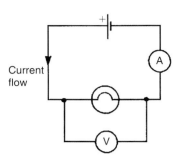

Figure 2.5

property of a conductor that limits current. The unit of resistance is the **ohm**; 1 ohm is defined as the resistance which will have a current of 1 ampere flowing through it when 1 volt is connected across it,

i.e. $\text{resistance } R = \dfrac{\text{Potential difference}}{\text{current}}$

2.5 Basic electrical measuring instruments

An **ammeter** is an instrument used to measure current and must be connected **in series** with the circuit. Figure 2.5 shows an ammeter connected in series with the lamp to measure the current flowing through it. Since all the current in the circuit passes through the ammeter it must have a very **low resistance**.

A **voltmeter** is an instrument used to measure p.d. and must be connected **in parallel** with the part of the circuit whose p.d. is required. In Fig. 2.5, a voltmeter is connected in parallel with the lamp to measure the p.d. across it. To avoid a significant current flowing through it a voltmeter must have a very **high resistance**.

An **ohmmeter** is an instrument for measuring resistance.

A **multimeter**, or universal instrument, may be used to measure voltage, current and resistance. An 'Avometer' and 'Fluke' are typical examples.

The **oscilloscope** may be used to observe waveforms and to measure voltages and currents. The display of an oscilloscope involves a spot of light moving across a screen. The amount by which the spot is deflected from its initial position depends on the p.d. applied to the terminals of the oscilloscope and the range selected. The displacement is calibrated in 'volts per cm'. For example, if the spot is deflected 3 cm and the volts/cm switch is on 10 V/cm then the magnitude of the p.d. is 3 cm × 10 V/cm, i.e. 30 V.

A **wattmeter** is an instrument for the measurement of power in an electrical circuit.

A **BM80** or a **420 MIT megger** or a **bridge megger** may be used to measure both continuity and insulation resistance. **Continuity testing** is the measurement of the resistance of a cable to discover if the cable is continuous, i.e. that it has no breaks or high resistance joints. **Insulation resistance testing** is the measurement of resistance of the insulation between cables, individual cables to earth or metal plugs and sockets, and so on. An insulation resistance in excess of 1 MΩ is normally acceptable.

A **tachometer** is an instrument that indicates the speed, usually in revolutions per minute, at which an engine shaft is rotating.

A **stroboscope** is a device for viewing a rotating object at regularly recurring intervals, by means of either (a) a rotating or vibrating shutter, or (b) a suitably designed lamp which flashes periodically. If the period between successive views is exactly the same as the time of one revolution of the revolving object, and the duration of the view very short, the object will appear to be stationary. (See Chapter 10 for more detail about electrical measuring instruments and measurements.)

2.6 Linear and non-linear devices

Figure 2.6 shows a circuit in which current I can be varied by the variable resistor R_2. For various settings of R_2, the current flowing in resistor R_1, displayed on the ammeter, and the p.d. across R_1, displayed on the voltmeter, are noted and a graph is plotted of p.d. against current. The result is shown in Fig. 2.7(a) where the straight line graph passing through the origin indicates that current is directly proportional to the p.d. Since the gradient, i.e. (p.d.)/(current) is constant, resistance R_1 is constant. A resistor is thus an example of a **linear device**.

If the resistor R_1 in Fig. 2.6 is replaced by a component such as a lamp then the graph shown in Fig. 2.7(b) results when values of p.d. are noted for various current

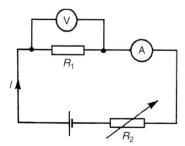

Figure 2.6

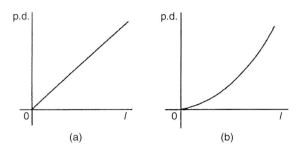

Figure 2.7

readings. Since the gradient is changing, the lamp is an example of a **non-linear device**.

2.7   Ohm's law

Ohm's law states that the current I flowing in a circuit is directly proportional to the applied voltage V and inversely proportional to the resistance R, provided the temperature remains constant. Thus,

$$I = \frac{V}{R} \quad \text{or} \quad V = IR \quad \text{or} \quad R = \frac{V}{I}$$

For a practical laboratory experiment on Ohm's law, see Chapter 24, page 406.

> **Problem 3.**   The current flowing through a resistor is 0.8 A when a p.d. of 20 V is applied. Determine the value of the resistance.

From Ohm's law,

$$\text{resistance } R = \frac{V}{I} = \frac{20}{0.8} = \frac{200}{8} = \mathbf{25\,\Omega}$$

2.8   Multiples and sub-multiples

Currents, voltages and resistances can often be very large or very small. Thus multiples and sub-multiples of units are often used, as stated in Chapter 1. The most common ones, with an example of each, are listed in Table 2.1.

> **Problem 4.**   Determine the p.d. which must be applied to a 2 kΩ resistor in order that a current of 10 mA may flow.

Resistance $R = 2\,k\Omega = 2 \times 10^3 = 2000\,\Omega$

Current $I = 10\,\text{mA} = 10 \times 10^{-3}\,\text{A}$

$$\text{or } \frac{10}{10^3}\,\text{A} \quad \text{or} \quad \frac{10}{1000}\,\text{A} = 0.01\,\text{A}$$

From Ohm's law, potential difference,

$$V = IR = (0.01)(2000) = \mathbf{20\,V}$$

> **Problem 5.**   A coil has a current of 50 mA flowing through it when the applied voltage is 12 V. What is the resistance of the coil?

$$\text{Resistance, } R = \frac{V}{I} = \frac{12}{50 \times 10^{-3}}$$

$$= \frac{12 \times 10^3}{50} = \frac{12\,000}{50} = \mathbf{240\,\Omega}$$

> **Problem 6.**   A 100 V battery is connected across a resistor and causes a current of 5 mA to flow. Determine the resistance of the resistor. If the

Table 2.1

Prefix	Name	Meaning	Example
M	mega	multiply by 1 000 000 (i.e. $\times 10^6$)	$2\,\text{M}\Omega = 2\,000\,000\,\text{ohms}$
k	kilo	multiply by 1000 (i.e. $\times 10^3$)	$10\,\text{kV} = 10\,000\,\text{volts}$
m	milli	divide by 1000 (i.e. $\times 10^{-3}$)	$25\,\text{mA} = \dfrac{25}{1000}\,\text{A}$ $= 0.025\,\text{amperes}$
μ	micro	divide by 1 000 000 (i.e. $\times 10^{-6}$)	$50\,\mu\text{V} = \dfrac{50}{1\,000\,000}\,\text{V}$ $= 0.000\,05\,\text{volts}$

voltage is now reduced to 25 V, what will be the new value of the current flowing?

$$\text{Resistance } R = \frac{V}{I} = \frac{100}{5 \times 10^{-3}} = \frac{100 \times 10^3}{5}$$

$$= 20 \times 10^3 = \mathbf{20\,k\Omega}$$

Current when voltage is reduced to 25 V,

$$I = \frac{V}{R} = \frac{25}{20 \times 10^3} = \frac{25}{20} \times 10^{-3} = \mathbf{1.25\,mA}$$

Problem 7. What is the resistance of a coil which draws a current of (a) 50 mA and (b) 200 μA from a 120 V supply?

(a) $\text{Resistance } R = \dfrac{V}{I} = \dfrac{120}{50 \times 10^{-3}}$

$$= \frac{120}{0.05} = \frac{12\,000}{5}$$

$$= \mathbf{2400\,\Omega} \text{ or } \mathbf{2.4\,k\Omega}$$

(b) $\text{Resistance } R = \dfrac{120}{200 \times 10^{-6}} = \dfrac{120}{0.0002}$

$$= \frac{1\,200\,000}{2} = \mathbf{600\,000\,\Omega}$$

$$\text{or } \mathbf{600\,k\Omega} \text{ or } \mathbf{0.6\,M\Omega}$$

Problem 8. The current/voltage relationship for two resistors A and B is as shown in Fig. 2.8. Determine the value of the resistance of each resistor.

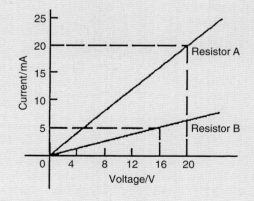

Figure 2.8

For resistor A,

$$R = \frac{V}{I} = \frac{20\,V}{20\,mA} = \frac{20}{0.02} = \frac{2000}{2}$$

$$= \mathbf{1000\,\Omega} \text{ or } \mathbf{1\,k\Omega}$$

For resistor B,

$$R = \frac{V}{I} = \frac{16\,V}{5\,mA} = \frac{16}{0.005} = \frac{16\,000}{5}$$

$$= \mathbf{3200\,\Omega} \text{ or } \mathbf{3.2\,k\Omega}$$

Now try the following exercise

Exercise 6 Further problems on Ohm's law

1. The current flowing through a heating element is 5 A when a p.d. of 35 V is applied across it. Find the resistance of the element. [7 Ω]

2. A 60 W electric light bulb is connected to a 240 V supply. Determine (a) the current flowing in the bulb and (b) the resistance of the bulb. [(a) 0.25 A (b) 960 Ω]

3. Graphs of current against voltage for two resistors P and Q are shown in Fig. 2.9. Determine the value of each resistor. [2 mΩ, 5 mΩ]

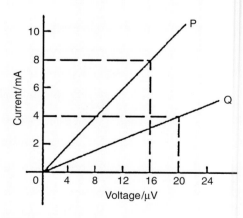

Figure 2.9

4. Determine the p.d. which must be applied to a 5 kΩ resistor such that a current of 6 mA may flow. [30 V]

5. A 20 V source of e.m.f. is connected across a circuit having a resistance of $400\,\Omega$. Calculate the current flowing.   [50 mA]

2.9   Conductors and insulators

A **conductor** is a material having a low resistance which allows electric current to flow in it. All metals are conductors and some examples include copper, aluminium, brass, platinum, silver, gold and carbon.

An **insulator** is a material having a high resistance which does not allow electric current to flow in it. Some examples of insulators include plastic, rubber, glass, porcelain, air, paper, cork, mica, ceramics and certain oils.

2.10   Electrical power and energy

Electrical power

Power P in an electrical circuit is given by the product of potential difference V and current I, as stated in Chapter 1. The unit of power is the **watt, W.**

Hence $P = V \times I$ watts   (1)

From Ohm's law, $V = IR$. Substituting for V in equation (1) gives:

$$P = (IR) \times I$$

i.e. $P = I^2 R$ watts

Also, from Ohm's law, $I = V/R$. Substituting for I in equation (1) gives:

$$P = V \times \frac{V}{R}$$

i.e. $P = \dfrac{V^2}{R}$ watts

There are thus three possible formulae which may be used for calculating power.

Problem 9.   A 100 W electric light bulb is connected to a 250 V supply. Determine (a) the current flowing in the bulb, and (b) the resistance of the bulb.

Power $P = V \times I$, from which, current $I = \dfrac{P}{V}$

(a)   Current $I = \dfrac{100}{250} = \dfrac{10}{25} = \dfrac{2}{5} = \mathbf{0.4\,A}$

(b)   Resistance $R = \dfrac{V}{I} = \dfrac{250}{0.4} = \dfrac{2500}{4} = \mathbf{625\,\Omega}$

Problem 10.   Calculate the power dissipated when a current of 4 mA flows through a resistance of $5\,k\Omega$.

$$\begin{aligned}
\textbf{Power } P &= I^2 R = (4 \times 10^{-3})^2 (5 \times 10^3) \\
&= 16 \times 10^{-6} \times 5 \times 10^3 \\
&= 80 \times 10^{-3} \\
&= \mathbf{0.08\,W} \text{ or } \mathbf{80\,mW}
\end{aligned}$$

Alternatively, since $I = 4 \times 10^{-3}$ and $R = 5 \times 10^3$ then from Ohm's law, voltage

$$V = IR = 4 \times 10^{-3} \times 5 \times 10^3 = 20\,V$$

Hence,

$$\begin{aligned}
\textbf{power } P &= V \times I = 20 \times 4 \times 10^{-3} \\
&= \mathbf{80\,mW}
\end{aligned}$$

Problem 11.   An electric kettle has a resistance of $30\,\Omega$. What current will flow when it is connected to a 240 V supply? Find also the power rating of the kettle.

$$\text{Current, } I = \frac{V}{R} = \frac{240}{30} = \mathbf{8\,A}$$

$$\text{Power, } P = VI = 240 \times 8 = 1920\,W$$

$$= \mathbf{1.92\,kW} = \text{power rating of kettle}$$

Problem 12.   A current of 5 A flows in the winding of an electric motor, the resistance of the winding being $100\,\Omega$. Determine (a) the p.d. across the winding, and (b) the power dissipated by the coil.

(a)   Potential difference across winding,

$$V = IR = 5 \times 100 = \mathbf{500\,V}$$

(b) Power dissipated by coil,

$$P = I^2 R = 5^2 \times 100$$

$$= \textbf{2500 W} \text{ or } \textbf{2.5 kW}$$

(Alternatively, $P = V \times I = 500 \times 5$

$$= \textbf{2500 W} \text{ or } \textbf{2.5 kW})$$

Problem 13. The hot resistance of a 240 V filament lamp is 960 Ω. Find the current taken by the lamp and its power rating.

From Ohm's law,

$$\text{current } I = \frac{V}{R} = \frac{240}{960}$$

$$= \frac{24}{96} = \frac{1}{4} \textbf{A} \text{ or } \textbf{0.25 A}$$

Power rating $P = VI = (240)\left(\frac{1}{4}\right) = \textbf{60 W}$

Electrical energy

> Electrical energy = power × time

If the power is measured in watts and the time in seconds then the unit of energy is watt-seconds or **joules**. If the power is measured in kilowatts and the time in hours then the unit of energy is **kilowatt-hours**, often called the '**unit of electricity**'. The 'electricity meter' in the home records the number of kilowatt-hours used and is thus an energy meter.

Problem 14. A 12 V battery is connected across a load having a resistance of 40 Ω. Determine the current flowing in the load, the power consumed and the energy dissipated in 2 minutes.

$$\text{Current } I = \frac{V}{R} = \frac{12}{40} = \textbf{0.3 A}$$

Power consumed, $P = VI = (12)(0.3) = \textbf{3.6 W}$

Energy dissipated = power × time

$$= (3.6 \text{ W})(2 \times 60 \text{ s})$$

$$= \textbf{432 J} \text{ (since } 1 \text{ J} = 1 \text{ Ws)}$$

Problem 15. A source of e.m.f. of 15 V supplies a current of 2 A for 6 minutes. How much energy is provided in this time?

Energy = power × time, and power = voltage × current. Hence

$$\text{energy} = VIt = 15 \times 2 \times (6 \times 60)$$

$$= 10\,800 \text{ Ws or J} = \textbf{10.8 kJ}$$

Problem 16. Electrical equipment in an office takes a current of 13 A from a 240 V supply. Estimate the cost per week of electricity if the equipment is used for 30 hours each week and 1 kWh of energy costs 12.5p.

$$\text{Power} = VI \text{ watts} = 240 \times 13$$

$$= 3120 \text{ W} = 3.12 \text{ kW}$$

Energy used per week = power × time

$$= (3.12 \text{ kW}) \times (30 \text{ h})$$

$$= 93.6 \text{ kWh}$$

Cost at 12.5p per kWh = $93.6 \times 12.5 = 1170$p. Hence **weekly cost of electricity = £11.70**

Problem 17. An electric heater consumes 3.6 MJ when connected to a 250 V supply for 40 minutes. Find the power rating of the heater and the current taken from the supply.

$$\text{Power} = \frac{\text{energy}}{\text{time}} = \frac{3.6 \times 10^6}{40 \times 60} \frac{\text{J}}{\text{s}} \text{ (or W)} = 1500 \text{ W}$$

i.e. Power rating of heater = **1.5 kW**.

$$\text{Power } P = VI$$

$$\text{thus } I = \frac{P}{V} = \frac{1500}{250} = 6 \text{ A}$$

Hence the current taken from the supply is **6 A**.

Problem 18. Determine the power dissipated by the element of an electric fire of resistance 20 Ω when a current of 10 A flows through it. If the fire is on for 6 hours determine the energy used and the cost if 1 unit of electricity costs 13p.

$$\text{Power } P = I^2 R = 10^2 \times 20$$

$$= 100 \times 20 = \textbf{2000 W} \text{ or } \textbf{2 kW}.$$

(Alternatively, from Ohm's law,

$$V = IR = 10 \times 20 = 200 \text{ V},$$

hence power

$$P = V \times I = 200 \times 10 = 2000\,\text{W} = 2\,\text{kW}).$$

Energy used in 6 hours
$$= \text{power} \times \text{time} = 2\,\text{kW} \times 6\,\text{h} = \textbf{12\,kWh}.$$
1 unit of electricity $= 1\,\text{kWh}$; hence the number of units used is 12. Cost of energy $= 12 \times 13 = \textbf{£1.56p}$

> **Problem 19.** A business uses two 3 kW fires for an average of 20 hours each per week, and six 150 W lights for 30 hours each per week. If the cost of electricity is 14 p per unit, determine the weekly cost of electricity to the business.

Energy $=$ power $\times$ time.
Energy used by one 3 kW fire in 20 hours
$$= 3\,\text{kW} \times 20\,\text{h} = 60\,\text{kWh}.$$
Hence weekly energy used by two 3 kW fires
$= 2 \times 60 = 120\,\text{kWh}.$
Energy used by one 150 W light for 30 hours
$= 150\,\text{W} \times 30\,\text{h} = 4500\,\text{Wh} = 4.5\,\text{kWh}.$
Hence weekly energy used by six 150 W lamps
$= 6 \times 4.5 = 27\,\text{kWh}.$
Total energy used per week $= 120 + 27 = 147\,\text{kWh}.$
1 unit of electricity $= 1\,\text{kWh}$ of energy. Thus weekly cost of energy at 14 p per kWh $= 14 \times 147 = 2058\,\text{p}$
$$= \textbf{£20.58}$$

Now try the following exercise

Exercise 7   Further problems on power and energy

1. The hot resistance of a 250 V filament lamp is 625 Ω. Determine the current taken by the lamp and its power rating.   [0.4 A, 100 W]

2. Determine the resistance of a coil connected to a 150 V supply when a current of (a) 75 mA (b) 300 μA flows through it.
   [(a) 2 kΩ (b) 0.5 MΩ]

3. Determine the resistance of an electric fire which takes a current of 12 A from a 240 V supply. Find also the power rating of the fire and the energy used in 20 h.
   [20 Ω, 2.88 kW, 57.6 kWh]

4. Determine the power dissipated when a current of 10 mA flows through an appliance having a resistance of 8 kΩ.   [0.8 W]

5. 85.5 J of energy are converted into heat in 9 s. What power is dissipated?   [9.5 W]

6. A current of 4 A flows through a conductor and 10 W is dissipated. What p.d. exists across the ends of the conductor?   [2.5 V]

7. Find the power dissipated when:
   (a) a current of 5 mA flows through a resistance of 20 kΩ
   (b) a voltage of 400 V is applied across a 120 kΩ resistor
   (c) a voltage applied to a resistor is 10 kV and the current flow is 4 m
   [(a) 0.5 W (b) 1.33 W (c) 40 W]

8. A battery of e.m.f. 15 V supplies a current of 2 A for 5 min. How much energy is supplied in this time?   [9 kJ]

9. A d.c. electric motor consumes 72 MJ when connected to 400 V supply for 2 h 30 min. Find the power rating of the motor and the current taken from the supply. [8 kW, 20 A]

10. A p.d. of 500 V is applied across the winding of an electric motor and the resistance of the winding is 50 Ω. Determine the power dissipated by the coil.   [5 kW]

11. In a household during a particular week three 2 kW fires are used on average 25 h each and eight 100 W light bulbs are used on average 35 h each. Determine the cost of electricity for the week if 1 unit of electricity costs 15 p.   [£26.70]

12. Calculate the power dissipated by the element of an electric fire of resistance 30 Ω when a current of 10 A flows in it. If the fire is on for 30 hours in a week determine the energy used. Determine also the weekly cost of energy if electricity costs 13.5p per unit.   [3 kW, 90 kWh, £12.15]

2.11   Main effects of electric current

The three main effects of an electric current are:
(a)   magnetic effect
(b)   chemical effect
(c)   heating effect

Some practical applications of the effects of an electric current include:

Magnetic effect: bells, relays, motors, generators, transformers, telephones, car-ignition and lifting magnets (see Chapter 8)

Chemical effect: primary and secondary cells and electroplating (see Chapter 4)

Heating effect: cookers, water heaters, electric fires, irons, furnaces, kettles and soldering irons

2.12   Fuses

If there is a fault in a piece of equipment then excessive current may flow. This will cause overheating and possibly a fire; **fuses** protect against this happening. Current from the supply to the equipment flows through the fuse. The fuse is a piece of wire which can carry a stated current; if the current rises above this value it will melt. If the fuse melts (blows) then there is an open circuit and no current can then flow – thus protecting the equipment by isolating it from the power supply. The fuse must be able to carry slightly more than the normal operating current of the equipment to allow for tolerances and small current surges. With some equipment there is a very large surge of current for a short time at switch on. If a fuse is fitted to withstand this large current there would be no protection against faults which cause the current to rise slightly above the normal value. Therefore special anti-surge fuses are fitted. These can stand 10 times the rated current for 10 milliseconds. If the surge lasts longer than this the fuse will blow.

A circuit diagram symbol for a fuse is shown in Fig. 2.4 on page 10.

Problem 20. If 5 A, 10 A and 13 A fuses are available, state which is most appropriate for the following appliances which are both connected to a 240 V supply: (a) Electric toaster having a power rating of 1 kW (b) Electric fire having a power rating of 3 kW.

Power $P = VI$, from which, current $I = \dfrac{P}{V}$

(a)   For the toaster,

$$\text{current } I = \frac{P}{V} = \frac{1000}{240} = \frac{100}{24} = 4.17\,\text{A}$$

Hence a **5 A fuse** is most appropriate

(b)   For the fire,

$$\text{current } I = \frac{P}{V} = \frac{3000}{240} = \frac{300}{24} = 12.5\,\text{A}$$

Hence a **13 A fuse** is most appropriate

Now try the following exercises

Exercise 8   Further problem on fuses

1.   A television set having a power rating of 120 W and electric lawnmower of power rating 1 kW are both connected to a 250 V supply. If 3 A, 5 A and 10 A fuses are available state which is the most appropriate for each appliance.   [3 A, 5 A]

2.13   Insulation and the dangers of constant high current flow

The use of insulation materials on electrical equipment, whilst being necessary, also has the effect of preventing heat loss, i.e. the heat is not able to dissipate, thus creating the possible danger of fire. In addition, the insulating material has a maximum temperature rating – this is heat it can withstand without being damaged. The current rating for all equipment and electrical components is therefore limited to keep the heat generated within safe limits. In addition, the maximum voltage present needs to be considered when choosing insulation.

Exercise 9   Short answer questions on the introduction to electric circuits

1.   Draw the preferred symbols for the following components used when drawing electrical circuit diagrams:
     (a) fixed resistor   (b) cell
     (c) filament lamp   (d) fuse
     (e) voltmeter

2.   State the unit of
     (a) current
     (b) potential difference
     (c) resistance

3.   State an instrument used to measure
     (a) current

(b) potential difference
(c) resistance

4. What is a multimeter?

5. State an instrument used to measure:
(a) engine rotational speed
(b) continuity and insulation testing
(c) electrical power

6. State Ohm's law

7. Give one example of
(a) a linear device
(b) a non-linear device

8. State the meaning of the following abbreviations of prefixes used with electrical units:
(a) k (b) μ (c) m (d) M

9. What is a conductor? Give four examples

10. What is an insulator? Give four examples

11. Complete the following statement:
'An ammeter has a . . . resistance and must be connected . . . with the load'

12. Complete the following statement:
'A voltmeter has a . . . resistance and must be connected . . . with the load'

13. State the unit of electrical power. State three formulae used to calculate power

14. State two units used for electrical energy

15. State the three main effects of an electric current and give two examples of each

16. What is the function of a fuse in an electrical circuit?

**Exercise 10   Multi-choice problems on the introduction to electric circuits
(Answers on page 420)**

1. 60 μs is equivalent to:
(a) 0.06   (b) 0.00006 s
(c) 1000 minutes   (d) 0.6 s

2. The current which flows when 0.1 coulomb is transferred in 10 ms is:
(a) 1 A   (b) 10 A
(c) 10 mA   (d) 100 mA

3. The p.d. applied to a 1 kΩ resistance in order that a current of 100 μA may flow is:

(a) 1 V   (b) 100 V   (c) 0.1 V
(d) 10 V

4. Which of the following formulae for electrical power is incorrect?

(a) VI (b) $\dfrac{V}{I}$ (c) I^2R (d) $\dfrac{V^2}{R}$

5. The power dissipated by a resistor of $4\,\Omega$ when a current of 5 A passes through it is:

(a) 6.25 W   (b) 20 W
(c) 80 W   (d) 100 W

6. Which of the following statements is true?
(a) Electric current is measured in volts
(b) 200 kΩ resistance is equivalent to 2 MΩ
(c) An ammeter has a low resistance and must be connected in parallel with a circuit
(d) An electrical insulator has a high resistance

7. A current of 3 A flows for 50 h through a 6 Ω resistor. The energy consumed by the resistor is:
(a) 0.9 kWh   (b) 2.7 kWh
(c) 9 kWh   (d) 27 kWh

8. What must be known in order to calculate the energy used by an electrical appliance?
(a) voltage and current
(b) current and time of operation
(c) power and time of operation
(d) current and resistance

9. Voltage drop is the:
(a) maximum potential
(b) difference in potential between two points
(c) voltage produced by a source
(d) voltage at the end of a circuit

10. A 240 V, 60 W lamp has a working resistance of:
(a) 1400 ohm   (b) 60 ohm
(c) 960 ohm   (d) 325 ohm

11. The largest number of 100 W electric light bulbs which can be operated from a 240 V supply fitted with a 13 A fuse is:

    (a) 2   (b) 7   (c) 31   (d) 18

12. The energy used by a 1.5 kW heater in 5 minutes is:

    (a) 5 J   (b) 450 J

    (c) 7500 J   (d) 450 000 J

13. When an atom loses an electron, the atom:

    (a) becomes positively charged
    (b) disintegrates
    (c) experiences no effect at all
    (d) becomes negatively charged

Chapter 3

Resistance variation

At the end of this chapter you should be able to:

- recognize three common methods of resistor construction
- appreciate that electrical resistance depends on four factors
- appreciate that resistance $R = \rho l/a$, where ρ is the resistivity
- recognize typical values of resistivity and its unit
- perform calculations using $R = \rho l/a$
- define the temperature coefficient of resistance, α
- recognize typical values for α
- perform calculations using $R_\theta = R_0(1 + \alpha\theta)$
- determine the resistance and tolerance of a fixed resistor from its colour code
- determine the resistance and tolerance of a fixed resistor from its letter and digit code

3.1 Resistor construction

There is a wide range of resistor types. Three of the most common methods of construction are:

(i) Wire wound resistors

A length of wire such as nichrome or manganin, whose resistive value per unit length is known, is cut to the desired value and wound around a ceramic former prior to being lacquered for protection. This type of resistor has a large physical size, which is a disadvantage; however, they can be made with a high degree of accuracy, and can have a **high power rating**.
Wire wound resistors are used in **power circuits** and **motor starters**.

(ii) Metal oxide resistors

With a metal oxide resistor a thin coating of platinum is deposited on a glass plate; it is then fired and a thin track etched out. It is then totally enclosed in an outer tube.

Metal oxide resistors are used in **electronic equipment**.

(iii) Carbon resistors

This type of resistor is made from a mixture of carbon black resin binder and a refractory powder that is pressed into shape and heated in a kiln to form a solid rod of standard length and width. The resistive value is predetermined by the ratio of the mixture. Metal end connections are crimped onto the rod to act as connecting points for electrical circuitry. This type of resistor is small and mass-produced cheaply; it has limited accuracy and a low power rating.
Carbon resistors are used in **electronic equipment**.

3.2 Resistance and resistivity

The resistance of an electrical conductor depends on four factors, these being: (a) the length of the conductor, (b) the cross-sectional area of the conductor, (c) the type of material and (d) the temperature of the material. Resistance, R, is directly proportional to length, l, of a

DOI: 10.1016/B978-0-08-089056-2.00003-6

conductor, i.e. $R \propto l$. Thus, for example, if the length of a piece of wire is doubled, then the resistance is doubled.

Resistance, R, is inversely proportional to cross-sectional area, a, of a conductor, i.e. $R \propto 1/a$. Thus, for example, if the cross-sectional area of a piece of wire is doubled then the resistance is halved.

Since $R \propto l$ and $R \propto 1/a$ then $R \propto l/a$. By inserting a constant of proportionality into this relationship the type of material used may be taken into account. The constant of proportionality is known as the **resistivity** of the material and is given the symbol ρ (Greek rho). Thus,

$$\text{resistance} \quad R = \frac{\rho l}{a} \text{ ohms}$$

ρ is measured in ohm metres (Ω m). The value of the resistivity is that resistance of a unit cube of the material measured between opposite faces of the cube.

Resistivity varies with temperature and some typical values of resistivities measured at about room temperature are given below:

Copper $1.7 \times 10^{-8} \Omega$ m (or $0.017 \mu\Omega$ m)

Aluminium $2.6 \times 10^{-8} \Omega$ m (or $0.026 \mu\Omega$ m)

Carbon (graphite) $10 \times 10^{-8} \Omega$ m ($0.10 \mu\Omega$ m)

Glass $1 \times 10^{10} \Omega$ m (or $10^4 \mu\Omega$ m)

Mica $1 \times 10^{13} \Omega$ m (or $10^7 \mu\Omega$ m)

Note that good conductors of electricity have a low value of resistivity and good insulators have a high value of resistivity.

Problem 1. The resistance of a 5 m length of wire is 600 Ω. Determine (a) the resistance of an 8 m length of the same wire, and (b) the length of the same wire when the resistance is 420 Ω.

(a) Resistance, R, is directly proportional to length, l, i.e. $R \propto l$. Hence, $600 \Omega \propto 5$ m or $600 = (k)(5)$, where k is the coefficient of proportionality.

Hence, $k = \dfrac{600}{5} = 120$

When the length l is 8 m, then resistance
$R = kl = (120)(8) = \mathbf{960\,\Omega}$

(b) When the resistance is 420 Ω, $420 = kl$, from which,

$$\text{length } l = \frac{420}{k} = \frac{420}{120} = \mathbf{3.5\,m}$$

Problem 2. A piece of wire of cross-sectional area 2 mm^2 has a resistance of 300 Ω. Find (a) the resistance of a wire of the same length and material if the cross-sectional area is 5 mm^2, (b) the cross-sectional area of a wire of the same length and material of resistance 750 Ω.

Resistance R is inversely proportional to cross-sectional area, a, i.e. $R \propto 1/a$

Hence $300 \Omega \propto \frac{1}{2}$ mm^2 or $300 = (k) (\frac{1}{2})$

from which, the coefficient of proportionality,
$$k = 300 \times 2 = 600$$

(a) When the cross-sectional area $a = 5$ mm^2 then
$$R = (k)(\tfrac{1}{5}) = (600)(\tfrac{1}{5}) = \mathbf{120\,\Omega}$$

(Note that resistance has decreased as the cross-sectional is increased.)

(b) When the resistance is 750 Ω then
$$750 = (k)\left(\frac{1}{a}\right)$$

from which

$$\text{cross-sectional area, } a = \frac{k}{750} = \frac{600}{750}$$
$$= \mathbf{0.8\,mm^2}$$

Problem 3. A wire of length 8 m and cross-sectional area 3 mm^2 has a resistance of 0.16 Ω. If the wire is drawn out until its cross-sectional area is 1 mm^2, determine the resistance of the wire.

Resistance R is directly proportional to length l, and inversely proportional to the cross-sectional area, a, i.e. $R \propto l/a$ or $R = k(l/a)$, where k is the coefficient of proportionality.
Since $R = 0.16$, $l = 8$ and $a = 3$, then $0.16 = (k)(8/3)$, from which $k = 0.16 \times 3/8 = 0.06$
If the cross-sectional area is reduced to 1/3 of its original area then the length must be tripled to 3×8, i.e. 24 m

$$\text{New resistance } R = k\left(\frac{l}{a}\right) = 0.06\left(\frac{24}{1}\right) = \mathbf{1.44\,\Omega}$$

Problem 4. Calculate the resistance of a 2 km length of aluminium overhead power cable if the cross-sectional area of the cable is $100\,\text{mm}^2$. Take the resistivity of aluminium to be $0.03 \times 10^{-6}\,\Omega\,\text{m}$.

Length $l = 2\,\text{km} = 2000\,\text{m}$,
area $a = 100\,\text{mm}^2 = 100 \times 10^{-6}\,\text{m}^2$
and resistivity $\rho = 0.03 \times 10^{-6}\,\Omega\,\text{m}$.

$$\text{Resistance } R = \frac{\rho l}{a}$$

$$= \frac{(0.03 \times 10^{-6}\,\Omega\,\text{m})(2000\,\text{m})}{(100 \times 10^{-6}\,\text{m}^2)}$$

$$= \frac{0.03 \times 2000}{100}\,\Omega = \mathbf{0.6\,\Omega}$$

Problem 5. Calculate the cross-sectional area, in mm^2, of a piece of copper wire, $40\,\text{m}$ in length and having a resistance of $0.25\,\Omega$. Take the resistivity of copper as $0.02 \times 10^{-6}\,\Omega\,\text{m}$.

Resistance $R = \rho l / a$ hence cross-sectional area

$$a = \frac{\rho l}{R} = \frac{(0.02 \times 10^{-6}\,\Omega\,\text{m})(40\,\text{m})}{0.25\,\Omega}$$

$$= 3.2 \times 10^{-6}\,\text{m}^2$$

$$= (3.2 \times 10^{-6}) \times 10^6\,\text{mm}^2 = \mathbf{3.2\,mm^2}$$

Problem 6. The resistance of $1.5\,\text{km}$ of wire of cross-sectional area $0.17\,\text{mm}^2$ is $150\,\Omega$. Determine the resistivity of the wire.

Resistance, $R = \rho l / a$ hence

$$\text{resistivity } \rho = \frac{Ra}{l}$$

$$= \frac{(150\,\Omega)(0.17 \times 10^{-6}\,\text{m}^2)}{(1500\,\text{m})}$$

$$= \mathbf{0.017 \times 10^{-6}\,\Omega\,m}$$

$$\text{or } \mathbf{0.017\,\mu\Omega\,m}$$

Problem 7. Determine the resistance of $1200\,\text{m}$ of copper cable having a diameter of $12\,\text{mm}$ if the resistivity of copper is $1.7 \times 10^{-8}\,\Omega\,\text{m}$.

Cross-sectional area of cable,

$$a = \pi r^2 = \pi \left(\frac{12}{2}\right)^2$$

$$= 36\pi\,\text{mm}^2 = 36\pi \times 10^{-6}\,\text{m}^2$$

$$\text{Resistance } R = \frac{\rho l}{a}$$

$$= \frac{(1.7 \times 10^{-8}\,\Omega\,\text{m})(1200\,\text{m})}{(36\pi \times 10^{-6}\,\text{m}^2)}$$

$$= \frac{1.7 \times 1200 \times 10^6}{10^8 \times 36\pi}\,\Omega$$

$$= \frac{1.7 \times 12}{36\pi}\,\Omega = \mathbf{0.180\,\Omega}$$

Now try the following exercise

Exercise 11 Further problems on resistance and resistivity

1. The resistance of a $2\,\text{m}$ length of cable is $2.5\,\Omega$. Determine (a) the resistance of a $7\,\text{m}$ length of the same cable and (b) the length of the same wire when the resistance is $6.25\,\Omega$.
     [(a) $8.75\,\Omega$ (b) $5\,\text{m}$]

2. Some wire of cross-sectional area $1\,\text{mm}^2$ has a resistance of $20\,\Omega$. Determine (a) the resistance of a wire of the same length and material if the cross-sectional area is $4\,\text{mm}^2$, and (b) the cross-sectional area of a wire of the same length and material if the resistance is $32\,\Omega$.
     [(a) $5\,\Omega$ (b) $0.625\,\text{mm}^2$]

3. Some wire of length $5\,\text{m}$ and cross-sectional area $2\,\text{mm}^2$ has a resistance of $0.08\,\Omega$. If the wire is drawn out until its cross-sectional area is $1\,\text{mm}^2$, determine the resistance of the wire.
     [$0.32\,\Omega$]

4. Find the resistance of $800\,\text{m}$ of copper cable of cross-sectional area $20\,\text{mm}^2$. Take the resistivity of copper as $0.02\,\mu\Omega\,\text{m}$.   [$0.8\,\Omega$]

5. Calculate the cross-sectional area, in mm^2, of a piece of aluminium wire $100\,\text{m}$ long and having a resistance of $2\,\Omega$. Take the resistivity of aluminium as $0.03 \times 10^{-6}\,\Omega\,\text{m}$.
     [$1.5\,\text{mm}^2$]

6. The resistance of $500\,\text{m}$ of wire of cross-sectional area $2.6\,\text{mm}^2$ is $5\,\Omega$. Determine the resistivity of the wire in $\mu\Omega\,\text{m}$.
     [$0.026\,\mu\Omega\,\text{m}$]

7. Find the resistance of 1 km of copper cable having a diameter of 10 mm if the resistivity of copper is $0.017 \times 10^{-6}\,\Omega\,\text{m}$.

[$0.216\,\Omega$]

3.3 Temperature coefficient of resistance

In general, as the temperature of a material increases, most conductors increase in resistance, insulators decrease in resistance, whilst the resistance of some special alloys remain almost constant.

The **temperature coefficient of resistance** of a material is the increase in the resistance of a $1\,\Omega$ resistor of that material when it is subjected to a rise of temperature of $1°C$. The symbol used for the temperature coefficient of resistance is α (Greek alpha). Thus, if some copper wire of resistance $1\,\Omega$ is heated through $1°C$ and its resistance is then measured as $1.0043\,\Omega$ then $\alpha = 0.0043\,\Omega/\Omega°C$ for copper. The units are usually expressed only as 'per $°C$', i.e. $\alpha = 0.0043/°C$ for copper. If the $1\,\Omega$ resistor of copper is heated through $100°C$ then the resistance at $100°C$ would be $1 + 100 \times 0.0043 = 1.43\,\Omega$. Some typical values of temperature coefficient of resistance measured at $0°C$ are given below:

Copper	$0.0043/°C$
Nickel	$0.0062/°C$
Constantan	0
Aluminium	$0.0038/°C$
Carbon	$-0.00048/°C$
Eureka	$0.00001/°C$

(Note that the negative sign for carbon indicates that its resistance falls with increase of temperature.)

If the resistance of a material at $0°C$ is known the resistance at any other temperature can be determined from:

$$R_\theta = R_0(1 + \alpha_0\theta)$$

where R_0 = resistance at $0°C$

R_θ = resistance at temperature $\theta°C$

α_0 = temperature coefficient of resistance at $0°C$

Problem 8. A coil of copper wire has a resistance of $100\,\Omega$ when its temperature is $0°C$. Determine its resistance at $70°C$ if the temperature coefficient of resistance of copper at $0°C$ is $0.0043/°C$.

Resistance $R_\theta = R_0(1 + \alpha_0\theta)$. Hence resistance at $100°C$,

$$R_{100} = 100[1 + (0.0043)(70)]$$
$$= 100[1 + 0.301]$$
$$= 100(1.301) = \mathbf{130.1\,\Omega}$$

Problem 9. An aluminium cable has a resistance of $27\,\Omega$ at a temperature of $35°C$. Determine its resistance at $0°C$. Take the temperature coefficient of resistance at $0°C$ to be $0.0038/°C$.

Resistance at $\theta°C$, $R_\theta = R_0(1 + \alpha_0\theta)$. Hence resistance at $0°C$,

$$R_0 = \frac{R_\theta}{(1 + \alpha_0\theta)} = \frac{27}{[1 + (0.0038)(35)]}$$
$$= \frac{27}{1 + 0.133}$$
$$= \frac{27}{1.133} = \mathbf{23.83\,\Omega}$$

Problem 10. A carbon resistor has a resistance of $1\,\text{k}\Omega$ at $0°C$. Determine its resistance at $80°C$. Assume that the temperature coefficient of resistance for carbon at $0°C$ is $-0.0005/°C$.

Resistance at temperature $\theta°C$,

$$R_\theta = R_0(1 + \alpha_0\theta)$$

i.e.

$$R_\theta = 1000[1 + (-0.0005)(80)]$$
$$= 1000[1 - 0.040] = 1000(0.96) = \mathbf{960\,\Omega}$$

If the resistance of a material at room temperature (approximately $20°C$), R_{20}, and the temperature coefficient of resistance at $20°C$, α_{20}, are known then the resistance R_θ at temperature $\theta°C$ is given by:

$$R_\theta = R_{20}[1 + \alpha_{20}(\theta - 20)]$$

Problem 11. A coil of copper wire has a resistance of $10\,\Omega$ at $20°C$. If the temperature coefficient of resistance of copper at $20°C$ is $0.004/°C$ determine the resistance of the coil when the temperature rises to $100°C$.

Resistance at $\theta°C$,

$$R_\theta = R_{20}[1 + \alpha_{20}(\theta - 20)]$$

Hence resistance at 100°C,

$$R_{100} = 10[1 + (0.004)(100 - 20)]$$

$$= 10[1 + (0.004)(80)]$$

$$= 10[1 + 0.32]$$

$$= 10(1.32) = \mathbf{13.2\,\Omega}$$

Problem 12. The resistance of a coil of aluminium wire at 18°C is 200 Ω. The temperature of the wire is increased and the resistance rises to 240 Ω. If the temperature coefficient of resistance of aluminium is 0.0039/°C at 18°C determine the temperature to which the coil has risen.

Let the temperature rise to $\theta°C$. Resistance at $\theta°C$,

$$R_\theta = R_{18}[1 + \alpha_{18}(\theta - 18)]$$

i.e.

$$240 = 200[1 + (0.0039)(\theta - 18)]$$

$$240 = 200 + (200)(0.0039)(\theta - 18)$$

$$240 - 200 = 0.78(\theta - 18)$$

$$40 = 0.78(\theta - 18)$$

$$\frac{40}{0.78} = \theta - 18$$

$$51.28 = \theta - 18, \text{ from which,}$$

$$\theta = 51.28 + 18 = 69.28°C$$

Hence the temperature of the coil increases to 69.28°C

If the resistance at 0°C is not known, but is known at some other temperature θ_1, then the resistance at any temperature can be found as follows:

$$R_1 = R_0(1 + \alpha_0\theta_1)$$

and

$$R_2 = R_0(1 + \alpha_0\theta_2)$$

Dividing one equation by the other gives:

$$\frac{R_1}{R_2} = \frac{1 + \alpha_0\theta_1}{1 + \alpha_0\theta_2}$$

where $R_2 =$ resistance at temperature θ_2

Problem 13. Some copper wire has a resistance of 200 Ω at 20°C. A current is passed through the wire and the temperature rises to 90°C. Determine the resistance of the wire at 90°C, correct to the nearest ohm, assuming that the temperature coefficient of resistance is 0.004/°C at 0°C.

$$R_{20} = 200\,\Omega, \alpha_0 = 0.004/°C$$

and

$$\frac{R_{20}}{R_{90}} = \frac{[1 + \alpha_0(20)]}{[1 + \alpha_0(90)]}$$

Hence

$$R_{90} = \frac{R_{20}[1 + 90\alpha_0]}{[1 + 20\alpha_0]}$$

$$= \frac{200[1 + 90(0.004)]}{[1 + 20(0.004)]}$$

$$= \frac{200[1 + 0.36]}{[1 + 0.08]}$$

$$= \frac{200(1.36)}{(1.08)} = \mathbf{251.85\,\Omega}$$

i.e. the resistance of the wire at 90°C is 252 Ω, correct to the nearest ohm

Now try the following exercise

Exercise 12 Further problems on the temperature coefficient of resistance

1. A coil of aluminium wire has a resistance of 50 Ω when its temperature is 0°C. Determine its resistance at 100°C if the temperature coefficient of resistance of aluminium at 0°C is 0.0038/°C   [69 Ω]

2. A copper cable has a resistance of 30 Ω at a temperature of 50°C. Determine its resistance at 0°C. Take the temperature coefficient of resistance of copper at 0°C as 0.0043/°C   [24.69 Ω]

3. The temperature coefficient of resistance for carbon at 0°C is −0.00048/°C. What is the significance of the minus sign? A carbon resistor has a resistance of 500 Ω at 0°C. Determine its resistance at 50°C.   [488 Ω]

4. A coil of copper wire has a resistance of $20\,\Omega$ at $18°C$. If the temperature coefficient of resistance of copper at $18°C$ is $0.004/°C$, determine the resistance of the coil when the temperature rises to $98°C$ [$26.4\,\Omega$]

5. The resistance of a coil of nickel wire at $20°C$ is $100\,\Omega$. The temperature of the wire is increased and the resistance rises to $130\,\Omega$. If the temperature coefficient of resistance of nickel is $0.006/°C$ at $20°C$, determine the temperature to which the coil has risen.   [$70°C$]

6. Some aluminium wire has a resistance of $50\,\Omega$ at $20°C$. The wire is heated to a temperature of $100°C$. Determine the resistance of the wire at $100°C$, assuming that the temperature coefficient of resistance at $0°C$ is $0.004/°C$.   [$64.8\,\Omega$]

7. A copper cable is $1.2\,km$ long and has a cross-sectional area of $5\,mm^2$. Find its resistance at $80°C$ if at $20°C$ the resistivity of copper is $0.02 \times 10^{-6}\,\Omega\,m$ and its temperature coefficient of resistance is $0.004/°C$.   [$5.95\,\Omega$]

3.4 Resistor colour coding and ohmic values

(a) Colour code for fixed resistors

The colour code for fixed resistors is given in Table 3.1

(i) For a **four-band fixed resistor** (i.e. resistance values with two significant figures): yellow-violet-orange-red indicates $47\,k\Omega$ with a tolerance of $\pm2\%$
(Note that the first band is the one nearest the end of the resistor)

(ii) For a **five-band fixed resistor** (i.e. resistance values with three significant figures): red-yellow-white-orange-brown indicates $249\,k\Omega$ with a tolerance of $\pm1\%$
(Note that the fifth band is 1.5 to 2 times wider than the other bands)

Problem 14. Determine the value and tolerance of a resistor having a colour coding of: orange-orange-silver-brown.

Table 3.1

Colour	Significant Figures	Multiplier	Tolerance
Silver	–	10^{-2}	$\pm10\%$
Gold	–	10^{-1}	$\pm5\%$
Black	0	1	–
Brown	1	10	$\pm1\%$
Red	2	10^2	$\pm2\%$
Orange	3	10^3	–
Yellow	4	10^4	–
Green	5	10^5	$\pm0.5\%$
Blue	6	10^6	$\pm0.25\%$
Violet	7	10^7	$\pm0.1\%$
Grey	8	10^8	–
White	9	10^9	–
None	–	–	$\pm20\%$

The first two bands, i.e. orange-orange, give 33 from Table 3.1.
The third band, silver, indicates a multiplier of 10^2 from Table 3.1, which means that the value of the resistor is $33 \times 10^{-2} = 0.33\,\Omega$
The fourth band, i.e. brown, indicates a tolerance of $\pm1\%$ from Table 3.1. Hence a colour coding of orange-orange-silver-brown represents a resistor of value **$0.33\,\Omega$ with a tolerance of $\pm1\%$**

Problem 15. Determine the value and tolerance of a resistor having a colour coding of: brown-black-brown.

The first two bands, i.e. brown-black, give 10 from Table 3.1.
The third band, brown, indicates a multiplier of 10 from Table 3.1, which means that the value of the resistor is $10 \times 10 = 100\,\Omega$
There is no fourth band colour in this case; hence, from Table 3.1, the tolerance is $\pm20\%$. Hence a colour coding of brown-black-brown represents a resistor of value **$100\,\Omega$ with a tolerance of $\pm20\%$**

Problem 16.   Between what two values should a resistor with colour coding brown-black-brown-silver lie?

From Table 3.1, brown-black-brown-silver indicates 10×10, i.e. $100\,\Omega$, with a tolerance of $\pm 10\%$
This means that the value could lie between

$$(100 - 10\% \text{ of } 100)\,\Omega$$

and $$(100 + 10\% \text{ of } 100)\,\Omega$$

i.e. brown-black-brown-silver indicates any value **between 90 Ω and 110 Ω**

Problem 17.   Determine the colour coding for a $47\,k\Omega$ having a tolerance of $\pm 5\%$.

From Table 3.1, $47\,k\Omega = 47 \times 10^3$ has a colour coding of yellow-violet-orange. With a tolerance of $\pm 5\%$, the fourth band will be gold.
Hence $47\,k\Omega \pm 5\%$ has a colour coding of:
yellow-violet-orange-gold

Problem 18.   Determine the value and tolerance of a resistor having a colour coding of: orange-green-red-yellow-brown.

Orange-green-red-yellow-brown is a five-band fixed resistor and from Table 3.1, indicates: $352 \times 10^4\,\Omega$ with a tolerance of $\pm 1\%$

$$352 \times 10^4\,\Omega = 3.52 \times 10^6\,\Omega, \text{i.e. } 3.52\,M\Omega$$

Hence   orange-green-red-yellow-brown   indicates **3.52 MΩ $\pm$ 1%**

(b) Letter and digit code for resistors

Another way of indicating the value of resistors is the letter and digit code shown in Table 3.2.
Tolerance is indicated as follows: $F = \pm 1\%$, $G = \pm 2\%$, $J = \pm 5\%$, $K = \pm 10\%$ and $M = \pm 20\%$
Thus, for example,

$$R33M = 0.33\,\Omega \pm 20\%$$

$$4R7K = 4.7\,\Omega \pm 10\%$$

$$390RJ = 390\,\Omega \pm 5\%$$

Problem 19.   Determine the value of a resistor marked as 6K8F.

Table 3.2

Resistance Value	Marked as:
0.47 Ω	R47
1 Ω	1R0
4.7 Ω	4R7
47 Ω	47R
100 Ω	100R
1 kΩ	1K0
10 kΩ	10K
10 MΩ	10M

From Table 3.2, 6K8F is equivalent to: **6.8 kΩ $\pm$ 1%**

Problem 20.   Determine the value of a resistor marked as 4M7M.

From Table 3.2, 4M7M is equivalent to: **4.7 MΩ $\pm$ 20%**

Problem 21.   Determine the letter and digit code for a resistor having a value of $68\,k\Omega \pm 10\%$.

From Table 3.2, $68\,k\Omega \pm 10\%$ has a letter and digit code of: **68 KK**

Now try the following exercises

Exercise 13   Further problems on resistor colour coding and ohmic values

1. Determine the value and tolerance of a resistor having a colour coding of: blue-grey-orange-red   [68 kΩ $\pm$ 2%]

2. Determine the value and tolerance of a resistor having a colour coding of: yellow-violet-gold
                [4.7 Ω $\pm$ 20%]

3. Determine the value and tolerance of a resistor having a colour coding of: blue-white-black-black-gold   [690 Ω $\pm$ 5%]

4. Determine the colour coding for a $51\,k\Omega$ four-band resistor having a tolerance of $\pm 2\%$
[green-brown-orange-red]

5. Determine the colour coding for a $1\,M\Omega$ four-band resistor having a tolerance of $\pm 10\%$
[brown-black-green-silver]

6. Determine the range of values expected for a resistor with colour coding: red-black-green-silver
[$1.8\,M\Omega$ to $2.2\,M\Omega$]

7. Determine the range of values expected for a resistor with colour coding: yellow-black-orange-brown
[$39.6\,k\Omega$ to $40.4\,k\Omega$]

8. Determine the value of a resistor marked as (a) R22G (b) 4K7F
[(a) $0.22\,\Omega \pm 2\%$ (b) $4.7\,k\Omega \pm 1\%$]

9. Determine the letter and digit code for a resistor having a value of $100\,k\Omega \pm 5\%$
[100 KJ]

10. Determine the letter and digit code for a resistor having a value of $6.8\,M\Omega \pm 20\%$
[6M8 M]

Exercise 14   Short answer questions on resistance variation

1. Name three types of resistor construction and state one practical application of each

2. Name four factors which can effect the resistance of a conductor

3. If the length of a piece of wire of constant cross-sectional area is halved, the resistance of the wire is ......

4. If the cross-sectional area of a certain length of cable is trebled, the resistance of the cable is ......

5. What is resistivity? State its unit and the symbol used

6. Complete the following:

   Good conductors of electricity have a ...... value of resistivity and good insulators have a ...... value of resistivity

7. What is meant by the 'temperature coefficient of resistance? State its units and the symbols used

8. If the resistance of a metal at $0°C$ is R_0, R_θ is the resistance at $\theta°C$ and α_0 is the temperature coefficient of resistance at $0°C$ then: $R_\theta = ...$

9. Explain briefly the colour coding on resistors

10. Explain briefly the letter and digit code for resistors

Exercise 15   Multi-choice questions on resistance variation
(Answers on page 420)

1. The unit of resistivity is:
   (a) ohms
   (b) ohm millimetre
   (c) ohm metre
   (d) ohm/metre

2. The length of a certain conductor of resistance $100\,\Omega$ is doubled and its cross-sectional area is halved. Its new resistance is:
   (a) $100\,\Omega$ (b) $200\,\Omega$
   (c) $50\,\Omega$ (d) $400\,\Omega$

3. The resistance of a $2\,km$ length of cable of cross-sectional area $2\,mm^2$ and resistivity of $2 \times 10^{-8}\,\Omega\,m$ is:
   (a) $0.02\,\Omega$ (b) $20\,\Omega$
   (c) $0.02\,m\Omega$ (d) $200\,\Omega$

4. A piece of graphite has a cross-sectional area of $10\,mm^2$. If its resistance is $0.1\,\Omega$ and its resistivity $10 \times 10^8\,\Omega\,m$, its length is:
   (a) $10\,km$ (b) $10\,cm$
   (c) $10\,mm$ (d) $10\,m$

5. The symbol for the unit of temperature coefficient of resistance is:
   (a) $\Omega/°C$ (b) Ω
   (c) $°C$ (d) $\Omega/\Omega°C$

6. A coil of wire has a resistance of $10\,\Omega$ at $0°C$. If the temperature coefficient of resistance for the wire is $0.004/°C$, its resistance at $100°C$ is:
   (a) $0.4\,\Omega$ (b) $1.4\,\Omega$
   (c) $14\,\Omega$ (d) $10\,\Omega$

7. A nickel coil has a resistance of $13\,\Omega$ at $50°C$. If the temperature coefficient of

resistance at 0°C is 0.006/°C, the resistance at 0°C is:

(a) 16.9 Ω (b) 10 Ω

(c) 43.3 Ω (d) 0.1 Ω

8. A colour coding of red-violet-black on a resistor indicates a value of:

(a) 27 Ω ±20%   (b) 270 Ω

(c) 270 Ω ±20%   (d) 27 Ω ±10%

9. A resistor marked as 4K7G indicates a value of:

(a) 47 Ω ±20%   (b) 4.7 k Ω ±20%

(c) 0.47 Ω ±10%   (d) 4.7 k Ω ±2%

Chapter 4

Batteries and alternative sources of energy

At the end of this chapter you should be able to:

- list practical applications of batteries
- understand electrolysis and its applications, including electroplating
- appreciate the purpose and construction of a simple cell
- explain polarisation and local action
- explain corrosion and its effects
- define the terms e.m.f., E, and internal resistance, r, of a cell
- perform calculations using $V = E - Ir$
- determine the total e.m.f. and total internal resistance for cells connected in series and in parallel
- distinguish between primary and secondary cells
- explain the construction and practical applications of the Leclanché, mercury, lead–acid and alkaline cells
- list the advantages and disadvantages of alkaline cells over lead–acid cells
- understand the term 'cell capacity' and state its unit
- understand the importance of safe battery disposal
- appreciate advantages of fuel cells and their likely future applications
- understand the implications of alternative energy sources and state five examples

4.1 Introduction to batteries

A battery is a device that **converts chemical energy to electricity**. If an appliance is placed between its terminals the current generated will power the device. Batteries are an indispensable item for many electronic devices and are essential for devices that require power when no mains power is available. For example, without the battery, there would be no mobile phones or laptop computers.

The battery is now over 200 years old and batteries are found almost everywhere in consumer and industrial products. Some **practical examples** where batteries are used include:

in laptops, in cameras, in mobile phones, in cars, in watches and clocks, for security equipment, in electronic meters, for smoke alarms, for meters used to read gas, water and electricity consumption at home, to power a camera for an endoscope looking internally at the body, and for transponders used for toll collection on highways throughout the world

Batteries tend to be split into two categories – **primary**, which are not designed to be electrically re-charged,

DOI: 10.1016/B978-0-08-089056-2.00004-8

i.e. are disposable (see Section 4.6), and **secondary batteries**, which are designed to be re-charged, such as those used in mobile phones (see Section 4.7).

In more recent years it has been necessary to design batteries with reduced size, but with increased lifespan and capacity.

If an application requires small size and high power then the 1.5 V battery is used. If longer lifetime is required then the 3 to 3.6 V battery is used. In the 1970s the 1.5 V **manganese battery** was gradually replaced by the **alkaline battery**. **Silver oxide batteries** were gradually introduced in the 1960s and are still the preferred technology for watch batteries today.

Lithium-ion batteries were introduced in the 1970s because of the need for longer lifetime applications. Indeed, some such batteries have been known to last well over 10 years before replacement, a characteristic that means that these batteries are still very much in demand today for digital cameras, and sometimes for watches and computer clocks. Lithium batteries are capable of delivering high currents but tend to be expensive.

More types of batteries and their uses are listed in Table 4.2 on page 37.

4.2 Some chemical effects of electricity

A material must contain **charged particles** to be able to conduct electric current. In **solids**, the current is carried by **electrons**. Copper, lead, aluminium, iron and carbon are some examples of solid conductors. In **liquids and gases**, the current is carried by the part of a molecule which has acquired an electric charge, called **ions**. These can possess a positive or negative charge, and examples include hydrogen ion H^+, copper ion Cu^{++} and hydroxyl ion OH^-. Distilled water contains no ions and is a poor conductor of electricity, whereas salt water contains ions and is a fairly good conductor of electricity.

Electrolysis is the decomposition of a liquid compound by the passage of electric current through it. Practical applications of electrolysis include the electroplating of metals (see below), the refining of copper and the extraction of aluminium from its ore.

An **electrolyte** is a compound which will undergo electrolysis. Examples include salt water, copper sulphate and sulphuric acid.

The **electrodes** are the two conductors carrying current to the electrolyte. The positive-connected electrode is called the **anode** and the negative-connected electrode the **cathode**.

When two copper wires connected to a battery are placed in a beaker containing a salt water solution, current will flow through the solution. Air bubbles appear around the wires as the water is changed into hydrogen and oxygen by electrolysis.

Electroplating uses the principle of electrolysis to apply a thin coat of one metal to another metal. Some practical applications include the tin-plating of steel, silver-plating of nickel alloys and chromium-plating of steel. If two copper electrodes connected to a battery are placed in a beaker containing copper sulphate as the electrolyte it is found that the cathode (i.e. the electrode connected to the negative terminal of the battery) gains copper whilst the anode loses copper.

4.3 The simple cell

The purpose of an **electric cell** is to convert chemical energy into electrical energy.

A **simple cell** comprises two dissimilar conductors (electrodes) in an electrolyte. Such a cell is shown in Fig. 4.1, comprising copper and zinc electrodes. An electric current is found to flow between the electrodes. Other possible electrode pairs exist, including zinc–lead and zinc–iron. The electrode potential (i.e. the p.d. measured between the electrodes) varies for each pair of metals. By knowing the e.m.f. of each metal with respect to some standard electrode, the e.m.f. of any pair of metals may be determined. The standard used is the hydrogen electrode. The **electrochemical series** is a way of listing elements in order of electrical potential, and Table 4.1 shows a number of elements in such a series.

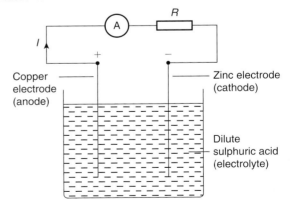

Figure 4.1

In a simple cell two faults exist – those due to **polarisation** and **local action**.

Table 4.1 Part of the electrochemical series

| Potassium |
| sodium |
| aluminium |
| zinc |
| iron |
| lead |
| hydrogen |
| copper |
| silver |
| carbon |

Polarisation

If the simple cell shown in Fig. 4.1 is left connected for some time, the current I decreases fairly rapidly. This is because of the formation of a film of hydrogen bubbles on the copper anode. This effect is known as the polarisation of the cell. The hydrogen prevents full contact between the copper electrode and the electrolyte and this increases the internal resistance of the cell. The effect can be overcome by using a chemical depolarising agent or depolariser, such as potassium dichromate which removes the hydrogen bubbles as they form. This allows the cell to deliver a steady current.

Local action

When commercial zinc is placed in dilute sulphuric acid, hydrogen gas is liberated from it and the zinc dissolves. The reason for this is that impurities, such as traces of iron, are present in the zinc which set up small primary cells with the zinc. These small cells are short-circuited by the electrolyte, with the result that localised currents flow causing corrosion. This action is known as local action of the cell. This may be prevented by rubbing a small amount of mercury on the zinc surface, which forms a protective layer on the surface of the electrode.

When two metals are used in a simple cell the electrochemical series may be used to predict the behaviour of the cell:

(i) The metal that is higher in the series acts as the negative electrode, and vice versa. For example,

the zinc electrode in the cell shown in Fig. 4.1 is negative and the copper electrode is positive.

(ii) The greater the separation in the series between the two metals the greater is the e.m.f. produced by the cell.

The electrochemical series is representative of the order of reactivity of the metals and their compounds:

(i) The higher metals in the series react more readily with oxygen and vice-versa.

(ii) When two metal electrodes are used in a simple cell the one that is higher in the series tends to dissolve in the electrolyte.

4.4 Corrosion

Corrosion is the gradual destruction of a metal in a damp atmosphere by means of simple cell action. In addition to the presence of moisture and air required for rusting, an electrolyte, an anode and a cathode are required for corrosion. Thus, if metals widely spaced in the electrochemical series, are used in contact with each other in the presence of an electrolyte, corrosion will occur. For example, if a brass valve is fitted to a heating system made of steel, corrosion will occur.

The **effects of corrosion** include the weakening of structures, the reduction of the life of components and materials, the wastage of materials and the expense of replacement.

Corrosion may be **prevented** by coating with paint, grease, plastic coatings and enamels, or by plating with tin or chromium. Also, iron may be galvanised, i.e., plated with zinc, the layer of zinc helping to prevent the iron from corroding.

4.5 E.m.f. and internal resistance of a cell

The **electromotive force (e.m.f.), E,** of a cell is the p.d. between its terminals when it is not connected to a load (i.e. the cell is on 'no load').

The e.m.f. of a cell is measured by using a **high resistance voltmeter** connected in parallel with the cell. The voltmeter must have a high resistance otherwise it will pass current and the cell will not be on 'no-load'. For example, if the resistance of a cell is $1\,\Omega$ and that of a voltmeter $1\,M\Omega$ then the equivalent resistance of the circuit is $1\,M\Omega + 1\,\Omega$, i.e. approximately $1\,M\Omega$, hence no current flows and the cell is not loaded.

The voltage available at the terminals of a cell falls when a load is connected. This is caused by the **internal resistance** of the cell which is the opposition of the material of the cell to the flow of current. The internal resistance acts in series with other resistances in the circuit. Figure 4.2 shows a cell of e.m.f. E volts and internal resistance, r, and XY represents the terminals of the cell.

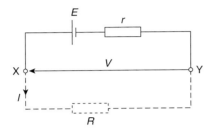

Figure 4.2

When a load (shown as resistance R) is not connected, no current flows and the terminal p.d., $V = E$. When R is connected a current I flows which causes a voltage drop in the cell, given by Ir. The p.d. available at the cell terminals is less than the e.m.f. of the cell and is given by:

$$V = E - Ir$$

Thus if a battery of e.m.f. 12 volts and internal resistance $0.01\,\Omega$ delivers a current of 100 A, the terminal p.d.,

$$V = 12 - (100)(0.01)$$
$$= 12 - 1 = 11\,\text{V}$$

When different values of potential difference V across a cell or power supply are measured for different values of current I, a graph may be plotted as shown in Fig. 4.3. Since the e.m.f. E of the cell or power supply is the p.d. across its terminals on no load (i.e. when $I = 0$), then E is as shown by the broken line.

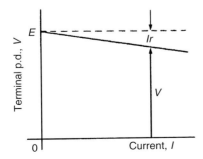

Figure 4.3

Since $V = E - Ir$ then the internal resistance may be calculated from

$$r = \frac{E - V}{I}$$

When a current is flowing in the direction shown in Fig. 4.2 the cell is said to be **discharging** ($E > V$). When a current flows in the opposite direction to that shown in Fig. 4.2 the cell is said to be **charging** ($V > E$). A **battery** is a combination of more than one cell. The cells in a battery may be connected in series or in parallel.

(i) **For cells connected in series:**

Total e.m.f. = sum of cell's e.m.f.s

Total internal resistance = sum of cell's internal resistances

(ii) **For cells connected in parallel:**

If each cell has the same e.m.f. and internal resistance:

Total e.m.f. = e.m.f. of one cell

Total internal resistance of n cells

$$= \frac{1}{n} \times \text{internal resistance of one cell}$$

Problem 1.   Eight cells, each with an internal resistance of $0.2\,\Omega$ and an e.m.f. of 2.2 V are connected (a) in series, (b) in parallel. Determine the e.m.f. and the internal resistance of the batteries so formed.

(a)   When connected in series, total e.m.f.

$$= \text{sum of cell's e.m.f.}$$
$$= 2.2 \times 8 = \textbf{17.6 V}$$

Total internal resistance

$$= \text{sum of cell's internal resistance}$$
$$= 0.2 \times 8 = \textbf{1.6 }\boldsymbol{\Omega}$$

(b)   When connected in parallel, total e.m.f

$$= \text{e.m.f. of one cell}$$
$$= \textbf{2.2 V}$$

Total internal resistance of 8 cells

$$= \frac{1}{8} \times \text{internal resistance of one cell}$$
$$= \frac{1}{8} \times 0.2 = \textbf{0.025 }\boldsymbol{\Omega}$$

Problem 2. A cell has an internal resistance of $0.02\,\Omega$ and an e.m.f. of 2.0 V. Calculate its terminal p.d. if it delivers (a) 5 A (b) 50 A.

(a) Terminal p.d. $V = E - Ir$ where $E =$ e.m.f. of cell, $I =$ current flowing and $r =$ internal resistance of cell

$E = 2.0\,\text{V}$, $I = 5\,\text{A}$ and $r = 0.02\,\Omega$

Hence **terminal p.d.**

$$V = 2.0 - (5)(0.02) = 2.0 - 0.1 = \mathbf{1.9\,V}$$

(b) When the current is 50 A, terminal p.d.,

$$V = E - Ir = 2.0 - 50(0.02)$$

i.e. $\qquad V = 2.0 - 1.0 = \mathbf{1.0\,V}$

Thus the terminal p.d. decreases as the current drawn increases.

Problem 3. The p.d. at the terminals of a battery is 25 V when no load is connected and 24 V when a load taking 10 A is connected. Determine the internal resistance of the battery.

When no load is connected the e.m.f. of the battery, E, is equal to the terminal p.d., V, i.e. $E = 25\,\text{V}$
When current $I = 10\,\text{A}$ and terminal p.d.

$$V = 24\,\text{V, then } V = E - Ir$$

i.e. $\qquad 24 = 25 - (10)r$

Hence, rearranging, gives

$$10r = 25 - 24 = 1$$

and the internal resistance,

$$\mathbf{r} = \frac{1}{10} = \mathbf{0.1\,\Omega}$$

Problem 4. Ten 1.5 V cells, each having an internal resistance of $0.2\,\Omega$, are connected in series to a load of $58\,\Omega$. Determine (a) the current flowing in the circuit and (b) the p.d. at the battery terminals.

(a) For ten cells, battery e.m.f., $E = 10 \times 1.5 = 15\,\text{V}$, and the total internal resistance, $r = 10 \times 0.2 = 2\,\Omega$.

When connected to a $58\,\Omega$ load the circuit is as shown in Fig. 4.4

$$\text{Current } I = \frac{\text{e.m.f.}}{\text{total resistance}}$$

$$= \frac{15}{58 + 2}$$

$$= \frac{15}{60} = \mathbf{0.25\,A}$$

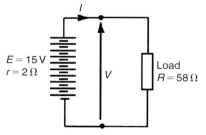

Figure 4.4

(b) P.d. at battery terminals, $V = E - Ir$

i.e. $V = 15 - (0.25)(2) = \mathbf{14.5\,V}$

Now try the following exercise

Exercise 16   Further problems on e.m.f. and internal resistance of a cell

1. Twelve cells, each with an internal resistance of $0.24\,\Omega$ and an e.m.f. of 1.5 V are connected (a) in series, (b) in parallel. Determine the e.m.f. and internal resistance of the batteries so formed.

    [(a) 18 V, $2.88\,\Omega$ (b) 1.5 V, $0.02\,\Omega$]

2. A cell has an internal resistance of $0.03\,\Omega$ and an e.m.f. of 2.2 V. Calculate its terminal p.d. if it delivers

    (a) 1 A   (b) 20 A   (c) 50 A

    [(a) 2.17 V (b) 1.6 V (c) 0.7 V]

3. The p.d. at the terminals of a battery is 16 V when no load is connected and 14 V when a load taking 8 A is connected. Determine the internal resistance of the battery.   [$0.25\,\Omega$]

4. A battery of e.m.f. 20 V and internal resistance $0.2\,\Omega$ supplies a load taking 10 A. Determine the p.d. at the battery terminals and the resistance of the load.   [18 V, $1.8\,\Omega$]

5. Ten 2.2 V cells, each having an internal resistance of 0.1 Ω are connected in series to a load of 21 Ω. Determine (a) the current flowing in the circuit, and (b) the p.d. at the battery terminals.   [(a) 1 A (b) 21 V]

6. For the circuits shown in Fig. 4.5 the resistors represent the internal resistance of the batteries. Find, in each case:
   (i) the total e.m.f. across *PQ*
   (ii) the total equivalent internal resistances of the batteries.
   [(i) (a) 6 V (b) 2 V (ii) (a) 4 Ω (b) 0.25 Ω]

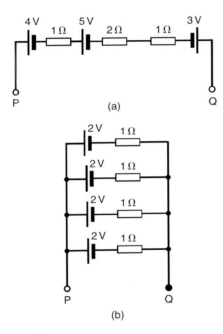

Figure 4.5

7. The voltage at the terminals of a battery is 52 V when no load is connected and 48.8 V when a load taking 80 A is connected. Find the internal resistance of the battery. What would be the terminal voltage when a load taking 20 A is connected?   [0.04 Ω, 51.2 V]

4.6 Primary cells

Primary cells cannot be recharged, that is, the conversion of chemical energy to electrical energy is irreversible and the cell cannot be used once the chemicals

are exhausted. Examples of primary cells include the Leclanché cell and the mercury cell.

Lechlanché cell

A typical dry Lechlanché cell is shown in Fig. 4.6. Such a cell has an e.m.f. of about 1.5 V when new, but this falls rapidly if in continuous use due to polarisation. The hydrogen film on the carbon electrode forms faster than can be dissipated by the depolariser. The Lechlanché cell is suitable only for intermittent use, applications including torches, transistor radios, bells, indicator circuits, gas lighters, controlling switch-gear, and so on. The cell is the most commonly used of primary cells, is cheap, requires little maintenance and has a shelf life of about 2 years.

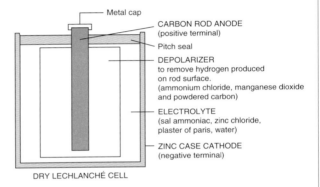

Figure 4.6

Mercury cell

A typical mercury cell is shown in Fig. 4.7. Such a cell has an e.m.f. of about 1.3 V which remains constant for a relatively long time. Its main advantages over the Lechlanché cell is its smaller size and its long shelf life. Typical practical applications include hearing aids, medical electronics, cameras and for guided missiles.

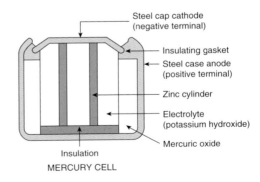

Figure 4.7

4.7 Secondary cells

Secondary cells can be recharged after use, that is, the conversion of chemical energy to electrical energy is reversible and the cell may be used many times. Examples of secondary cells include the lead–acid cell and the nickel cadmium and nickel–metal cells. Practical applications of such cells include car batteries, telephone circuits and for traction purposes – such as milk delivery vans and fork lift trucks.

Lead–acid cell

A typical lead–acid cell is constructed of:

(i)   A container made of glass, ebonite or plastic.

(ii) **Lead plates**

    (a) the negative plate (cathode) consists of spongy lead

    (b) the positive plate (anode) is formed by pressing lead peroxide into the lead grid.

    The plates are interleaved as shown in the plan view of Fig. 4.8 to increase their effective cross-sectional area and to minimise internal resistance.

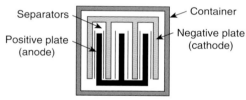

PLAN VIEW OF LEAD–ACID CELL

Figure 4.8

(iii) **Separators** made of glass, celluloid or wood.

(iv) An **electrolyte** which is a mixture of sulphuric acid and distilled water.

The relative density (or specific gravity) of a lead–acid cell, which may be measured using a hydrometer, varies between about 1.26 when the cell is fully charged to about 1.19 when discharged. The terminal p.d. of a lead–acid cell is about 2 V.

When a cell supplies current to a load it is said to be **discharging**. During discharge:

(i)   the lead peroxide (positive plate) and the spongy lead (negative plate) are converted into lead sulphate, and

(ii) the oxygen in the lead peroxide combines with hydrogen in the electrolyte to form water. The electrolyte is therefore weakened and the relative density falls.

The terminal p.d. of a lead–acid cell when fully discharged is about 1.8 V. A cell is **charged** by connecting a d.c. supply to its terminals, the positive terminal of the cell being connected to the positive terminal of the supply. The charging current flows in the reverse direction to the discharge current and the chemical action is reversed. During charging:

(i)   the lead sulphate on the positive and negative plates is converted back to lead peroxide and lead respectively, and

(ii) the water content of the electrolyte decreases as the oxygen released from the electrolyte combines with the lead of the positive plate. The relative density of the electrolyte thus increases.

The colour of the positive plate when fully charged is dark brown and when discharged is light brown. The colour of the negative plate when fully charged is grey and when discharged is light grey.

Nickel cadmium and nickel–metal cells

In both types the positive plate is made of nickel hydroxide enclosed in finely perforated steel tubes, the resistance being reduced by the addition of pure nickel or graphite. The tubes are assembled into nickel–steel plates.

In the nickel–metal cell, (sometimes called the **Edison cell** or **nife cell**), the negative plate is made of iron oxide, with the resistance being reduced by a little mercuric oxide, the whole being enclosed in perforated steel tubes and assembled in steel plates. In the nickel cadmium cell the negative plate is made of cadmium. The electrolyte in each type of cell is a solution of potassium hydroxide which does not undergo any chemical change and thus the quantity can be reduced to a minimum. The plates are separated by insulating rods and assembled in steel containers which are then enclosed in a non-metallic crate to insulate the cells from one another. The average discharge p.d. of an alkaline cell is about 1.2 V.

Advantages of a nickel cadmium cell or a nickel–metal cell over a lead–acid cell include:

(i)   More robust construction

(ii) Capable of withstanding heavy charging and discharging currents without damage

Table 4.2

Type of battery	Common uses	Hazardous component	Disposal recycling options
Wet cell (i.e. a primary cell that has a liquid electrolyte)			
Lead acid batteries	Electrical energy supply for vehicles including cars, trucks, boats, tractors and motorcycles. Small sealed lead acid batteries are used for emergency lighting and uninterruptible power supplies	Sulphuric acid and lead	Recycle – most petrol stations and garages accept old car batteries, and council waste facilities have collection points for lead acid batteries
Dry cell: Non-chargeable – single use (for example, AA, AAA, C, D, lantern and miniature watch sizes)			
Zinc carbon	Torches, clocks, shavers, radios, toys and smoke alarms	Zinc	Not classed as hazardous waste – can be disposed with household waste
Zinc chloride	Torches, clocks, shavers, radios, toys and smoke alarms	Zinc	Not classed as hazardous waste – can be disposed with household waste
Alkaline manganese	Personal stereos and radio/cassette players	Manganese	Not classed as hazardous waste – can be disposed with household waste
Primary button cells (i.e. a small flat battery shaped like a 'button' used in small electronic devices)			
Mercuric oxide	Hearing aids, pacemakers and cameras	Mercury	Recycle at council waste facility, if available
Zinc air	Hearing aids, pagers and cameras	Zinc	Recycle at council waste facility, if available
Silver oxide	Calculators, watches and cameras	Silver	Recycle at council waste facility, if available
Lithium	Computers, watches and cameras	Lithium (explosive and flammable)	Recycle at council waste facility, if available
Dry cell rechargeable – secondary batteries			
Nickel cadmium (NiCd)	Mobile phones, cordless power tools, laptop computers, shavers, motorised toys, personal stereos	Cadmium	Recycle at council waste facility, if available
Nickel–metal hydride (NiMH)	Alternative to NiCd batteries, but longer life	Nickel	Recycle at council waste facility, if available
Lithium-ion (Li-ion)	Alternative to NiCd and NiMH batteries, but greater energy storage capacity	Lithium	Recycle at council waste facility, if available

(iii)   Has a longer life

(iv)   For a given capacity is lighter in weight

(v)   Can be left indefinitely in any state of charge or discharge without damage

(vi)   Is not self-discharging

Disadvantages of nickel cadmium and nickel–metal cells over a lead–acid cell include:

(i)   Is relatively more expensive

(ii)   Requires more cells for a given e.m.f.

(iii)   Has a higher internal resistance

(iv)   Must be kept sealed

(v)   Has a lower efficiency

Nickel cells may be used in extremes of temperature, in conditions where vibration is experienced or where duties require long idle periods or heavy discharge currents. Practical examples include traction and marine work, lighting in railway carriages, military portable radios and for starting diesel and petrol engines. See also Table 4.2, page 37.

4.8   Cell capacity

The **capacity** of a cell is measured in ampere-hours (Ah). A fully charged 50 Ah battery rated for 10 h discharge can be discharged at a steady current of 5 A for 10 h, but if the load current is increased to 10 A then the battery is discharged in 3–4 h, since the higher the discharge current, the lower is the effective capacity of the battery. Typical discharge characteristics for a lead–acid cell are shown in Fig. 4.9

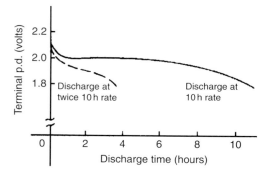

Figure 4.9

4.9   Safe disposal of batteries

Battery disposal has become a topical subject in the UK because of greater awareness of the dangers and implications of depositing up to 300 million batteries per annum – a waste stream of over 20 000 tonnes – into landfill sites.

Certain batteries contain substances which can be a hazard to humans, wildlife and the environment, as well a posing a fire risk. Other batteries can be recycled for their metal content.

Waste batteries are a concentrated source of toxic heavy metals such as mercury, lead and cadmium. If batteries containing heavy metals are disposed of incorrectly, the metals can leach out and pollute the soil and groundwater, endangering humans and wildlife. Long-term exposure to cadmium, a known human carcinogen (i.e. a substance producing cancerous growth), can cause liver and lung disease. Mercury can cause damage to the human brain, spinal system, kidneys and liver. Sulphuric acid in lead acid batteries can cause severe skin burns or irritation upon contact. It is increasingly important to correctly dispose of all types of batteries.

Table 4.2 lists types of batteries, their common uses, their hazardous components and disposal recycling options.

Battery disposal has become more regulated since the Landfill Regulations 2002 and Hazardous Waste Regulations 2005. From the Waste Electrical and Electronic Equipment (WEEE) Regulations 2006, commencing July 2007 all producers (manufacturers and importers) of electrical and electronic equipment will be responsible for the cost of collection, treatment and recycling of obligated WEEE generated in the UK.

4.10   Fuel cells

A **fuel cell** is an electrochemical energy conversion device, similar to a battery, but differing from the latter in that it is designed for continuous replenishment of the reactants consumed, i.e. it produces electricity from an external source of fuel and oxygen, as opposed to the limited energy storage capacity of a battery. Also, the electrodes within a battery react and change as a battery is charged or discharged, whereas a fuel cells' electrodes are catalytic (i.e. not permanently changed) and relatively stable.

Typical reactants used in a fuel cell are hydrogen on the anode side and oxygen on the cathode side (i.e. a **hydrogen cell**). Usually, reactants flow in and reaction products flow out. Virtually continuous long-term operation is feasible as long as these flows are maintained.

Fuel cells are very attractive in modern applications for their high efficiency and ideally emission-free use, in contrast to currently more modern fuels such as methane or natural gas that generate carbon dioxide. The only by-product of a fuel cell operating on pure hydrogen is water vapour.

Currently, fuel cells are a very expensive alternative to internal combustion engines. However, continued research and development is likely to make fuel cell vehicles available at market prices within a few years.

Fuel cells are very useful as power sources in remote locations, such as spacecraft, remote weather stations, and in certain military applications. A fuel cell running on hydrogen can be compact, lightweight and has no moving parts.

4.11 Alternative and renewable energy sources

Alternative energy refers to energy sources which could replace coal, traditional gas and oil, all of which increase the atmospheric carbon when burned as fuel. **Renewable energy** implies that it is derived from a source which is automatically replenished or one that is effectively infinite so that it is not depleted as it is used. Coal, gas and oil are not renewable because, although the fields may last for generations, their time span is finite and will eventually run out.

There are many means of harnessing energy which have less damaging impacts on our environment and include the following:

1. **Solar energy** is one of the most resourceful sources of energy for the future. The reason for this is that the total energy received each year from the sun is around 35 000 times the total energy used by man. However, about one third of this energy is either absorbed by the outer atmosphere or reflected back into space. Solar energy could be used to run cars, power plants and space ships. **Solar panels** on roofs capture heat in water storage systems. **Photovoltaic cells**, when suitably positioned, convert sunlight to electricity.

2. **Wind power** is another alternative energy source that can be used without producing by-products that are harmful to nature. The fins of a windmill rotate in a vertical plane which is kept vertical to the wind by means of a tail fin and as wind flow crosses the blades of the windmill it is forced to rotate and can be used to generate electricity (see Chapter 9). Like solar power, harnessing the wind is highly dependent upon weather and location. The average wind velocity of Earth is around 9 m/s, and the power that could be produced when a windmill is facing a wind of 10 m.p.h. (i.e. around 4.5 m/s) is around 50 watts.

3. **Hydroelectricity** is achieved by the damming of rivers and utilising the potential energy in the water. As the water stored behind a dam is released at high pressure, its kinetic energy is transferred onto turbine blades and used to generate electricity. The system has enormous initial costs but has relatively low maintenance costs and provides power quite cheaply.

4. **Tidal power** utilises the natural motion of the tides to fill reservoirs which are then slowly discharged through electricity-producing turbines.

5. **Geothermal energy** is obtained from the internal heat of the planet and can be used to generate steam to run a steam turbine which, in turn, generates electricity. The radius of the Earth is about 4000 miles with an internal core temperature of around 4000°C at the centre. Drilling 3 miles from the surface of the Earth, a temperature of 100°C is encountered; this is sufficient to boil water to run a steam-powered electric power plant. Although drilling 3 miles down is possible, it is not easy. Fortunately, however, volcanic features called **geothermal hotspots** are found all around the world. These are areas which transmit excess internal heat from the interior of the Earth to the outer crust which can be used to generate electricity.

Now try the following exercises

Exercise 17   Short answer questions on the chemical effects of electricity

1. Define a battery

2. State five practical applications of batteries

3. State advantages of lithium-ion batteries over alkaline batteries

4. What is electrolysis?

5. What is an electrolyte?

6. Conduction in electrolytes is due to ......

7. A positive-connected electrode is called the ...... and the negative-connected electrode the ......

8. State two practical applications of electrolysis

9. The purpose of an electric cell is to convert ...... to ......

10. Make a labelled sketch of a simple cell

11. What is the electrochemical series?

12. With reference to a simple cell, explain briefly what is meant by (a) polarisation (b) local action

13. What is corrosion? Name two effects of corrosion and state how they may be prevented

14. What is meant by the e.m.f. of a cell? How may the e.m.f. of a cell be measured?

15. Define internal resistance

16. If a cell has an e.m.f. of E volts, an internal resistance of r ohms and supplies a current I amperes to a load, the terminal p.d. V volts is given by: $V = ...$

17. Name the two main types of cells

18. Explain briefly the difference between primary and secondary cells

19. Name two types of primary cells

20. Name two types of secondary cells

21. State three typical applications of primary cells

22. State three typical applications of secondary cells

23. In what unit is the capacity of a cell measured?

24. Why is safe disposal of batteries important?

25. Name any six types of battery and state three common applications for each

26. What is a 'fuel cell'? How does it differ from a battery?

27. State the advantages of fuel cells

28. State three practical applications of fuel cells

29. What is meant by (a) alternative energy (b) renewable energy

30. State five alternative energy sources and briefly describe each

Exercise 18 Multi-choice questions on the chemical effects of electricity
(Answers on page 420)

1. A battery consists of:
   (a) a cell   (b) a circuit
   (c) a generator   (d) a number of cells

2. The terminal p.d. of a cell of e.m.f. 2 V and internal resistance $0.1\,\Omega$ when supplying a current of 5 A will be:
   (a) 1.5 V   (b) 2 V
   (c) 1.9 V   (d) 2.5 V

3. Five cells, each with an e.m.f. of 2 V and internal resistance $0.5\,\Omega$ are connected in series. The resulting battery will have:
   (a) an e.m.f. of 2 V and an internal resistance of $0.5\,\Omega$
   (b) an e.m.f. of 10 V and an internal resistance of $2.5\,\Omega$
   (c) an e.m.f. of 2 V and an internal resistance of $0.1\,\Omega$
   (d) an e.m.f. of 10 V and an internal resistance of $0.1\,\Omega$

4. If the five cells of question 3 are connected in parallel the resulting battery will have:
   (a) an e.m.f. of 2 V and an internal resistance of $0.5\,\Omega$
   (b) an e.m.f. of 10 V and an internal resistance of $2.5\,\Omega$
   (c) an e.m.f. of 2 V and an internal resistance of $0.1\,\Omega$
   (d) an e.m.f. of 10 V and an internal resistance of $0.1\,\Omega$

5. Which of the following statements is false?
   (a) A Leclanché cell is suitable for use in torches
   (b) A nickel–cadmium cell is an example of a primary cell

(c) When a cell is being charged its terminal p.d. exceeds the cell e.m.f.

(d) A secondary cell may be recharged after use

6. Which of the following statements is false? When two metal electrodes are used in a simple cell, the one that is higher in the electrochemical series:
   (a) tends to dissolve in the electrolyte
   (b) is always the negative electrode
   (c) reacts most readily with oxygen
   (d) acts as an anode

7. Five 2 V cells, each having an internal resistance of $0.2\,\Omega$ are connected in series to a load of resistance $14\,\Omega$. The current flowing in the circuit is:
   (a) 10 A (b) 1.4 A
   (c) 1.5 A (d) $\frac{2}{3}$ A

8. For the circuit of question 7, the p.d. at the battery terminals is:
   (a) 10 V (b) $9\frac{1}{3}$ V
   (c) 0 V (d) $10\frac{2}{3}$ V

9. Which of the following statements is true?
   (a) The capacity of a cell is measured in volts
   (b) A primary cell converts electrical energy into chemical energy

(c) Galvanising iron helps to prevent corrosion

(d) A positive electrode is termed the cathode

10. The greater the internal resistance of a cell:
    (a) the greater the terminal p.d.
    (b) the less the e.m.f.
    (c) the greater the e.m.f.
    (d) the less the terminal p.d.

11. The negative pole of a dry cell is made of:
    (a) carbon
    (b) copper
    (c) zinc
    (d) mercury

12. The energy of a secondary cell is usually renewed:
    (a) by passing a current through it
    (b) it cannot be renewed at all
    (c) by renewing its chemicals
    (d) by heating it

13. Which of the following statements is true?
    (a) A zinc carbon battery is rechargeable and is not classified as hazardous
    (b) A nickel cadmium battery is not rechargeable and is classified as hazardous
    (c) A lithium battery is used in watches and is not rechargeable
    (d) An alkaline manganese battery is used in torches and is classified as hazardous

Revision Test 1

This revision test covers the material contained in Chapters 1 to 4. *The marks for each question are shown in brackets at the end of each question.*

1. An electromagnet exerts a force of 15 N and moves a soft iron armature through a distance of 12 mm in 50 ms. Determine the power consumed. (5)

2. A d.c. motor consumes 47.25 MJ when connected to a 250 V supply for 1 hour 45 minutes. Determine the power rating of the motor and the current taken from the supply. (5)

3. A 100 W electric light bulb is connected to a 200 V supply. Calculate (a) the current flowing in the bulb, and (b) the resistance of the bulb. (4)

4. Determine the charge transferred when a current of 5 mA flows for 10 minutes. (2)

5. A current of 12 A flows in the element of an electric fire of resistance 25 Ω. Determine the power dissipated by the element. If the fire is on for 5 hours every day, calculate for a one week period (a) the energy used, and (b) cost of using the fire if electricity cost 13.5p per unit. (6)

6. Calculate the resistance of 1200 m of copper cable of cross-sectional area 15 mm^2. Take the resistivity of copper as 0.02 $\mu\Omega$m (5)

7. At a temperature of 40°C, an aluminium cable has a resistance of 25 Ω. If the temperature coefficient of resistance at 0°C is 0.0038/°C, calculate its resistance at 0°C (5)

8. (a) Determine the values of the resistors with the following colour coding:

   (i) red-red-orange-silver

   (ii) orange-orange-black-blue-green

   (b) What is the value of a resistor marked as 47 KK? (6)

9. Four cells, each with an internal resistance of 0.40 Ω and an e.m.f. of 2.5 V are connected in series to a load of 38.4 Ω. (a) Determine the current flowing in the circuit and the p.d. at the battery terminals. (b) If the cells are connected in parallel instead of in series, determine the current flowing and the p.d. at the battery terminals. (10)

10. (a) State six typical applications of primary cells

    (b) State six typical applications of secondary cells

    (c) State the advantages of a fuel cell over a conventional battery and state three practical applications. (12)

11. Name five alternative, renewable energy sources, and give a brief description of each. (15)

Chapter 5

Series and parallel networks

At the end of this chapter you should be able to:

- calculate unknown voltages, current and resistances in a series circuit
- understand voltage division in a series circuit
- calculate unknown voltages, currents and resistances in a parallel network
- calculate unknown voltages, currents and resistances in series-parallel networks
- understand current division in a two-branch parallel network
- appreciate the loading effect of a voltmeter
- understand the difference between potentiometers and rheostats
- perform calculations to determine load currents and voltages in potentiometers and rheostats
- understand and perform calculations on relative and absolute voltages
- state three causes of short circuits in electrical circuits
- describe the advantages and disadvantages of series and parallel connection of lamps

5.1 Series circuits

Figure 5.1 shows three resistors R_1, R_2 and R_3 connected end to end, i.e. in series, with a battery source of V volts. Since the circuit is closed a current I will flow and the p.d. across each resistor may be determined from the voltmeter readings V_1, V_2 and V_3.

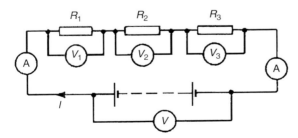

Figure 5.1

In a series circuit

(a) the current I is the same in all parts of the circuit and hence the same reading is found on each of the ammeters shown, and

(b) the sum of the voltages V_1, V_2 and V_3 is equal to the total applied voltage, V,

i.e. $$V = V_1 + V_2 + V_3$$

From Ohm's law: $V_1 = IR_1$, $V_2 = IR_2$, $V_3 = IR_3$ and $V = IR$ where R is the total circuit resistance. Since $V = V_1 + V_2 + V_3$ then $IR = IR_1 + IR_2 + IR_3$. Dividing throughout by I gives

$$R = R_1 + R_2 + R_3$$

Thus for a series circuit, the total resistance is obtained by adding together the values of the separate resistances.

DOI: 10.1016/B978-0-08-089056-2.00005-X

Problem 1. For the circuit shown in Fig. 5.2, determine (a) the battery voltage V, (b) the total resistance of the circuit, and (c) the values of resistors R_1, R_2 and R_3, given that the p.d.'s across R_1, R_2 and R_3 are 5 V, 2 V and 6 V respectively.

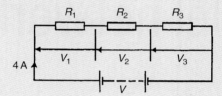

Figure 5.2

(a) Battery voltage $V = V_1 + V_2 + V_3$
$$= 5 + 2 + 6 = \mathbf{13\,V}$$

(b) Total circuit resistance $R = \dfrac{V}{I} = \dfrac{13}{4} = \mathbf{3.25\,\Omega}$

(c) Resistance $R_1 = \dfrac{V_1}{I} = \dfrac{5}{4} = \mathbf{1.25\,\Omega}$

Resistance $R_2 = \dfrac{V_2}{I} = \dfrac{2}{4} = \mathbf{0.5\,\Omega}$

Resistance $R_3 = \dfrac{V_3}{I} = \dfrac{6}{4} = \mathbf{1.5\,\Omega}$

(Check: $R_1 + R_2 + R_3 = 1.25 + 0.5 + 1.5$
$$= 3.25\,\Omega = R)$$

Problem 2. For the circuit shown in Fig. 5.3, determine the p.d. across resistor R_3. If the total resistance of the circuit is 100 Ω, determine the current flowing through resistor R_1. Find also the value of resistor R_2.

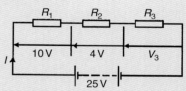

Figure 5.3

P.d. across R_3, $V_3 = 25 - 10 - 4 = \mathbf{11\,V}$

Current $I = \dfrac{V}{R} = \dfrac{25}{100} = \mathbf{0.25\,A}$,

which is the current flowing in each resistor

Resistance $R_2 = \dfrac{V_2}{I} = \dfrac{4}{0.25} = \mathbf{16\,\Omega}$

Problem 3. A 12 V battery is connected in a circuit having three series-connected resistors having resistances of 4 Ω, 9 Ω and 11 Ω. Determine the current flowing through, and the p.d. across the 9 Ω resistor. Find also the power dissipated in the 11 Ω resistor.

The circuit diagram is shown in Fig. 5.4

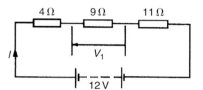

Figure 5.4

Total resistance $R = 4 + 9 + 11 = 24\,\Omega$

Current $I = \dfrac{V}{R} = \dfrac{12}{24} = \mathbf{0.5\,A}$,

which is the current in the 9 Ω resistor.
P.d. across the 9 Ω resistor,

$$V_1 = I \times 9 = 0.5 \times 9 = \mathbf{4.5\,V}$$

Power dissipated in the 11 Ω resistor,

$$P = I^2 R = (0.5)^2 (11)$$
$$= (0.25)(11) = \mathbf{2.75\,W}$$

5.2 Potential divider

The voltage distribution for the circuit shown in Fig. 5.5(a) is given by:

$$V_1 = \left(\frac{R_1}{R_1 + R_2}\right) V \text{ and } V_2 = \left(\frac{R_2}{R_1 + R_2}\right) V$$

The circuit shown in Fig. 5.5(b) is often referred to as a **potential divider** circuit. Such a circuit can consist of a number of similar elements in series connected across a voltage source, voltages being taken from connections between the elements. Frequently the divider consists of two resistors as shown in Fig. 5.5(b), where

$$V_{\text{OUT}} = \left(\frac{R_2}{R_1 + R_2}\right) V_{\text{IN}}$$

A potential divider is the simplest way of producing a source of lower e.m.f. from a source of higher e.m.f., and is the basic operating mechanism of the **potentiometer**,

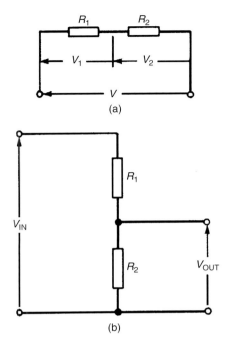

(a)

(b)

Figure 5.5

a measuring device for accurately measuring potential differences (see page 135).

Problem 4. Determine the value of voltage V shown in Fig. 5.6

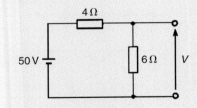

Figure 5.6

Figure 5.6 may be redrawn as shown in Fig. 5.7, and

$$\text{voltage } V = \left(\frac{6}{6+4}\right)(50) = \mathbf{30\,V}$$

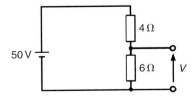

Figure 5.7

Problem 5. Two resistors are connected in series across a 24 V supply and a current of 3 A flows in the circuit. If one of the resistors has a resistance of $2\,\Omega$ determine (a) the value of the other resistor, and (b) the p.d. across the $2\,\Omega$ resistor. If the circuit is connected for 50 hours, how much energy is used?

The circuit diagram is shown in Fig. 5.8

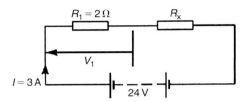

Figure 5.8

(a) Total circuit resistance

$$R = \frac{V}{I} = \frac{24}{3} = 8\,\Omega$$

Value of unknown resistance,

$$R_x = 8 - 2 = \mathbf{6\,\Omega}$$

(b) P.d. across $2\,\Omega$ resistor,

$$V_1 = IR_1 = 3 \times 2 = \mathbf{6\,V}$$

Alternatively, from above,

$$V_1 = \left(\frac{R_1}{R_1 + R_x}\right)V$$

$$= \left(\frac{2}{2+6}\right)(24) = 6\,V$$

Energy used $=$ power $\times$ time

$$= (V \times I) \times t$$

$$= (24 \times 3\,\text{W})(50\,\text{h})$$

$$= 3600\,\text{Wh} = \mathbf{3.6\,kWh}$$

Now try the following exercise

Exercise 19   Further problems on series circuits

1. The p.d.'s measured across three resistors connected in series are 5 V, 7 V and 10 V, and the

supply current is 2 A. Determine (a) the supply voltage, (b) the total circuit resistance, and (c) the values of the three resistors.

[(a) 22 V (b) 11 Ω (c) 2.5 Ω, 3.5 Ω, 5 Ω]

2. For the circuit shown in Fig. 5.9, determine the value of V_1. If the total circuit resistance is 36 Ω determine the supply current and the value of resistors R_1, R_2 and R_3

[10 V, 0.5 A, 20 Ω, 10 Ω, 6 Ω]

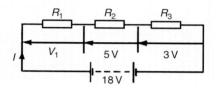

Figure 5.9

3. When the switch in the circuit in Fig. 5.10 is closed the reading on voltmeter 1 is 30 V and that on voltmeter 2 is 10 V. Determine the reading on the ammeter and the value of resistor R_x [4 A, 2.5 Ω]

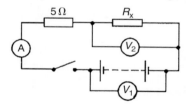

Figure 5.10

4. Calculate the value of voltage V in Fig. 5.11

[45 V]

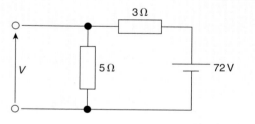

Figure 5.11

5. Two resistors are connected in series across an 18 V supply and a current of 5 A flows. If one of the resistors has a value of 2.4 Ω determine (a) the value of the other resistor and (b) the p.d. across the 2.4 Ω resistor.

[(a) 1.2 Ω (b) 12 V]

6. An arc lamp takes 9.6 A at 55 V. It is operated from a 120 V supply. Find the value of the stabilising resistor to be connected in series.

[6.77 Ω]

7. An oven takes 15 A at 240 V. It is required to reduce the current to 12 A. Find (a) the resistor which must be connected in series, and (b) the voltage across the resistor.

[(a) 4 Ω (b) 48 V]

5.3 Parallel networks

Figure 5.12 shows three resistors, R_1, R_2 and R_3 connected across each other, i.e. in parallel, across a battery source of V volts.

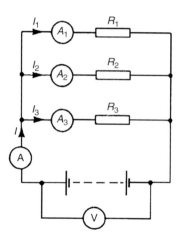

Figure 5.12

In a parallel circuit:

(a) the sum of the currents I_1, I_2 and I_3 is equal to the total circuit current, I,

i.e. $$I = I_1 + I_2 + I_3 \qquad \text{and}$$

(b) the source p.d., V volts, is the same across each of the resistors.

From Ohm's law:

$$I_1 = \frac{V}{R_1}, \quad I_2 = \frac{V}{R_2}, \quad I_3 = \frac{V}{R_3} \quad \text{and} \quad I = \frac{V}{R}$$

where R is the total circuit resistance. Since

$$I = I_1 + I_2 + I_3 \text{ then } \frac{V}{R} = \frac{V}{R_1} + \frac{V}{R_2} + \frac{V}{R_3}$$

Dividing throughout by V gives:

$$\frac{1}{R} = \frac{1}{R_1} + \frac{1}{R_2} + \frac{1}{R_3}$$

This equation must be used when finding the total resistance R of a parallel circuit. For the special case of **two resistors in parallel**

$$\frac{1}{R} = \frac{1}{R_1} + \frac{1}{R_2} = \frac{R_2 + R_1}{R_1 R_2}$$

Hence $\qquad R = \dfrac{R_1 R_2}{R_1 + R_2} \quad \left(\text{i.e. } \dfrac{\text{product}}{\text{sum}}\right)$

Problem 6. For the circuit shown in Fig. 5.13, determine (a) the reading on the ammeter, and (b) the value of resistor R_2.

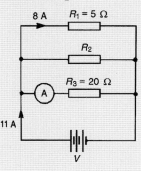

Figure 5.13

P.d. across R_1 is the same as the supply voltage V. Hence supply voltage, $V = 8 \times 5 = 40\,\text{V}$

(a) Reading on ammeter,

$$I = \frac{V}{R_3} = \frac{40}{20} = 2\,\text{A}$$

(b) Current flowing through $R_2 = 11 - 8 - 2 = 1\,\text{A}$. Hence

$$R_2 = \frac{V}{I_2} = \frac{40}{1} = 40\,\Omega$$

Problem 7. Two resistors, of resistance $3\,\Omega$ and $6\,\Omega$, are connected in parallel across a battery having a voltage of $12\,\text{V}$. Determine (a) the total circuit resistance and (b) the current flowing in the $3\,\Omega$ resistor.

The circuit diagram is shown in Fig. 5.14

(a) The total circuit resistance R is given by

$$\frac{1}{R} = \frac{1}{R_1} + \frac{1}{R_2} = \frac{1}{3} + \frac{1}{6} = \frac{2+1}{6} = \frac{3}{6}$$

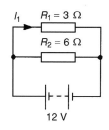

Figure 5.14

Since $\dfrac{1}{R} = \dfrac{3}{6}$ then $\mathbf{R = 2\,\Omega}$

(Alternatively,

$$R = \frac{R_1 R_2}{R_1 + R_2} = \frac{3 \times 6}{3 + 6} = \frac{18}{9} = \mathbf{2\,\Omega})$$

(b) Current in the $3\,\Omega$ resistance,

$$I_1 = \frac{V}{R_1} = \frac{12}{3} = \mathbf{4\,A}$$

Problem 8. For the circuit shown in Fig. 5.15, find (a) the value of the supply voltage V and (b) the value of current I.

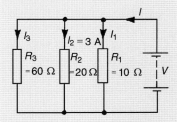

Figure 5.15

(a) P.d. across $20\,\Omega$ resistor $= I_2 R_2 = 3 \times 20 = 60\,\text{V}$, hence supply voltage $\mathbf{V = 60\,V}$ since the circuit is connected in parallel

(b) Current $I_1 = \dfrac{V}{R_1} = \dfrac{60}{10} = 6\,\text{A}$, $\quad I_2 = 3\,\text{A}$

and $\qquad I_3 = \dfrac{V}{R_3} = \dfrac{60}{60} = 1\,\text{A}$

Current $I = I_1 + I_2 + I_3$ hence
$\qquad\qquad I = 6 + 3 + 1 = \mathbf{10\,A}$.
Alternatively,

$$\frac{1}{R} = \frac{1}{60} + \frac{1}{20} + \frac{1}{10} = \frac{1+3+6}{60} = \frac{10}{60}$$

Hence total resistance

$$R = \frac{60}{10} = 6\,\Omega, \text{ and current}$$

$$I = \frac{V}{R} = \frac{60}{6} = \mathbf{10\,A}$$

Problem 9. Given four $1\,\Omega$ resistors, state how they must be connected to give an overall resistance of (a) $\frac{1}{4}\,\Omega$ (b) $1\,\Omega$ (c) $1\frac{1}{3}\,\Omega$ (d) $2\frac{1}{2}\,\Omega$, all four resistors being connected in each case.

(a) **All four in parallel** (see Fig. 5.16), since

$$\frac{1}{R} = \frac{1}{1} + \frac{1}{1} + \frac{1}{1} + \frac{1}{1} = \frac{4}{1} \text{ i.e. } R = \frac{1}{4}\,\Omega$$

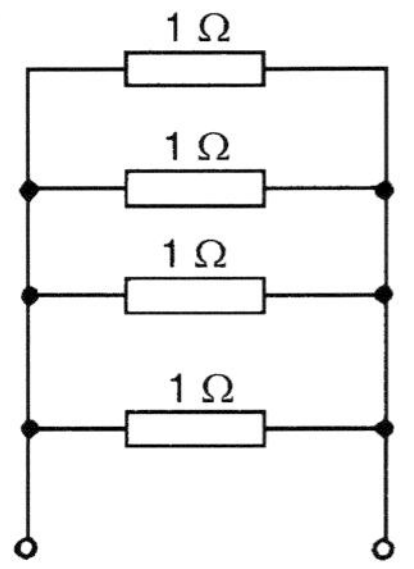

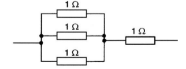

Figure 5.16

(b) **Two in series, in parallel with another two in series** (see Fig. 5.17), since $1\,\Omega$ and $1\,\Omega$ in series gives $2\,\Omega$, and $2\,\Omega$ in parallel with $2\,\Omega$ gives

$$\frac{2 \times 2}{2 + 2} = \frac{4}{4} = 1\,\Omega$$

Figure 5.17

(c) **Three in parallel, in series with one** (see Fig. 5.18), since for the three in parallel,

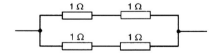

Figure 5.18

$$\frac{1}{R} = \frac{1}{1} + \frac{1}{1} + \frac{1}{1} = \frac{3}{1}$$

i.e. $R = \frac{1}{3}\,\Omega$ and $\frac{1}{3}\,\Omega$ in series with $1\,\Omega$ gives $1\frac{1}{3}\,\Omega$

(d) **Two in parallel, in series with two in series** (see Fig. 5.19), since for the two in parallel

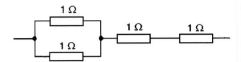

Figure 5.19

$$R = \frac{1 \times 1}{1 + 1} = \frac{1}{2}\,\Omega$$

and $\frac{1}{2}\,\Omega$, $1\,\Omega$ and $1\,\Omega$ in series gives $2\frac{1}{2}\,\Omega$

Problem 10. Find the equivalent resistance for the circuit shown in Fig. 5.20

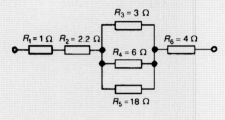

Figure 5.20

R_3, R_4 and R_5 are connected in parallel and their equivalent resistance R is given by

$$\frac{1}{R} = \frac{1}{3} + \frac{1}{6} + \frac{1}{18} = \frac{6 + 3 + 1}{18} = \frac{10}{18}$$

hence $R = (18/10) = 1.8\,\Omega$. The circuit is now equivalent to four resistors in series and the **equivalent circuit resistance** $= 1 + 2.2 + 1.8 + 4 = \mathbf{9\,\Omega}$

Problem 11. Resistances of $10\,\Omega$, $20\,\Omega$ and $30\,\Omega$ are connected (a) in series and (b) in parallel to a $240\,V$ supply. Calculate the supply current in each case.

(a) The series circuit is shown in Fig. 5.21

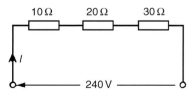

Figure 5.21

The equivalent resistance
$R_T = 10\,\Omega + 20\,\Omega + 30\,\Omega = 60\,\Omega$

Supply current $I = \frac{V}{R_T} = \frac{240}{60} = \mathbf{4\,A}$

(b) The parallel circuit is shown in Fig. 5.22.
The equivalent resistance R_T of $10\,\Omega$, $20\,\Omega$
and $30\,\Omega$ resistance's connected in parallel is

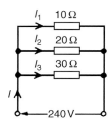

Figure 5.22

given by:

$$\frac{1}{R_T} = \frac{1}{10} + \frac{1}{20} + \frac{1}{30} = \frac{6+3+2}{60} = \frac{11}{60}$$

hence $R_T = \dfrac{60}{11}\,\Omega$

Supply current

$$I = \frac{V}{R_T} = \frac{240}{\frac{60}{11}} = \frac{240 \times 11}{60} = \mathbf{44\,A}$$

(Check:

$$I_1 = \frac{V}{R_1} = \frac{240}{10} = 24\,A,$$

$$I_2 = \frac{V}{R_2} = \frac{240}{20} = 12\,A$$

$$\text{and } I_3 = \frac{V}{R_3} = \frac{240}{30} = 8\,A$$

For a parallel circuit $I = I_1 + I_2 + I_3$
$= 24 + 12 + 8 = \mathbf{44\,A}$, as above)

5.4 Current division

For the circuit shown in Fig. 5.23, the total circuit
resistance, R_T is given by

$$R_T = \frac{R_1 R_2}{R_1 + R_2}$$

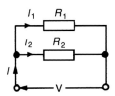

Figure 5.23

and

$$V = IR_T = I\left(\frac{R_1 R_2}{R_1 + R_2}\right)$$

Current

$$I_1 = \frac{V}{R_1} = \frac{I}{R_1}\left(\frac{R_1 R_2}{R_1 + R_2}\right)$$

$$= \left(\frac{R_2}{R_1 + R_2}\right)(I)$$

Similarly,

current

$$I_2 = \frac{V}{R_2} = \frac{I}{R_2}\left(\frac{R_1 R_2}{R_1 + R_2}\right)$$

$$= \left(\frac{R_1}{R_1 + R_2}\right)(I)$$

Summarising, with reference to Fig. 5.23

$$I_1 = \left(\frac{R_2}{R_1 + R_2}\right)(I)$$

and

$$I_2 = \left(\frac{R_1}{R_1 + R_2}\right)(I)$$

Problem 12. For the series-parallel arrangement
shown in Fig. 5.24, find (a) the supply current,
(b) the current flowing through each resistor and
(c) the p.d. across each resistor.

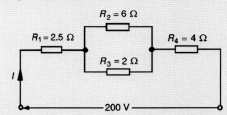

Figure 5.24

(a) The equivalent resistance R_x of R_2 and R_3 in
parallel is:

$$R_x = \frac{6 \times 2}{6+2} = 1.5\,\Omega$$

The equivalent resistance R_T of R_1, R_x and R_4 in
series is:

$$R_T = 2.5 + 1.5 + 4 = 8\,\Omega$$

Supply current

$$I = \frac{V}{R_T} = \frac{200}{8} = \mathbf{25\,A}$$

(b) The current flowing through R_1 and R_4 is 25 A. The current flowing through R_2

$$= \left(\frac{R_3}{R_2 + R_3}\right) I = \left(\frac{2}{6+2}\right) 25$$
$$= 6.25\,\text{A}$$

The current flowing through R_3

$$= \left(\frac{R_2}{R_2 + R_3}\right) I$$
$$= \left(\frac{6}{6+2}\right) 25 = 18.75\,\text{A}$$

(Note that the currents flowing through R_2 and R_3 must add up to the total current flowing into the parallel arrangement, i.e. 25 A)

(c) The equivalent circuit of Fig. 5.24 is shown in Fig. 5.25

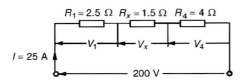

Figure 5.25

p.d. across R_1, i.e.

$$V_1 = IR_1 = (25)(2.5) = \textbf{62.5\,V}$$

p.d. across R_x, i.e.

$$V_x = IR_x = (25)(1.5) = \textbf{37.5\,V}$$

p.d. across R_4, i.e.

$$V_4 = IR_4 = (25)(4) = \textbf{100\,V}$$

Hence the p.d. across R_2

$$= \text{p.d. across } R_3 = \textbf{37.5\,V}$$

Problem 13. For the circuit shown in Fig. 5.26 calculate (a) the value of resistor R_x such that the

total power dissipated in the circuit is 2.5 kW, (b) the current flowing in each of the four resistors.

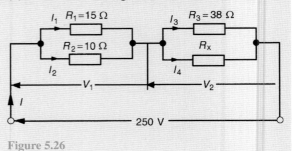

Figure 5.26

(a) Power dissipated $P = VI$ watts, hence
$$2500 = (250)(I)$$

i.e.
$$I = \frac{2500}{250} = 10\,\text{A}$$

From Ohm's law,

$$R_T = \frac{V}{I} = \frac{250}{10} = 25\,\Omega,$$

where R_T is the equivalent circuit resistance. The equivalent resistance of R_1 and R_2 in parallel is

$$\frac{15 \times 10}{15 + 10} = \frac{150}{25} = 6\,\Omega$$

The equivalent resistance of resistors R_3 and R_x in parallel is equal to $25\,\Omega - 6\,\Omega$, i.e. $19\,\Omega$. There are three methods whereby R_x can be determined.

Method 1

The voltage $V_1 = IR$, where R is $6\,\Omega$, from above, i.e. $V_1 = (10)(6) = 60\,\text{V}$. Hence

$$V_2 = 250\,\text{V} - 60\,\text{V} = 190\,\text{V}$$
$$= \text{p.d. across } R_3$$
$$= \text{p.d. across } R_x$$
$$I_3 = \frac{V_2}{R_3} = \frac{190}{38} = 5\,\text{A}.$$

Thus $I_4 = 5\,\text{A}$ also, since $I = 10\,\text{A}$. Thus

$$\mathbf{R_x} = \frac{V_2}{I_4} = \frac{190}{5} = \textbf{38}\,\boldsymbol{\Omega}$$

Method 2

Since the equivalent resistance of R_3 and R_x in parallel is $19\,\Omega$,

$$19 = \frac{38R_x}{38 + R_x} \quad \left(\text{i.e. } \frac{\text{product}}{\text{sum}}\right)$$

Hence

$$19(38 + R_x) = 38R_x$$

$$722 + 19R_x = 38R_x$$

$$722 = 38R_x - 19R_x = 19R_x$$

$$= 19R_x$$

Thus $$\mathbf{R_x} = \frac{722}{19} = \mathbf{38\,\Omega}$$

Method 3

When two resistors having the same value are connected in parallel the equivalent resistance is always half the value of one of the resistors. Thus, in this case, since $R_T = 19\,\Omega$ and $R_3 = 38\,\Omega$, then $R_x = 38\,\Omega$ could have been deduced on sight.

(b) Current $I_1 = \left(\dfrac{R_2}{R_1 + R_2}\right) I$

$$= \left(\frac{10}{15 + 10}\right)(10)$$

$$= \left(\frac{2}{5}\right)(10) = \mathbf{4\,A}$$

Current $I_2 = \left(\dfrac{R_1}{R_1 + R_2}\right) I = \left(\dfrac{15}{15 + 10}\right)(10)$

$$= \left(\frac{3}{5}\right)(10) = \mathbf{6\,A}$$

From part (a), method 1, $\mathbf{I_3 = I_4 = 5\,A}$

Problem 14.   For the arrangement shown in Fig. 5.27, find the current I_x.

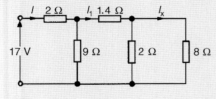

Figure 5.27

Commencing at the right-hand side of the arrangement shown in Fig. 5.27, the circuit is gradually reduced in stages as shown in Fig. 5.28(a)–(d).
From Fig. 5.28(d),

$$I = \frac{17}{4.25} = 4\,A$$

From Fig. 5.28(b),

$$I_1 = \left(\frac{9}{9+3}\right)(I) = \left(\frac{9}{12}\right)(4) = 3\,A$$

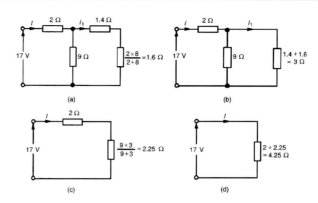

Figure 5.28

From Fig. 5.27

$$I_x = \left(\frac{2}{2+8}\right)(I_1) = \left(\frac{2}{10}\right)(3) = \mathbf{0.6\,A}$$

For a practical laboratory experiment on series-parallel dc circuits, see Chapter 24, page 407.

Now try the following exercise

Exercise 20   Further problems on parallel networks

1. Resistances of $4\,\Omega$ and $12\,\Omega$ are connected in parallel across a 9 V battery. Determine (a) the equivalent circuit resistance, (b) the supply current, and (c) the current in each resistor.

    [(a) $3\,\Omega$ (b) 3 A (c) 2.25 A, 0.75 A]

2. For the circuit shown in Fig. 5.29 determine (a) the reading on the ammeter, and (b) the value of resistor R.   [2.5 A, 2.5 Ω]

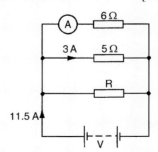

Figure 5.29

3. Find the equivalent resistance when the following resistances are connected (a) in series (b) in parallel (i) $3\,\Omega$ and $2\,\Omega$ (ii) $20\,k\Omega$ and

40 kΩ (iii) 4 Ω, 8 Ω and 16 Ω (iv) 800 Ω, 4 kΩ and 1500 Ω.

[(a) (i) 5 Ω   (ii) 60 kΩ
(iii) 28 Ω   (iv) 6.3 Ω
(b) (i) 1.2 Ω   (ii) 13.33 kΩ
(iii) 2.29 Ω (iv) 461.54 Ω]

4. Find the total resistance between terminals A and B of the circuit shown in Fig. 5.30(a).
[8 Ω]

5. Find the equivalent resistance between terminals C and D of the circuit shown in Fig. 5.30(b).
[27.5 Ω]

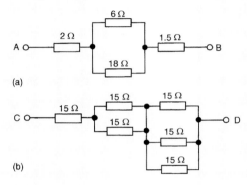

(a)

(b)

Figure 5.30

6. Resistors of 20 Ω, 20 Ω and 30 Ω are connected in parallel. What resistance must be added in series with the combination to obtain a total resistance of 10 Ω. If the complete circuit expends a power of 0.36 kW, find the total current flowing.
[2.5 Ω, 6 A]

7. (a) Calculate the current flowing in the 30 Ω resistor shown in Fig. 5.31. (b) What additional value of resistance would have to be placed in parallel with the 20 Ω and 30 Ω resistors to change the supply current to 8 A, the supply voltage remaining constant.
[(a) 1.6 A (b) 6 Ω]

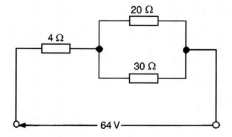

Figure 5.31

8. For the circuit shown in Fig. 5.32, find (a) V_1, (b) V_2, without calculating the current flowing.
[(a) 30 V (b) 42 V]

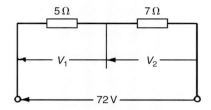

Figure 5.32

9. Determine the currents and voltages indicated in the circuit shown in Fig. 5.33.
$[I_1 = 5\,A, I_2 = 2.5\,A, I_3 = 1\frac{2}{3}\,A, I_4 = \frac{5}{6}\,A$
$I_5 = 3\,A, I_6 = 2\,A, V_1 = 20\,V, V_2 = 5\,V,$
$V_3 = 6\,V]$

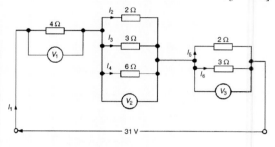

Figure 5.33

10. Find the current I in Fig. 5.34.   [1.8 A]

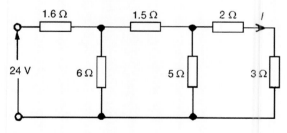

Figure 5.34

11. A resistor of 2.4 Ω is connected in series with another of 3.2 Ω. What resistance must be placed across the one of 2.4 Ω so that the total resistance of the circuit shall be 5 Ω?
[7.2 Ω]

12. A resistor of 8 Ω is connected in parallel with one of 12 Ω and the combination is connected in series with one of 4 Ω. A p.d. of 10 V is applied to the circuit. The 8 Ω resistor is now

placed across the $4\,\Omega$ resistor. Find the p.d. required to send the same current through the $8\,\Omega$ resistor.   [30 V]

5.5   Loading effect

Loading effect is the terminology used when a measuring instrument such as an oscilloscope or voltmeter is connected across a component and the current drawn by the instrument upsets the circuit under test. The best way of demonstrating loading effect is by a numerical example.

In the simple circuit of Fig. 5.35, the voltage across each of the resistors can be calculated using voltage division, or by inspection. In this case, the voltage shown as V should be 20 V.

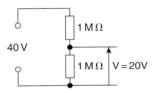

Figure 5.35

Using a voltmeter having a resistance of, say, $600\,\text{k}\Omega$, places $600\,\text{k}\Omega$ in parallel with the $1\,\text{M}\Omega$ resistor, as shown in Fig. 5.36.

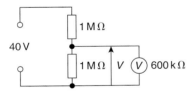

Figure 5.36

Resistance of parallel section

$$= \frac{1 \times 10^6 \times 600 \times 10^3}{(1 \times 10^6 + 600 \times 10^3)}$$

$$= 375\,\text{k}\Omega \text{ (using product/sum)}$$

The voltage V now equals

$$= \frac{375 \times 10^3}{(1 \times 10^6 + 375 \times 10^3)} \times 40$$

$$= \mathbf{10.91\,V} \text{ (by voltage division)}$$

The voltmeter has loaded the circuit by drawing current for its operation, and by so doing, reduces the voltage

across the $1\,\text{M}\Omega$ resistor from the correct value of 20 V to 10.91 V.

Using a Fluke (or multimeter) which has a set internal resistance of, say, $10\,\text{M}\Omega$, as shown in Fig. 5.37, produces a much better result and the loading effect is minimal, as shown below.

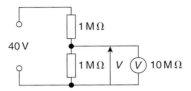

Figure 5.37

Resistance of parallel section

$$= \frac{1 \times 10^6 \times 10 \times 10^6}{(1 \times 10^6 + 10 \times 10^6)} = 0.91\,\text{M}\Omega$$

The voltage V now equals

$$= \frac{0.91 \times 10^6}{(0.91 \times 10^6 + 1 \times 10^6)} \times 40 = \mathbf{19.06\,V}$$

When taking measurements, it is vital that the loading effect is understood and kept in mind at all times. An incorrect voltage reading may be due to this loading effect rather than the equipment under investigation being defective. Ideally, **the resistance of a voltmeter should be infinite**.

5.6   Potentiometers and rheostats

It is frequently desirable to be able to **vary the value of a resistor** in a circuit. A simple example of this is the volume control of a radio or television set.

Voltages and currents may be varied in electrical circuits by using **potentiometers** and **rheostats**.

Potentiometers

When a variable resistor uses **three terminals**, it is known as a **potentiometer**. The potentiometer provides an adjustable voltage divider circuit, which is useful as a means of obtaining **various voltages** from a fixed potential difference. Consider the potentiometer circuit shown in Fig. 5.38 incorporating a lamp and supply voltage V.

In the circuit of Fig. 5.38, the input voltage is applied across points A and B at the ends of the potentiometer, while the output is tapped off between the sliding contact S and the fixed end B. It will be seen that with the slider at the far left-hand end of the resistor, the full voltage

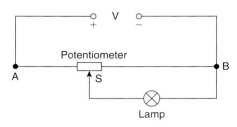

Figure 5.38

will appear across the lamp, and as the slider is moved towards point B the lamp brightness will reduce. When S is at the far right of the potentiometer, the lamp is short-circuited, no current will flow through it, and the lamp will be fully off.

> **Problem 15.** Calculate the volt drop across the $60\,\Omega$ load in the circuit shown in Fig. 5.39, when the slider S is at the halfway point of the $200\,\Omega$ potentiometer.

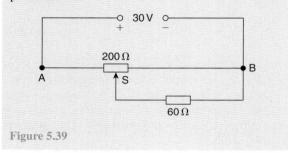

Figure 5.39

With the slider halfway, the equivalent circuit is shown in Fig. 5.40.

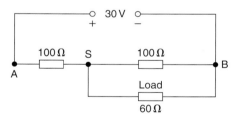

Figure 5.40

For the parallel resistors, total resistance,

$$R_P = \frac{100 \times 60}{100 + 60} = \frac{100 \times 60}{160} = 37.5\,\Omega$$

$$\text{(or use } \frac{1}{R_P} = \frac{1}{100} + \frac{1}{60} \text{ to determine } R_P)$$

The equivalent circuit is now as shown in Fig. 5.41. The volt drop across the $37.5\,\Omega$ resistor in Fig. 5.41 is the same as the volt drop across both of the parallel resistors in Fig. 5.40.

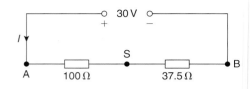

Figure 5.41

There are two methods for determining the volt drop V_{SB}:

Method 1

Total circuit resistance,
$$R_T = 100 + 37.5 = 137.5\,\Omega$$

Hence, supply current, $\quad I = \dfrac{30}{137.5} = 0.2182\,A$

Thus, volt drop, $\qquad V_{SB} = I \times 37.5 = 0.2182 \times 37.5$

$$= \mathbf{8.18\,V}$$

Method 2

By the principle of voltage division,

$$V_{SB} = \left(\frac{37.5}{100 + 37.5}\right)(30) = 8.18\,V$$

Hence, **the volt drop across the $60\,\Omega$ load of Fig. 5.39 is 8.18 V**.

Rheostats

A variable resistor where only **two terminals** are used, one fixed and one sliding, is known as a **rheostat**. The rheostat circuit, shown in Fig. 5.42, similar in construction to the potentiometer, is used to **control current flow**. The rheostat also acts as a dropping resistor, reducing the voltage across the load, but is more effective at controlling current.

For this reason **the resistance of the rheostat should be greater than that of the load**, otherwise it will have little or no effect. Typical uses are in a train set or Scalextric. Another practical example is in varying the brilliance of the panel lighting controls in a car.

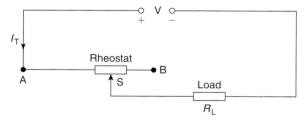

Figure 5.42

The rheostat resistance is connected in series with the load circuit, R_L, with the slider arm tapping off an amount of resistance (i.e. that between A and S) to provide the current flow required. With the slider at the far left-hand end, the load receives maximum current; with the slider at the far right-hand end, minimum current flows. The current flowing can be calculated by finding the total resistance of the circuit (i.e. $R_T = R_{AS} + R_L$), then by applying Ohm's law, $I_T = \dfrac{V}{R_{AS} + R_L}$

Calculations involved with the rheostat circuit are simpler than those for the potentiometer circuit.

Problem 16. In the circuit of Fig. 5.43, calculate the current flowing in the $100\,\Omega$ load, when the sliding point S is 2/3 of the way from A to B.

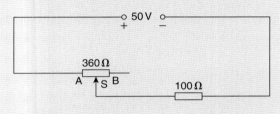

Figure 5.43

Resistance, $\qquad R_{AS} = \dfrac{2}{3} \times 360 = 240\,\Omega$

Total circuit resistance, $R_T = R_{AS} + R_L = 240 + 100$
$$= 340\,\Omega$$

Current flowing in load, $I = \dfrac{V}{R_T} = \dfrac{50}{340}$
$$= \mathbf{0.147\,A \ or \ 147\,mA}$$

Summary

A **potentiometer** (a) has three terminals, and (b) is used for voltage control.
A **rheostat** (a) has two terminals, and (b) is used for current control.

A rheostat is not suitable if the load resistance is higher than the rheostat resistance; rheostat resistance must be higher than the load resistance to be able to influence current flow.

Now try the following exercise

Exercise 21   Further problems on potentiometers and rheostats

1. For the circuit shown in Fig. 5.44, AS is 3/5 of AB. Determine the voltage across the $120\,\Omega$

load. Is this a potentiometer or a rheostat circuit?

[44.44 V, potentiometer]

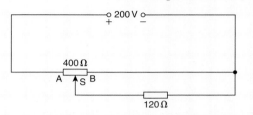

Figure 5.44

2. For the circuit shown in Fig. 5.45, calculate the current flowing in the $25\,\Omega$ load and the voltage drop across the load when (a) AS is half of AB, and (b) point S coincides with point B. Is this a potentiometer or a rheostat?

[(a) 0.545 A, 13.64 V
(b) 0.286 A, 7.14 V rheostat]

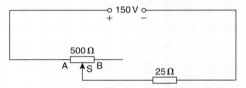

Figure 5.45

3. For the circuit shown in Fig. 5.46, calculate the voltage across the $600\,\Omega$ load when point S splits AB in the ratio 1:3.   [136.4 V]

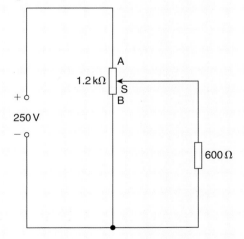

Figure 5.46

4. For the circuit shown in Fig. 5.47, the slider S is set at halfway. Calculate the voltage drop across the $120\,\Omega$ load.   [9.68 V]

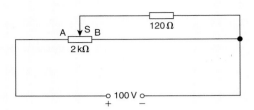

Figure 5.47

5. For the potentiometer circuit shown in Fig. 5.48, AS is 60% of AB. Calculate the voltage across the 70 Ω load. [63.40 V]

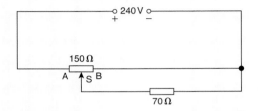

Figure 5.48

5.7 Relative and absolute voltages

In an electrical circuit, the voltage at any point can be quoted as being 'with reference to' (w.r.t.) any other point in the circuit. Consider the circuit shown in Fig. 5.49. The total resistance,

$$R_T = 30 + 50 + 5 + 15 = 100 \, \Omega \text{ and}$$

$$\text{current, } I = \frac{200}{100} = 2 \, A$$

If a voltage at point A is quoted with reference to point B then the voltage is written as V_{AB}. This is known as a 'relative voltage'. In the circuit shown in Fig. 5.49, the voltage at A w.r.t. B is $I \times 50$, i.e. $2 \times 50 = 100$ V and is written as $V_{AB} = 100$ V.

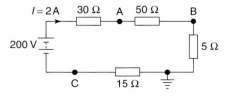

Figure 5.49

It must also be indicated whether the voltage at A w.r.t. B is closer to the positive or the negative terminal of the supply source. Point A is nearer to the

positive terminal than B so is written as $V_{AB} = 100$ V or $V_{AB} = +100$ V or $V_{AB} = 100$ V +ve.

If no positive or negative is included, then the voltage is always taken to be positive.

If the voltage at B w.r.t. A is required, then V_{BA} is negative and written as $V_{BA} = -100$ V or $V_{BA} = 100$ V −ve. If the reference point is changed to the **earth point** then any voltage taken w.r.t. the earth is known as an '**absolute potential**'. If the absolute voltage of A in Fig. 5.49 is required, then this will be the sum of the voltages across the 50 Ω and 5 Ω resistors, i.e. $100 + 10 = 110$ V and is written as $V_A = 110$ V or $V_A = +110$ V or $V_A = 110$ V +ve, positive since moving from the earth point to point A is moving towards the positive terminal of the source. If the voltage is negative w.r.t. earth then this must be indicated; for example, $V_C = 30$ V negative w.r.t. earth, and is written as $V_C = -30$ V or $V_C = 30$ V −ve.

Problem 17. For the circuit shown in Fig. 5.50, calculate (a) the voltage drop across the 4 kΩ resistor, (b) the current through the 5 kΩ resistor, (c) the power developed in the 1.5 kΩ resistor, (d) the voltage at point X w.r.t. earth, and (e) the absolute voltage at point X.

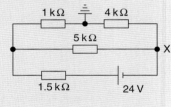

Figure 5.50

(a) Total circuit resistance, $R_T = [(1+4)k\Omega$ in parallel with $5 \, k\Omega]$ in series with $1.5 \, k\Omega$

i.e. $$R_T = \frac{5 \times 5}{5 + 5} + 1.5 = 4 \, k\Omega$$

Total circuit current, $I_T = \dfrac{V}{R_T} = \dfrac{24}{4 \times 10^3} = 6 \, mA$

By current division, current in top branch

$$= \left(\frac{5}{5+1+4}\right) \times 6 = 3 \, mA$$

Hence, **volt drop across 4 kΩ resistor**

$$= 3 \times 10^{-3} \times 4 \times 10^3 = \textbf{12 V}$$

(b) **Current through the 5 kΩ resistor**

$$= \left(\frac{1+4}{5+1+4}\right) \times 6 = \textbf{3 mA}$$

(c)   **Power in the 1.5 kΩ resistor**
$$= I_T^2 \, R = (6 \times 10^{-3})^2 (1.5 \times 10^3) = \mathbf{54 \, mW}$$

(d)   The voltage at the earth point is 0 volts. The volt drop across the $4 \, k\Omega$ is 12 V, from part (a). Since moving from the earth point to point X is moving towards the negative terminal of the voltage source, the voltage at point X w.r.t. earth is **−12 V**

(e)   The 'absolute voltage at point X' means the 'voltage at point X w.r.t. earth', hence **the absolute voltage at point X is −12 V**. Questions (d) and (e) mean the same thing.

Now try the following exercise

Exercise 22   Further problems on relative and absolute voltages

1.   For the circuit of Fig. 5.51, calculate (a) the absolute voltage at points A, B and C, (b) the voltage at A relative to B and C, and (c) the voltage at D relative to B and A.
[(a) +40 V, +29.6 V, +24 V (b) +10.4 V, +16 V (c) −5.6 V, −16 V]

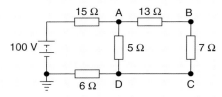

Figure 5.51

2.   For the circuit shown in Fig. 5.52, calculate (a) the voltage drop across the 7 Ω resistor, (b) the current through the 30 Ω resistor, (c) the power developed in the 8 Ω resistor, (d) the voltage at point X w.r.t. earth, and (e) the absolute voltage at point X.
[(a) 1.68 V (b) 0.16 A (c) 460.8 mW (d) +2.88 V (e) +2.88 V]

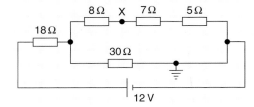

Figure 5.52

3.   In the bridge circuit of Fig. 5.53 calculate (a) the absolute voltages at points A and B, and (b) the voltage at A relative to B.
[(a) 10 V, 10 V (b) 0 V]

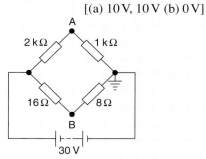

Figure 5.53

5.8   Earth potential and short circuits

The earth, and hence the sea, is at a potential of zero volts. Items connected to the earth (or sea), i.e. circuit wiring and electrical components, are said to be earthed or at earth potential. This means that there is no difference of potential between the item and earth. A ships' hull, being immersed in the sea, is at earth potential and therefore at zero volts. Earth faults, or short circuits, are caused by low resistance between the current-carrying conductor and earth. This occurs when the insulation resistance of the circuit wiring decreases, and is normally caused by:

1.   Dampness.

2.   Insulation becoming hard or brittle with age or heat.

3.   Accidental damage.

5.9   Wiring lamps in series and in parallel

Series connection

Figure 5.54 shows three lamps, each rated at 240 V, connected in series across a 240 V supply.

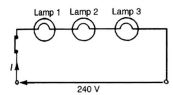

Figure 5.54

(i) Each lamp has only $(240/3)$ V, i.e. 80 V across it and thus each lamp glows dimly.

(ii) If another lamp of similar rating is added in series with the other three lamps then each lamp now has $(240/4)$ V, i.e. 60 V across it and each now glows even more dimly.

(iii) If a lamp is removed from the circuit or if a lamp develops a fault (i.e. an open circuit) or if the switch is opened, then the circuit is broken, no current flows, and the remaining lamps will not light up.

(iv) Less cable is required for a series connection than for a parallel one.

The series connection of lamps is usually limited to decorative lighting such as for Christmas tree lights.

Parallel connection

Figure 5.55 shows three similar lamps, each rated at 240 V, connected in parallel across a 240 V supply.

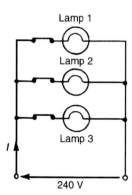

Figure 5.55

(i) Each lamp has 240 V across it and thus each will glow brilliantly at their rated voltage.

(ii) If any lamp is removed from the circuit or develops a fault (open circuit) or a switch is opened, the remaining lamps are unaffected.

(iii) The addition of further similar lamps in parallel does not affect the brightness of the other lamps.

(iv) More cable is required for parallel connection than for a series one.

The parallel connection of lamps is the most widely used in electrical installations.

Problem 18. If three identical lamps are connected in parallel and the combined resistance is 150 Ω, find the resistance of one lamp.

Let the resistance of one lamp be R, then

$$\frac{1}{150} = \frac{1}{R} + \frac{1}{R} + \frac{1}{R} = \frac{3}{R}$$

from which, $R = 3 \times 150 = \mathbf{450\,\Omega}$

Problem 19. Three identical lamps A, B and C are connected in series across a 150 V supply. State (a) the voltage across each lamp, and (b) the effect of lamp C failing.

(a) Since each lamp is identical and they are connected in series there is $150/3$ V, i.e. **50 V** across each.

(b) If lamp C fails, i.e. open circuits, no current will flow and **lamps A and B will not operate**.

___

Now try the following exercises

1. If four identical lamps are connected in parallel and the combined resistance is 100 Ω, find the resistance of one lamp.   [400 Ω]

2. Three identical filament lamps are connected (a) in series, (b) in parallel across a 210 V supply. State for each connection the p.d. across each lamp.   [(a) 70 V (b) 210 V]

1. Name three characteristics of a series circuit

2. Show that for three resistors R_1, R_2 and R_3 connected in series the equivalent resistance R is given by $R = R_1 + R_2 + R_3$

3. Name three characteristics of a parallel network

4. Show that for three resistors R_1, R_2 and R_3 connected in parallel the equivalent

resistance R is given by

$$\frac{1}{R} = \frac{1}{R_1} + \frac{1}{R_2} + \frac{1}{R_3}$$

5. Explain the potential divider circuit

6. Describe, using a circuit diagram, the method of operation of a potentiometer

7. State the main use of a potentiometer

8. Describe, using a circuit diagram, the method of operation of a rheostat

9. State the main use of a rheostat

10. Explain the difference between relative and absolute voltages

11. State three causes of short circuits in electrical circuits

12. Compare the merits of wiring lamps in (a) series (b) parallel

Exercise 25 Multi-choice questions on series and parallel networks
(Answers on page 420)

1. If two $4\,\Omega$ resistors are connected in series the effective resistance of the circuit is:
   (a) $8\,\Omega$ (b) $4\,\Omega$ (c) $2\,\Omega$ (d) $1\,\Omega$

2. If two $4\,\Omega$ resistors are connected in parallel the effective resistance of the circuit is:
   (a) $8\,\Omega$ (b) $4\,\Omega$ (c) $2\,\Omega$ (d) $1\,\Omega$

3. With the switch in Fig. 5.56 closed, the ammeter reading will indicate:
   (a) $1\,A$ (b) $75\,A$ (c) $\frac{1}{3}\,A$ (d) $3\,A$

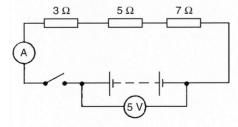

Figure 5.56

4. The effect of connecting an additional parallel load to an electrical supply source is to increase the
   (a) resistance of the load
   (b) voltage of the source
   (c) current taken from the source
   (d) p.d. across the load

5. The equivalent resistance when a resistor of $\frac{1}{3}\,\Omega$ is connected in parallel with a $\frac{1}{4}\,\Omega$ resistance is:
   (a) $\frac{1}{7}\,\Omega$ (b) $7\,\Omega$ (c) $\frac{1}{12}\,\Omega$ (d) $\frac{3}{4}\,\Omega$

6. With the switch in Fig. 5.57 closed the ammeter reading will indicate:
   (a) $108\,A$ (b) $\frac{1}{3}\,A$ (c) $3\,A$ (d) $4\frac{3}{5}\,A$

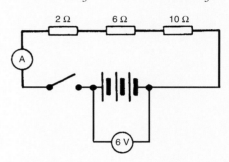

Figure 5.57

7. A $6\,\Omega$ resistor is connected in parallel with the three resistors of Fig. 5.57. With the switch closed the ammeter reading will indicate:
   (a) $\frac{3}{4}\,A$ (b) $4\,A$ (c) $\frac{1}{4}\,A$ (d) $1\frac{1}{3}\,A$

8. A $10\,\Omega$ resistor is connected in parallel with a $15\,\Omega$ resistor and the combination in series with a $12\,\Omega$ resistor. The equivalent resistance of the circuit is:
   (a) $37\,\Omega$ (b) $18\,\Omega$ (c) $27\,\Omega$ (d) $4\,\Omega$

9. When three $3\,\Omega$ resistors are connected in parallel, the total resistance is:
   (a) $3\,\Omega$ (b) $9\,\Omega$
   (c) $1\,\Omega$ (d) $0.333\,\Omega$

10. The total resistance of two resistors R_1 and R_2 when connected in parallel is given by:
    (a) $R_1 + R_2$ (b) $\dfrac{1}{R_1} + \dfrac{1}{R_2}$
    (c) $\dfrac{R_1 + R_2}{R_1 R_2}$ (d) $\dfrac{R_1 R_2}{R_1 + R_2}$

11. If in the circuit shown in Fig. 5.58, the reading on the voltmeter is 5 V and the reading on the ammeter is 25 mA, the resistance of resistor R is:
   (a) 0.005 Ω   (b) 5 Ω
   (c) 125 Ω   (d) 200 Ω

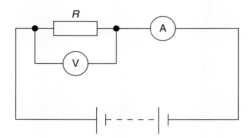

Figure 5.58

12. A variable resistor has a range of 0 to 5 kΩ. If the slider is set at halfway, the value of current flowing through a 750 Ω load, when connected to a 100 V supply and used as a potentiometer, is:
   (a) 25 mA   (b) 40 mA
   (c) 17.39 mA   (d) 20 mA

Chapter 6

Capacitors and capacitance

At the end of this chapter you should be able to:

- appreciate some applications of capacitors
- describe an electrostatic field
- appreciate Coulomb's law
- define electric field strength E and state its unit
- define capacitance and state its unit
- describe a capacitor and draw the circuit diagram symbol
- perform simple calculations involving $C = Q/V$ and $Q = It$
- define electric flux density D and state its unit
- define permittivity, distinguishing between ε_0, ε_r and ε
- perform simple calculations involving

$$D = \frac{Q}{A}, \quad E = \frac{V}{d} \quad \text{and} \quad \frac{D}{E} = \varepsilon_0 \varepsilon_r$$

- understand that for a parallel plate capacitor,

$$C = \frac{\varepsilon_0 \varepsilon_r A (n-1)}{d}$$

- perform calculations involving capacitors connected in parallel and in series
- define dielectric strength and state its unit
- state that the energy stored in a capacitor is given by $W = \frac{1}{2}CV^2$ joules
- describe practical types of capacitor
- understand the precautions needed when discharging capacitors

6.1 Introduction to capacitors

A capacitor is an electrical device that is used to store electrical energy. Next to the resistor, the capacitor is the most commonly encountered component in electrical circuits. Capacitors are used extensively in electrical and electronic circuits. For example, capacitors are used to smooth rectified a.c. outputs, they are used in telecommunication equipment – such as radio receivers – for tuning to the required frequency, they are used in time delay circuits, in electrical filters, in oscillator circuits, and in magnetic resonance imaging (MRI) in medical body scanners, to name but a few practical applications.

DOI: 10.1016/B978-0-08-089056-2.00006-1

6.2 Electrostatic field

Figure 6.1 represents two parallel metal plates, A and B, charged to different potentials. If an electron that has a negative charge is placed between the plates, a force will act on the electron tending to push it away from the negative plate B towards the positive plate, A. Similarly, a positive charge would be acted on by a force tending to move it toward the negative plate. Any region such as that shown between the plates in Fig. 6.1, in which an electric charge experiences a force, is called an **electrostatic field**. The direction of the field is defined as that of the force acting on a positive charge placed in the field. In Fig. 6.1, the direction of the force is from the positive plate to the negative plate. Such a field may be represented in magnitude and direction by **lines of electric force** drawn between the charged surfaces. The closeness of the lines is an indication of the field strength. Whenever a p.d. is established between two points, an electric field will always exist.

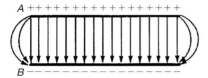

Figure 6.1

Figure 6.2(a) shows a typical field pattern for an isolated point charge, and Fig. 6.2(b) shows the field pattern for adjacent charges of opposite polarity. Electric lines of force (often called electric flux lines) are continuous and start and finish on point charges; also, the lines cannot cross each other. When a charged body is placed close to an uncharged body, an induced charge of opposite sign appears on the surface of the uncharged body. This is because lines of force from the charged body terminate on its surface.

The concept of field lines or lines of force is used to illustrate the properties of an electric field. However, it should be remembered that they are only aids to the imagination.

The **force of attraction or repulsion** between two electrically charged bodies is proportional to the magnitude of their charges and inversely proportional to the square of the distance separating them, i.e.

$$\text{force} \propto \frac{q_1 q_2}{d^2}$$

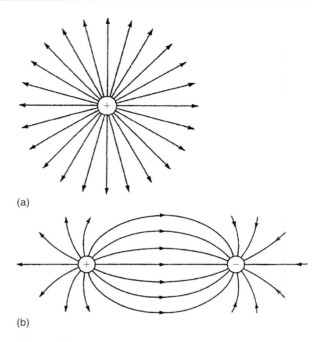

(a)

(b)

Figure 6.2

or

$$\text{force} = k \frac{q_1 q_2}{d^2}$$

where constant $k \approx 9 \times 10^9$. This is known as **Coulomb's law**.

Hence the force between two charged spheres in air with their centres 16 mm apart and each carrying a charge of $+1.6\,\mu\text{C}$ is given by:

$$\text{force} = k \frac{q_1 q_2}{d^2} \approx (9 \times 10^9) \frac{(1.6 \times 10^{-6})^2}{(16 \times 10^{-3})^2}$$

$$= \textbf{90 newtons}$$

6.3 Electric field strength

Figure 6.3 shows two parallel conducting plates separated from each other by air. They are connected to opposite terminals of a battery of voltage V volts. There is therefore an electric field in the space between the plates. If the plates are close together, the electric lines of force will be straight and parallel and equally spaced, except near the edge where fringing will occur (see Fig. 6.1). Over the area in which there is negligible fringing,

$$\text{Electric field strength, } E = \frac{V}{d} \text{ volts/metre}$$

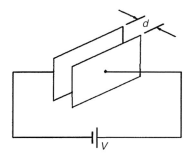

Figure 6.3

where d is the distance between the plates. Electric field strength is also called **potential gradient**.

6.4 Capacitance

Static electric fields arise from electric charges, electric field lines beginning and ending on electric charges. Thus the presence of the field indicates the presence of equal positive and negative electric charges on the two plates of Fig. 6.3. Let the charge be $+Q$ coulombs on one plate and $-Q$ coulombs on the other. The property of this pair of plates which determines how much charge corresponds to a given p.d. between the plates is called their capacitance:

$$\text{capacitance } C = \frac{Q}{V}$$

The **unit of capacitance** is the **farad** F (or more usually $\mu F = 10^{-6}\,F$ or $pF = 10^{-12}\,F$), which is defined as the capacitance when a p.d. of one volt appears across the plates when charged with one coulomb.

6.5 Capacitors

Every system of electrical conductors possesses capacitance. For example, there is capacitance between the conductors of overhead transmission lines and also between the wires of a telephone cable. In these examples the capacitance is undesirable but has to be accepted, minimised or compensated for. There are other situations where capacitance is a desirable property.

Devices specially constructed to possess capacitance are called **capacitors** (or condensers, as they used to be called). In its simplest form a capacitor consists of two plates which are separated by an insulating material known as a **dielectric**. A capacitor has the ability to store a quantity of static electricity.

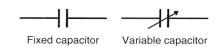

Fixed capacitor   Variable capacitor

Figure 6.4

The symbols for a fixed capacitor and a variable capacitor used in electrical circuit diagrams are shown in Fig. 6.4

The **charge Q** stored in a capacitor is given by:

$$Q = I \times t \text{ coulombs}$$

where I is the current in amperes and t the time in seconds.

> **Problem 1.**   (a) Determine the p.d. across a $4\,\mu F$ capacitor when charged with $5\,mC$. (b) Find the charge on a $50\,pF$ capacitor when the voltage applied to it is $2\,kV$.

(a) $C = 4\,\mu F = 4 \times 10^{-6}\,F$ and
    $Q = 5\,mC = 5 \times 10^{-3}\,C$.

Since $C = \dfrac{Q}{V}$ then $V = \dfrac{Q}{C} = \dfrac{5 \times 10^{-3}}{4 \times 10^{-6}}$

$$= \frac{5 \times 10^{6}}{4 \times 10^{3}} = \frac{5000}{4}$$

Hence p.d. $V = 1250\,V$ or $1.25\,kV$

(b) $C = 50\,pF = 50 \times 10^{-12}\,F$ and

    $V = 2\,kV = 2000\,V$

$$Q = CV = 50 \times 10^{-12} \times 2000$$

$$= \frac{5 \times 2}{10^{8}} = 0.1 \times 10^{-6}$$

Hence, charge $Q = 0.1\,\mu C$

> **Problem 2.**   A direct current of $4\,A$ flows into a previously uncharged $20\,\mu F$ capacitor for $3\,ms$. Determine the p.d. between the plates.

$I = 4\,A$, $C = 20\,\mu F = 20 \times 10^{-6}\,F$ and
$t = 3\,ms = 3 \times 10^{-3}\,s$.
$Q = It = 4 \times 3 \times 10^{-3}\,C$.

$$V = \frac{Q}{C} = \frac{4 \times 3 \times 10^{-3}}{20 \times 10^{-6}}$$

$$= \frac{12 \times 10^{6}}{20 \times 10^{3}} = 0.6 \times 10^{3} = 600\,V$$

Hence, the p.d. between the plates is $600\,V$

Problem 3. A $5\,\mu\text{F}$ capacitor is charged so that the p.d. between its plates is 800 V. Calculate how long the capacitor can provide an average discharge current of 2 mA.

$C = 5\,\mu\text{F} = 5 \times 10^{-6}\,\text{F}$, $V = 800\,\text{V}$ and
$I = 2\,\text{mA} = 2 \times 10^{-3}\,\text{A}$.

$Q = CV = 5 \times 10^{-6} \times 800 = 4 \times 10^{-3}\,\text{C}$
Also, $Q = It$. Thus,

$$t = \frac{Q}{I} = \frac{4 \times 10^{-3}}{2 \times 10^{-3}} = 2\,\text{s}$$

Hence, the capacitor can provide an average discharge current of 2 mA for 2 s.

Now try the following exercise

Exercise 26 Further problems on capacitors and capacitance

1. Find the charge on a $10\,\mu\text{F}$ capacitor when the applied voltage is 250 V. [2.5 mC]

2. Determine the voltage across a 1000 pF capacitor to charge it with $2\,\mu\text{C}$. [2 kV]

3. The charge on the plates of a capacitor is 6 mC when the potential between them is 2.4 kV. Determine the capacitance of the capacitor. [2.5 μF]

4. For how long must a charging current of 2 A be fed to a $5\,\mu\text{F}$ capacitor to raise the p.d. between its plates by 500 V. [1.25 ms]

5. A direct current of 10 A flows into a previously uncharged $5\,\mu\text{F}$ capacitor for 1 ms. Determine the p.d. between the plates. [2 kV]

6. A $16\,\mu\text{F}$ capacitor is charged at a constant current of $4\,\mu\text{A}$ for 2 min. Calculate the final p.d. across the capacitor and the corresponding charge in coulombs. [30 V, 480 μC]

7. A steady current of 10 A flows into a previously uncharged capacitor for 1.5 ms when the p.d. between the plates is 2 kV. Find the capacitance of the capacitor. [7.5 μF]

6.6 Electric flux density

Unit flux is defined as emanating from a positive charge of 1 coulomb. Thus electric flux ψ is measured in coulombs, and for a charge of Q coulombs, the flux $\psi = Q$ coulombs.

Electric flux density D is the amount of flux passing through a defined area A that is perpendicular to the direction of the flux:

$$\text{electric flux density, } D = \frac{Q}{A} \text{ coulombs/metre}^2$$

Electric flux density is also called **charge density**, σ.

6.7 Permittivity

At any point in an electric field, the electric field strength E maintains the electric flux and produces a particular value of electric flux density D at that point. For a field established in **vacuum** (or for practical purposes in air), the ratio D/E is a constant ε_0, i.e.

$$\frac{D}{E} = \varepsilon_0$$

where ε_0 is called the **permittivity of free space** or the free space constant. The value of ε_0 is $8.85 \times 10^{-12}\,\text{F/m}$.

When an insulating medium, such as mica, paper, plastic or ceramic, is introduced into the region of an electric field the ratio of D/E is modified:

$$\frac{D}{E} = \varepsilon_0 \varepsilon_r$$

where ε_r, the **relative permittivity** of the insulating material, indicates its insulating power compared with that of vacuum:

relative permittivity,

$$\varepsilon_r = \frac{\text{flux density in material}}{\text{flux density in vacuum}}$$

ε_r has no unit. Typical values of ε_r include air, 1.00; polythene, 2.3; mica, 3–7; glass, 5–10; water, 80; ceramics, 6–1000.

The product $\varepsilon_0 \varepsilon_r$ is called the **absolute permittivity**, ε, i.e.

$$\varepsilon = \varepsilon_0 \varepsilon_r$$

The insulating medium separating charged surfaces is called a **dielectric**. Compared with conductors, dielectric materials have very high resistivities. They are therefore used to separate conductors at different potentials, such as capacitor plates or electric power lines.

> **Problem 4.** Two parallel rectangular plates measuring 20 cm by 40 cm carry an electric charge of 0.2 μC. Calculate the electric flux density. If the plates are spaced 5 mm apart and the voltage between them is 0.25 kV determine the electric field strength.

Area $= 20\,cm \times 40\,cm = 800\,cm^2 = 800 \times 10^{-4}\,m^2$ and charge $Q = 0.2\,\mu C = 0.2 \times 10^{-6}\,C$,
Electric flux density

$$D = \frac{Q}{A} = \frac{0.2 \times 10^{-6}}{800 \times 10^{-4}} = \frac{0.2 \times 10^4}{800 \times 10^6}$$

$$= \frac{2000}{800} \times 10^{-6} = \mathbf{2.5\,\mu C/m^2}$$

Voltage $V = 0.25\,kV = 250\,V$ and plate spacing, $d = 5\,mm = 5 \times 10^{-3}\,m$.
Electric field strength

$$E = \frac{V}{d} = \frac{250}{5 \times 10^{-3}} = \mathbf{50\,kV/m}$$

> **Problem 5.** The flux density between two plates separated by mica of relative permittivity 5 is $2\,\mu C/m^2$. Find the voltage gradient between the plates.

Flux density $D = 2\,\mu C/m^2 = 2 \times 10^{-6}\,C/m^2$,
$\varepsilon_0 = 8.85 \times 10^{-12}\,F/m$ and $\varepsilon_r = 5$.
$D/E = \varepsilon_0\varepsilon_r$, hence **voltage gradient**,

$$E = \frac{D}{\varepsilon_0\varepsilon_r} = \frac{2 \times 10^{-6}}{8.85 \times 10^{-12} \times 5}\,V/m$$

$$= \mathbf{45.2\,kV/m}$$

> **Problem 6.** Two parallel plates having a p.d. of 200 V between them are spaced 0.8 mm apart. What is the electric field strength? Find also the electric flux density when the dielectric between the plates is (a) air, and (b) polythene of relative permittivity 2.3.

Electric field strength

$$E = \frac{V}{d} = \frac{200}{0.8 \times 10^{-3}} = \mathbf{250\,kV/m}$$

(a) For air: $\varepsilon_r = 1$ and $\dfrac{D}{E} = \varepsilon_0\varepsilon_r$

Hence **electric flux density**

$$D = E\varepsilon_0\varepsilon_r$$

$$= (250 \times 10^3 \times 8.85 \times 10^{-12} \times 1)\,C/m^2$$

$$= \mathbf{2.213\,\mu C/m^2}$$

(b) For polythene, $\varepsilon_r = 2.3$

Electric flux density

$$D = E\varepsilon_0\varepsilon_r$$

$$= (250 \times 10^3 \times 8.85 \times 10^{-12} \times 2.3)\,C/m^2$$

$$= \mathbf{5.089\,\mu C/m^2}$$

Now try the following exercise

> **Exercise 27 Further problems on electric field strength, electric flux density and permittivity**
>
> (Where appropriate take ε_0 as $8.85 \times 10^{-12}\,F/m$)
>
> 1. A capacitor uses a dielectric 0.04 mm thick and operates at 30 V. What is the electric field strength across the dielectric at this voltage? [750 kV/m]
>
> 2. A two-plate capacitor has a charge of 25 C. If the effective area of each plate is $5\,cm^2$ find the electric flux density of the electric field. [$50\,kC/m^2$]
>
> 3. A charge of 1.5 μC is carried on two parallel rectangular plates each measuring 60 mm by 80 mm. Calculate the electric flux density. If the plates are spaced 10 mm apart and the voltage between them is 0.5 kV determine the electric field strength. [$312.5\,\mu C/m^2$, 50 kV/m]
>
> 4. Two parallel plates are separated by a dielectric and charged with 10 μC. Given that the

area of each plate is $50\,cm^2$, calculate the electric flux density in the dielectric separating the plates.

[$2\,mC/m^2$]

5. The electric flux density between two plates separated by polystyrene of relative permittivity 2.5 is $5\,\mu C/m^2$. Find the voltage gradient between the plates. [$226\,kV/m$]

6. Two parallel plates having a p.d. of $250\,V$ between them are spaced 1 mm apart. Determine the electric field strength. Find also the electric flux density when the dielectric between the plates is (a) air and (b) mica of relative permittivity 5.

[$250\,kV/m$ (a) $2.213\,\mu C/m^2$
(b) $11.063\,\mu C/m^2$]

6.8 The parallel plate capacitor

For a parallel plate capacitor, as shown in Fig. 6.5(a), experiments show that capacitance C is proportional to the area A of a plate, inversely proportional to the plate spacing d (i.e. the dielectric thickness) and depends on the nature of the dielectric:

$$\text{Capacitance, } C = \frac{\varepsilon_0 \varepsilon_r A}{d} \text{ farads}$$

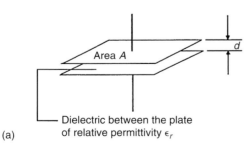

Area A

d

Dielectric between the plate
(a) of relative permittivity ϵ_r

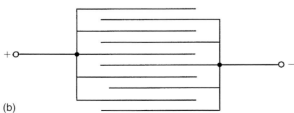

$+\circ$ $\circ\,-$

(b)

Figure 6.5

where $\varepsilon_0 = 8.85 \times 10^{-12}\,F/m$ (constant)

ε_r = relative permittivity

A = area of one of the plates, in m^2, and

d = thickness of dielectric in m

Another method used to increase the capacitance is to interleave several plates as shown in Fig. 6.5(b). Ten plates are shown, forming nine capacitors with a capacitance nine times that of one pair of plates. If such an arrangement has n plates then capacitance $C \propto (n-1)$. Thus capacitance

$$C = \frac{\varepsilon_0 \varepsilon_r A (n-1)}{d} \text{ farads}$$

Problem 7. (a) A ceramic capacitor has an effective plate area of $4\,cm^2$ separated by 0.1 mm of ceramic of relative permittivity 100. Calculate the capacitance of the capacitor in picofarads. (b) If the capacitor in part (a) is given a charge of $1.2\,\mu C$ what will be the p.d. between the plates?

(a) Area $A = 4\,cm^2 = 4 \times 10^{-4}\,m^2$,

$d = 0.1\,mm = 0.1 \times 10^{-3}\,m$,

$\varepsilon_0 = 8.85 \times 10^{-12}\,F/m$ and $\varepsilon_r = 100$

Capacitance,

$$C = \frac{\varepsilon_0 \varepsilon_r A}{d} \text{ farads}$$

$$= \frac{8.85 \times 10^{-12} \times 100 \times 4 \times 10^{-4}}{0.1 \times 10^{-3}}\,F$$

$$= \frac{8.85 \times 4}{10^{10}}\,F$$

$$= \frac{8.85 \times 4 \times 10^{12}}{10^{10}}\,pF = \mathbf{3540\,pF}$$

(b) $Q = CV$ thus

$$V = \frac{Q}{C} = \frac{1.2 \times 10^{-6}}{3540 \times 10^{-12}}\,V = \mathbf{339\,V}$$

Problem 8. A waxed paper capacitor has two parallel plates, each of effective area $800\,cm^2$. If the capacitance of the capacitor is $4425\,pF$ determine the effective thickness of the paper if its relative permittivity is 2.5

$A = 800\,cm^2 = 800 \times 10^{-4}\,m^2 = 0.08\,m^2$,

$C = 4425\,pF = 4425 \times 10^{-12}\,F$, $\varepsilon_0 = 8.85 \times 10^{-12}\,F/m$

and $\varepsilon_r = 2.5$. Since

$$C = \frac{\varepsilon_0 \varepsilon_A A}{d} \quad \text{then} \quad d = \frac{\varepsilon_0 \varepsilon_r A}{C}$$

i.e.
$$d = \frac{8.85 \times 10^{-12} \times 2.5 \times 0.08}{4425 \times 10^{-12}}$$
$$= 0.0004 \, \text{m}$$

Hence, the thickness of the paper is 0.4 mm.

Problem 9. A parallel plate capacitor has nineteen interleaved plates each 75 mm by 75 mm separated by mica sheets 0.2 mm thick. Assuming the relative permittivity of the mica is 5, calculate the capacitance of the capacitor.

$n = 19$ thus $n - 1 = 18$, $A = 75 \times 75 = 5625 \, \text{mm}^2 = 5625 \times 10^{-6} \, \text{m}^2$, $\varepsilon_r = 5$, $\varepsilon_0 = 8.85 \times 10^{-12} \, \text{F/m}$ and $d = 0.2 \, \text{mm} = 0.2 \times 10^{-3} \, \text{m}$. Capacitance,

$$C = \frac{\varepsilon_0 \varepsilon_r A (n - 1)}{d}$$
$$= \frac{8.85 \times 10^{-12} \times 5 \times 5625 \times 10^{-6} \times 18}{0.2 \times 10^{-3}} \, \text{F}$$
$$= \mathbf{0.0224 \, \mu F \text{ or } 22.4 \, nF}$$

Now try the following exercise

Exercise 28   Further problems on parallel plate capacitors

(Where appropriate take ε_0 as $8.85 \times 10^{-12} \, \text{F/m}$)

1. A capacitor consists of two parallel plates each of area $0.01 \, \text{m}^2$, spaced 0.1 mm in air. Calculate the capacitance in picofarads.   [885 pF]

2. A waxed paper capacitor has two parallel plates, each of effective area $0.2 \, \text{m}^2$. If the capacitance is 4000 pF determine the effective thickness of the paper if its relative permittivity is 2   [0.885 mm]

3. Calculate the capacitance of a parallel plate capacitor having 5 plates, each 30 mm by 20 mm and separated by a dielectric 0.75 mm thick having a relative permittivity of 2.3.   [65.14 pF]

4. How many plates has a parallel plate capacitor having a capacitance of 5 nF, if each plate is 40 mm by 40 mm and each dielectric is 0.102 mm thick with a relative permittivity of 6.   [7]

5. A parallel plate capacitor is made from 25 plates, each 70 mm by 120 mm interleaved with mica of relative permittivity 5. If the capacitance of the capacitor is 3000 pF determine the thickness of the mica sheet.   [2.97 mm]

6. A capacitor is constructed with parallel plates and has a value of 50 pF. What would be the capacitance of the capacitor if the plate area is doubled and the plate spacing is halved?   [200 pF]

7. The capacitance of a parallel plate capacitor is 1000 pF. It has 19 plates, each 50 mm by 30 mm separated by a dielectric of thickness 0.40 mm. Determine the relative permittivity of the dielectric.   [1.67]

8. The charge on the square plates of a multi-plate capacitor is $80 \, \mu\text{C}$ when the potential between them is 5 kV. If the capacitor has twenty-five plates separated by a dielectric of thickness 0.102 mm and relative permittivity 4.8, determine the width of a plate.   [40 mm]

9. A capacitor is to be constructed so that its capacitance is 4250 pF and to operate at a p.d. of 100 V across its terminals. The dielectric is to be polythene ($\varepsilon_r = 2.3$) which, after allowing a safety factor, has a dielectric strength of 20 MV/m. Find (a) the thickness of the polythene needed, and (b) the area of a plate.   [(a) 0.005 mm (b) 10.44 cm^2]

6.9   Capacitors connected in parallel and series

(a) Capacitors connected in parallel

Figure 6.6 shows three capacitors, C_1, C_2 and C_3, connected in parallel with a supply voltage V applied across the arrangement.

When the charging current I reaches point A it divides, some flowing into C_1, some flowing into C_2 and some into C_3. Hence the total charge $Q_T (= I \times t)$ is divided between the three capacitors. The capacitors

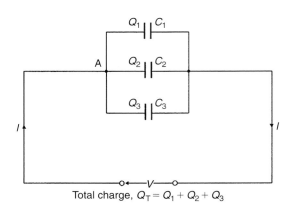

Total charge, $Q_T = Q_1 + Q_2 + Q_3$

Figure 6.6

each store a charge and these are shown as Q_1, Q_2 and Q_3 respectively. Hence

$$Q_T = Q_1 + Q_2 + Q_3$$

But $Q_T = CV$, $Q_1 = C_1 V$, $Q_2 = C_2 V$ and $Q_3 = C_3 V$. Therefore $CV = C_1 V + C_2 V + C_3 V$ where C is the total equivalent circuit capacitance, i.e.

$$C = C_1 + C_2 + C_3$$

It follows that for n parallel-connected capacitors,

$$C = C_1 + C_2 + C_3 \cdots\cdots + C_n$$

i.e. the equivalent capacitance of a group of parallel-connected capacitors is the sum of the capacitances of the individual capacitors. (Note that this formula is similar to that used for **resistors** connected in **series**).

(b) Capacitors connected in series

Figure 6.7 shows three capacitors, C_1, C_2 and C_3, connected in series across a supply voltage V. Let the p.d. across the individual capacitors be V_1, V_2 and V_3 respectively as shown.

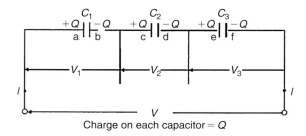

Charge on each capacitor = Q

Figure 6.7

Let the charge on plate 'a' of capacitor C_1 be $+Q$ coulombs. This induces an equal but opposite charge

of $-Q$ coulombs on plate 'b'. The conductor between plates 'b' and 'c' is electrically isolated from the rest of the circuit so that an equal but opposite charge of $+Q$ coulombs must appear on plate 'c', which, in turn, induces an equal and opposite charge of $-Q$ coulombs on plate 'd', and so on.

Hence when capacitors are connected in series the charge on each is the same. In a series circuit:

$$V = V_1 + V_2 + V_3$$

Since $V = \dfrac{Q}{C}$ then $\dfrac{Q}{C} = \dfrac{Q}{C_1} + \dfrac{Q}{C_2} + \dfrac{Q}{C_3}$

where C is the total equivalent circuit capacitance, i.e.

$$\frac{1}{C} = \frac{1}{C_1} + \frac{1}{C_2} + \frac{1}{C_3}$$

It follows that for n series-connected capacitors:

$$\frac{1}{C} = \frac{1}{C_1} + \frac{1}{C_2} + \frac{1}{C_3} + \cdots + \frac{1}{C_n}$$

i.e. for series-connected capacitors, the reciprocal of the equivalent capacitance is equal to the sum of the reciprocals of the individual capacitances. (Note that this formula is similar to that used for **resistors** connected in **parallel**.)

For the special case of **two capacitors in series**:

$$\frac{1}{C} = \frac{1}{C_1} + \frac{1}{C_2} = \frac{C_2 + C_1}{C_1 C_2}$$

Hence

$$C = \frac{C_1 C_2}{C_1 + C_2} \quad \left(\text{i.e.} \ \frac{\text{product}}{\text{sum}} \right)$$

Problem 10. Calculate the equivalent capacitance of two capacitors of $6\,\mu$F and $4\,\mu$F connected (a) in parallel and (b) in series.

(a)   In parallel, equivalent capacitance,
$C = C_1 + C_2 = 6\,\mu\text{F} + 4\,\mu\text{F} = \mathbf{10\,\mu F}$

(b)   In series, equivalent capacitance C is given by:

$$C = \frac{C_1 C_2}{C_1 + C_2}$$

This formula is used for the special case of **two** capacitors in series. Thus

$$C = \frac{6 \times 4}{6 + 4} = \frac{24}{10} = \mathbf{2.4\,\mu F}$$

Problem 11.   What capacitance must be connected in series with a $30\,\mu\text{F}$ capacitor for the equivalent capacitance to be $12\,\mu\text{F}$?

Let $C = 12\,\mu\text{F}$ (the equivalent capacitance), $C_1 = 30\,\mu\text{F}$ and C_2 be the unknown capacitance. For two capacitors in series

$$\frac{1}{C} = \frac{1}{C_1} + \frac{1}{C_2}$$

Hence

$$\frac{1}{C_2} = \frac{1}{C} - \frac{1}{C_1} = \frac{C_1 - C}{CC_1}$$

and

$$C_2 = \frac{CC_1}{C_1 - C} = \frac{12 \times 30}{30 - 12} = \frac{360}{18} = 20\,\mu\text{F}$$

Problem 12.   Capacitances of $1\,\mu\text{F}$, $3\,\mu\text{F}$, $5\,\mu\text{F}$ and $6\,\mu\text{F}$ are connected in parallel to a direct voltage supply of $100\,\text{V}$. Determine (a) the equivalent circuit capacitance, (b) the total charge, and (c) the charge on each capacitor.

(a)   The equivalent capacitance C for four capacitors in parallel is given by:

$$C = C_1 + C_2 + C_3 + C_4$$

i.e. $C = 1 + 3 + 5 + 6 = 15\,\mu\text{F}$

(b)   Total charge $Q_T = CV$ where C is the equivalent circuit capacitance i.e.

$$Q_T = 15 \times 10^{-6} \times 100 = 1.5 \times 10^{-3}\,C$$
$$= 1.5\,\text{mC}$$

(c)   The charge on the $1\,\mu\text{F}$ capacitor
$$Q_1 = C_1 V = 1 \times 10^{-6} \times 100 = 0.1\,\text{mC}$$
The charge on the $3\,\mu\text{F}$ capacitor
$$Q_2 = C_2 V = 3 \times 10^{-6} \times 100 = 0.3\,\text{mC}$$
The charge on the $5\,\mu\text{F}$ capacitor
$$Q_3 = C_3 V = 5 \times 10^{-6} \times 100 = 0.5\,\text{mC}$$
The charge on the $6\,\mu\text{F}$ capacitor
$$Q_4 = C_4 V = 6 \times 10^{-6} \times 100 = 0.6\,\text{mC}$$
[Check: In a parallel circuit

$$Q_T = Q_1 + Q_2 + Q_3 + Q_4$$
$$Q_1 + Q_2 + Q_3 + Q_4 = 0.1 + 0.3 + 0.5 + 0.6$$
$$= 1.5\,\text{mC} = Q_T]$$

Problem 13.   Capacitances of $3\,\mu\text{F}$, $6\,\mu\text{F}$ and $12\,\mu\text{F}$ are connected in series across a $350\,\text{V}$ supply. Calculate (a) the equivalent circuit capacitance, (b) the charge on each capacitor, and (c) the p.d. across each capacitor.

The circuit diagram is shown in Fig. 6.8.

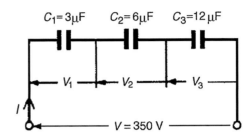

Figure 6.8

(a)   The equivalent circuit capacitance C for three capacitors in series is given by:

$$\frac{1}{C} = \frac{1}{C_1} + \frac{1}{C_2} + \frac{1}{C_3}$$

i.e. $\dfrac{1}{C} = \dfrac{1}{3} + \dfrac{1}{6} + \dfrac{1}{12} = \dfrac{4 + 2 + 1}{12} = \dfrac{7}{12}$

Hence the equivalent circuit capacitance

$$C = \frac{12}{7} = 1\frac{5}{7}\,\mu\text{F}\ \text{or } 1.714\,\mu\text{F}$$

(b)   Total charge $Q_T = CV$, hence

$$Q_T = \frac{12}{7} \times 10^{-6} \times 350$$
$$= 600\,\mu\text{C or } 0.6\,\text{mC}$$

Since the capacitors are connected in series 0.6 mC is the charge on each of them.

(c)   The voltage across the $3\,\mu\text{F}$ capacitor,

$$V_1 = \frac{Q}{C_1}$$
$$= \frac{0.6 \times 10^{-3}}{3 \times 10^{-6}} = 200\,\text{V}$$

The voltage across the $6\,\mu\text{F}$ capacitor,

$$V_2 = \frac{Q}{C_2}$$
$$= \frac{0.6 \times 10^{-3}}{6 \times 10^{-6}} = 100\,\text{V}$$

The voltage across the $12\,\mu F$ capacitor,

$$V_3 = \frac{Q}{C_3}$$

$$= \frac{0.6 \times 10^{-3}}{12 \times 10^{-6}} = \mathbf{50\,V}$$

[Check: In a series circuit $V = V_1 + V_2 + V_3$. $V_1 + V_2 + V_3 = 200 + 100 + 50 = 350\,V = $ supply voltage]

In practice, capacitors are rarely connected in series unless they are of the same capacitance. The reason for this can be seen from the above problem where the lowest valued capacitor (i.e. $3\,\mu F$) has the highest p.d. across it (i.e. $200\,V$) which means that if all the capacitors have an identical construction they must all be rated at the highest voltage.

Problem 14. For the arrangement shown in Fig. 6.9 find (a) the equivalent capacitance of the circuit, (b) the voltage across QR, and (c) the charge on each capacitor.

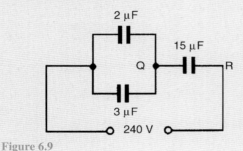

Figure 6.9

(a) $2\,\mu F$ in parallel with $3\,\mu F$ gives an equivalent capacitance of $2\,\mu F + 3\,\mu F = 5\,\mu F$. The circuit is now as shown in Fig. 6.10.

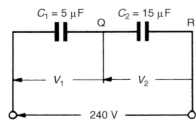

Figure 6.10

The **equivalent capacitance** of $5\,\mu F$ in series with $15\,\mu F$ is given by

$$\frac{5 \times 15}{5 + 15}\,\mu F = \frac{75}{20}\,\mu F = \mathbf{3.75\,\mu F}$$

(b) The charge on each of the capacitors shown in Fig. 6.10 will be the same since they are connected in series. Let this charge be Q coulombs.

Then $\qquad Q = C_1 V_1 = C_2 V_2$

i.e. $\qquad 5V_1 = 15V_2$

$$V_1 = 3V_2 \qquad\qquad (1)$$

Also $\quad V_1 + V_2 = 240\,V$

Hence $\quad 3V_2 + V_2 = 240\,V$ from equation (1)

Thus $\qquad V_2 = 60\,V$ and $V_1 = 180\,V$

Hence the voltage across QR is 60 V

(c) The charge on the $15\,\mu F$ capacitor is

$$C_2 V_2 = 15 \times 10^{-6} \times 60 = \mathbf{0.9\,mC}$$

The charge on the $2\,\mu F$ capacitor is

$$2 \times 10^{-6} \times 180 = \mathbf{0.36\,mC}$$

The charge on the $3\,\mu F$ capacitor is

$$3 \times 10^{-6} \times 180 = \mathbf{0.54\,mC}$$

Now try the following exercise

Exercise 29 Further problems on capacitors in parallel and series

1. Capacitors of $2\,\mu F$ and $6\,\mu F$ are connected (a) in parallel and (b) in series. Determine the equivalent capacitance in each case.
   [(a) $8\,\mu F$ (b) $1.5\,\mu F$]

2. Find the capacitance to be connected in series with a $10\,\mu F$ capacitor for the equivalent capacitance to be $6\,\mu F$. [$15\,\mu F$]

3. What value of capacitance would be obtained if capacitors of $0.15\,\mu F$ and $0.10\,\mu F$ are connected (a) in series and (b) in parallel?
   [(a) $0.06\,\mu F$ (b) $0.25\,\mu F$]

4. Two $6\,\mu F$ capacitors are connected in series with one having a capacitance of $12\,\mu F$. Find the total equivalent circuit capacitance. What

capacitance must be added in series to obtain a capacitance of $1.2\,\mu\text{F}$?

[$2.4\,\mu\text{F}$, $2.4\,\mu\text{F}$]

5. Determine the equivalent capacitance when the following capacitors are connected (a) in parallel and (b) in series:

    (i) $2\,\mu\text{F}$, $4\,\mu\text{F}$ and $8\,\mu\text{F}$

    (ii) $0.02\,\mu\text{F}$, $0.05\,\mu\text{F}$ and $0.10\,\mu\text{F}$

    (iii) $50\,\text{pF}$ and $450\,\text{pF}$

    (iv) $0.01\,\mu\text{F}$ and $200\,\text{pF}$

    [(a)   (i) $14\,\mu\text{F}$ (ii) $0.17\,\mu\text{F}$

            (iii) $500\,\text{pF}$ (iv) $0.0102\,\mu\text{F}$

      (b)   (i) $1.143\,\mu\text{F}$ (ii) $0.0125\,\mu\text{F}$

            (iii) $45\,\text{pF}$ (iv) $196.1\,\text{pF}$]

6. For the arrangement shown in Fig. 6.11 find (a) the equivalent circuit capacitance and (b) the voltage across a $4.5\,\mu\text{F}$ capacitor.

[(a) $1.2\,\mu\text{F}$ (b) $100\,\text{V}$]

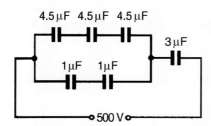

Figure 6.11

7. Three $12\,\mu\text{F}$ capacitors are connected in series across a $750\,\text{V}$ supply. Calculate (a) the equivalent capacitance, (b) the charge on each capacitor, and (c) the p.d. across each capacitor.   [(a) $4\,\mu\text{F}$ (b) $3\,\text{mC}$ (c) $250\,\text{V}$]

8. If two capacitors having capacitances of $3\,\mu\text{F}$ and $5\,\mu\text{F}$ respectively are connected in series across a $240\,\text{V}$ supply, determine (a) the p.d. across each capacitor and (b) the charge on each capacitor.

[(a) $150\,\text{V}$, $90\,\text{V}$ (b) $0.45\,\text{mC}$ on each]

9. In Fig. 6.12 capacitors P, Q and R are identical and the total equivalent capacitance of the circuit is $3\,\mu\text{F}$. Determine the values of P, Q and R [$4.2\,\mu\text{F}$ each]

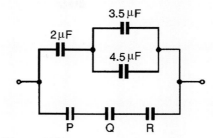

Figure 6.12

10. Capacitances of $4\,\mu\text{F}$, $8\,\mu\text{F}$ and $16\,\mu\text{F}$ are connected in parallel across a $200\,\text{V}$ supply. Determine (a) the equivalent capacitance, (b) the total charge, and (c) the charge on each capacitor.   [(a) $28\,\mu\text{F}$ (b) $5.6\,\text{mC}$

(c) $0.8\,\text{mC}$, $1.6\,\text{mC}$, $3.2\,\text{mC}$]

11. A circuit consists of two capacitors P and Q in parallel, connected in series with another capacitor R. The capacitances of P, Q and R are $4\,\mu\text{F}$, $12\,\mu\text{F}$ and $8\,\mu\text{F}$ respectively. When the circuit is connected across a $300\,\text{V}$ d.c. supply find (a) the total capacitance of the circuit, (b) the p.d. across each capacitor, and (c) the charge on each capacitor.

[(a) $5.33\,\mu\text{F}$ (b) $100\,\text{V}$ across P, $100\,\text{V}$

across Q, $200\,\text{V}$ across R (c) $0.4\,\text{mC}$ on P,

$1.2\,\text{mC}$ on Q, $1.6\,\text{mC}$ on R]

12. For the circuit shown in Fig. 6.13, determine (a) the total circuit capacitance, (b) the total energy in the circuit, and (c) the charges in the capacitors shown as C_1 and C_2

[(a) $0.857\,\mu\text{F}$ (b) $1.071\,\text{mJ}$

(c) $42.85\,\mu\text{C}$ on each]

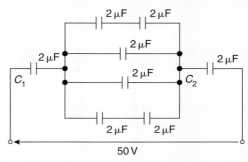

Figure 6.13

6.10 Dielectric strength

The maximum amount of field strength that a dielectric can withstand is called the dielectric strength of the material. Dielectric strength,

$$E_m = \frac{V_m}{d}$$

Problem 15. A capacitor is to be constructed so that its capacitance is $0.2\,\mu\text{F}$ and to take a p.d. of $1.25\,\text{kV}$ across its terminals. The dielectric is to be mica which, after allowing a safety factor of 2, has a dielectric strength of $50\,\text{MV/m}$. Find (a) the thickness of the mica needed, and (b) the area of a plate assuming a two-plate construction. (Assume ε_r for mica to be 6.)

(a) Dielectric strength,

$$E = \frac{V}{d}$$

i.e. $\quad d = \dfrac{V}{E} = \dfrac{1.25 \times 10^3}{50 \times 10^6}\,\text{m}$

$$= 0.025\,\text{mm}$$

(b) Capacitance,

$$C = \frac{\varepsilon_0 \varepsilon_r A}{d}$$

hence

area $A = \dfrac{Cd}{\varepsilon_0 \varepsilon_r} = \dfrac{0.2 \times 10^{-6} \times 0.025 \times 10^{-3}}{8.85 \times 10^{-12} \times 6}\,\text{m}^2$

$$= 0.09416\,\text{m}^2 = \mathbf{941.6\,cm^2}$$

6.11 Energy stored in capacitors

The energy, W, stored by a capacitor is given by

$$W = \frac{1}{2}CV^2 \text{ joules}$$

Problem 16. (a) Determine the energy stored in a $3\,\mu\text{F}$ capacitor when charged to $400\,\text{V}$. (b) Find also the average power developed if this energy is dissipated in a time of $10\,\mu\text{s}$.

(a) **Energy stored**

$$W = \frac{1}{2}CV^2 \text{ joules} = \frac{1}{2} \times 3 \times 10^{-6} \times 400^2$$

$$= \frac{3}{2} \times 16 \times 10^{-2} = \mathbf{0.24\,J}$$

(b) **Power** $= \dfrac{\text{energy}}{\text{time}} = \dfrac{0.24}{10 \times 10^{-6}}\,\text{W} = \mathbf{24\,kW}$

Problem 17. A $12\,\mu\text{F}$ capacitor is required to store $4\,\text{J}$ of energy. Find the p.d. to which the capacitor must be charged.

Energy stored

$$W = \frac{1}{2}CV^2$$

hence $\quad V^2 = \dfrac{2W}{C}$

and $\quad$ p.d. $V = \sqrt{\dfrac{2W}{C}} = \sqrt{\dfrac{2 \times 4}{12 \times 10^{-6}}}$

$$= \sqrt{\dfrac{2 \times 10^6}{3}} = \mathbf{816.5\,V}$$

Problem 18. A capacitor is charged with $10\,\text{mC}$. If the energy stored is $1.2\,\text{J}$ find (a) the voltage and (b) the capacitance.

Energy stored $W = \frac{1}{2}CV^2$ and $C = Q/V$. Hence

$$W = \frac{1}{2}\left(\frac{Q}{V}\right)V^2$$

$$= \frac{1}{2}QV$$

from which $\quad V = \dfrac{2W}{Q}$

$$Q = 10\,\text{mC} = 10 \times 10^{-3}\,\text{C}$$

and $\quad W = 1.2\,\text{J}$

(a) Voltage

$$V = \frac{2W}{Q} = \frac{2 \times 1.2}{10 \times 10^{-3}} = \mathbf{0.24\,kV \text{ or } 240\,V}$$

(b) Capacitance

$$C = \frac{Q}{V} = \frac{10 \times 10^{-3}}{240}\,\text{F} = \frac{10 \times 10^6}{240 \times 10^3}\,\mu\text{F}$$

$$= \mathbf{41.67\,\mu F}$$

Now try the following exercise

Exercise 30   Further problems on energy stored in capacitors

(Assume $\varepsilon_0 = 8.85 \times 10^{-12}$ F/m)

1. When a capacitor is connected across a 200 V supply the charge is $4\,\mu$C. Find (a) the capacitance and (b) the energy stored.
    [(a) $0.02\,\mu$F (b) 0.4 mJ]

2. Find the energy stored in a $10\,\mu$F capacitor when charged to 2 kV.   [20 J]

3. A 3300 pF capacitor is required to store 0.5 mJ of energy. Find the p.d. to which the capacitor must be charged.   [550 V]

4. A capacitor is charged with 8 mC. If the energy stored is 0.4 J find (a) the voltage and (b) the capacitance.   [(a) 100 V (b) $80\,\mu$F]

5. A capacitor, consisting of two metal plates each of area $50\,\text{cm}^2$ and spaced 0.2 mm apart in air, is connected across a 120 V supply. Calculate (a) the energy stored, (b) the electric flux density and (c) the potential gradient.
    [(a) $1.593\,\mu$J (b) $5.31\,\mu\text{C/m}^2$ (c) 600 kV/m]

6. A bakelite capacitor is to be constructed to have a capacitance of $0.04\,\mu$F and to have a steady working potential of 1 kV maximum. Allowing a safe value of field stress of 25 MV/m find (a) the thickness of bakelite required, (b) the area of plate required if the relative permittivity of bakelite is 5, (c) the maximum energy stored by the capacitor, and (d) the average power developed if this energy is dissipated in a time of $20\,\mu$s.
    [(a) 0.04 mm (b) $361.6\,\text{cm}^2$
    (c) 0.02 J (d) 1 kW]

6.12   Practical types of capacitor

Practical types of capacitor are characterized by the material used for their dielectric. The main types include: variable air, mica, paper, ceramic, plastic, titanium oxide and electrolytic.

1. **Variable air capacitors.** These usually consist of two sets of metal plates (such as aluminium), one

fixed, the other variable. The set of moving plates rotate on a spindle as shown by the end view of Fig. 6.14.

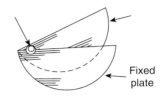

Fixed plate

Figure 6.14

As the moving plates are rotated through half a revolution, the meshing, and therefore the capacitance, varies from a minimum to a maximum value. Variable air capacitors are used in radio and electronic circuits where very low losses are required, or where a variable capacitance is needed. The maximum value of such capacitors is between 500 pF and 1000 pF.

2. **Mica capacitors.** A typical older type construction is shown in Fig. 6.15.

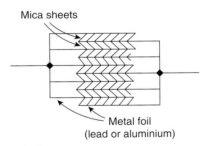

Mica sheets

Metal foil
(lead or aluminium)

Figure 6.15

Usually the whole capacitor is impregnated with wax and placed in a bakelite case. Mica is easily obtained in thin sheets and is a good insulator.

However, mica is expensive and is not used in capacitors above about $0.2\,\mu$F. A modified form of mica capacitor is the silvered mica type. The mica is coated on both sides with a thin layer of silver which forms the plates. Capacitance is stable and less likely to change with age. Such capacitors have a constant capacitance with change of temperature, a high working voltage rating and a long service life and are used in high frequency circuits with fixed values of capacitance up to about 1000 pF.

3. **Paper capacitors.** A typical paper capacitor is shown in Fig. 6.16 where the length of the roll corresponds to the capacitance required.

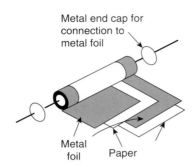

Figure 6.16

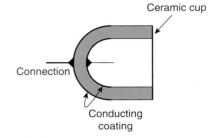

Figure 6.18

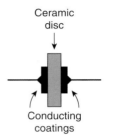

Figure 6.19

The whole is usually impregnated with oil or wax to exclude moisture, and then placed in a plastic or aluminium container for protection. Paper capacitors are made in various working voltages up to about 150 kV and are used where loss is not very important. The maximum value of this type of capacitor is between 500 pF and 10 μF. Disadvantages of paper capacitors include variation in capacitance with temperature change and a shorter service life than most other types of capacitor.

4. **Ceramic capacitors**. These are made in various forms, each type of construction depending on the value of capacitance required. For high values, a tube of ceramic material is used as shown in the cross-section of Fig. 6.17. For smaller values the cup construction is used as shown in Fig. 6.18, and for still smaller values the disc construction shown in Fig. 6.19 is used. Certain ceramic materials have a very high permittivity and this enables capacitors of high capacitance to be made which are of small physical size with a high working voltage rating. Ceramic capacitors are available in the range 1 pF to 0.1 μF and may be used in high frequency electronic circuits subject to a wide range of temperatures.

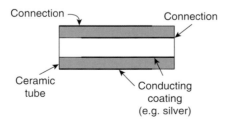

Figure 6.17

5. **Plastic capacitors**. Some plastic materials such as polystyrene and Teflon can be used as dielectrics. Construction is similar to the paper capacitor but using a plastic film instead of paper. Plastic capacitors operate well under conditions of high

temperature, provide a precise value of capacitance, a very long service life and high reliability.

6. **Titanium oxide capacitors** have a very high capacitance with a small physical size when used at a low temperature.

7. **Electrolytic capacitors**. Construction is similar to the paper capacitor with aluminium foil used for the plates and with a thick absorbent material, such as paper, impregnated with an electrolyte (ammonium borate), separating the plates. The finished capacitor is usually assembled in an aluminium container and hermetically sealed. Its operation depends on the formation of a thin aluminium oxide layer on the positive plate by electrolytic action when a suitable direct potential is maintained between the plates. This oxide layer is very thin and forms the dielectric. (The absorbent paper between the plates is a conductor and does not act as a dielectric.) Such capacitors **must always be used on d.c.** and must be connected with the correct polarity; if this is not done the capacitor will be destroyed since the oxide layer will be destroyed. Electrolytic capacitors are manufactured with working voltage from 6 V to 600 V, although accuracy is generally not very high. These capacitors possess a much larger capacitance than other types of capacitors of similar dimensions due to the oxide film being only a few microns thick. The fact that they can be used only on d.c. supplies limit their usefulness.

6.13   Discharging capacitors

When a capacitor has been disconnected from the supply it may still be charged and it may retain this charge for some considerable time. Thus precautions must be taken to ensure that the capacitor is automatically discharged after the supply is switched off. This is done by connecting a high value resistor across the capacitor terminals.

Now try the following exercises

Exercise 31   **Short answer questions on capacitors and capacitance**

1. What is a capacitor?

2. State five practical applications of capacitors

3. Explain the term 'electrostatics'

4. Complete the statements:
    Like charges ...... ; unlike charges ......

5. How can an 'electric field' be established between two parallel metal plates?

6. What is capacitance?

7. State the unit of capacitance

8. Complete the statement:
    $$\text{Capacitance} = \frac{......}{......}$$

9. Complete the statements:
    (a) $1\,\mu\text{F} = ...\text{F}$ (b) $1\,\text{pF} = ...\text{F}$

10. Complete the statement:
    $$\text{Electric field strength } E = \frac{......}{......}$$

11. Complete the statement:
    $$\text{Electric flux density } D = \frac{......}{......}$$

12. Draw the electrical circuit diagram symbol for a capacitor

13. Name two practical examples where capacitance is present, although undesirable

14. The insulating material separating the plates of a capacitor is called the ......

15. 10 volts applied to a capacitor results in a charge of 5 coulombs. What is the capacitance of the capacitor?

16. Three $3\,\mu\text{F}$ capacitors are connected in parallel. The equivalent capacitance is. ...

17. Three $3\,\mu\text{F}$ capacitors are connected in series. The equivalent capacitance is. ...

18. State a disadvantage of series-connected capacitors

19. Name three factors upon which capacitance depends

20. What does 'relative permittivity' mean?

21. Define 'permittivity of free space'

22. What is meant by the 'dielectric strength' of a material?

23. State the formula used to determine the energy stored by a capacitor

24. Name five types of capacitor commonly used

25. Sketch a typical rolled paper capacitor

26. Explain briefly the construction of a variable air capacitor

27. State three advantages and one disadvantage of mica capacitors

28. Name two disadvantages of paper capacitors

29. Between what values of capacitance are ceramic capacitors normally available

30. What main advantages do plastic capacitors possess?

31. Explain briefly the construction of an electrolytic capacitor

32. What is the main disadvantage of electrolytic capacitors?

33. Name an important advantage of electrolytic capacitors

34. What safety precautions should be taken when a capacitor is disconnected from a supply?

Exercise 32   Multi-choice questions on capacitors and capacitance

(Answers on page 420)

1. Electrostatics is a branch of electricity concerned with
    (a) energy flowing across a gap between conductors
    (b) charges at rest
    (c) charges in motion
    (d) energy in the form of charges

2. The capacitance of a capacitor is the ratio
    (a) charge to p.d. between plates
    (b) p.d. between plates to plate spacing
    (c) p.d. between plates to thickness of dielectric
    (d) p.d. between plates to charge

3. The p.d. across a $10\,\mu F$ capacitor to charge it with $10\,mC$ is
    (a) $10\,V$ (b) $1\,kV$
    (c) $1\,V$ (d) $10\,V$

4. The charge on a $10\,pF$ capacitor when the voltage applied to it is $10\,kV$ is
    (a) $100\,\mu C$ (b) $0.1\,C$
    (c) $0.1\,\mu C$ (d) $0.01\,\mu C$

5. Four $2\,\mu F$ capacitors are connected in parallel. The equivalent capacitance is
    (a) $8\,\mu F$ (b) $0.5\,\mu F$
    (c) $2\,\mu F$ (d) $6\,\mu F$

6. Four $2\,\mu F$ capacitors are connected in series. The equivalent capacitance is
    (a) $8\,\mu F$ (b) $0.5\,\mu F$
    (c) $2\,\mu F$ (d) $6\,\mu F$

7. State which of the following is false.
    The capacitance of a capacitor
    (a) is proportional to the cross-sectional area of the plates

    (b) is proportional to the distance between the plates
    (c) depends on the number of plates
    (d) is proportional to the relative permittivity of the dielectric

8. Which of the following statement is false?
    (a) An air capacitor is normally a variable type
    (b) A paper capacitor generally has a shorter service life than most other types of capacitor
    (c) An electrolytic capacitor must be used only on a.c. supplies
    (d) Plastic capacitors generally operate satisfactorily under conditions of high temperature

9. The energy stored in a $10\,\mu F$ capacitor when charged to $500\,V$ is
    (a) $1.25\,mJ$ (b) $0.025\,\mu J$
    (c) $1.25\,J$ (d) $1.25\,C$

10. The capacitance of a variable air capacitor is at maximum when
    (a) the movable plates half overlap the fixed plates
    (b) the movable plates are most widely separated from the fixed plates
    (c) both sets of plates are exactly meshed
    (d) the movable plates are closer to one side of the fixed plate than to the other

11. When a voltage of $1\,kV$ is applied to a capacitor, the charge on the capacitor is $500\,nC$. The capacitance of the capacitor is:
    (a) $2 \times 10^9\,F$ (b) $0.5\,pF$
    (c) $0.5\,mF$ (d) $0.5\,nF$

Chapter 7

Magnetic circuits

At the end of this chapter you should be able to:

- appreciate some applications of magnets
- describe the magnetic field around a permanent magnet
- state the laws of magnetic attraction and repulsion for two magnets in close proximity
- define magnetic flux, Φ, and magnetic flux density, B, and state their units
- perform simple calculations involving $B = \Phi/A$
- define magnetomotive force, F_m, and magnetic field strength, H, and state their units
- perform simple calculations involving $F_m = NI$ and $H = NI/l$
- define permeability, distinguishing between μ_0, μ_r and μ
- understand the B–H curves for different magnetic materials
- appreciate typical values of μ_r
- perform calculations involving $B = \mu_0 \mu_r H$
- define reluctance, S, and state its units
- perform calculations involving

$$S = \frac{\text{m.m.f.}}{\Phi} = \frac{l}{\mu_0 \mu_r A}$$

- perform calculations on composite series magnetic circuits
- compare electrical and magnetic quantities
- appreciate how a hysteresis loop is obtained and that hysteresis loss is proportional to its area

7.1 Introduction to magnetism and magnetic circuits

The study of magnetism began in the thirteenth century with many eminent scientists and physicists such as William Gilbert, Hans Christian Oersted, Michael Faraday, James Maxwell, André Ampère and Wilhelm Weber all having some input on the subject since. The association between electricity and magnetism is a fairly recent finding in comparison with the very first understanding of basic magnetism.

Today, magnets have **many varied practical applications**. For example, they are used in motors and generators, telephones, relays, loudspeakers, computer hard drives and floppy disks, anti-lock brakes, cameras, fishing reels, electronic ignition systems, keyboards, t.v. and radio components and in transmission equipment.

DOI: 10.1016/B978-0-08-089056-2.00007-3

The full theory of magnetism is one of the most complex of subjects; this chapter provides an introduction to the topic.

7.2 Magnetic fields

A **permanent magnet** is a piece of ferromagnetic material (such as iron, nickel or cobalt) which has properties of attracting other pieces of these materials. A permanent magnet will position itself in a north and south direction when freely suspended. The north-seeking end of the magnet is called the **north pole, N**, and the south-seeking end the **south pole, S**.

The area around a magnet is called the **magnetic field** and it is in this area that the effects of the **magnetic force** produced by the magnet can be detected. A magnetic field cannot be seen, felt, smelt or heard and therefore is difficult to represent. Michael Faraday suggested that the magnetic field could be represented pictorially, by imagining the field to consist of **lines of magnetic flux**, which enables investigation of the distribution and density of the field to be carried out.

The distribution of a magnetic field can be investigated by using some iron filings. A bar magnet is placed on a flat surface covered by, say, cardboard, upon which is sprinkled some iron filings. If the cardboard is gently tapped the filings will assume a pattern similar to that shown in Fig. 7.1. If a number of magnets of different strength are used, it is found that the stronger the field the closer are the lines of magnetic flux and vice versa. Thus a magnetic field has the property of exerting a force, demonstrated in this case by causing the iron filings to move into the pattern shown. The strength of the magnetic field decreases as we move away from the magnet. It should be realised, of course, that the magnetic field is three dimensional in its effect, and not acting in one plane as appears to be the case in this experiment.

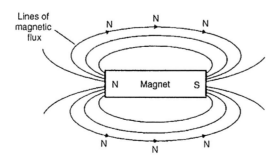

Figure 7.1

If a compass is placed in the magnetic field in various positions, the direction of the lines of flux may be determined by noting the direction of the compass pointer. The direction of a magnetic field at any point is taken as that in which the north-seeking pole of a compass needle points when suspended in the field. The direction of a line of flux is from the north pole to the south pole on the outside of the magnet and is then assumed to continue through the magnet back to the point at which it emerged at the north pole. Thus such lines of flux always form complete closed loops or paths, they never intersect and always have a definite direction.

The laws of magnetic attraction and repulsion can be demonstrated by using two bar magnets. In Fig. 7.2(a), **with unlike poles adjacent, attraction takes place**. Lines of flux are imagined to contract and the magnets try to pull together. The magnetic field is strongest in between the two magnets, shown by the lines of flux being close together. In Fig. 7.2(b), **with similar poles adjacent (i.e. two north poles), repulsion occurs**, i.e. the two north poles try to push each other apart, since magnetic flux lines running side by side in the same direction repel.

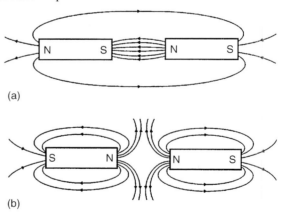

(a)

(b)

Figure 7.2

7.3 Magnetic flux and flux density

Magnetic flux is the amount of magnetic field (or the number of lines of force) produced by a magnetic source. The symbol for magnetic flux is Φ (Greek letter 'phi'). The unit of magnetic flux is the **weber, Wb**.

Magnetic flux density is the amount of flux passing through a defined area that is perpendicular to the direction of the flux:

$$\text{Magnetic flux density} = \frac{\text{magnetic flux}}{\text{area}}$$

The symbol for magnetic flux density is B. The unit of magnetic flux density is the tesla, T, where $1\,T = 1\,Wb/m^2$. Hence

$$B = \frac{\Phi}{A} \text{ tesla}$$

where $A(m^2)$ is the area

Problem 1. A magnetic pole face has a rectangular section having dimensions 200 mm by 100 mm. If the total flux emerging from the pole is 150 μWb, calculate the flux density.

Flux $\Phi = 150\,\mu Wb = 150 \times 10^{-6}\,Wb$
Cross-sectional area $A = 200 \times 100 = 20\,000\,mm^2$
$$= 20\,000 \times 10^{-6}\,m^2.$$

$$\text{Flux density, } B = \frac{\Phi}{A} = \frac{150 \times 10^{-6}}{20\,000 \times 10^{-6}}$$

$$= \textbf{0.0075\,T or 7.5\,mT}$$

Problem 2. The maximum working flux density of a lifting electromagnet is 1.8 T and the effective area of a pole face is circular in cross-section. If the total magnetic flux produced is 353 mWb, determine the radius of the pole face.

Flux density $B = 1.8\,T$ and
flux $\Phi = 353\,mWb = 353 \times 10^{-3}\,Wb$.
Since $B = \Phi/A$, cross-sectional area $A = \Phi/B$

i.e. $A = \dfrac{353 \times 10^{-3}}{1.8}\,m^2 = 0.1961\,m^2$

The pole face is circular, hence area $= \pi r^2$, where r is the radius. Hence $\pi r^2 = 0.1961$ from which, $r^2 = 0.1961/\pi$ and radius $r = \sqrt{(0.1961/\pi)} = 0.250\,m$ i.e. **the radius of the pole face is 250 mm**.

7.4 Magnetomotive force and magnetic field strength

Magnetomotive force (m.m.f.) is the cause of the existence of a magnetic flux in a magnetic circuit,

$$\text{m.m.f. } F_m = NI \text{ amperes}$$

where N is the number of conductors (or turns) and I is the current in amperes. The unit of m.m.f is sometimes expressed as 'ampere-turns'. However since 'turns' have no dimensions, the S.I. unit of m.m.f. is the ampere.

Magnetic field strength (or **magnetising force**),

$$H = \frac{NI}{l} \text{ ampere per metre}$$

where l is the mean length of the flux path in metres. Thus

$$\text{m.m.f. } = NI = Hl \text{ amperes}$$

Problem 3. A magnetising force of 8000 A/m is applied to a circular magnetic circuit of mean diameter 30 cm by passing a current through a coil wound on the circuit. If the coil is uniformly wound around the circuit and has 750 turns, find the current in the coil.

$H = 8000\,A/m$, $l = \pi d = \pi \times 30 \times 10^{-2}\,m$ and $N = 750$ turns. Since $H = NI/l$, then

$$I = \frac{Hl}{N} = \frac{8000 \times \pi \times 30 \times 10^{-2}}{750}$$

Thus, **current $I = 10.05\,A$**

Now try the following exercise

---

1. What is the flux density in a magnetic field of cross-sectional area $20\,cm^2$ having a flux of 3 mWb?   [1.5 T]

2. Determine the total flux emerging from a magnetic pole face having dimensions 5 cm by 6 cm, if the flux density is 0.9 T
    [2.7 mWb]

3. The maximum working flux density of a lifting electromagnet is 1.9 T and the effective area of a pole face is circular in cross-section. If the total magnetic flux produced is 611 mWb determine the radius of the pole face.
    [32 cm]

4. A current of 5 A is passed through a 1000-turn coil wound on a circular magnetic circuit of radius 120 mm. Calculate (a) the magnetomotive force, and (b) the magnetic field strength.
    [(a) 5000 A (b) 6631 A/m]

5. An electromagnet of square cross-section produces a flux density of 0.45 T. If the magnetic

flux is $720\,\mu\text{Wb}$ find the dimensions of the electromagnet cross-section.

[4 cm by 4 cm]

6. Find the magnetic field strength applied to a magnetic circuit of mean length 50 cm when a coil of 400 turns is applied to it carrying a current of 1.2 A [960 A/m]

7. A solenoid 20 cm long is wound with 500 turns of wire. Find the current required to establish a magnetising force of 2500 A/m inside the solenoid. [1 A]

8. A magnetic field strength of 5000 A/m is applied to a circular magnetic circuit of mean diameter 250 mm. If the coil has 500 turns find the current in the coil. [7.85 A]

7.5 Permeability and B–H curves

For air, or any non-magnetic medium, the ratio of magnetic flux density to magnetising force is a constant, i.e. $B/H =$ a constant. This constant is μ_0, the **permeability of free space** (or the magnetic space constant) and is equal to $4\pi \times 10^{-7}$ H/m, i.e. **for air, or any non-magnetic medium**, the ratio

$$\frac{B}{H} = \mu_0$$

(Although all non-magnetic materials, including air, exhibit slight magnetic properties, these can effectively be neglected.)
For all media other than free space,

$$\frac{B}{H} = \mu_0 \mu_r$$

where μ_r is the relative permeability, and is defined as

$$\mu_r = \frac{\textbf{flux density in material}}{\textbf{flux density in a vacuum}}$$

μ_r varies with the type of magnetic material and, since it is a ratio of flux densities, it has no unit. From its definition, μ_r for a vacuum is 1.
$\boldsymbol{\mu_0 \mu_r = \mu}$, called the **absolute permeability**
By plotting measured values of flux density B against magnetic field strength H, a **magnetisation curve** (or **B–H curve**) is produced. For non-magnetic materials this is a straight line. Typical curves for four magnetic materials are shown in Fig. 7.3

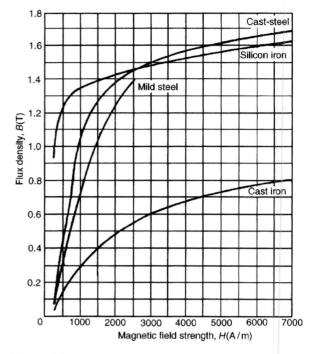

Figure 7.3

The **relative permeability** of a ferromagnetic material is proportional to the slope of the B–H curve and thus varies with the magnetic field strength. The approximate range of values of relative permeability μ_r for some common magnetic materials are:

Cast iron $\mu_r = 100\text{–}250$
Mild steel $\mu_r = 200\text{–}800$
Silicon iron $\mu_r = 1000\text{–}5000$
Cast steel $\mu_r = 300\text{–}900$
Mumetal $\mu_r = 200\text{–}5000$
Stalloy $\mu_r = 500\text{–}6000$

Problem 4. A flux density of 1.2 T is produced in a piece of cast steel by a magnetising force of 1250 A/m. Find the relative permeability of the steel under these conditions.

For a magnetic material: $B = \mu_0 \mu_r H$

i.e. $\mu_r = \dfrac{B}{\mu_0 H} = \dfrac{1.2}{(4\pi \times 10^{-7})(1250)} = \textbf{764}$

Problem 5. Determine the magnetic field strength and the m.m.f. required to produce a flux density of 0.25 T in an air gap of length 12 mm.

For air: $B = \mu_0 H$ (since $\mu_r = 1$)

Magnetic field strength,

$$H = \frac{B}{\mu_0} = \frac{0.25}{4\pi \times 10^{-7}} = \mathbf{198\,940\,A/m}$$

m.m.f. $= Hl = 198\,940 \times 12 \times 10^{-3} = \mathbf{2387\,A}$

Problem 6. A coil of 300 turns is wound uniformly on a ring of non-magnetic material. The ring has a mean circumference of 40 cm and a uniform cross-sectional area of 4 cm². If the current in the coil is 5 A, calculate (a) the magnetic field strength, (b) the flux density and (c) the total magnetic flux in the ring.

(a) Magnetic field strength

$$H = \frac{NI}{l} = \frac{300 \times 5}{40 \times 10^{-2}}$$

$$= \mathbf{3750\,A/m}$$

(b) For a non-magnetic material $\mu_r = 1$, thus flux density $B = \mu_0 H$

i.e $B = 4\pi \times 10^{-7} \times 3750$

$$= \mathbf{4.712\,mT}$$

(c) Flux $\Phi = BA = (4.712 \times 10^{-3})(4 \times 10^{-4})$

$$= \mathbf{1.885\,\mu Wb}$$

Problem 7. An iron ring of mean diameter 10 cm is uniformly wound with 2000 turns of wire. When a current of 0.25 A is passed through the coil a flux density of 0.4 T is set up in the iron. Find (a) the magnetising force and (b) the relative permeability of the iron under these conditions.

$l = \pi d = \pi \times 10\,\text{cm} = \pi \times 10 \times 10^{-2}\,\text{m}$,
$N = 2000$ turns, $I = 0.25\,\text{A}$ and $B = 0.4\,\text{T}$

(a) $H = \dfrac{NI}{l} = \dfrac{2000 \times 0.25}{\pi \times 10 \times 10^{-2}}$

$$= \mathbf{1592\,A/m}$$

(b) $B = \mu_0 \mu_r H$, hence

$$\mu_r = \frac{B}{\mu_0 H} = \frac{0.4}{(4\pi \times 10^{-7})(1592)} = \mathbf{200}$$

Problem 8. A uniform ring of cast iron has a cross-sectional area of 10 cm² and a mean circumference of 20 cm. Determine the m.m.f. necessary to produce a flux of 0.3 mWb in the ring. The magnetisation curve for cast iron is shown on page 80.

$A = 10\,\text{cm}^2 = 10 \times 10^{-4}\,\text{m}^2$,　$l = 20\,\text{cm} = 0.2\,\text{m}$　and
$\Phi = 0.3 \times 10^{-3}\,\text{Wb}$.

Flux density $B = \dfrac{\Phi}{A} = \dfrac{0.3 \times 10^{-3}}{10 \times 10^{-4}} = 0.3\,\text{T}$

From the magnetisation curve for cast iron on page 80, when $B = 0.3\,\text{T}$, $H = 1000\,\text{A/m}$, hence
m.m.f. $= Hl = 1000 \times 0.2 = \mathbf{200\,A}$
A tabular method could have been used in this problem. Such a solution is shown below in Table 7.1.

Problem 9. From the magnetisation curve for cast iron, shown on page 80, derive the curve of μ_r against H.

$B = \mu_0 \mu_r H$, hence

$$\mu_r = \frac{B}{\mu_0 H} = \frac{1}{\mu_0} \times \frac{B}{H}$$

$$= \frac{10^7}{4\pi} \times \frac{B}{H}$$

A number of co-ordinates are selected from the B–H curve and μ_r is calculated for each as shown in Table 7.2. μ_r is plotted against H as shown in Fig. 7.4. The curve demonstrates the change that occurs in the relative permeability as the magnetising force increases.

Table 7.1

Part of circuit	Material	Φ(Wb)	$A(m^2)$	$B = \dfrac{\Phi}{A}$(T)	H from graph	$l(m)$	m.m.f. = Hl(A)
Ring	Cast iron	0.3×10^{-3}	10×10^{-4}	0.3	1000	0.2	200

Table 7.2

$B(T)$	0.04	0.13	0.17	0.30	0.41	0.49	0.60	0.68	0.73	0.76	0.79
$H(A/m)$	200	400	500	1000	1500	2000	3000	4000	5000	6000	7000
$\mu_r = \dfrac{10^7}{4\pi} \times \dfrac{B}{H}$	159	259	271	239	218	195	159	135	116	101	90

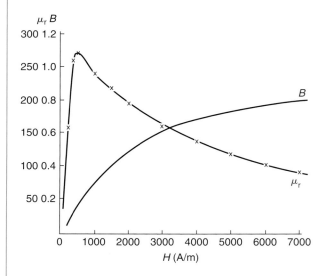

Figure 7.4

Now try the following exercise

Exercise 34   **Further problems on magnetic circuits**

(Where appropriate, assume $\mu_0 = 4\pi \times 10^{-7}$ H/m)

1. Find the magnetic field strength and the magnetomotive force needed to produce a flux density of 0.33 T in an air gap of length 15 mm.
   [(a) 262 600 A/m (b) 3939 A]

2. An air gap between two pole pieces is 20 mm in length and the area of the flux path across the gap is 5 cm². If the flux required in the air gap is 0.75 mWb find the m.m.f. necessary.
   [23 870 A]

3. (a) Determine the flux density produced in an air-cored solenoid due to a uniform magnetic field strength of 8000 A/m. (b) Iron having a relative permeability of 150 at 8000 A/m is inserted into the solenoid of part (a). Find the flux density now in the solenoid.
   [(a) 10.05 mT (b) 1.508 T]

4. Find the relative permeability of a material if the absolute permeability is 4.084×10^{-4} H/m. [325]

5. Find the relative permeability of a piece of silicon iron if a flux density of 1.3 T is produced by a magnetic field strength of 700 A/m.
   [1478]

6. A steel ring of mean diameter 120 mm is uniformly wound with 1500 turns of wire. When a current of 0.30 A is passed through the coil a flux density of 1.5 T is set up in the steel. Find the relative permeability of the steel under these conditions. [1000]

7. A uniform ring of cast steel has a cross-sectional area of 5 cm² and a mean circumference of 15 cm. Find the current required in a coil of 1200 turns wound on the ring to produce a flux of 0.8 mWb. (Use the magnetisation curve for cast steel shown on page 80.)
   [0.60 A]

8. (a) A uniform mild steel ring has a diameter of 50 mm and a cross-sectional area of 1 cm². Determine the m.m.f. necessary to produce a flux of 50 μWb in the ring. (Use the B–H curve for mild steel shown on page 80.) (b) If a coil of 440 turns is wound uniformly around the ring in Part (a) what current would be required to produce the flux? [(a) 110 A (b) 0.25 A]

9. From the magnetisation curve for mild steel shown on page 80, derive the curve of relative permeability against magnetic field strength. From your graph determine (a) the value of μ_r when the magnetic field strength is 1200 A/m, and (b) the value of the magnetic field strength when μ_r is 500. [(a) 590–600 (b) 2000]

7.6 Reluctance

Reluctance S (or R_M) is the 'magnetic resistance' of a magnetic circuit to the presence of magnetic flux.
Reluctance,

$$S = \frac{F_M}{\Phi} = \frac{NI}{\Phi} = \frac{Hl}{BA} = \frac{l}{(B/H)A} = \frac{l}{\mu_0\mu_r A}$$

The unit of reluctance is $1/H$ (or H^{-1}) or A/Wb.
Ferromagnetic materials have a low reluctance and can be used as **magnetic screens** to prevent magnetic fields affecting materials within the screen.

Problem 10.   Determine the reluctance of a piece of mumetal of length 150 mm and cross-sectional area 1800 mm^2 when the relative permeability is 4000. Find also the absolute permeability of the mumetal.

Reluctance,

$$\begin{aligned} S &= \frac{l}{\mu_0\mu_r A} \\ &= \frac{150 \times 10^{-3}}{(4\pi \times 10^{-7})(4000)(1800 \times 10^{-6})} \\ &= \mathbf{16\,580/H} \end{aligned}$$

Absolute permeability,

$$\begin{aligned} \boldsymbol{\mu} &= \mu_0\mu_r = (4\pi \times 10^{-7})(4000) \\ &= \mathbf{5.027 \times 10^{-3}\,H/m} \end{aligned}$$

Problem 11.   A mild steel ring has a radius of 50 mm and a cross-sectional area of 400 mm^2. A current of 0.5 A flows in a coil wound uniformly around the ring and the flux produced is 0.1 mWb. If the relative permeability at this value of current is 200 find (a) the reluctance of the mild steel and (b) the number of turns on the coil.

$l = 2\pi r = 2 \times \pi \times 50 \times 10^{-3}$ m, $A = 400 \times 10^{-6}$ m^2,
$I = 0.5$ A, $\Phi = 0.1 \times 10^{-3}$ Wb and $\mu_r = 200$

(a) **Reluctance,**

$$\begin{aligned} S &= \frac{l}{\mu_0\mu_r A} \\ &= \frac{2 \times \pi \times 50 \times 10^{-3}}{(4\pi \times 10^{-7})(200)(400 \times 10^{-6})} \\ &= \mathbf{3.125 \times 10^6/H} \end{aligned}$$

(b) $S = \dfrac{\text{m.m.f.}}{\Phi}$ from which

m.m.f. $= S\Phi$ i.e. $NI = S\Phi$

Hence, number of terms

$$\begin{aligned} N &= \frac{S\Phi}{I} = \frac{3.125 \times 10^6 \times 0.1 \times 10^{-3}}{0.5} \\ &= \mathbf{625\,turns} \end{aligned}$$

Now try the following exercise

Exercise 35   Further problems on magnetic circuits

(Where appropriate, assume $\mu_0 = 4\pi \times 10^{-7}$ H/m)

1. Part of a magnetic circuit is made from steel of length 120 mm, cross-sectional area 15 cm^2 and relative permeability 800. Calculate (a) the reluctance and (b) the absolute permeability of the steel.

    [(a) 79 580 /H (b) 1 mH/m]

2. A mild steel closed magnetic circuit has a mean length of 75 mm and a cross-sectional area of 320.2 mm^2. A current of 0.40 A flows in a coil wound uniformly around the circuit and the flux produced is 200 μWb. If the relative permeability of the steel at this value of current is 400 find (a) the reluctance of the material and (b) the number of turns of the coil.

    [(a) 466 000 /H (b) 233]

7.7 Composite series magnetic circuits

For a series magnetic circuit having n parts, the **total reluctance S** is given by: $S = S_1 + S_2 + \cdots + S_n$ (This is similar to resistors connected in series in an electrical circuit).

Problem 12.   A closed magnetic circuit of cast steel contains a 6 cm long path of cross-sectional area 1 cm^2 and a 2 cm path of cross-sectional area 0.5 cm^2. A coil of 200 turns is wound around the 6 cm length of the circuit and a current of 0.4 A flows. Determine the flux density in the 2 cm path, if the relative permeability of the cast steel is 750.

For the 6 cm long path:

$$\text{Reluctance } S_1 = \frac{l_1}{\mu_0 \mu_r A_1}$$

$$= \frac{6 \times 10^{-2}}{(4\pi \times 10^{-7})(750)(1 \times 10^{-4})}$$

$$= 6.366 \times 10^5/\text{H}$$

For the 2 cm long path:

$$\text{Reluctance } S_2 = \frac{l_2}{\mu_0 \mu_r A_2}$$

$$= \frac{2 \times 10^{-2}}{(4\pi \times 10^{-7})(750)(0.5 \times 10^{-4})}$$

$$= 4.244 \times 10^5/\text{H}$$

Total circuit reluctance $S = S_1 + S_2$

$$= (6.366 + 4.244) \times 10^5$$

$$= 10.61 \times 10^5/\text{H}$$

$$S = \frac{\text{m.m.f.}}{\Phi} \text{ i.e. } \Phi = \frac{\text{m.m.f.}}{S} = \frac{NI}{S}$$

$$= \frac{200 \times 0.4}{10.61 \times 10^5} = 7.54 \times 10^{-5} \text{Wb}$$

Flux density in the 2 cm path,

$$B = \frac{\Phi}{A} = \frac{7.54 \times 10^{-5}}{0.5 \times 10^{-4}} = \textbf{1.51 T}$$

Problem 13. A silicon iron ring of cross-sectional area 5 cm^2 has a radial air gap of 2 mm cut into it. If the mean length of the silicon iron path is 40 cm calculate the magnetomotive force to produce a flux of 0.7 mWb. The magnetisation curve for silicon is shown on page 80.

There are two parts to the circuit – the silicon iron and the air gap. The total m.m.f. will be the sum of the m.m.f.'s of each part.

For the silicon iron:

$$B = \frac{\Phi}{A} = \frac{0.7 \times 10^{-3}}{5 \times 10^{-4}} = 1.4 \text{ T}$$

From the B–H curve for silicon iron on page 80, when $B = 1.4$ T, $H = 1650$ A/m. Hence the m.m.f. for the iron path $= Hl = 1650 \times 0.4 = 660$ A

For the air gap:

The flux density will be the same in the air gap as in the iron, i.e. 1.4 T (This assumes no leakage or fringing occurring). For air,

$$H = \frac{B}{\mu_0} = \frac{1.4}{4\pi \times 10^{-7}} = 1\,114\,000 \text{ A/m}$$

Hence the m.m.f. for the air gap
$= Hl = 1\,114\,000 \times 2 \times 10^{-3} = 2228$ A.
Total m.m.f. to produce a flux of 0.6 mWb
$= 660 + 2228 = \textbf{2888 A}$.

A tabular method could have been used as shown in Table 7.3 at top of next page.

Problem 14. Figure 7.5 shows a ring formed with two different materials – cast steel and mild steel.

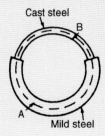

Cast steel

B

A

Mild steel

Figure 7.5

The dimensions are:

	mean length	cross-sectional area
Mild steel	400 mm	500 mm²
Cast steel	300 mm	312.5 mm²

Find the total m.m.f. required to cause a flux of $500\,\mu\text{Wb}$ in the magnetic circuit. Determine also the total circuit reluctance.

A tabular solution is shown in Table 7.4 on page 85.

$$\left.\begin{array}{r}\textbf{Total circuit}\\\textbf{reluctance}\end{array}\right\} S = \frac{\text{m.m.f.}}{\Phi}$$

$$= \frac{2000}{500 \times 10^{-6}} = \textbf{4} \times \textbf{10}^6/\textbf{H}$$

Problem 15. A section through a magnetic circuit of uniform cross-sectional area 2 cm^2 is

Table 7.3

Part of circuit	Material	Φ(Wb)	$A(m^2)$	$B(T)$	$H(A/m)$	$l(m)$	m.m.f. $=Hl(A)$
Ring	Silicon iron	0.7×10^{-3}	5×10^{-4}	1.4	1650 (from graph)	0.4	660
Air gap	Air	0.7×10^{-3}	5×10^{-4}	1.4	$\dfrac{1.4}{4\pi \times 10^{-7}}$ $= 1\,114\,000$	2×10^{-3}	2228
						Total:	**2888 A**

Table 7.4

Part of circuit	Material	Φ(Wb)	$A(m^2)$	$B(T)$ $(=\Phi/A)$	$H(A/m)$ (from graphs page 80)	$l(m)$	m.m.f. $=Hl(A)$
A	Mild steel	500×10^{-6}	500×10^{-6}	1.0	1400	400×10^{-3}	560
B	Cast steel	500×10^{-6}	312.5×10^{-6}	1.6	4800	300×10^{-3}	1440
						Total:	**2000 A**

shown in Fig. 7.6. The cast steel core has a mean length of 25 cm. The air gap is 1 mm wide and the coil has 5000 turns. The B–H curve for cast steel is shown on page 80. Determine the current in the coil to produce a flux density of 0.80 T in the air gap, assuming that all the flux passes through both parts of the magnetic circuit.

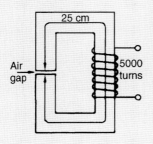

Figure 7.6

For the cast steel core, when $B = 0.80\,T$, $H = 750\,A/m$ (from page 80).

Reluctance of core $S_1 = \dfrac{l_1}{\mu_0 \mu_r A_1}$ and

since $B = \mu_0 \mu_r H$, then $\mu_r = \dfrac{B}{\mu_0 H}$

$$S_1 = \frac{l_1}{\mu_0 \left(\dfrac{B}{\mu_0 H} \right) A_1} = \frac{l_1 H}{B A_1}$$

$$= \frac{(25 \times 10^{-2})(750)}{(0.8)(2 \times 10^{-4})} = 1\,172\,000/H$$

For the air gap:

Reluctance, $S_2 = \dfrac{l_2}{\mu_0 \mu_r A_2}$

$\qquad\qquad = \dfrac{l_2}{\mu_0 A_2}$ (since $\mu_r = 1$ for air)

$\qquad\qquad = \dfrac{1 \times 10^{-3}}{(4\pi \times 10^{-7})(2 \times 10^{-4})}$

$\qquad\qquad = 3\,979\,000/H$

Total circuit reluctance

$$S = S_1 + S_2 = 1\,172\,000 + 3\,979\,000$$

$$= 5\,151\,000/H$$

Flux $\Phi = BA = 0.80 \times 2 \times 10^{-4} = 1.6 \times 10^{-4}\,Wb$

$$S = \frac{m.m.f.}{\Phi}$$

thus

$$m.m.f. = S\Phi \text{ hence } NI = S\Phi$$

and

$$\text{current } I = \frac{S\Phi}{N} = \frac{(5\,151\,000)(1.6 \times 10^{-4})}{5000}$$

$$= 0.165\,A$$

Now try the following exercise

Exercise 36   Further problems on composite series magnetic circuits

1.   A magnetic circuit of cross-sectional area $0.4\,cm^2$ consists of one part 3 cm long, of material having relative permeability 1200, and a second part 2 cm long of material having relative permeability 750. With a 100 turn coil carrying 2 A, find the value of flux existing in the circuit.   [0.195 mWb]

2.   (a) A cast steel ring has a cross-sectional area of $600\,mm^2$ and a radius of 25 mm. Determine the m.m.f. necessary to establish a flux of 0.8 mWb in the ring. Use the B–H curve for cast steel shown on page 80. (b) If a radial air gap 1.5 mm wide is cut in the ring of part (a) find the m.m.f. now necessary to maintain the same flux in the ring.
        [(a) 270 A (b)1860 A]

3.   A closed magnetic circuit made of silicon iron consists of a 40 mm long path of cross-sectional area $90\,mm^2$ and a 15 mm long path of cross-sectional area $70\,mm^2$. A coil of 50 turns is wound around the 40 mm length of the circuit and a current of 0.39 A flows. Find the flux density in the 15 mm length path if the relative permeability of the silicon iron at this value of magnetising force is 3000.
        [1.59 T]

4.   For the magnetic circuit shown in Fig. 7.7 find the current I in the coil needed to produce a flux of 0.45 mWb in the air gap. The silicon iron magnetic circuit has a uniform cross-sectional area of $3\,cm^2$ and its magnetisation curve is as shown on page 80.   [0.83 A]

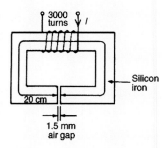

Figure 7.7

5.   A ring forming a magnetic circuit is made from two materials; one part is mild steel of mean length 25 cm and cross-sectional area $4\,cm^2$, and the remainder is cast iron of mean length 20 cm and cross-sectional area $7.5\,cm^2$. Use a tabular approach to determine the total m.m.f. required to cause a flux of 0.30 mWb in the magnetic circuit. Find also the total reluctance of the circuit. Use the magnetisation curves shown on page 80.
        [550 A, 1.83×10^6/H]

6.   Figure 7.8 shows the magnetic circuit of a relay. When each of the air gaps are 1.5 mm wide find the m.m.f. required to produce a flux density of 0.75 T in the air gaps. Use the B–H curves shown on page 80.   [2970 A]

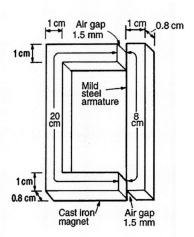

Figure 7.8

7.8 Comparison between electrical and magnetic quantities

Electrical circuit	Magnetic circuit
e.m.f. E (V)	m.m.f. F_m (A)
current I (A)	flux Φ (Wb)
resistance R (Ω)	reluctance S (H^{-1})
$I = \dfrac{E}{R}$	$\Phi = \dfrac{\text{m.m.f.}}{S}$
$R = \dfrac{\rho l}{A}$	$S = \dfrac{l}{\mu_0 \mu_r A}$

7.9 Hysteresis and hysteresis loss

Hysteresis loop

Let a ferromagnetic material which is completely demagnetised, i.e. one in which $B = H = 0$ be subjected to increasing values of magnetic field strength H and the corresponding flux density B measured. The resulting relationship between B and H is shown by the curve Oab in Fig. 7.9. At a particular value of H, shown as Oy, it becomes difficult to increase the flux density any further. The material is said to be saturated. Thus **by** is the **saturation flux density**.

If the value of H is now reduced it is found that the flux density follows curve **bc**. When H is reduced to zero, flux remains in the iron. This **remanent flux density** or **remanence** is shown as **Oc** in Fig. 7.9. When H is increased in the opposite direction, the flux density decreases until, at a value shown as **Od**, the flux density has been reduced to zero. The magnetic field strength **Od** required to remove the residual magnetism, i.e. reduce B to zero, is called the **coercive force**.

Further increase of H in the reverse direction causes the flux density to increase in the reverse direction until saturation is reached, as shown by curve **de**. If H is varied backwards from **Ox** to **Oy**, the flux density follows the curve **efgb**, similar to curve **bcde**.

It is seen from Fig. 7.9 that the flux density changes lag behind the changes in the magnetic field strength. This effect is called **hysteresis**. The closed figure **bcdefgb** is called the **hysteresis loop** (or the B/H loop).

Hysteresis loss

A disturbance in the alignment of the domains (i.e. groups of atoms) of a ferromagnetic material causes energy to be expended in taking it through a cycle of magnetisation. This energy appears as heat in the specimen and is called the **hysteresis loss**.

The energy loss associated with hysteresis is proportional to the area of the hysteresis loop.

The area of a hysteresis loop varies with the type of material. The area, and thus the energy loss, is much greater for hard materials than for soft materials.

Figure 7.10 shows typical hysteresis loops for:

(a) **hard material**, which has a high remanence Oc and a large coercivity **Od**

(b) **soft steel**, which has a large remanence and small coercivity

(c) **ferrite**, this being a ceramic-like magnetic substance made from oxides of iron, nickel, cobalt, magnesium, aluminium and manganese; the hysteresis of ferrite is very small.

For a.c.-excited devices the hysteresis loop is repeated every cycle of alternating current. Thus a hysteresis loop with a large area (as with hard steel) is often unsuitable since the energy loss would be considerable. Silicon steel has a narrow hysteresis loop, and thus small hysteresis loss, and is suitable for transformer cores and rotating machine armatures.

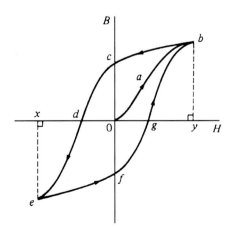

Figure 7.9

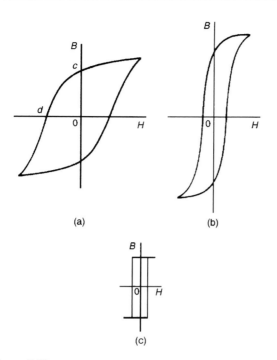

(a)

(b)

(c)

Figure 7.10

Now try the following exercises

Exercise 37   Short answer questions on magnetic circuits

1. State six practical applications of magnets

2. What is a permanent magnet?

3. Sketch the pattern of the magnetic field associated with a bar magnet. Mark the direction of the field.

4. Define magnetic flux

5. The symbol for magnetic flux is ... and the unit of flux is the ...

6. Define magnetic flux density

7. The symbol for magnetic flux density is ... and the unit of flux density is ...

8. The symbol for m.m.f. is ... and the unit of m.m.f. is the ...

9. Another name for the magnetising force is ...... ; its symbol is ... and its unit is ...

10. Complete the statement:
$$\frac{\text{flux density}}{\text{magnetic field strength}} = \dots$$

11. What is absolute permeability?

12. The value of the permeability of free space is ...

13. What is a magnetisation curve?

14. The symbol for reluctance is ... and the unit of reluctance is ...

15. Make a comparison between magnetic and electrical quantities

16. What is hysteresis?

17. Draw a typical hysteresis loop and on it identify:
    (a) saturation flux density
    (b) remanence
    (c) coercive force

18. State the units of (a) remanence (b) coercive force

19. How is magnetic screening achieved?

20. Complete the statement: magnetic materials have a ... reluctance; non-magnetic materials have a ... reluctance

21. What loss is associated with hysteresis?

Exercise 38   Multi-choice questions on magnetic circuits
(Answers on page 420)

1. The unit of magnetic flux density is the:
   (a) weber   (b) weber per metre
   (c) ampere per metre   (d) tesla

2. The total flux in the core of an electrical machine is 20 mWb and its flux density is 1 T. The cross-sectional area of the core is:
   (a) $0.05\,\text{m}^2$ (b) $0.02\,\text{m}^2$
   (c) $20\,\text{m}^2$ (d) $50\,\text{m}^2$

3. If the total flux in a magnetic circuit is 2 mWb and the cross-sectional area of the circuit is 10 cm^2, the flux density is:
    (a) 0.2 T   (b) 2 T
    (c) 20 T   (d) 20 mT

    Questions 4 to 8 refer to the following data:
    A coil of 100 turns is wound uniformly on a wooden ring. The ring has a mean circumference of 1 m and a uniform cross-sectional area of 10 cm^2. The current in the coil is 1 A.

4. The magnetomotive force is:
    (a) 1 A   (b) 10 A
    (c) 100 A   (d) 1000 A

5. The magnetic field strength is:
    (a) 1 A/m   (b) 10 A/m
    (c) 100 A/m   (d) 1000 A/m

6. The magnetic flux density is:
    (a) 800 T   (b) 8.85×10^{-10} T
    (c) $4\pi \times 10^{-7}$ T   (d) $40\pi\,\mu$T

7. The magnetic flux is:
    (a) $0.04\pi\,\mu$Wb   (b) 0.01 Wb
    (c) $8.85\,\mu$Wb   (d) $4\pi\,\mu$Wb

8. The reluctance is:
    (a) $\dfrac{10^8}{4\pi}\,H^{-1}$ (b) $1000\,H^{-1}$
    (c) $\dfrac{2.5}{\pi} \times 10^9\,H^{-1}$ (d) $\dfrac{10^8}{8.85}\,H^{-1}$

9. Which of the following statements is false?
    (a) For non-magnetic materials reluctance is high
    (b) Energy loss due to hysteresis is greater for harder magnetic materials than for softer magnetic materials

(c) The remanence of a ferrous material is measured in ampere/metre
(d) Absolute permeability is measured in henrys per metre

10. The current flowing in a 500 turn coil wound on an iron ring is 4 A. The reluctance of the circuit is 2×10^6 H. The flux produced is:
    (a) 1 Wb   (b) 1000 Wb
    (c) 1 mWb   (d) $62.5\,\mu$Wb

11. A comparison can be made between magnetic and electrical quantities. From the following list, match the magnetic quantities with their equivalent electrical quantities.
    (a) current   (b) reluctance
    (c) e.m.f.   (d) flux
    (e) m.m.f.   (f) resistance

12. The effect of an air gap in a magnetic circuit is to:
    (a) increase the reluctance
    (b) reduce the flux density
    (c) divide the flux
    (d) reduce the magnetomotive force

13. Two bar magnets are placed parallel to each other and about 2 cm apart, such that the south pole of one magnet is adjacent to the north pole of the other. With this arrangement, the magnets will:
    (a) attract each other
    (b) have no effect on each other
    (c) repel each other
    (d) lose their magnetism

Revision Test 2

This revision test covers the material contained in Chapters 5 to 7. *The marks for each question are shown in brackets at the end of each question.*

1. Resistances of $5\,\Omega$, $7\,\Omega$, and $8\,\Omega$ are connected in series. If a $10\,V$ supply voltage is connected across the arrangement determine the current flowing through and the p.d. across the $7\,\Omega$ resistor. Calculate also the power dissipated in the $8\,\Omega$ resistor. (6)

2. For the series-parallel network shown in Fig. RT2.1, find (a) the supply current, (b) the current flowing through each resistor, (c) the p.d. across each resistor, (d) the total power dissipated in the circuit, (e) the cost of energy if the circuit is connected for 80 hours. Assume electrical energy costs 14p per unit. (15)

3. The charge on the plates of a capacitor is $8\,mC$ when the potential between them is $4\,kV$. Determine the capacitance of the capacitor. (2)

4. Two parallel rectangular plates measuring $80\,mm$ by $120\,mm$ are separated by $4\,mm$ of mica and carry an electric charge of $0.48\,\mu C$. The voltage between the plates is $500\,V$. Calculate (a) the electric flux density (b) the electric field strength, and (c) the capacitance of the capacitor, in picofarads, if the relative permittivity of mica is 5. (7)

5. A $4\,\mu F$ capacitor is connected in parallel with a $6\,\mu F$ capacitor. This arrangement is then connected in series with a $10\,\mu F$ capacitor. A supply p.d. of $250\,V$ is connected across the circuit. Find (a) the equivalent capacitance of the circuit, (b) the voltage across the $10\,\mu F$ capacitor, and (c) the charge on each capacitor. (7)

6. A coil of 600 turns is wound uniformly on a ring of non-magnetic material. The ring has a uniform cross-sectional area of $200\,mm^2$ and a mean circumference of $500\,mm$. If the current in the coil is $4\,A$, determine (a) the magnetic field strength,

(b) the flux density, and (c) the total magnetic flux in the ring. (5)

7. A mild steel ring of cross-sectional area $4\,cm^2$ has a radial air gap of $3\,mm$ cut into it. If the mean length of the mild steel path is $300\,mm$, calculate the magnetomotive force to produce a flux of $0.48\,mWb$. (Use the B–H curve on page 80) (8)

8. In the circuit shown in Fig. RT2.2, the slider S is at the half-way point.

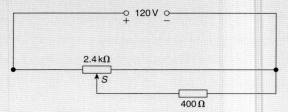

Figure RT2.2

(a) Calculate the p.d. across and the current flowing in the $400\,\Omega$ load resistor.
(b) Is the circuit a potentiometer or a rheostat? (5)

9. For the circuit shown in Fig. RT2.3, calculate the current flowing in the $50\,\Omega$ load and the voltage drop across the load when

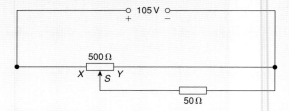

Figure RT2.3

(a) XS is 3/5 of XY
(b) point S coincides with point Y (5)

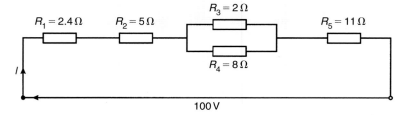

Figure RT2.1

Chapter 8

Electromagnetism

At the end of this chapter you should be able to:

- understand that magnetic fields are produced by electric currents
- apply the screw rule to determine direction of magnetic field
- recognize that the magnetic field around a solenoid is similar to a magnet
- apply the screw rule or grip rule to a solenoid to determine magnetic field direction
- recognize and describe practical applications of an electromagnet, i.e. electric bell, relay, lifting magnet, telephone receiver
- appreciate factors upon which the force F on a current-carrying conductor depends
- perform calculations using $F = BIl$ and $F = BIl \sin \theta$
- recognize that a loudspeaker is a practical application of force F
- use Fleming's left-hand rule to pre-determine direction of force in a current-carrying conductor
- describe the principle of operation of a simple d.c. motor
- describe the principle of operation and construction of a moving coil instrument
- appreciate that force F on a charge in a magnetic field is given by $F = QvB$
- perform calculations using $F = QvB$

8.1 Magnetic field due to an electric current

Magnetic fields can be set up not only by permanent magnets, as shown in Chapter 7, but also by electric currents.

Let a piece of wire be arranged to pass vertically through a horizontal sheet of cardboard on which is placed some iron filings, as shown in Fig. 8.1(a). If a current is now passed through the wire, then the iron filings will form a definite circular field pattern with the wire at the centre, when the cardboard is gently tapped. By placing a compass in different positions the lines of flux are seen to have a definite direction as shown in Fig. 8.1(b).

If the current direction is reversed, the direction of the lines of flux is also reversed. The effect on both the iron filings and the compass needle disappears when

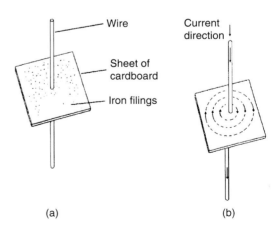

Figure 8.1

the current is switched off. The magnetic field is thus produced by the electric current. The magnetic flux

DOI: 10.1016/B978-0-08-089056-2.00008-5

produced has the same properties as the flux produced by a permanent magnet. If the current is increased the strength of the field increases and, as for the permanent magnet, the field strength decreases as we move away from the current-carrying conductor.

In Fig. 8.1, the effect of only a small part of the magnetic field is shown. If the whole length of the conductor is similarly investigated it is found that the magnetic field round a straight conductor is in the form of concentric cylinders as shown in Fig. 8.2, the field direction depending on the direction of the current flow.

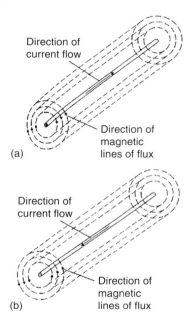

Direction of current flow

Direction of magnetic lines of flux

(a)

Direction of current flow

Direction of magnetic lines of flux

(b)

Figure 8.2

When dealing with magnetic fields formed by electric current it is usual to portray the effect as shown in Fig. 8.3. The convention adopted is:

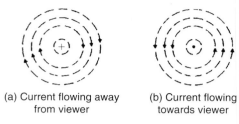

(a) Current flowing away from viewer

(b) Current flowing towards viewer

Figure 8.3

(i)   Current flowing away from the viewer, i.e. into the paper, is indicated by $\oplus$. This may be thought of as the feathered end of the shaft of an arrow. See Fig. 8.3(a).

(ii) Current flowing towards the viewer, i.e. out of the paper, is indicated by $\odot$. This may be thought of as the point of an arrow. See Fig. 8.3(b).

The direction of the magnetic lines of flux is best remembered by the **screw rule** which states that:

If a normal right-hand thread screw is screwed along the conductor in the direction of the current, the direction of rotation of the screw is in the direction of the magnetic field.

For example, with current flowing away from the viewer (Fig. 8.3(a)) a right-hand thread screw driven into the paper has to be rotated clockwise. Hence the direction of the magnetic field is clockwise.

A magnetic field set up by a long coil, or **solenoid**, is shown in Fig. 8.4(a) and is seen to be similar to that of a bar magnet. If the solenoid is wound on an iron bar, as shown in Fig. 8.4(b), an even stronger magnetic field is produced, the iron becoming magnetised and behaving like a permanent magnet. The direction of the magnetic field produced by the current I in the solenoid may be found by either of two methods, i.e. the screw rule or the grip rule.

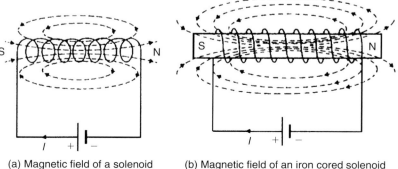

(a) Magnetic field of a solenoid

(b) Magnetic field of an iron cored solenoid

Figure 8.4

(a) **The screw rule** states that if a normal right-hand thread screw is placed along the axis of the solenoid and is screwed in the direction of the current it moves in the direction of the magnetic field **inside** the solenoid. The direction of the magnetic field **inside** the solenoid is from south to north. Thus in Figs 8.4(a) and (b) the north pole is to the right.

(b) **The grip rule** states that if the coil is gripped with the **right** hand, with the fingers pointing in the direction of the current, then the thumb, outstretched parallel to the axis of the solenoid, points in the direction of the magnetic field **inside** the solenoid.

Problem 1. Figure 8.5 shows a coil of wire wound on an iron core connected to a battery. Sketch the magnetic field pattern associated with the current-carrying coil and determine the polarity of the field.

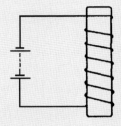

Figure 8.5

The magnetic field associated with the solenoid in Fig. 8.5 is similar to the field associated with a bar magnet and is as shown in Fig. 8.6. The polarity of the field is determined either by the screw rule or by the grip rule. Thus the north pole is at the bottom and the south pole at the top.

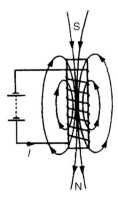

Figure 8.6

8.2 Electromagnets

The solenoid is very important in electromagnetic theory since the magnetic field inside the solenoid is practically uniform for a particular current, and is also versatile, inasmuch that a variation of the current can alter the strength of the magnetic field. An electromagnet, based on the solenoid, provides the basis of many items of electrical equipment, examples of which include electric bells, relays, lifting magnets and telephone receivers.

(i) Electric bell

There are various types of electric bell, including the single-stroke bell, the trembler bell, the buzzer and a continuously ringing bell, but all depend on the attraction exerted by an electromagnet on a soft iron armature. A typical single stroke bell circuit is shown in Fig. 8.7. When the push button is operated a current passes through the coil. Since the iron-cored coil is energised the soft iron armature is attracted to the electromagnet. The armature also carries a striker which hits the gong. When the circuit is broken the coil becomes demagnetised and the spring steel strip pulls the armature back to its original position. The striker will only operate when the push button is operated.

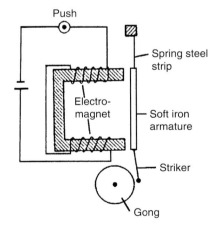

Figure 8.7

(ii) Relay

A relay is similar to an electric bell except that contacts are opened or closed by operation instead of a gong being struck. A typical simple relay is shown in Fig. 8.8, which consists of a coil wound on a soft iron core. When the coil is energised the hinged soft iron armature is

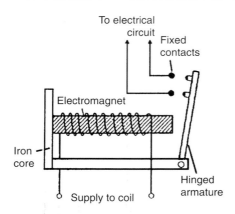

Figure 8.8

attracted to the electromagnet and pushes against two fixed contacts so that they are connected together, thus closing some other electrical circuit.

(iii) Lifting magnet

Lifting magnets, incorporating large electromagnets, are used in iron and steel works for lifting scrap metal. A typical robust lifting magnet, capable of exerting large attractive forces, is shown in the elevation and plan view of Fig. 8.9 where a coil, C, is wound round a central core, P, of the iron casting. Over the face of the electromagnet is placed a protective non-magnetic sheet of material, R. The load, Q, which must be of magnetic material is lifted when the coils are energised, the magnetic flux paths, M, being shown by the broken lines.

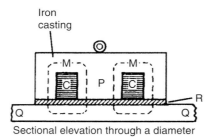

Sectional elevation through a diameter

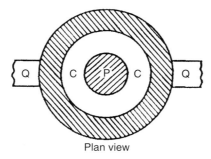

Plan view

Figure 8.9

(iv) Telephone receiver

Whereas a transmitter or microphone changes sound waves into corresponding electrical signals, a telephone receiver converts the electrical waves back into sound waves. A typical telephone receiver is shown in Fig. 8.10 and consists of a permanent magnet with coils wound on its poles. A thin, flexible diaphragm of magnetic material is held in position near to the magnetic poles but not touching them. Variation in current from the transmitter varies the magnetic field and the diaphragm consequently vibrates. The vibration produces sound variations corresponding to those transmitted.

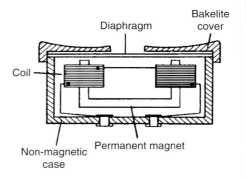

Figure 8.10

8.3 Force on a current-carrying conductor

If a current-carrying conductor is placed in a magnetic field produced by permanent magnets, then the fields due to the current-carrying conductor and the permanent magnets interact and cause a force to be exerted on the conductor. The force on the current-carrying conductor in a magnetic field depends upon:

(a) the flux density of the field, B teslas,

(b) the strength of the current, I amperes,

(c) the length of the conductor perpendicular to the magnetic field, l metres, and

(d) the directions of the field and the current.

When the magnetic field, the current and the conductor are mutually at right angles then:

$$\text{Force } F = BIl \text{ newtons}$$

When the conductor and the field are at an angle $\theta°$ to each other then:

$$\text{Force } F = BIl \sin \theta \text{ newtons}$$

Since when the magnetic field, current and conductor are mutually at right angles, $F = BIl$, the magnetic flux density B may be defined by $B = (F)/(Il)$, i.e. the flux density is 1 T if the force exerted on 1 m of a conductor when the conductor carries a current of 1 A is 1 N.

Loudspeaker

A simple application of the above force is the moving coil loudspeaker. The loudspeaker is used to convert electrical signals into sound waves.

Figure 8.11 shows a typical loudspeaker having a magnetic circuit comprising a permanent magnet and soft iron pole pieces so that a strong magnetic field is available in the short cylindrical air gap. A moving coil, called the voice or speech coil, is suspended from the end of a paper or plastic cone so that it lies in the gap. When an electric current flows through the coil it produces a force which tends to move the cone backwards and forwards according to the direction of the current. The cone acts as a piston, transferring this force to the air, and producing the required sound waves.

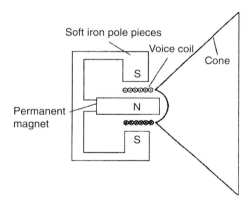

Soft iron pole pieces

Voice coil

Cone

Permanent magnet

Figure 8.11

Problem 2. A conductor carries a current of 20 A and is at right-angles to a magnetic field having a flux density of 0.9 T. If the length of the conductor in the field is 30 cm, calculate the force acting on the conductor. Determine also the value of the force if the conductor is inclined at an angle of 30° to the direction of the field.

$B = 0.9\,\text{T}$, $I = 20\,\text{A}$ and $l = 30\,\text{cm} = 0.30\,\text{m}$

Force $F = BIl = (0.9)(20)(0.30)$ newtons when the conductor is at right-angles to the field, as shown in Fig. 8.12(a), i.e. $F = 5.4\,\text{N}$.

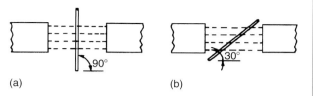

(a)   (b)

Figure 8.12

When the conductor is inclined at 30° to the field, as shown in Fig. 8.12(b), then

$$\text{Force } F = BIl \sin\theta$$

$$= (0.9)(20)(0.30)\sin 30°$$

i.e. $\textbf{F} = \textbf{2.7 N}$

If the current-carrying conductor shown in Fig. 8.3(a) is placed in the magnetic field shown in Fig. 8.13(a), then the two fields interact and cause a force to be exerted on the conductor as shown in Fig. 8.13(b). The field is strengthened above the conductor and weakened below, thus tending to move the conductor downwards. This is the basic principle of operation of the electric motor (see Section 8.4) and the moving-coil instrument (see Section 8.5).

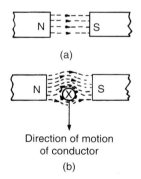

(a)

Direction of motion
of conductor

(b)

Figure 8.13

The direction of the force exerted on a conductor can be pre-determined by using **Fleming's left-hand rule** (often called the motor rule) which states:

Let the thumb, first finger and second finger of the left hand be extended such that they are all at right-angles to each other (as shown in Fig. 8.14). If the first finger points in the direction of the magnetic field, the second finger points in the direction of the current, then the thumb will point in the direction of the motion of the conductor.

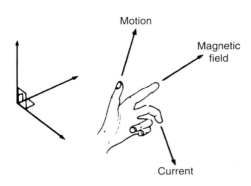

Figure 8.14

Summarising:

First finger – Field

SeCond finger – Current

ThuMb – Motion

Problem 3. Determine the current required in a 400 mm length of conductor of an electric motor, when the conductor is situated at right-angles to a magnetic field of flux density 1.2 T, if a force of 1.92 N is to be exerted on the conductor. If the conductor is vertical, the current flowing downwards and the direction of the magnetic field is from left to right, what is the direction of the force?

Force $= 1.92$ N, $l = 400$ mm $= 0.40$ m and $B = 1.2$ T. Since $F = BIl$, then $I = F/Bl$ hence

$$\text{current } I = \frac{1.92}{(1.2)(0.4)} = 4\,\text{A}$$

If the current flows downwards, the direction of its magnetic field due to the current alone will be clockwise when viewed from above. The lines of flux will reinforce (i.e. strengthen) the main magnetic field at the back of the conductor and will be in opposition in the front (i.e. weaken the field). **Hence the force on the conductor will be from back to front (i.e. toward the viewer).** This direction may also have been deduced using Fleming's left-hand rule.

Problem 4. A conductor 350 mm long carries a current of 10 A and is at right-angles to a magnetic field lying between two circular pole faces each of radius 60 mm. If the total flux between the pole faces is 0.5 mWb, calculate the magnitude of the force exerted on the conductor.

$l = 350$ mm $= 0.35$ m, $I = 10$ A, area of pole face $A = \pi r^2 = \pi(0.06)^2$ m^2 and $\Phi = 0.5$ mWb $= 0.5 \times 10^{-3}$ Wb

Force $F = BIl$,   and $B = \dfrac{\Phi}{A}$ hence

$$\text{force } F = \frac{\Phi}{A}Il$$

$$= \frac{(0.5 \times 10^{-3})}{\pi(0.06)^2}(10)(0.35)\text{ newtons}$$

i.e.   **force $= 0.155$ N**

Problem 5. With reference to Fig. 8.15 determine (a) the direction of the force on the conductor in Fig. 8.15(a), (b) the direction of the force on the conductor in Fig. 8.15(b), (c) the direction of the current in Fig. 8.15(c), (d) the polarity of the magnetic system in Fig. 8.15(d).

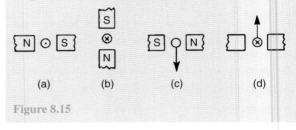

Figure 8.15

(a)   The direction of the main magnetic field is from north to south, i.e. left to right. The current is flowing towards the viewer, and using the screw rule, the direction of the field is anticlockwise. Hence either by Fleming's left-hand rule, or by sketching the interacting magnetic field as shown in Fig. 8.16(a), the direction of the force on the conductor is seen to be upward.

(b)   Using a similar method to part (a) it is seen that the force on the conductor is to the right – see Fig. 8.16(b).

(c)   Using Fleming's left-hand rule, or by sketching as in Fig. 8.16(c), it is seen that the current is toward the viewer, i.e. out of the paper.

(d)   Similar to part (c), the polarity of the magnetic system is as shown in Fig. 8.16(d).

Problem 6. A coil is wound on a rectangular former of width 24 mm and length 30 mm. The former is pivoted about an axis passing through the middle of the two shorter sides and is placed in a uniform magnetic field of flux density 0.8 T, the axis being perpendicular to the field. If the coil carries a current of 50 mA, determine the force on each coil side (a) for a single-turn coil, (b) for a coil wound with 300 turns.

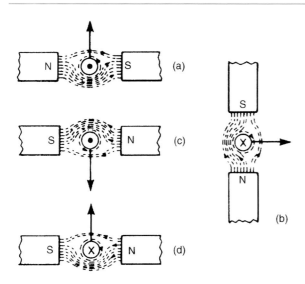

Figure 8.16

(a) Flux density $B = 0.8\,T$, length of conductor lying at right-angles to field $l = 30\,mm = 30 \times 10^{-3}\,m$ and current $I = 50\,mA = 50 \times 10^{-3}\,A$. For a single-turn coil, force on each coil side

$$F = BIl = 0.8 \times 50 \times 10^{-3} \times 30 \times 10^{-3}$$
$$= \mathbf{1.2 \times 10^{-3}\,N}\ \text{or}\ \mathbf{0.0012\,N}$$

(b) When there are 300 turns on the coil there are effectively 300 parallel conductors each carrying a current of 50 mA. Thus the total force produced by the current is 300 times that for a single-turn coil. Hence force on coil side,
$$F = 300\ BIl = 300 \times 0.0012 = \mathbf{0.36\,N}$$

Now try the following exercise

Exercise 39   **Further problems on the force on a current-carrying conductor**

1. A conductor carries a current of 70 A at right-angles to a magnetic field having a flux density of 1.5 T. If the length of the conductor in the field is 200 mm calculate the force acting on the conductor. What is the force when the conductor and field are at an angle of 45°?
[21.0 N, 14.8 N]

2. Calculate the current required in a 240 mm length of conductor of a d.c. motor when the conductor is situated at right-angles to the magnetic field of flux density 1.25 T, if a force of 1.20 N is to be exerted on the conductor.
[4.0 A]

3. A conductor 30 cm long is situated at right-angles to a magnetic field. Calculate the flux density of the magnetic field if a current of 15 A in the conductor produces a force on it of 3.6 N.
[0.80 T]

4. A conductor 300 mm long carries a current of 13 A and is at right-angles to a magnetic field between two circular pole faces, each of diameter 80 mm. If the total flux between the pole faces is 0.75 mWb calculate the force exerted on the conductor.
[0.582 N]

5. (a) A 400 mm length of conductor carrying a current of 25 A is situated at right-angles to a magnetic field between two poles of an electric motor. The poles have a circular cross-section. If the force exerted on the conductor is 80 N and the total flux between the pole faces is 1.27 mWb, determine the diameter of a pole face.

   (b) If the conductor in part (a) is vertical, the current flowing downwards and the direction of the magnetic field is from left to right, what is the direction of the 80 N force?
[(a) 14.2 mm (b) towards the viewer]

6. A coil is wound uniformly on a former having a width of 18 mm and a length of 25 mm. The former is pivoted about an axis passing through the middle of the two shorter sides and is placed in a uniform magnetic field of flux density 0.75 T, the axis being perpendicular to the field. If the coil carries a current of 120 mA, determine the force exerted on each coil side, (a) for a single-turn coil, (b) for a coil wound with 400 turns.
[(a) $2.25 \times 10^{-3}\,N$ (b) 0.9 N]

8.4 Principle of operation of a simple d.c. motor

A rectangular coil which is free to rotate about a fixed axis is shown placed inside a magnetic field produced by permanent magnets in Fig. 8.17. A direct current is fed

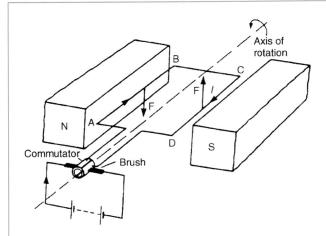

Figure 8.17

into the coil via carbon brushes bearing on a commutator, which consists of a metal ring split into two halves separated by insulation. When current flows in the coil a magnetic field is set up around the coil which interacts with the magnetic field produced by the magnets. This causes a force F to be exerted on the current-carrying conductor which, by Fleming's left-hand rule, is downwards between points A and B and upward between C and D for the current direction shown. This causes a torque and the coil rotates anticlockwise. When the coil has turned through $90°$ from the position shown in Fig. 8.17 the brushes connected to the positive and negative terminals of the supply make contact with different halves of the commutator ring, thus reversing the direction of the current flow in the conductor. If the current is not reversed and the coil rotates past this position the forces acting on it change direction and it rotates in the opposite direction thus never making more than half a revolution. The current direction is reversed every time the coil swings through the vertical position and thus

the coil rotates anticlockwise for as long as the current flows. This is the principle of operation of a d.c. motor which is thus a device that takes in electrical energy and converts it into mechanical energy.

8.5 Principle of operation of a moving-coil instrument

A moving-coil instrument operates on the motor principle. When a conductor carrying current is placed in a magnetic field, a force F is exerted on the conductor, given by $F = BIl$. If the flux density B is made constant (by using permanent magnets) and the conductor is a fixed length (say, a coil) then the force will depend only on the current flowing in the conductor.

In a moving-coil instrument a coil is placed centrally in the gap between shaped pole pieces as shown by the front elevation in Fig. 8.18(a). (The air gap is kept as small as possible, although for clarity it is shown exaggerated in Fig. 8.18). The coil is supported by steel pivots, resting in jewel bearings, on a cylindrical iron core. Current is led into and out of the coil by two phosphor bronze spiral hairsprings which are wound in opposite directions to minimise the effect of temperature change and to limit the coil swing (i.e. to **control** the movement) and return the movement to zero position when no current flows. Current flowing in the coil produces forces as shown in Fig. 8.18(b), the directions being obtained by Fleming's left-hand rule. The two forces, F_A and F_B, produce a torque which will move the coil in a clockwise direction, i.e. move the pointer from left to right. Since force is proportional to current the scale is linear.

When the aluminium frame, on which the coil is wound, is rotated between the poles of the magnet,

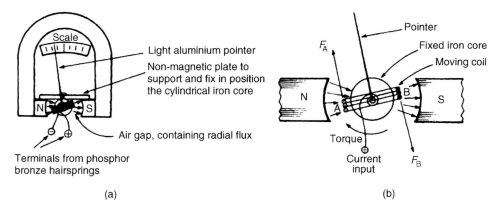

(a)

(b)

Figure 8.18

small currents (called eddy currents) are induced into the frame, and this provides automatically the necessary **damping** of the system due to the reluctance of the former to move within the magnetic field. The moving-coil instrument will measure only direct current or voltage and the terminals are marked positive and negative to ensure that the current passes through the coil in the correct direction to deflect the pointer 'up the scale'.

The range of this sensitive instrument is extended by using shunts and multipliers (see Chapter 10).

8.6 Force on a charge

When a charge of Q coulombs is moving at a velocity of v m/s in a magnetic field of flux density B teslas, the charge moving perpendicular to the field, then the magnitude of the force F exerted on the charge is given by:

$$F = QvB \text{ newtons}$$

Problem 7. An electron in a television tube has a charge of 1.6×10^{-19} coulombs and travels at 3×10^{7} m/s perpendicular to a field of flux density $18.5\,\mu$T. Determine the force exerted on the electron in the field.

From above, force $F = QvB$ newtons, where $Q =$ charge in coulombs $= 1.6 \times 10^{-19}$ C, $v =$ velocity of charge $= 3 \times 10^{7}$ m/s, and $B =$ flux density $= 18.5 \times 10^{-6}$ T. Hence force on electron,

$$F = 1.6 \times 10^{-19} \times 3 \times 10^{7} \times 18.5 \times 10^{-6}$$
$$= 1.6 \times 3 \times 18.5 \times 10^{-18}$$
$$= 88.8 \times 10^{-18} = \mathbf{8.88 \times 10^{-17}\,N}$$

Now try the following exercises

Exercise 40 Further problems on the force on a charge

1. Calculate the force exerted on a charge of 2×10^{-18} C travelling at 2×10^{6} m/s perpendicular to a field of density 2×10^{-7} T
    $[8 \times 10^{-19}$ N]

2. Determine the speed of a 10^{-19} C charge travelling perpendicular to a field of flux density 10^{-7} T, if the force on the charge is 10^{-20} N
    $[10^{6}$ m/s]

Exercise 41 Short answer questions on electromagnetism

1. The direction of the magnetic field around a current-carrying conductor may be remembered using the ...... rule

2. Sketch the magnetic field pattern associated with a solenoid connected to a battery and wound on an iron bar. Show the direction of the field

3. Name three applications of electromagnetism

4. State what happens when a current-carrying conductor is placed in a magnetic field between two magnets

5. The force on a current-carrying conductor in a magnetic field depends on four factors. Name them

6. The direction of the force on a conductor in a magnetic field may be predetermined using Fleming's ...... rule

7. State three applications of the force on a current-carrying conductor

8. Figure 8.19 shows a simplified diagram of a section through the coil of a moving-coil instrument. For the direction of current flow shown in the coil determine the direction that the pointer will move

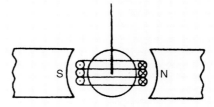

Figure 8.19

9. Explain, with the aid of a sketch, the action of a simplified d.c. motor

10. Sketch and label the movement of a moving-coil instrument. Briefly explain the principle of operation of such an instrument

Exercise 42 Multi-choice questions on electromagnetism
(Answers on page 420)

1. A conductor carries a current of 10 A at right-angles to a magnetic field having a flux density of 500 mT. If the length of the conductor in the field is 20 cm, the force on the conductor is:
   (a) 100 kN   (b) 1 kN
   (c) 100 N   (d) 1 N

2. If a conductor is horizontal, the current flowing from left to right and the direction of the surrounding magnetic field is from above to below, the force exerted on the conductor is:
   (a) from left to right
   (b) from below to above
   (c) away from the viewer
   (d) towards the viewer

3. For the current-carrying conductor lying in the magnetic field shown in Fig. 8.20(a), the direction of the force on the conductor is:
   (a) to the left   (b) upwards
   (c) to the right   (d) downwards

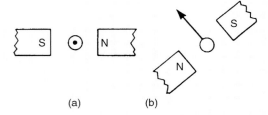

(a)   (b)

Figure 8.20

4. For the current-carrying conductor lying in the magnetic field shown in Fig. 8.20(b), the direction of the current in the conductor is:
   (a) towards the viewer
   (b) away from the viewer

5. Figure 8.21 shows a rectangular coil of wire placed in a magnetic field and free to rotate about axis AB. If the current flows into the coil at C, the coil will:

   (a) commence to rotate anti-clockwise
   (b) commence to rotate clockwise
   (c) remain in the vertical position
   (d) experience a force towards the north pole

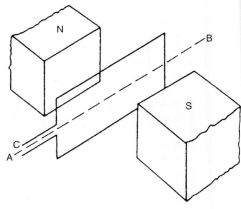

Figure 8.21

6. The force on an electron travelling at 10^7 m/s in a magnetic field of density 10μT is 1.6×10^{-17} N. The electron has a charge of:
   (a) 1.6×10^{-28} C   (b) 1.6×10^{-15} C
   (c) 1.6×10^{-19} C   (d) 1.6×10^{-25} C

7. An electric bell depends for its action on:
   (a) a permanent magnet
   (b) reversal of current
   (c) a hammer and a gong
   (d) an electromagnet

8. A relay can be used to:
   (a) decrease the current in a circuit
   (b) control a circuit more readily
   (c) increase the current in a circuit
   (d) control a circuit from a distance

9. There is a force of attraction between two current-carrying conductors when the current in them is:
   (a) in opposite directions
   (b) in the same direction
   (c) of different magnitude
   (d) of the same magnitude

10. The magnetic field due to a current-carrying conductor takes the form of:
    (a) rectangles
    (b) concentric circles
    (c) wavy lines
    (d) straight lines radiating outwards

Chapter 9

Electromagnetic induction

At the end of this chapter you should be able to:

- understand how an e.m.f. may be induced in a conductor
- state Faraday's laws of electromagnetic induction
- state Lenz's law
- use Fleming's right-hand rule for relative directions
- appreciate that the induced e.m.f., $E = Blv$ or $E = Blv \sin \theta$
- calculate induced e.m.f. given B, l, v and θ and determine relative directions
- understand and perform calculations on rotation of a loop in a magnetic field
- define inductance L and state its unit
- define mutual inductance
- appreciate that e.m.f.

$$E = -N \frac{d\Phi}{dt} = -L \frac{dI}{dt}$$

- calculate induced e.m.f. given N, t, L, change of flux or change of current
- appreciate factors which affect the inductance of an inductor
- draw the circuit diagram symbols for inductors
- calculate the energy stored in an inductor using $W = \frac{1}{2}LI^2$ joules
- calculate inductance L of a coil, given $L = \dfrac{N\Phi}{I}$ and $L = \dfrac{N^2}{S}$
- calculate mutual inductance using $E_2 = -M \dfrac{dI_1}{dt}$ and $M = \dfrac{N_1 N_2}{S}$

9.1 Introduction to electromagnetic induction

When a conductor is moved across a magnetic field so as to cut through the lines of force (or flux), an electromotive force (e.m.f.) is produced in the conductor. If the conductor forms part of a closed circuit then the e.m.f. produced causes an electric current to flow round the circuit. Hence an e.m.f. (and thus current) is 'induced' in

the conductor as a result of its movement across the magnetic field. This effect is known as '**electromagnetic induction**'.

Figure 9.1(a) shows a coil of wire connected to a centre-zero galvanometer, which is a sensitive ammeter with the zero-current position in the centre of the scale.

(a) When the magnet is moved at constant speed towards the coil (Fig. 9.1(a)), a deflection is noted

DOI: 10.1016/B978-0-08-089056-2.00009-7

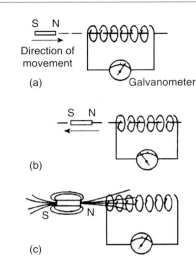

Figure 9.1

on the galvanometer showing that a current has been produced in the coil.

(b) When the magnet is moved at the same speed as in (a) but away from the coil the same deflection is noted but is in the opposite direction (see Fig. 9.1(b)).

(c) When the magnet is held stationary, even within the coil, no deflection is recorded.

(d) When the coil is moved at the same speed as in (a) and the magnet held stationary the same galvanometer deflection is noted.

(e) When the relative speed is, say, doubled, the galvanometer deflection is doubled.

(f) When a stronger magnet is used, a greater galvanometer deflection is noted.

(g) When the number of turns of wire of the coil is increased, a greater galvanometer deflection is noted.

Figure 9.1(c) shows the magnetic field associated with the magnet. As the magnet is moved towards the coil, the magnetic flux of the magnet moves across, or cuts, the coil. **It is the relative movement of the magnetic flux and the coil that causes an e.m.f. and thus current, to be induced in the coil**. This effect is known as electromagnetic induction. The laws of electromagnetic induction stated in Section 9.2 evolved from experiments such as those described above.

9.2 Laws of electromagnetic induction

Faraday's laws of electromagnetic induction state:

(i) *An induced e.m.f. is set up whenever the magnetic field linking that circuit changes.*

(ii) *The magnitude of the induced e.m.f. in any circuit is proportional to the rate of change of the magnetic flux linking the circuit.*

Lenz's law states:

The direction of an induced e.m.f. is always such that it tends to set up a current opposing the motion or the change of flux responsible for inducing that e.m.f.

An alternative method to Lenz's law of determining relative directions is given by **Fleming's Right-hand rule** (often called the gene**R**ator rule) which states:

Let the thumb, first finger and second finger of the right hand be extended such that they are all at right angles to each other (as shown in Fig. 9.2). If the first finger points in the direction of the magnetic field and the thumb points in the direction of motion of the conductor relative to the magnetic field, then the second finger will point in the direction of the induced e.m.f.

Summarising:

First finger – **F**ield

Thu**M**b – **M**otion

S**E**cond finger – **E**.m.f.

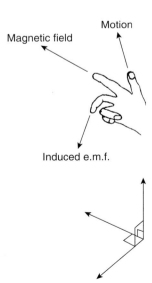

Figure 9.2

In a generator, conductors forming an electric circuit are made to move through a magnetic field. By Faraday's law an e.m.f. is induced in the conductors and thus a source of e.m.f. is created. A generator converts mechanical energy into electrical energy. (The action of a simple a.c. generator is described in Chapter 14).

The induced e.m.f. E set up between the ends of the conductor shown in Fig. 9.3 is given by:

$$E = Blv \text{ volts}$$

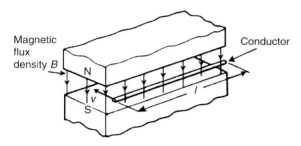

Figure 9.3

where B, the flux density, is measured in teslas, l, the length of conductor in the magnetic field, is measured in metres, and v, the conductor velocity, is measured in metres per second.

If the conductor moves at an angle $\theta°$ to the magnetic field (instead of at 90° as assumed above) then

$$E = Blv \sin \theta \text{ volts}$$

Problem 1. A conductor 300 mm long moves at a uniform speed of 4 m/s at right-angles to a uniform magnetic field of flux density 1.25 T. Determine the current flowing in the conductor when (a) its ends are open-circuited, (b) its ends are connected to a load of 20 Ω resistance.

When a conductor moves in a magnetic field it will have an e.m.f. induced in it but this e.m.f. can only produce a current if there is a closed circuit. Induced e.m.f.

$$E = Blv = (1.25)\left(\frac{300}{1000}\right)(4) = 1.5 \text{ V}$$

(a) If the ends of the conductor are open circuited **no current will flow** even though 1.5 V has been induced.

(b) From Ohm's law,

$$I = \frac{E}{R} = \frac{1.5}{20} = \textbf{0.075 A} \text{ or } \textbf{75 mA}$$

Problem 2. At what velocity must a conductor 75 mm long cut a magnetic field of flux density 0.6 T if an e.m.f. of 9 V is to be induced in it? Assume the conductor, the field and the direction of motion are mutually perpendicular.

Induced e.m.f. $E = Blv$, hence velocity $v = E/Bl$
Thus

$$v = \frac{9}{(0.6)(75 \times 10^{-3})}$$
$$= \frac{9 \times 10^3}{0.6 \times 75}$$
$$= \textbf{200 m/s}$$

Problem 3. A conductor moves with a velocity of 15 m/s at an angle of (a) 90° (b) 60° and (c) 30° to a magnetic field produced between two square-faced poles of side length 2 cm. If the flux leaving a pole face is 5 μWb, find the magnitude of the induced e.m.f. in each case.

$v = 15$ m/s, length of conductor in magnetic field, $l = 2$ cm $= 0.02$ m, $A = 2 \times 2$ cm$^2 = 4 \times 10^{-4}$ m^2 and $\Phi = 5 \times 10^{-6}$ Wb

(a) $E_{90} = Blv \sin 90°$
$$= \left(\frac{\Phi}{A}\right) lv \sin 90°$$
$$= \left(\frac{5 \times 10^{-6}}{4 \times 10^{-4}}\right)(0.02)(15)(1)$$
$$= \textbf{3.75 mV}$$

(b) $E_{60} = Blv \sin 60° = E_{90} \sin 60°$
$$= 3.75 \sin 60° = \textbf{3.25 mV}$$

(c) $E_{30} = Blv \sin 30° = E_{90} \sin 30°$
$$= 3.75 \sin 30° = \textbf{1.875 mV}$$

Problem 4. The wing span of a metal aeroplane is 36 m. If the aeroplane is flying at 400 km/h, determine the e.m.f. induced between its wing tips. Assume the vertical component of the earth's magnetic field is 40 μT.

Induced e.m.f. across wing tips, $E = Blv$
$B = 40 \mu T = 40 \times 10^{-6}$ T, $l = 36$ m and

$$v = 400 \frac{\text{km}}{\text{h}} \times 1000 \frac{\text{m}}{\text{km}} \times \frac{1 \text{h}}{60 \times 60 \text{s}}$$

$$= \frac{(400)(1000)}{3600}$$

$$= \frac{4000}{36} \text{m/s}$$

Hence

$$E = Blv = (40 \times 10^{-6})(36)\left(\frac{4000}{36}\right)$$

$$= \mathbf{0.16\,V}$$

Problem 5. The diagrams shown in Fig. 9.4 represents the generation of e.m.f.'s. Determine (i) the direction in which the conductor has to be moved in Fig. 9.4(a), (ii) the direction of the induced e.m.f. in Fig. 9.4(b), (iii) the polarity of the magnetic system in Fig. 9.4(c).

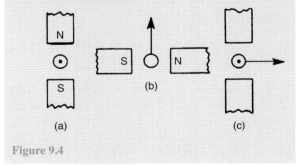

Figure 9.4

The direction of the e.m.f., and thus the current due to the e.m.f. may be obtained by either Lenz's law or Fleming's <u>R</u>ight-hand rule (i.e. Gene<u>R</u>ator rule).

(i) Using Lenz's law: The field due to the magnet and the field due to the current-carrying conductor are shown in Fig. 9.5(a) and are seen to reinforce to the left of the conductor. Hence the force on the conductor is to the right. However Lenz's law states that the direction of the induced e.m.f. is always such as to oppose the effect producing it. **Thus the conductor will have to be moved to the left**.

(ii) Using Fleming's right-hand rule:

First finger – <u>F</u>ield,

i.e. N → S, or right to left;

Thu<u>M</u>b – <u>M</u>otion, i.e. upwards;

S<u>E</u>cond finger – <u>E</u>.m.f.

i.e. **towards the viewer or out of the paper**, as shown in Fig. 9.5(b)

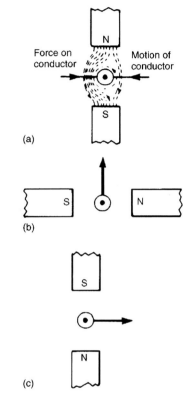

Figure 9.5

(iii) The polarity of the magnetic system of Fig. 9.4(c) is shown in Fig. 9.5(c) and is obtained using Fleming's right-hand rule.

Now try the following exercise

Exercise 43   Further problems on induced e.m.f.

1. A conductor of length 15 cm is moved at 750 mm/s at right-angles to a uniform flux density of 1.2 T. Determine the e.m.f. induced in the conductor. [0.135 V]

2. Find the speed that a conductor of length 120 mm must be moved at right-angles to a magnetic field of flux density 0.6 T to induce in it an e.m.f. of 1.8 V. [25 m/s]

3. A 25 cm long conductor moves at a uniform speed of 8 m/s through a uniform magnetic field of flux density 1.2 T. Determine the current flowing in the conductor when (a) its ends are open-circuited, (b) its ends are connected to a load of 15 ohms resistance.

[(a) 0 (b) 0.16 A]

4. A straight conductor 500 mm long is moved with constant velocity at right-angles both to its length and to a uniform magnetic field. Given that the e.m.f. induced in the conductor is 2.5 V and the velocity is 5 m/s, calculate the flux density of the magnetic field. If the conductor forms part of a closed circuit of total resistance 5 ohms, calculate the force on the conductor. [1 T, 0.25 N]

5. A car is travelling at 80 km/h. Assuming the back axle of the car is 1.76 m in length and the vertical component of the earth's magnetic field is 40 μT, find the e.m.f. generated in the axle due to motion. [1.56 mV]

6. A conductor moves with a velocity of 20 m/s at an angle of (a) 90° (b) 45° (c) 30°, to a magnetic field produced between two square-faced poles of side length 2.5 cm. If the flux on the pole face is 60 mWb, find the magnitude of the induced e.m.f. in each case.

[(a) 48 V (b) 33.9 V (c) 24 V]

7. A conductor 400 mm long is moved at 70° to a 0.85 T magnetic field. If it has a velocity of 115 km/h, calculate (a) the induced voltage, and (b) force acting on the conductor if connected to an 8 Ω resistor.

[(a) 10.21 V (b) 0.408 N]

9.3 Rotation of a loop in a magnetic field

Figure 9.6 shows a view of a looped conductor whose sides are moving across a magnetic field.

The left-hand side is moving in an upward direction (check using Fleming's right-hand rule), with length l cutting the lines of flux which are travelling from left to right. By definition, the induced e.m.f. will be equal to $Blv \sin \theta$ and flowing into the page.

The right-hand side is moving in a downward direction (again, check using Fleming's right-hand rule), with

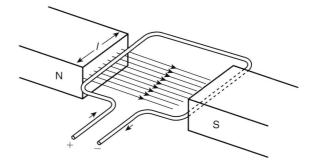

Figure 9.6

length l cutting the same lines of flux as above. The induced e.m.f. will also be equal to $Blv \sin \theta$ but flowing out of the page.

Therefore the total e.m.f. for the loop conductor = $2Blv \sin \theta$

Now consider a coil made up of a number of turns N

The total e.m.f. E for the loop conductor is now given by:

$$E = 2NBlv \sin \theta$$

Problem 6. A rectangular coil of sides 12 cm and 8 cm is rotated in a magnetic field of flux density 1.4 T, the longer side of the coil actually cutting this flux. The coil is made up of 80 turns and rotates at 1200 rev/min. (a) Calculate the maximum generated e.m.f. (b) If the coil generates 90 V, at what speed will the coil rotate?

(a) Generated e.m.f. $E = 2NBLv \sin \theta$

where number of turns, $N = 80$, flux density, $B = 1.4$ T,

length of conductor in magnetic field, $l = 12$ cm
$= 0.12$ m,

velocity, $v = \omega r = \left(\dfrac{1200}{60} \times 2\pi \text{ rad/s} \right) \left(\dfrac{0.08}{2} \text{ m} \right)$
$= 1.6\pi$ m/s,

and for maximum e.m.f. induced, $\theta = 90°$, from which, $\sin \theta = 1$

Hence, **maximum e.m.f. induced,**

$E = 2NBlv \sin \theta$

$= 2 \times 80 \times 1.4 \times 0.12 \times 1.6\pi \times 1$

$= \textbf{135.1 volts}$

(b) Since $\quad E = 2NBlv \sin \theta$

then $\quad\quad 90 = 2 \times 80 \times 1.4 \times 0.12 \times v \times 1$

from which, $v = \dfrac{90}{2 \times 80 \times 1.4 \times 0.12} = 3.348$ m/s

$v = \omega r$ hence, angular velocity, $\omega = \dfrac{v}{r} = \dfrac{3.348}{\dfrac{0.08}{2}}$

$= 83.7\,\text{rad/s}$

Speed of coil in rev/min $= \dfrac{83.7 \times 60}{2\pi}$

$= \mathbf{799\,rev/min}$

An **alternative method** of determining (b) is by **direct proportion**.

Since $E = 2NBlv\sin\theta$, then with N, B, l and θ being constant, $\boldsymbol{E \propto v}$

If from (a), 135.1 V is produced by a speed of 1200 rev/min,

then 1 V would be produced by a speed of $\dfrac{1200}{135.1} = 8.88\,\text{rev/min}$

Hence, 90 V would be produced by a speed of $90 \times 8.88 = \mathbf{799\,rev/min}$

Now try the following exercise

Exercise 44   Further problems on induced e.m.f. in a coil

1. A rectangular coil of sides 8 cm by 6 cm is rotating in a magnetic field such that the longer sides cut the magnetic field. Calculate the maximum generated e.m.f. if there are 60 turns on the coil, the flux density is 1.6 T and the coil rotates at 1500 rev/min.   [72.38 V]

2. A generating coil on a former 100 mm long has 120 turns and rotates in a 1.4 T magnetic field. Calculate the maximum e.m.f. generated if the coil, having a diameter of 60 mm, rotates at 450 rev/min.   [47.50 V]

3. If the coils in problems 1 and 2 generates 60 V, calculate (a) the new speed for each coil, and (b) the flux density required if the speed is unchanged.
   [(a) 1243 rev/min, 568 rev/min
   (b) 1.33 T, 1.77 T]

9.4   Inductance

Inductance is the name given to the property of a circuit whereby there is an e.m.f. induced into the circuit by the change of flux linkages produced by a current change.

When the e.m.f. is induced in the same circuit as that in which the current is changing, the property is called **self inductance, L**. When the e.m.f. is induced in a circuit by a change of flux due to current changing in an adjacent circuit, the property is called **mutual inductance, M**. The unit of inductance is the **henry, H**.

A circuit has an inductance of one henry when an e.m.f. of one volt is induced in it by a current changing at the rate of one ampere per second
Induced e.m.f. in a coil of N turns,

$$E = -N\frac{d\Phi}{dt}\ \text{volts}$$

where $d\Phi$ is the change in flux in Webers, and dt is the time taken for the flux to change in seconds (i.e. $\frac{d\Phi}{dt}$ is the rate of change of flux).

Induced e.m.f. in a coil of inductance L henrys,

$$E = -L\frac{dI}{dt}\ \text{volts}$$

where dI is the change in current in amperes and dt is the time taken for the current to change in seconds (i.e. $\frac{dI}{dt}$ is the rate of change of current). The minus sign in each of the above two equations remind us of its direction (given by Lenz's law).

Problem 7. Determine the e.m.f. induced in a coil of 200 turns when there is a change of flux of 25 mWb linking with it in 50 ms.

Induced e.m.f. $E = -N\dfrac{d\Phi}{dt} = -(200)\left(\dfrac{25 \times 10^{-3}}{50 \times 10^{-3}}\right)$

$= \mathbf{-100\,volts}$

Problem 8. A flux of 400 μWb passing through a 150-turn coil is reversed in 40 ms. Find the average e.m.f. induced.

Since the flux reverses, the flux changes from $+400\,\mu\text{Wb}$ to $-400\,\mu\text{Wb}$, a total change of flux of 800 μWb.

Induced e.m.f. $E = -N\dfrac{d\Phi}{dt} = -(150)\left(\dfrac{800 \times 10^{-6}}{40 \times 10^{-3}}\right)$

$= -\dfrac{150 \times 800 \times 10^{3}}{40 \times 10^{6}}$

Hence, **the average e.m.f. induced, E = −3 volts**

Problem 9. Calculate the e.m.f. induced in a coil of inductance 12 H by a current changing at the rate of 4 A/s.

Induced e.m.f. $E = -L\dfrac{\mathrm{d}I}{\mathrm{d}t} = -(12)(4)$

$$= -48\,\text{volts}$$

Problem 10. An e.m.f. of 1.5 kV is induced in a coil when a current of 4 A collapses uniformly to zero in 8 ms. Determine the inductance of the coil.

Change in current, $\mathrm{d}I = (4-0) = 4\,\text{A}$, $\mathrm{d}t = 8\,\text{ms} = 8 \times 10^{-3}\,\text{s}$,

$$\dfrac{\mathrm{d}I}{\mathrm{d}t} = \dfrac{4}{8 \times 10^{-3}} = \dfrac{4000}{8}$$

$$= 500\,\text{A/s}$$

and $\qquad E = 1.5\,\text{kV} = 1500\,\text{V}$

Since $\qquad |E| = L\dfrac{\mathrm{d}I}{\mathrm{d}t}$

inductance, $L = \dfrac{|E|}{(\mathrm{d}I/\mathrm{d}t)} = \dfrac{1500}{500} = \mathbf{3\,H}$

(Note that $|E|$ means the 'magnitude of E' which disregards the minus sign)

Problem 11. An average e.m.f. of 40 V is induced in a coil of inductance 150 mH when a current of 6 A is reversed. Calculate the time taken for the current to reverse.

$|E| = 40\,\text{V}$, $L = 150\,\text{mH} = 0.15\,\text{H}$ and change in current, $\mathrm{d}I = 6 - (-6) = 12\,\text{A}$ (since the current is reversed).

Since $|E| = \dfrac{\mathrm{d}I}{\mathrm{d}t}$

time $\mathrm{d}t = \dfrac{L\,\mathrm{d}I}{|E|} = \dfrac{(0.15)(12)}{40}$

$$= \mathbf{0.045\,s}\text{ or }\mathbf{45\,ms}$$

Now try the following exercise

Exercise 45 Further problems on inductance

1. Find the e.m.f. induced in a coil of 200 turns when there is a change of flux of 30 mWb linking with it in 40 ms. [−150 V]

2. An e.m.f. of 25 V is induced in a coil of 300 turns when the flux linking with it changes by 12 mWb. Find the time, in milliseconds, in which the flux makes the change. [144 ms]

3. An ignition coil having 10 000 turns has an e.m.f. of 8 kV induced in it. What rate of change of flux is required for this to happen? [0.8 Wb/s]

4. A flux of 0.35 mWb passing through a 125-turn coil is reversed in 25 ms. Find the magnitude of the average e.m.f. induced. [3.5 V]

5. Calculate the e.m.f. induced in a coil of inductance 6 H by a current changing at a rate of 15 A/s. [−90 V]

9.5 Inductors

A component called an inductor is used when the property of inductance is required in a circuit. The basic form of an inductor is simply a coil of wire. Factors which affect the inductance of an inductor include:

(i) the number of turns of wire – the more turns the higher the inductance

(ii) the cross-sectional area of the coil of wire – the greater the cross-sectional area the higher the inductance

(iii) the presence of a magnetic core – when the coil is wound on an iron core the same current sets up a more concentrated magnetic field and the inductance is increased

(iv) the way the turns are arranged – a short thick coil of wire has a higher inductance than a long thin one.

Two examples of practical inductors are shown in Fig. 9.7, and the standard electrical circuit diagram symbols for air-cored and iron-cored inductors are shown in Fig. 9.8.

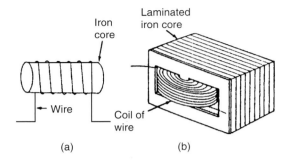

Figure 9.7

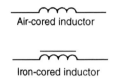

Figure 9.8

An iron-cored inductor is often called a **choke** since, when used in a.c. circuits, it has a choking effect, limiting the current flowing through it.

Inductance is often undesirable in a circuit. To reduce inductance to a minimum the wire may be bent back on itself, as shown in Fig. 9.9, so that the magnetising effect of one conductor is neutralised by that of the adjacent conductor. The wire may be coiled around an insulator, as shown, without increasing the inductance. Standard resistors may be non-inductively wound in this manner.

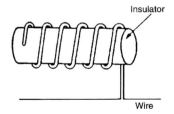

Figure 9.9

9.6 Energy stored

An inductor possesses an ability to store energy. The energy stored, W, in the magnetic field of an inductor is given by:

$$W = \frac{1}{2}LI^2 \text{ joules}$$

Problem 12. An 8 H inductor has a current of 3 A flowing through it. How much energy is stored in the magnetic field of the inductor?

Energy stored,

$$W = \frac{1}{2}LI^2 = \frac{1}{2}(8)(3)^2 = \textbf{36 joules}$$

Now try the following exercise

Exercise 46 Further problems on energy stored

1. An inductor of 20 H has a current of 2.5 A flowing in it. Find the energy stored in the magnetic field of the inductor. [62.5 J]

2. Calculate the value of the energy stored when a current of 30 mA is flowing in a coil of inductance 400 mH. [0.18 mJ]

3. The energy stored in the magnetic field of an inductor is 80 J when the current flowing in the inductor is 2 A. Calculate the inductance of the coil. [40 H]

9.7 Inductance of a coil

If a current changing from 0 to I amperes, produces a flux change from 0 to Φ webers, then $dI = I$ and $d\Phi = \Phi$. Then, from Section 9.3,

$$\text{induced e.m.f. } E = \frac{N\Phi}{t} = \frac{LI}{t}$$

from which, **inductance of coil,**

$$L = \frac{N\Phi}{I} \text{ henrys}$$

Since $E = -L\dfrac{dI}{dt} = -N\dfrac{d\Phi}{dt}$ then $L = N\dfrac{d\Phi}{dt}\left(\dfrac{dt}{dI}\right)$

i.e. $L = N\dfrac{d\Phi}{dI}$

From Chapter 7, m.m.f. $= \Phi S$ from which, $\Phi = \dfrac{\text{m.m.f}}{S}$

Substituting into $L = N\dfrac{\mathrm{d}\Phi}{\mathrm{d}I}$ gives

$$L = N\frac{\mathrm{d}}{\mathrm{d}I}\left(\frac{\text{m.m.f.}}{S}\right)$$

i.e. $$L = \frac{N}{S}\frac{\mathrm{d}(NI)}{\mathrm{d}I} \quad \text{since m.m.f.} = NI$$

i.e. $$L = \frac{N^2}{S}\frac{\mathrm{d}I}{\mathrm{d}I} \quad \text{and since } \frac{\mathrm{d}I}{\mathrm{d}I} = 1,$$

$$L = \frac{N^2}{S} \text{ henrys}$$

Problem 13. Calculate the coil inductance when a current of 4 A in a coil of 800 turns produces a flux of 5 mWb linking with the coil.

For a coil, inductance

$$L = \frac{N\Phi}{I} = \frac{(800)(5 \times 10^{-3})}{4} = \mathbf{1\,H}$$

Problem 14. A flux of 25 mWb links with a 1500 turn coil when a current of 3 A passes through the coil. Calculate (a) the inductance of the coil, (b) the energy stored in the magnetic field, and (c) the average e.m.f. induced if the current falls to zero in 150 ms.

(a) **Inductance,**

$$L = \frac{N\Phi}{I} = \frac{(1500)(25 \times 10^{-3})}{3} = \mathbf{12.5\,H}$$

(b) **Energy stored,**

$$W = \frac{1}{2}LI^2 = \frac{1}{2}(12.5)(3)^2 = \mathbf{56.25\,J}$$

(c) **Induced e.m.f.,**

$$E = -L\frac{\mathrm{d}I}{\mathrm{d}t} = -(12.5)\left(\frac{3-0}{150 \times 10^{-3}}\right)$$
$$= \mathbf{-250\,V}$$

(Alternatively,

$$E = -N\frac{\mathrm{d}\Phi}{\mathrm{d}t}$$
$$= -(1500)\left(\frac{25 \times 10^{-3}}{150 \times 10^{-3}}\right)$$
$$= \mathbf{-250\,V}$$

since if the current falls to zero so does the flux)

Problem 15. When a current of 1.5 A flows in a coil the flux linking with the coil is 90 μWb. If the coil inductance is 0.60 H, calculate the number of turns of the coil.

For a coil, $L = \dfrac{N\Phi}{I}$

Thus $$N = \frac{LI}{\Phi} = \frac{(0.6)(1.5)}{90 \times 10^{-6}} = \mathbf{10\,000\,turns}$$

Problem 16. A 750 turn coil of inductance 3 H carries a current of 2 A. Calculate the flux linking the coil and the e.m.f. induced in the coil when the current collapses to zero in 20 ms.

Coil inductance, $L = \dfrac{N\Phi}{I}$ from which,

flux $$\Phi = \frac{LI}{N} = \frac{(3)(2)}{750} = 8 \times 10^{-3} = \mathbf{8\,mWb}$$

Induced e.m.f.

$$E = -L\frac{\mathrm{d}I}{\mathrm{d}t} = -(3)\left(\frac{2-0}{20 \times 10^{-3}}\right)$$
$$= \mathbf{-300\,V}$$

(Alternatively,

$$E = -N\frac{\mathrm{d}\Phi}{\mathrm{d}t} = -(750)\left(\frac{8 \times 10^{-3}}{20 \times 10^{-3}}\right)$$
$$= \mathbf{-300\,V})$$

Problem 17. A silicon iron ring is wound with 800 turns, the ring having a mean diameter of 120 mm and a cross-sectional area of 400 mm². If when carrying a current of 0.5 A the relative permeability is found to be 3000, calculate (a) the self-inductance of the coil, (b) the induced e.m.f. if the current is reduced to zero in 80 ms.

The ring is shown sketched in Fig. 9.10.

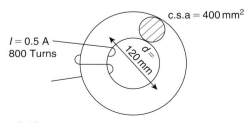

Figure 9.10

(a) Inductance, $L = \dfrac{N^2}{S}$ and from Chapter 7,

reluctance, $S = \dfrac{l}{\mu_0 \mu_r A}$

i.e. $S = \dfrac{\pi \times 120 \times 10^{-3}}{4\pi \times 10^{-7} \times 3000 \times 400 \times 10^{-6}}$

$= 250 \times 10^3 \text{ A/Wb}$

Hence, **self-inductance**, $L = \dfrac{N^2}{S} = \dfrac{800^2}{250 \times 10^3}$

$= \mathbf{2.56\,H}$

(b) **Induced e.m.f.**, $E = -L\dfrac{dI}{dt} = -(2.56)\dfrac{(0.5 - 0)}{80 \times 10^{-3}}$

$= \mathbf{-16\,V}$

Now try the following exercise

Exercise 47   Further problems on the inductance of a coil

1. A flux of 30 mWb links with a 1200 turn coil when a current of 5 A is passing through the coil. Calculate (a) the inductance of the coil, (b) the energy stored in the magnetic field, and (c) the average e.m.f. induced if the current is reduced to zero in 0.20 s.
   [(a) 7.2 H (b) 90 J (c) 180 V]

2. An e.m.f. of 2 kV is induced in a coil when a current of 5 A collapses uniformly to zero in 10 ms. Determine the inductance of the coil.
   [4 H]

3. An average e.m.f. of 60 V is induced in a coil of inductance 160 mH when a current of 7.5 A is reversed. Calculate the time taken for the current to reverse.
   [40 ms]

4. A coil of 2500 turns has a flux of 10 mWb linking with it when carrying a current of 2 A. Calculate the coil inductance and the e.m.f. induced in the coil when the current collapses to zero in 20 ms.
   [12.5 H, 1.25 kV]

5. Calculate the coil inductance when a current of 5 A in a coil of 1000 turns produces a flux of 8 mWb linking with the coil.
   [1.6 H]

6. A coil is wound with 600 turns and has a self inductance of 2.5 H. What current must flow to set up a flux of 20 mWb?
   [4.8 A]

7. When a current of 2 A flows in a coil, the flux linking with the coil is 80 μWb. If the coil inductance is 0.5 H, calculate the number of turns of the coil.
   [12 500]

8. A coil of 1200 turns has a flux of 15 mWb linking with it when carrying a current of 4 A. Calculate the coil inductance and the e.m.f. induced in the coil when the current collapses to zero in 25 ms.
   [4.5 H, 720 V]

9. A coil has 300 turns and an inductance of 4.5 mH. How many turns would be needed to produce a 0.72 mH coil assuming the same core is used?
   [48 turns]

10. A steady current of 5 A when flowing in a coil of 1000 turns produces a magnetic flux of 500 μWb. Calculate the inductance of the coil. The current of 5 A is then reversed in 12.5 ms. Calculate the e.m.f. induced in the coil.
    [0.1 H, 80 V]

11. An iron ring has a cross-sectional area of 500 mm² and a mean length of 300 mm. It is wound with 100 turns and its relative permeability is 1600. Calculate (a) the current required to set up a flux of 500 μWb in the coil, (b) the inductance of the system, and (c) the induced e.m.f. if the field collapses in 1 ms.
    [(a) 1.492 A (b) 33.51 mH (c) −50 V]

9.8   Mutual inductance

Mutually induced e.m.f. in the second coil,

$$E_2 = -M\dfrac{dI_1}{dt} \text{ volts}$$

where M is the **mutual inductance** between two coils, in henrys, and (dI_1/dt) is the rate of change of current in the first coil.

The phenomenon of mutual inductance is used in **transformers** (see Chapter 21, page 333)

Another expression for M

Let an iron ring have two coils, A and B, wound on it. If the fluxes Φ_1 and Φ_2 are produced from currents I_1 and I_2 in coils A and B respectively, then the reluctance could be expressed as:

$$S = \dfrac{I_1 N_1}{\Phi_1} = \dfrac{I_2 N_2}{\Phi_2}$$

If the flux in coils A and B are the same and produced from the current I_1 in coil A only, assuming 100% coupling, then the mutual inductance can be expressed as:

$$M = \frac{N_2 \Phi_1}{I_1}$$

Multiplying by $\left(\dfrac{N_1}{N_1}\right)$ gives:

$$M = \frac{N_2 \Phi_1 N_1}{I_1 N_1}$$

However,
$$S = \frac{I_1 N_1}{\Phi_1}$$

Thus, **mutual inductance**, $M = \dfrac{N_1 N_2}{S}$

Problem 18. Calculate the mutual inductance between two coils when a current changing at 200 A/s in one coil induces an e.m.f. of 1.5 V in the other.

Induced e.m.f. $|E_2| = M\, dI_1/dt$, i.e. $1.5 = M(200)$. Thus **mutual inductance**,

$$M = \frac{1.5}{200} = 0.0075\,\text{H or } 7.5\,\text{mH}$$

Problem 19. The mutual inductance between two coils is 18 mH. Calculate the steady rate of change of current in one coil to induce an e.m.f. of 0.72 V in the other.

Induced e.m.f. $|E_2| = M \dfrac{dI_1}{dt}$

Hence rate of change of current,

$$\frac{dI_1}{dt} = \frac{|E_2|}{M} = \frac{0.72}{0.018} = 40\,\text{A/s}$$

Problem 20. Two coils have a mutual inductance of 0.2 H. If the current in one coil is changed from 10 A to 4 A in 10 ms, calculate (a) the average induced e.m.f. in the second coil, (b) the change of flux linked with the second coil if it is wound with 500 turns.

(a) Induced e.m.f.

$$|E_2| = -M\frac{dI_1}{dt}$$
$$= -(0.2)\left(\frac{10-4}{10 \times 10^{-3}}\right) = -120\,\text{V}$$

(b) Induced e.m.f.

$$|E_2| = N\frac{d\Phi}{dt}, \text{ hence } d\Phi = \frac{|E_2|dt}{N}$$

Thus the change of flux,

$$d\Phi = \frac{(120)(10 \times 10^{-3})}{500} = 2.4\,\text{mWb}$$

Problem 21. In the device shown in Fig. 9.11, when the current in the primary coil of 1000 turns increases linearly from 1 A to 6 A in 200 ms, an e.m.f. of 15 V is induced into the secondary coil of 480 turns, which is left open circuited. Determine (a) the mutual inductance of the two coils, (b) the reluctance of the former, and (c) the self-inductance of the primary coil.

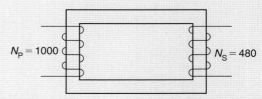

Figure 9.11

(a) $E_S = M\dfrac{dI_p}{dt}$ from which,

mutual inductance, $M = \dfrac{E_S}{\dfrac{dI_P}{dt}} = \dfrac{15}{\left(\dfrac{6-1}{200 \times 10^{-3}}\right)}$

$$= \frac{15}{25} = 0.60\,\text{H}$$

(b) $M = \dfrac{N_P N_S}{S}$ from which,

reluctance, $S = \dfrac{N_P N_S}{M} = \dfrac{(1000)(480)}{0.60}$

$$= 800\,000\,\text{A/Wb or } 800\,\text{kA/Wb}$$

(c) Primary self-inductance, $L_P = \dfrac{N_P^2}{S} = \dfrac{(1000)^2}{800\,000}$

$$= 1.25\,\text{H}$$

Now try the following exercises

Exercise 48 **Further problems on mutual inductance**

1. The mutual inductance between two coils is 150 mH. Find the magnitude of the e.m.f. induced in one coil when the current in the other is increasing at a rate of 30 A/s.

[4.5 V]

2. Determine the mutual inductance between two coils when a current changing at 50 A/s in one coil induces an e.m.f. of 80 mV in the other.

[1.6 mH]

3. Two coils have a mutual inductance of 0.75 H. Calculate the magnitude of the e.m.f. induced in one coil when a current of 2.5 A in the other coil is reversed in 15 ms. [250 V]

4. The mutual inductance between two coils is 240 mH. If the current in one coil changes from 15 A to 6 A in 12 ms, calculate (a) the average e.m.f. induced in the other coil, (b) the change of flux linked with the other coil if it is wound with 400 turns.

[(a) −180 V (b) 5.4 mWb]

5. A mutual inductance of 0.06 H exists between two coils. If a current of 6 A in one coil is reversed in 0.8 s calculate (a) the average e.m.f. induced in the other coil, (b) the number of turns on the other coil if the flux change linking with the other coil is 5 mWb.

[(a) −0.9 V (b) 144]

6. When the current in the primary coil of 400 turns of a magnetic circuit increases linearly from 10 mA to 35 mA in 100 ms, an e.m.f. of 75 mV is induced into the secondary coil of 240 turns, which is left open circuited. Determine (a) the mutual inductance of the two coils, (b) the reluctance of the former, and (c) the self-inductance of the secondary coil.

[(a) 0.30 H (b) 320 kA/Wb (c) 0.18 H]

Exercise 49 **Short answer questions on electromagnetic induction**

1. What is electromagnetic induction?

2. State Faraday's laws of electromagnetic induction

3. State Lenz's law

4. Explain briefly the principle of the generator

5. The direction of an induced e.m.f. in a generator may be determined using Fleming's . . . . . . rule

6. The e.m.f. E induced in a moving conductor may be calculated using the formula $E = Blv$. Name the quantities represented and their units

7. The total e.m.f., E, for a loop conductor with N turns is given by: $E = \ldots\ldots\ldots\ldots$

8. What is self-inductance? State its symbol

9. State and define the unit of inductance

10. When a circuit has an inductance L and the current changes at a rate of (di/dt) then the induced e.m.f. E is given by $E = \ldots\ldots$ volts

11. If a current of I amperes flowing in a coil of N turns produces a flux of Φ webers, the coil inductance L is given by $L = \ldots\ldots$ henrys

12. The energy W stored by an inductor is given by $W = \ldots\ldots$ joules

13. If the number of turns of a coil is N and its reluctance is S, then the inductance, L, is given by: $L = \ldots\ldots\ldots$

14. What is mutual inductance? State its symbol

15. The mutual inductance between two coils is M. The e.m.f. E_2 induced in one coil by the current changing at (dI_1/dt) in the other is given by $E_2 = \ldots\ldots$ volts

16. Two coils wound on an iron ring of reluctance S have N_A and N_B turns respectively. The mutual inductance, M, is given by: $M = \ldots\ldots\ldots$

Exercise 50 **Multi-choice questions on electromagnetic induction**
(Answers on page 420)

1. A current changing at a rate of 5 A/s in a coil of inductance 5 H induces an e.m.f. of:

(a) 25 V in the same direction as the applied voltage

(b) 1 V in the same direction as the applied voltage

(c) 25 V in the opposite direction to the applied voltage

(d) 1 V in the opposite direction to the applied voltage

2. A bar magnet is moved at a steady speed of 1.0 m/s towards a coil of wire which is connected to a centre-zero galvanometer. The magnet is now withdrawn along the same path at 0.5 m/s. The deflection of the galvanometer is in the:

(a) same direction as previously, with the magnitude of the deflection doubled

(b) opposite direction as previously, with the magnitude of the deflection halved

(c) same direction as previously, with the magnitude of the deflection halved

(d) opposite direction as previously, with the magnitude of the deflection doubled

3. When a magnetic flux of 10 Wb links with a circuit of 20 turns in 2 s, the induced e.m.f. is:

(a) 1 V   (b) 4 V

(c) 100 V   (d) 400 V

4. A current of 10 A in a coil of 1000 turns produces a flux of 10 mWb linking with the coil. The coil inductance is:

(a) 10^6 H   (b) 1 H

(c) 1 µH   (d) 1 mH

5. An e.m.f. of 1 V is induced in a conductor moving at 10 cm/s in a magnetic field of 0.5 T. The effective length of the conductor in the magnetic field is:

(a) 20 cm   (b) 5 m

(c) 20 m   (d) 50 m

6. Which of the following is false?

(a) Fleming's left-hand rule or Lenz's law may be used to determine the direction of an induced e.m.f.

(b) An induced e.m.f. is set up whenever the magnetic field linking that circuit changes

(c) The direction of an induced e.m.f. is always such as to oppose the effect producing it

(d) The induced e.m.f. in any circuit is proportional to the rate of change of the magnetic flux linking the circuit

7. The effect of inductance occurs in an electrical circuit when:

(a) the resistance is changing

(b) the flux is changing

(c) the current is changing

8. Which of the following statements is false? The inductance of an inductor increases:

(a) with a short, thick coil

(b) when wound on an iron core

(c) as the number of turns increases

(d) as the cross-sectional area of the coil decreases

9. The mutual inductance between two coils, when a current changing at 20 A/s in one coil induces an e.m.f. of 10 mV in the other, is:

(a) 0.5 H   (b) 200 mH

(c) 0.5 mH   (d) 2 H

10. A strong permanent magnet is plunged into a coil and left in the coil. What is the effect produced on the coil after a short time?

(a) There is no effect

(b) The insulation of the coil burns out

(c) A high voltage is induced

(d) The coil winding becomes hot

11. Self-inductance occurs when:

(a) the current is changing

(b) the circuit is changing

(c) the flux is changing

(d) the resistance is changing

12. Faraday's laws of electromagnetic induction are related to:

(a) the e.m.f. of a chemical cell

(b) the e.m.f. of a generator

(c) the current flowing in a conductor

(d) the strength of a magnetic field

Chapter 10

Electrical measuring instruments and measurements

At the end of this chapter you should be able to:

- recognize the importance of testing and measurements in electric circuits
- appreciate the essential devices comprising an analogue instrument
- explain the operation of an attraction and a repulsion type of moving-iron instrument
- explain the operation of a moving-coil rectifier instrument
- compare moving-coil, moving-iron and moving-coil rectifier instruments
- calculate values of shunts for ammeters and multipliers for voltmeters
- understand the advantages of electronic instruments
- understand the operation of an ohmmeter/megger
- appreciate the operation of multimeters/Avometers /Flukes
- understand the operation of a wattmeter
- appreciate instrument 'loading' effect
- understand the operation of an oscilloscope for d.c. and a.c. measurements
- calculate periodic time, frequency, peak-to-peak values from waveforms on an oscilloscope
- appreciate virtual test and measuring instruments
- recognize harmonics present in complex waveforms
- determine ratios of powers, currents and voltages in decibels
- understand null methods of measurement for a Wheatstone bridge and d.c. potentiometer
- understand the operation of a.c. bridges
- understand the operation of a Q-meter
- appreciate the most likely source of errors in measurements
- appreciate calibration accuracy of instruments

DOI: 10.1016/B978-0-08-089056-2.00010-3

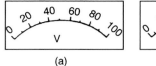
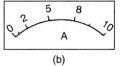

(a)   (b)

Figure 10.1

10.1 Introduction

Tests and measurements are important in designing, evaluating, maintaining and servicing electrical circuits and equipment. In order to detect electrical quantities such as current, voltage, resistance or power, it is necessary to transform an electrical quantity or condition into a visible indication. This is done with the aid of instruments (or meters) that indicate the magnitude of quantities either by the position of a pointer moving over a graduated scale (called an analogue instrument) or in the form of a decimal number (called a digital instrument).

The digital instrument has, in the main, become the instrument of choice in recent years; in particular, computer-based instruments are rapidly replacing items of conventional test equipment, with the virtual storage test instrument, the **digital storage oscilloscope**, being the most common. This is explained later in this chapter, but before that some analogue instruments, which are still used in some installations, are explored.

10.2 Analogue instruments

All analogue electrical indicating instruments require three essential devices:

(a) A deflecting or operating device. A mechanical force is produced by the current or voltage which causes the pointer to deflect from its zero position.

(b) A controlling device. The controlling force acts in opposition to the deflecting force and ensures that the deflection shown on the meter is always the same for a given measured quantity. It also prevents the pointer always going to the maximum deflection. There are two main types of controlling device – spring control and gravity control.

(c) A damping device. The damping force ensures that the pointer comes to rest in its final position quickly and without undue oscillation. There are three main types of damping used – eddy-current damping, air-friction damping and fluid-friction damping.

There are basically **two types of scale** – linear and non-linear. A linear scale is shown in Fig. 10.1(a), where the divisions or graduations are evenly spaced. The voltmeter shown has a range 0–100 V, i.e. a full-scale deflection (f.s.d.) of 100 V. A non-linear scale is shown in Fig. 10.1(b) where the scale is cramped at the

beginning and the graduations are uneven throughout the range. The ammeter shown has a f.s.d. of 10 A.

10.3 Moving-iron instrument

(a) An attraction type of moving-iron instrument is shown diagrammatically in Fig. 10.2(a). When current flows in the solenoid, a pivoted soft-iron disc is attracted towards the solenoid and the movement causes a pointer to move across a scale.

(b) In the repulsion type moving-iron instrument shown diagrammatically in Fig. 10.2(b), two pieces of iron are placed inside the solenoid, one being fixed, and the other attached to the spindle carrying the pointer. When current passes through the solenoid, the two pieces of iron are magnetised in the same direction and therefore repel each other. The pointer thus moves across the scale. The force moving the pointer is, in each type, proportional to I^2 and because of this the

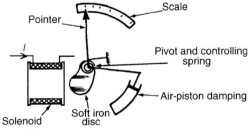

(a)   ATTRACTION TYPE

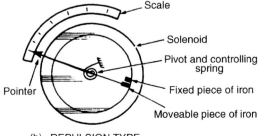

(b)   REPULSION TYPE

Figure 10.2

direction of current does not matter. The moving-iron instrument can be used on d.c. or a.c.; the scale, however, is non-linear.

10.4 The moving-coil rectifier instrument

A moving-coil instrument, which measures only d.c., may be used in conjunction with a bridge rectifier circuit as shown in Fig. 10.3 to provide an indication of alternating currents and voltages (see Chapter 14). The average value of the full wave rectified current is 0.637 I_m. However, a meter being used to measure a.c. is usually calibrated in r.m.s. values. For sinusoidal quantities the indication is $(0.707 I_m)/(0.637 I_m)$ i.e. 1.11 times the mean value. Rectifier instruments have scales calibrated in r.m.s. quantities and it is assumed by the manufacturer that the a.c. is sinusoidal.

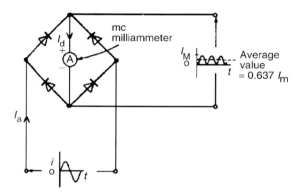

Figure 10.3

10.5 Comparison of moving-coil, moving-iron and moving-coil rectifier instruments

See Table at top of next page. (For the principle of operation of a moving-coil instrument, see Chapter 8, page 98.)

10.6 Shunts and multipliers

An **ammeter**, which measures current, has a low resistance (ideally zero) and must be connected in series with the circuit.

A **voltmeter**, which measures p.d., has a high resistance (ideally infinite) and must be connected in parallel with the part of the circuit whose p.d. is required.

There is no difference between the basic instrument used to measure current and voltage since both use a milliammeter as their basic part. This is a sensitive instrument which gives f.s.d. for currents of only a few milliamperes. When an ammeter is required to measure currents of larger magnitude, a proportion of the current is diverted through a low-value resistance connected in parallel with the meter. Such a diverting resistor is called a **shunt**.

From Fig. 10.4(a), $V_{PQ} = V_{RS}$.

Hence $I_a r_a = I_s R_s$. Thus the value of the shunt,

$$R_s = \frac{I_a r_a}{I_s} \text{ ohms}$$

The milliammeter is converted into a voltmeter by connecting a high value resistance (called a **multiplier**) in series with it as shown in Fig. 10.4(b). From Fig. 10.4(b),

$$V = V_a + V_M = I r_a + I R_M$$

Thus the value of the multiplier,

$$R_M = \frac{V - I r_a}{I} \text{ ohms}$$

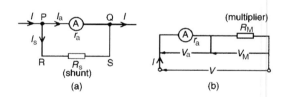

Figure 10.4

Problem 1. A moving-coil instrument gives a f.s.d. when the current is 40 mA and its resistance is 25 Ω. Calculate the value of the shunt to be connected in parallel with the meter to enable it to be used as an ammeter for measuring currents up to 50 A.

The circuit diagram is shown in Fig. 10.5, where r_a = resistance of instrument = 25 Ω, R_s = resistance

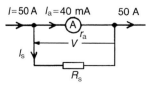

Figure 10.5

Type of instrument	Moving-coil	Moving-iron	Moving-coil rectifier
Suitable for measuring	Direct current and voltage	Direct and alternating currents and voltage (reading in r.m.s. value)	Alternating current and voltage (reads average value but scale is adjusted to give r.m.s. value for sinusoidal waveforms)
Scale	Linear	Non-linear	Linear
Method of control	Hairsprings	Hairsprings	Hairsprings
Method of damping	Eddy current	Air	Eddy current
Frequency limits	—	20–200 Hz	20–100 kHz
Advantages	1. Linear scale 2. High sensitivity 3. Well shielded from stray magnetic fields 4. Low power consumption	1. Robust construction 2. Relatively cheap 3. Measures dc and ac 4. In frequency range 20–100 Hz reads r.m.s. correctly regardless of supply wave-form	1. Linear scale 2. High sensitivity 3. Well shielded from stray magnetic fields 4. Lower power consumption 5. Good frequency range
Disadvantages	1. Only suitable for dc 2. More expensive than moving iron type 3. Easily damaged	1. Non-linear scale 2. Affected by stray magnetic fields 3. Hysteresis errors in dc circuits 4. Liable to temperature errors 5. Due to the inductance of the solenoid, readings can be affected by variation of frequency	1. More expensive than moving iron type 2. Errors caused when supply is non-sinusoidal

of shunt, I_a = maximum permissible current flowing in instrument = 40 mA = 0.04 A, I_s = current flowing in shunt and I = total circuit current required to give f.s.d. = 50 A.

Since $I = I_a + I_s$ then $I_s = I - I_a$

i.e. $I_s = 50 - 0.04 = 49.96$ A

$V = I_a r_a = I_s R_s$, hence

$R_s = \dfrac{I_a r_a}{I_s} = \dfrac{(0.04)(25)}{49.96} = 0.02002\,\Omega$

$= \mathbf{20.02\,m\Omega}$

Thus for the moving-coil instrument to be used as an ammeter with a range 0–50 A, a resistance of value 20.02 mΩ needs to be connected in parallel with the instrument.

Problem 2. A moving-coil instrument having a resistance of 10 Ω, gives a f.s.d. when the current is 8 mA. Calculate the value of the multiplier to be connected in series with the instrument so that it can be used as a voltmeter for measuring p.d.s. up to 100 V.

The circuit diagram is shown in Fig. 10.6, where r_a = resistance of instrument = 10 Ω, R_M = resistance

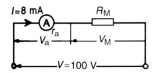

Figure 10.6

of multiplier I = total permissible instrument current = 8 mA = 0.008 A, V = total p.d. required to give f.s.d. = 100 V

$$V = V_a + V_M = Ir_a + IR_M$$

i.e. $100 = (0.008)(10) + (0.008)R_M$

or $100 - 0.08 = 0.008 R_M$, thus

$$R_M = \frac{99.92}{0.008} = 12\,490\,\Omega = \mathbf{12.49\,k\Omega}$$

Hence for the moving-coil instrument to be used as a voltmeter with a range 0–100 V, a resistance of value 12.49 kΩ needs to be connected in series with the instrument.

Now try the following exercise

Exercise 51   Further problems on shunts and multipliers

1. A moving-coil instrument gives f.s.d. for a current of 10 mA. Neglecting the resistance of the instrument, calculate the approximate value of series resistance needed to enable the instrument to measure up to (a) 20 V (b) 100 V (c) 250 V.   [(a) 2 kΩ (b) 10 kΩ (c) 25 kΩ]

2. A meter of resistance 50 Ω has a f.s.d. of 4 mA. Determine the value of shunt resistance required in order that f.s.d. should be (a) 15 mA (b) 20 A (c) 100 A.
    [(a) 18.18 Ω (b) 10.00 mΩ (c) 2.00 mΩ]

3. A moving-coil instrument having a resistance of 20 Ω, gives a f.s.d. when the current is 5 mA. Calculate the value of the multiplier to be connected in series with the instrument so that it can be used as a voltmeter for measuring p.d.'s up to 200 V.   [39.98 kΩ]

4. A moving-coil instrument has a f.s.d. of 20 mA and a resistance of 25 Ω. Calculate the

values of resistance required to enable the instrument to be used (a) as a 0–10 A ammeter, and (b) as a 0–100 V voltmeter. State the mode of resistance connection in each case.
[(a) 50.10 mΩ in parallel
(b) 4.975 kΩ in series]

5. A meter has a resistance of 40 Ω and registers a maximum deflection when a current of 15 mA flows. Calculate the value of resistance that converts the movement into (a) an ammeter with a maximum deflection of 50 A, and (b) a voltmeter with a range 0–250 V.
[(a) 12.00 mΩ in parallel
(b) 16.63 kΩ in series]

10.7   Electronic instruments

Electronic measuring instruments have advantages over instruments such as the moving-iron or moving-coil meters, in that they have a much higher input resistance (some as high as 1000 MΩ) and can handle a much wider range of frequency (from d.c. up to MHz).

The digital voltmeter (DVM) is one which provides a digital display of the voltage being measured. Advantages of a DVM over analogue instruments include higher accuracy and resolution, no observational or parallex errors (see Section 10.22) and a very high input resistance, constant on all ranges.

A digital multimeter is a DVM with additional circuitry which makes it capable of measuring a.c. voltage, d.c. and a.c. current and resistance.

Instruments for a.c. measurements are generally calibrated with a sinusoidal alternating waveform to indicate r.m.s. values when a sinusoidal signal is applied to the instrument. Some instruments, such as the moving-iron and electro-dynamic instruments, give a true r.m.s. indication. With other instruments the indication is either scaled up from the mean value (such as with the rectified moving-coil instrument) or scaled down from the peak value.

Sometimes quantities to be measured have complex waveforms (see Section 10.15), and whenever a quantity is non-sinusoidal, errors in instrument readings can occur if the instrument has been calibrated for sine waves only. Such waveform errors can be largely eliminated by using electronic instruments.

10.8   The ohmmeter

An **ohmmeter** is an instrument for measuring electrical resistance. A simple ohmmeter circuit is shown in Fig. 10.7(a). Unlike the ammeter or voltmeter, the ohmmeter circuit does not receive the energy necessary for its operation from the circuit under test. In the ohmmeter this energy is supplied by a self-contained source of voltage, such as a battery. Initially, terminals XX are short-circuited and R adjusted to give f.s.d. on the milliammeter. If current I is at a maximum value and voltage E is constant, then resistance $R = E/I$ is at a minimum value. Thus f.s.d. on the milliammeter is made zero on the resistance scale. When terminals XX are open circuited no current flows and $R (= E/O)$ is infinity, ∞.

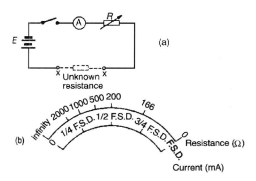

Figure 10.7

The milliammeter can thus be calibrated directly in ohms. A cramped (non-linear) scale results and is 'back to front', as shown in Fig. 10.7(b). When calibrated, an unknown resistance is placed between terminals XX and its value determined from the position of the pointer on the scale. An ohmmeter designed for measuring low values of resistance is called a **continuity tester**. An ohmmeter designed for measuring high values of resistance (i.e. megohms) is called an **insulation resistance tester** (e.g. '**Megger**').

10.9   Multimeters

Instruments are manufactured that combine a moving-coil meter with a number of shunts and series multipliers, to provide a range of readings on a single scale graduated to read current and voltage. If a battery is incorporated then resistance can also be measured. Such instruments are called **multimeters** or **universal instruments** or **multirange instruments**. An 'Avometer' is a typical example. A particular range may be selected either by the use of separate terminals or by a selector switch. Only one measurement can be performed at a time. Often such instruments can be used in a.c. as well as d.c. circuits when a rectifier is incorporated in the instrument.

Digital Multimeters (DMM) are now almost universally used, the **Fluke Digital Multimeter** being an industry leader for performance, accuracy, resolution, ruggedness, reliability and safety. These instruments measure d.c. currents and voltages, resistance and continuity, a.c. (r.m.s.) currents and voltages, temperature, and much more.

10.10   Wattmeters

A **wattmeter** is an instrument for measuring electrical power in a circuit. Figure 10.8 shows typical connections of a wattmeter used for measuring power supplied to a load. The instrument has two coils:

(i)   a current coil, which is connected in series with the load, like an ammeter, and

(ii)   a voltage coil, which is connected in parallel with the load, like a voltmeter.

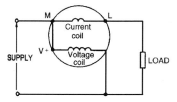

Figure 10.8

10.11   Instrument 'loading' effect

Some measuring instruments depend for their operation on power taken from the circuit in which measurements are being made. Depending on the 'loading' effect of the instrument (i.e. the current taken to enable it to operate), the prevailing circuit conditions may change.

The resistance of voltmeters may be calculated since each have a stated sensitivity (or 'figure of merit'), often stated in 'kΩ per volt' of f.s.d. A voltmeter should have as high a resistance as possible (– ideally infinite). In a.c. circuits the impedance of the instrument varies with frequency and thus the loading effect of the instrument can change.

Problem 3. Calculate the power dissipated by the voltmeter and by resistor R in Fig. 10.9 when (a) $R = 250\,\Omega$ (b) $R = 2\,M\Omega$. Assume that the voltmeter sensitivity (sometimes called figure of merit) is $10\,k\Omega/V$.

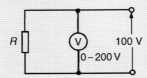

Figure 10.9

(a) Resistance of voltmeter, R_v = sensitivity × f.s.d. Hence, $R_v = (10\ k\Omega/V) \times (200\ V) = 2000\,k\Omega = 2\,M\Omega$. Current flowing in voltmeter,

$$I_v = \frac{V}{R_v} = \frac{100}{2 \times 10^6} = 50 \times 10^{-6}\,A$$

Power dissipated by voltmeter

$$= VI_v = (100)(50 \times 10^{-6}) = \mathbf{5\,mW}.$$

When $R = 250\,\Omega$, current in resistor,

$$I_R = \frac{V}{R} = \frac{100}{250} = \mathbf{0.4\,A}$$

Power dissipated in load resistor $R = VI_R = (100)(0.4) = \mathbf{40\,W}$. Thus the power dissipated in the voltmeter is insignificant in comparison with the power dissipated in the load.

(b) When $R = 2\,M\Omega$, current in resistor,

$$I_R = \frac{V}{R} = \frac{100}{2 \times 10^6} = 50 \times 10^{-6}\,A$$

Power dissipated in load resistor $R = VI_R = 100 \times 50 \times 10^{-6} = \mathbf{5\,mW}$. In this case the higher load resistance reduced the power dissipated such that the voltmeter is using as much power as the load.

Problem 4. An ammeter has a f.s.d. of $100\,mA$ and a resistance of $50\,\Omega$. The ammeter is used to measure the current in a load of resistance $500\,\Omega$ when the supply voltage is $10\,V$. Calculate (a) the ammeter reading expected (neglecting its resistance), (b) the actual current in the circuit, (c) the power dissipated in the ammeter, and (d) the power dissipated in the load.

From Fig. 10.10,

(a) expected ammeter reading $= V/R = 10/500$
$$= \mathbf{20\,mA}.$$

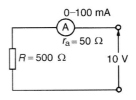

Figure 10.10

(b) Actual ammeter reading
$$= V/(R + r_a) = 10/(500 + 50)$$
$$= \mathbf{18.18\,mA}.$$

Thus the ammeter itself has caused the circuit conditions to change from $20\,mA$ to $18.18\,mA$.

(c) Power dissipated in the ammeter
$$= I^2 r_a = (18.18 \times 10^{-3})^2(50) = \mathbf{16.53\,mW}.$$

(d) Power dissipated in the load resistor
$$= I^2 R = (18.18 \times 10^{-3})^2(500) = \mathbf{165.3\,mW}.$$

Problem 5. A voltmeter having a f.s.d. of $100\,V$ and a sensitivity of $1.6\,k\Omega/V$ is used to measure voltage V_1 in the circuit of Fig. 10.11. Determine (a) the value of voltage V_1 with the voltmeter not connected, and (b) the voltage indicated by the voltmeter when connected between A and B.

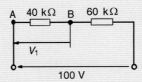

Figure 10.11

(a) By voltage division,

$$V_1 = \left(\frac{40}{40 + 60}\right)100 = \mathbf{40\,V}$$

(b) The resistance of a voltmeter having a $100\,V$ f.s.d. and sensitivity $1.6\,k\Omega/V$ is $100\,V \times 1.6\,k\Omega/V = 160\,k\Omega$. When the voltmeter is connected across the $40\,k\Omega$ resistor the circuit is as shown in Fig. 10.12(a) and the equivalent resistance of the parallel network is given by

$$\left(\frac{40 \times 160}{40 + 160}\right)k\Omega$$

i.e. $$\left(\frac{40 \times 160}{200}\right)k\Omega = 32\,k\Omega$$

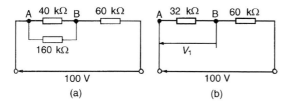

Figure 10.12

The circuit is now effectively as shown in Fig. 10.12(b). Thus the voltage indicated on the voltmeter is

$$\left(\frac{32}{32+60}\right)100\,\text{V} = \mathbf{34.78\,V}$$

A considerable error is thus caused by the loading effect of the voltmeter on the circuit. The error is reduced by using a voltmeter with a higher sensitivity.

Problem 6.　(a) A current of 20 A flows through a load having a resistance of 2 Ω. Determine the power dissipated in the load. (b) A wattmeter, whose current coil has a resistance of 0.01 Ω is connected as shown in Fig. 10.13. Determine the wattmeter reading.

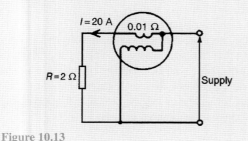

Figure 10.13

(a)　Power dissipated in the load, $P = I^2 R = (20)^2(2)$
$$= \mathbf{800\,W}$$

(b)　With the wattmeter connected in the circuit the total resistance R_T is $2 + 0.01 = 2.01\,\Omega$. The wattmeter reading is thus $I^2 R_T = (20)^2(2.01)$
$$= \mathbf{804\,W}$$

Now try the following exercise

Exercise 52　**Further problems on instrument 'loading' effects**

1.　A 0–1 A ammeter having a resistance of 50 Ω is used to measure the current flowing in a 1 kΩ

resistor when the supply voltage is 250 V. Calculate: (a) the approximate value of current (neglecting the ammeter resistance), (b) the actual current in the circuit, (c) the power dissipated in the ammeter, (d) the power dissipated in the 1 kΩ resistor.　　[(a) 0.250 A
(b) 0.238 A (c) 2.832 W (d) 56.64 W]

2.　(a) A current of 15 A flows through a load having a resistance of 4 Ω. Determine the power dissipated in the load. (b) A wattmeter, whose current coil has a resistance of 0.02 Ω is connected (as shown in Fig. 10.13) to measure the power in the load. Determine the wattmeter reading assuming the current in the load is still 15 A.　　[(a) 900 W (b) 904.5 W]

3.　A voltage of 240 V is applied to a circuit consisting of an 800 Ω resistor in series with a 1.6 kΩ resistor. What is the voltage across the 1.6 kΩ resistor? The p.d. across the 1.6 kΩ resistor is measured by a voltmeter of f.s.d. 250 V and sensitivity 100 Ω/V. Determine the voltage indicated.　　[160 V; 156.7 V]

4.　A 240 V supply is connected across a load resistance R. Also connected across R is a voltmeter having a f.s.d. of 300 V and a figure of merit (i.e. sensitivity) of 8 kΩ/V. Calculate the power dissipated by the voltmeter and by the load resistance if (a) $R = 100\,\Omega$ (b) $R = 1\,\text{M}\Omega$. Comment on the results obtained.
　　[(a) 24 mW, 576 W (b) 24 mW, 57.6 mW]

10.12　The oscilloscope

The oscilloscope is basically a graph-displaying device – it draws a graph of an electrical signal. In most applications the graph shows how signals change over time. From the graph it is possible to:

• determine the time and voltage values of a signal

• calculate the frequency of an oscillating signal

• see the 'moving parts' of a circuit represented by the signal

• tell if a malfunctioning component is distorting the signal

• find out how much of a signal is d.c. or a.c.

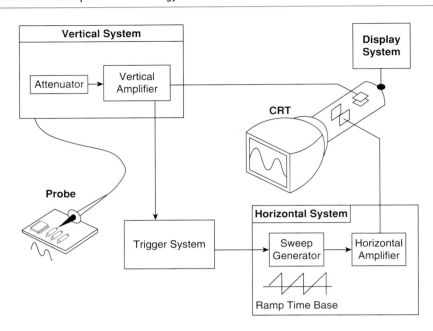

Figure 10.14

• tell how much of the signal is noise and whether the noise is changing with time

Oscilloscopes are used by everyone from television repair technicians to physicists. They are indispensable for anyone designing or repairing electronic equipment. The usefulness of an oscilloscope is not limited to the world of electronics. With the proper transducer (i.e. a device that creates an electrical signal in response to physical stimuli, such as sound, mechanical stress, pressure, light or heat), an oscilloscope can measure any kind of phenomena. An automobile engineer uses an oscilloscope to measure engine vibrations; a medical researcher uses an oscilloscope to measure brain waves, and so on.

Oscilloscopes are available in both analogue and digital types. An **analogue oscilloscope** works by directly applying a voltage being measured to an electron beam moving across the oscilloscope screen. The voltage deflects the beam up or down proportionally, tracing the waveform on the screen. This gives an immediate picture of the waveform.

In contrast, a **digital oscilloscope** samples the waveform and uses an analogue to digital converter (see Section 19.11, page 307) to convert the voltage being measured into digital information. It then uses this digital information to reconstruct the waveform on the screen.

For many applications either an analogue or digital oscilloscope is appropriate. However, each type does

possess some unique characteristics making it more or less suitable for specific tasks.

Analogue oscilloscopes are often preferred when it is important to display rapidly varying signals in 'real time' (i.e. as they occur).

Digital oscilloscopes allow the capture and viewing of events that happen only once. They can process the digital waveform data or send the data to a computer for processing. Also, they can store the digital waveform data for later viewing and printing. Digital storage oscilloscopes are explained in Section 10.14.

Analogue oscilloscopes

When an oscilloscope probe is connected to a circuit, the voltage signal travels through the probe to the vertical system of the oscilloscope. Figure 10.14 shows a simple block diagram that shows how an analogue oscilloscope displays a measured signal.

Depending on how the vertical scale (volts/division control) is set, an attenuator reduces the signal voltage or an amplifier increases the signal voltage. Next, the signal travels directly to the vertical deflection plates of the cathode ray tube (CRT). Voltage applied to these deflection plates causes a glowing dot to move. (An electron beam hitting phosphor inside the CRT creates the glowing dot.) A positive voltage causes the dot to move up while a negative voltage causes the dot to move down.

The signal also travels to the trigger system to start or trigger a 'horizontal sweep'. Horizontal sweep is a term referring to the action of the horizontal system causing the glowing dot to move across the screen. Triggering the horizontal system causes the horizontal time base to move the glowing dot across the screen from left to right within a specific time interval. Many sweeps in rapid sequence cause the movement of the glowing dot to blend into a solid line. At higher speeds, the dot may sweep across the screen up to 500 000 times each second.

Together, the horizontal sweeping action (i.e. the X direction) and the vertical deflection action (i.e. the Y direction), traces a graph of the signal on the screen. The trigger is necessary to stabilise a repeating signal. It ensures that the sweep begins at the same point of a repeating signal, resulting in a clear picture.

In conclusion, to use an analogue oscilloscope, three basic settings to accommodate an incoming signal need to be adjusted:

- the attenuation or amplification of the signal – use the volts/division control to adjust the amplitude of the signal before it is applied to the vertical deflection plates

- the time base – use the time/division control to set the amount of time per division represented horizontally across the screen

- the triggering of the oscilloscope – use the trigger level to stabilise a repeating signal, as well as triggering on a single event.

Also, adjusting the focus and intensity controls enable a sharp, visible display to be created.

(i) With **direct voltage measurements**, only the Y amplifier 'volts/cm' switch on the oscilloscope is used. With no voltage applied to the Y plates the position of the spot trace on the screen is noted. When a direct voltage is applied to the Y plates the new position of the spot trace is an indication of the magnitude of the voltage. For example, in Fig. 10.15(a), with no voltage applied to the Y plates, the spot trace is in the centre of the screen (initial position) and then the spot trace moves 2.5 cm to the final position shown, on application of a d.c. voltage. With the 'volts/cm' switch on 10 volts/cm the magnitude of the direct voltage is 2.5 cm × 10 volts/cm, i.e. 25 volts.

(ii) With **alternating voltage measurements**, let a sinusoidal waveform be displayed on an oscilloscope screen as shown in Fig. 10.15(b). If the time/cm switch is on, say, 5 ms/cm then the

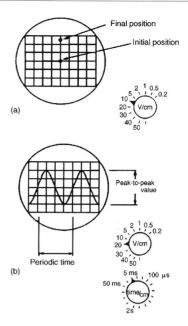

Figure 10.15

periodic time T of the sinewave is 5 ms/cm × 4 cm, i.e. **20 ms** or **0.02 s**. Since frequency

$$f = \frac{1}{T}, \ \textbf{frequency} = \frac{1}{0.02} = \textbf{50 Hz}$$

If the 'volts/cm' switch is on, say, 20 volts/cm then the **amplitude** or **peak value** of the sinewave shown is 20 volts/cm × 2 cm, i.e. 40 V. Since

$$\text{r.m.s. voltage} = \frac{\text{peak voltage}}{\sqrt{2}} \ (\text{see Chapter 14}),$$

$$\textbf{r.m.s. voltage} = \frac{40}{\sqrt{2}} = \textbf{28.28 volts}$$

Double beam oscilloscopes are useful whenever two signals are to be compared simultaneously. The c.r.o. demands reasonable skill in adjustment and use. However its greatest advantage is in observing the shape of a waveform – a feature not possessed by other measuring instruments.

Digital oscilloscopes

Some of the systems that make up digital oscilloscopes are the same as those in analogue oscilloscopes; however, digital oscilloscopes contain additional data processing systems – as shown in the block diagram of Fig. 10.16. With the added systems, the digital oscilloscope collects data for the entire waveform and then displays it.

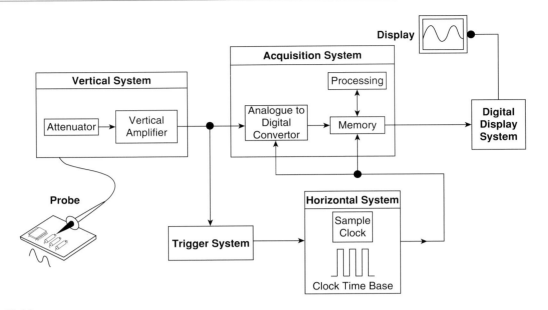

Figure 10.16

When a digital oscilloscope probe is attached to a circuit, the vertical system adjusts the amplitude of the signal, just as in the analogue oscilloscope. Next, the analogue to digital converter (ADC) in the acquisition system samples the signal at discrete points in time and converts the signals' voltage at these points to digital values called *sample points*. The horizontal systems' sample clock determines how often the ADC takes a sample. The rate at which the clock 'ticks' is called the sample rate and is measured in samples per second.

The sample points from the ADC are stored in memory as *waveform points*. More than one sample point may make up one waveform point.

Together, the waveform points make up one waveform *record*. The number of waveform points used to make a waveform record is called a *record length*. The trigger system determines the start and stop points of the record. The display receives these record points after being stored in memory.

Depending on the capabilities of an oscilloscope, additional processing of the sample points may take place, enhancing the display. Pre-trigger may be available, allowing events to be seen before the trigger point.

Fundamentally, with a digital oscilloscope as with an analogue oscilloscope, there is a need to adjust vertical, horizontal, and trigger settings to take a measurement.

> **Problem 7.** For the oscilloscope square voltage waveform shown in Fig. 10.17 determine (a) the

periodic time, (b) the frequency, and (c) the peak-to-peak voltage. The 'time/cm' (or timebase control) switch is on $100\,\mu s/cm$ and the 'volts/cm' (or signal amplitude control) switch is on $20\,V/cm$.

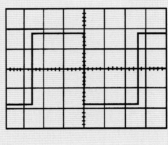

Figure 10.17

(*In Figs. 10.17 to 10.20 assume that the squares shown are 1 cm by 1 cm*)

(a) The width of one complete cycle is 5.2 cm. Hence the periodic time,
$$T = 5.2\,cm \times 100 \times 10^{-6}\,s/cm = \mathbf{0.52\ ms}.$$

(b) Frequency, $f = \dfrac{1}{T} = \dfrac{1}{0.52 \times 10^{-3}} = \mathbf{1.92\,kHz}$.

(c) The peak-to-peak height of the display is 3.6 cm, hence the peak-to-peak voltage
$$= 3.6\,cm \times 20\,V/cm = \mathbf{72\,V}$$

Problem 8. For the oscilloscope display of a pulse waveform shown in Fig. 10.18 the 'time/cm' switch is on 50 ms/cm and the 'volts/cm' switch is on 0.2 V/cm. Determine (a) the periodic time, (b) the frequency, (c) the magnitude of the pulse voltage.

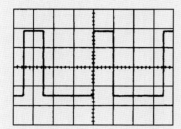

Figure 10.18

(a) The width of one complete cycle is 3.5 cm. Hence the periodic time,
$$T = 3.5\,\text{cm} \times 50\,\text{ms/cm} = \textbf{175\,ms}.$$

(b) Frequency, $f = \dfrac{1}{T} = \dfrac{1}{0.52 \times 10^{-3}} = \textbf{5.71\,Hz}.$

(c) The height of a pulse is 3.4 cm hence the magnitude of the pulse voltage
$$= 3.4\,\text{cm} \times 0.2\,\text{V/cm} = \textbf{0.68\,V}$$

Problem 9. A sinusoidal voltage trace displayed by an oscilloscope is shown in Fig. 10.19. If the 'time/cm' switch is on 500 µs/cm and the 'volts/cm' switch is on 5 V/cm, find, for the waveform, (a) the frequency, (b) the peak-to-peak voltage, (c) the amplitude, (d) the r.m.s. value.

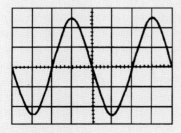

Figure 10.19

(a) The width of one complete cycle is 4 cm. Hence the periodic time, T is 4 cm × 500 µs/cm, i.e. 2 ms.

Frequency, $f = \dfrac{1}{T} = \dfrac{1}{2 \times 10^{-3}} = \textbf{500\,Hz}$

(b) The peak-to-peak height of the waveform is 5 cm. Hence the peak-to-peak voltage
$$= 5\,\text{cm} \times 5\,\text{V/cm} = \textbf{25\,V}.$$

(c) Amplitude $= \frac{1}{2} \times 25\,\text{V} = \textbf{12.5\,V}$

(d) The peak value of voltage is the amplitude, i.e. 12.5 V, and r.m.s.
$$\text{voltage} = \frac{\text{peak voltage}}{\sqrt{2}} = \frac{12.5}{\sqrt{2}} = \textbf{8.84\,V}$$

Problem 10. For the double-beam oscilloscope displays shown in Fig. 10.20 determine (a) their frequency, (b) their r.m.s. values, (c) their phase difference. The 'time/cm' switch is on 100 µs/cm and the 'volts/cm' switch on 2 V/cm.

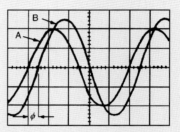

Figure 10.20

(a) The width of each complete cycle is 5 cm for both waveforms. Hence the periodic time, T, of each waveform is 5 cm × 100 µs/cm, i.e. 0.5 ms. Frequency of each waveform,
$$f = \frac{1}{T} = \frac{1}{0.5 \times 10^{-3}} = \textbf{2\,kHz}$$

(b) The peak value of waveform A is 2 cm × 2 V/cm = **4 V**, hence the r.m.s. value of waveform A
$$= 4/(\sqrt{2}) = \textbf{2.83\,V}$$

The peak value of waveform B is 2.5 cm × 2 V/cm = 5 V, hence the r.m.s. value of waveform B
$$= 5/(\sqrt{2}) = \textbf{3.54\,V}$$

(c)   Since 5 cm represents 1 cycle, then 5 cm represents 360°, i.e. 1 cm represents $360/5 = 72°$. The phase angle $\phi = 0.5$ cm

$$= 0.5 \text{ cm} \times 72°/\text{cm} = 36°.$$

Hence waveform A leads waveform B by 36°.

Now try the following exercise

Exercise 53   Further problems on the cathode ray oscilloscope

1.   For the square voltage waveform displayed on an oscilloscope shown in Fig. 10.21, find (a) its frequency, (b) its peak-to-peak voltage.
   [(a) 41.7 Hz (b) 176 V]

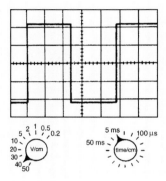

Figure 10.21

2.   For the pulse waveform shown in Fig. 10.22, find (a) its frequency, (b) the magnitude of the pulse voltage.   [(a) 0.56 Hz (b) 8.4 V]

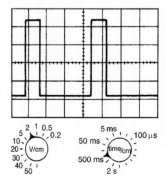

Figure 10.22

3.   For the sinusoidal waveform shown in Fig. 10.23, determine (a) its frequency,

(b) the peak-to-peak voltage, (c) the r.m.s. voltage.
   [(a) 7.14 Hz (b) 220 V (c) 77.78 V]

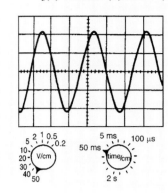

Figure 10.23

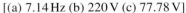

10.13   Virtual test and measuring instruments

Computer-based instruments are rapidly replacing items of conventional test equipment in many of today's test and measurement applications. Probably the most commonly available virtual test instrument is the digital storage oscilloscope (DSO). Because of the processing power available from the PC coupled with the mass storage capability, a computer-based virtual DSO is able to provide a variety of additional functions, such as spectrum analysis and digital display of both frequency and voltage. In addition, the ability to save waveforms and captured measurement data for future analysis or for comparison purposes can be extremely valuable, particularly where evidence of conformance with standards or specifications is required.

Unlike a conventional oscilloscope (which is primarily intended for waveform display) a computer-based virtual oscilloscope effectively combines several test instruments in one single package. The functions and available measurements from such an instrument usually includes:

- real time or stored waveform display

- precise time and voltage measurement (using adjustable cursors)

- digital display of voltage

- digital display of frequency and/or periodic time

- accurate measurement of phase angle

- frequency spectrum display and analysis

- data logging (stored waveform data can be exported in formats that are compatible with conventional spreadsheet packages, e.g. as .xls files)

- ability to save/print waveforms and other information in graphical format (e.g. as .jpg or .bmp files).

Virtual instruments can take various forms including:

- internal hardware in the form of a conventional PCI expansion card

- external hardware unit which is connected to the PC by means of either a conventional 25-pin parallel port connector or by means of a serial USB connector

The software (and any necessary drivers) is invariably supplied on CD-ROM or can be downloaded from the manufacturer's web site. Some manufacturers also supply software drivers together with sufficient accompanying documentation in order to allow users to control virtual test instruments from their own software developed using popular programming languages such as VisualBASIC or C++.

10.14   Virtual digital storage oscilloscopes

Several types of virtual DSO are currently available. These can be conveniently arranged into three different categories according to their application:

- Low-cost DSO

- High-speed DSO

- High-resolution DSO

Unfortunately, there is often some confusion between the last two categories. A high-speed DSO is designed for examining waveforms that are rapidly changing. Such an instrument does not necessarily provide high-resolution measurement. Similarly, a high-resolution DSO is useful for displaying waveforms with a high degree of precision but it may not be suitable for examining fast waveforms. The difference between these two types of DSO should become a little clearer later on.

Low-cost DSO are primarily designed for low frequency signals (typically signals up to around 20 kHz) and are usually able to sample their signals at rates

of between 10K and 100K samples per second. Resolution is usually limited to either 8-bits or 12-bits (corresponding to 256 and 4096 discrete voltage levels respectively).

High-speed DSOs are rapidly replacing CRT-based oscilloscopes. They are invariably dual-channel instruments and provide all the features associated with a conventional 'scope including trigger selection, timebase and voltage ranges, and an ability to operate in X-Y mode.

Additional features available with a computer-based instrument include the ability to capture transient signals (as with a conventional digital storage 'scope') and save waveforms for future analysis. The ability to analyse a signal in terms of its frequency spectrum is yet another feature that is only possible with a DSO (see later).

Upper frequency limit

The upper signal frequency limit of a DSO is determined primarily by the rate at which it can sample an incoming signal. Typical sampling rates for different types of virtual instrument are:

Type of DSO	Typical sampling rate
Low-cost DSO	20 K to 100 K per second
High-speed DSO	100 M to 1000 M per second
High-resolution DSO	20 M to 100 M per second

In order to display waveforms with reasonable accuracy it is normally suggested that the sampling rate should be *at least* twice and *preferably more* than five times the highest signal frequency. Thus, in order to display a 10 MHz signal with any degree of accuracy a sampling rate of 50M samples per second will be required.

The 'five times rule' merits a little explanation. When sampling signals in a digital to analogue converter we usually apply the Nyquist criterion that the sampling frequency must be at least twice the highest analogue signal frequency. Unfortunately, this no longer applies in the case of a DSO where we need to sample at an even faster rate if we are to accurately display the signal. In practice we would need a minimum of about five points within a single cycle of a sampled waveform in order to reproduce it with approximate fidelity. Hence the sampling rate should be at least five times that of highest signal frequency in order to display a waveform reasonably faithfully.

A special case exists with dual-channel DSOs. Here the sampling rate may be shared between the two channels. Thus an effective sampling rate of 20M samples per second might equate to 10M samples per second for *each* of the two channels. In such a case the upper frequency limit would not be 4 MHz but only a mere 2 MHz.

The approximate bandwidth required to display different types of signals with reasonable precision is given in the table below:

Signal	Bandwidth required (approx)
Low-frequency and power	d.c. to 10 kHz
Audio frequency (general)	d.c. to 20 kHz
Audio frequency (high-quality)	d.c. to 50 kHz
Square and pulse waveforms (up to 5 kHz)	d.c. to 100 kHz
Fast pulses with small rise-times	d.c. to 1 MHz
Video	d.c. to 10 MHz
Radio (LF, MF and HF)	d.c. to 50 MHz

The general rule is that, for sinusoidal signals, the bandwidth should ideally be at least double that of the highest signal frequency whilst for square wave and pulse signals, the bandwidth should be at least ten times that of the highest signal frequency.

It is worth noting that most manufacturers define the bandwidth of an instrument as the frequency at which a sine wave input signal will fall to 0.707 of its true amplitude (i.e. the −3 dB point). To put this into context, at the cut-off frequency the displayed trace will be in error by a whopping 29%!

Resolution

The relationship between resolution and signal accuracy (not bandwidth) is simply that the more bits used in the conversion process the more discrete voltage levels

can be resolved by the DSO. The relationship is as follows:

$$x = 2^n$$

where x is the number of discrete voltage levels and n is the number of bits. Thus, each time we use an additional bit in the conversion process we double the resolution of the DSO, as shown in the table below:

Number of bits, n	Number of discrete voltage levels, x
8-bit	256
10-bit	1024
12-bit	4096
16-bit	65 536

Buffer memory capacity

A DSO stores its captured waveform samples in a buffer memory. Hence, for a given sampling rate, the size of this memory buffer will determine for how long the DSO can capture a signal before its buffer memory becomes full.

The relationship between sampling rate and buffer memory capacity is important. A DSO with a high sampling rate but small memory will only be able to use its full sampling rate on the top few time base ranges.

To put this into context, it's worth considering a simple example. Assume that we need to display 10 000 cycles of a 10 MHz square wave. This signal will occur in a time frame of 1 ms. If applying the 'five times rule' we would need a bandwidth of at least 50 MHz to display this signal accurately.

To reconstruct the square wave we would need a minimum of about five samples per cycle so a minimum sampling rate would be 5 × 10 MHz = 50M samples per second. To capture data at the rate of 50M samples per second for a time interval of 1 ms requires a memory that can store 50 000 samples. If each sample uses 16-bits we would require 100 kbyte of extremely fast memory.

Accuracy

The measurement resolution or measurement accuracy of a DSO (in terms of the smallest voltage change that can be measured) depends on the actual range that is selected. So, for example, on the 1 V range an 8-bit DSO is able to detect a voltage change of one two hundred and fifty sixth of a volt or (1/256) V or about 4 mV. For most measurement applications this will prove to be perfectly adequate as it amounts to an accuracy of about 0.4% of full-scale.

Figure 10.24 depicts a PicoScope software display showing multiple windows providing conventional oscilloscope waveform display, spectrum analyser display, frequency display, and voltmeter display.

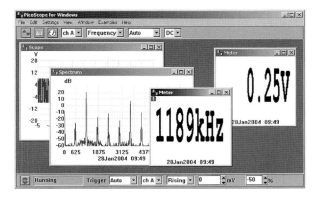

Figure 10.24

Adjustable cursors make it possible to carry out extremely accurate measurements. In Fig. 10.25, the peak value of the (nominal 10 V peak) waveform is measured at precisely 9625 mV (9.625 V). The time to reach the peak value (from 0 V) is measured as 246.7 μs (0.2467 ms).

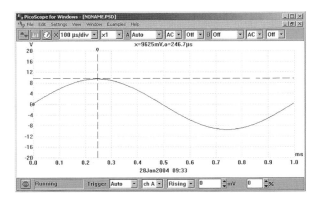

Figure 10.25

The addition of a second time cursor makes it possible to measure the time accurately between two events. In Fig. 10.26, event 'o' occurs 131 ns before the trigger point whilst event 'x' occurs 397 ns after the trigger point. The elapsed time between these two events is

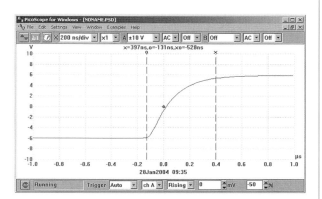

Figure 10.26

528 ns. The two cursors can be adjusted by means of the mouse (or other pointing device) or, more accurately, using the PC's cursor keys.

Autoranging

Autoranging is another very useful feature that is often provided with a virtual DSO. If you regularly use a conventional 'scope for a variety of measurements you will know only too well how many times you need to make adjustments to the vertical sensitivity of the instrument.

High-resolution DSO

High-resolution DSOs are used for precision applications where it is necessary to faithfully reproduce a waveform and also to be able to perform an accurate analysis of noise floor and harmonic content. Typical applications include small signal work and high-quality audio.

Unlike the low-cost DSO, which typically has 8-bit resolution and poor d.c. accuracy, these units are usually accurate to better than 1% and have either 12-bit or 16-bit resolution. This makes them ideal for audio, noise and vibration measurements.

The increased resolution also allows the instrument to be used as a spectrum analyser with very wide dynamic range (up to 100 dB). This feature is ideal for performing noise and distortion measurements on low-level analogue circuits.

Bandwidth alone is not enough to ensure that a DSO can accurately capture a high frequency signal. The goal of manufacturers is to achieve a flat frequency response. This response is sometimes referred to as a Maximally Flat Envelope Delay (MFED). A frequency response of this type delivers excellent pulse fidelity with minimum overshoot, undershoot and ringing.

It is important to remember that, if the input signal is not a pure sine wave it will contain a number of higher frequency harmonics. For example, a square wave will contain odd harmonics that have levels that become progressively reduced as their frequency increases. Thus, to display a 1 MHz square wave accurately you need to take into account the fact that there will be signal components present at 3 MHz, 5 MHz, 7 MHz, 9 MHz, 11 MHz, and so on.

Spectrum analysis

The technique of Fast Fourier Transformation (FFT) calculated using software algorithms using data captured by a virtual DSO has made it possible to produce frequency spectrum displays. Such displays can be to investigate the harmonic content of waveforms as well as the relationship between several signals within a composite waveform.

Figure 10.27 shows the frequency spectrum of the 1 kHz sine wave signal from a low-distortion signal generator. Here the virtual DSO has been set to capture samples at a rate of 4096 per second within a frequency range of d.c. to 12.2 kHz. The display clearly shows the second harmonic (at a level of −50 dB or −70 dB relative to the fundamental), plus further harmonics at 3 kHz, 5 kHz and 7 kHz (all of which are greater than 75 dB down on the fundamental).

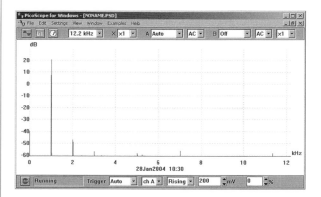

Figure 10.27

Problem 11. Figure 10.28 shows the frequency spectrum of a signal at 1184 kHz displayed by a high-speed virtual DSO. Determine (a) the harmonic relationship between the signals marked 'o' and 'x', (b) the difference in amplitude (expressed in dB) between the signals marked 'o'

and 'x', and (c) the amplitude of the second harmonic relative to the fundamental signal 'o'.

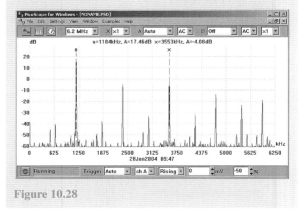

Figure 10.28

(a) The signal x is at a frequency of 3553 kHz. This is three times the frequency of the signal at 'o' which is at 1184 kHz. Thus, **x is the third harmonic of the signal 'o'**

(b) The signal at 'o' has an amplitude of +17.46 dB whilst the signal at 'x' has an amplitude of −4.08 dB. Thus, **the difference in level** = $(+17.46) − (−4.08) = $ **21.54 dB**

(c) **The amplitude of the second harmonic** (shown at approximately 2270 kHz) = **−5 dB**

10.15 Waveform harmonics

(i) Let an instantaneous voltage v be represented by $v = V_m \sin 2\pi ft$ volts. This is a waveform which varies sinusoidally with time t, has a frequency f, and a maximum value V_m. Alternating voltages are usually assumed to have wave-shapes which are sinusoidal where only one frequency is present. If the waveform is not sinusoidal it is called a **complex wave**, and, whatever its shape, it may be split up mathematically into components called the **fundamental** and a number of **harmonics**. This process is called harmonic analysis. The fundamental (or first harmonic) is sinusoidal and has the supply frequency, f; the other harmonics are also sine waves having frequencies which are integer multiples of f. Thus, if the supply frequency is 50 Hz, then the third harmonic frequency is 150 Hz, the fifth 250 Hz, and so on.

(ii) A complex waveform comprising the sum of the fundamental and a third harmonic of about half the amplitude of the fundamental is shown in Fig. 10.29(a), both waveforms being initially in phase with each other. If further odd harmonic waveforms of the appropriate amplitudes are added, a good approximation to a square wave results. In Fig. 10.29(b), the third harmonic is shown having an initial phase displacement from the fundamental. The positive and negative half cycles of each of the complex waveforms shown in Figs 10.29(a) and (b) are identical in shape, and this is a feature of waveforms containing the fundamental and only odd harmonics.

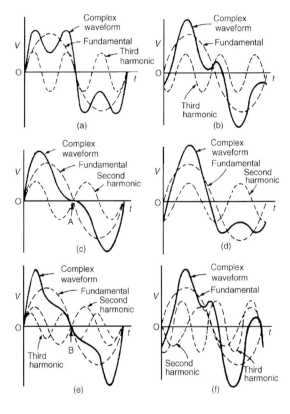

Figure 10.29

(iii)   A complex waveform comprising the sum of the fundamental and a second harmonic of about half the amplitude of the fundamental is shown in Fig. 10.29(c), each waveform being initially in phase with each other. If further even harmonics of appropriate amplitudes are added a good approximation to a triangular wave results. In Fig. 10.29(c), the negative cycle, if reversed, appears as a mirror image of the positive cycle about point A. In Fig. 10.29(d) the second harmonic is shown with an initial phase

displacement from the fundamental and the positive and negative half cycles are dissimilar.

(iv)   A complex waveform comprising the sum of the fundamental, a second harmonic and a third harmonic is shown in Fig. 10.29(e), each waveform being initially 'in-phase'. The negative half cycle, if reversed, appears as a mirror image of the positive cycle about point B. In Fig. 10.29(f), a complex waveform comprising the sum of the fundamental, a second harmonic and a third harmonic are shown with initial phase displacement. The positive and negative half cycles are seen to be dissimilar.

The features mentioned relative to Figs 10.29(a) to (f) make it possible to recognize the harmonics present in a complex waveform displayed on a CRO.

10.16   Logarithmic ratios

In electronic systems, the ratio of two similar quantities measured at different points in the system, are often expressed in logarithmic units. By definition, if the ratio of two powers P_1 and P_2 is to be expressed in **decibel (dB) units** then the number of decibels, X, is given by:

$$X = 10\lg\left(\frac{P_2}{P_1}\right)\text{dB} \qquad (1)$$

Thus, when the power ratio, $P_2/P_1 = 1$ then the decibel power ratio $= 10\lg 1 = 0$, when the power ratio, $P_2/P_1 = 100$ then the decibel power ratio $= 10\lg 100 = +20$ (i.e. a power gain), and when the power ratio, $P_2/P_1 = 1/100$ then the decibel power ratio $= 10\lg 1/100 = -20$ (i.e. a power loss or attenuation).

Logarithmic units may also be used for voltage and current ratios. Power, P, is given by $P = I^2R$ or $P = V^2/R$. Substituting in equation (1) gives:

$$X = 10\lg\left(\frac{I_2^2 R_2}{I_1^2 R_1}\right)\text{dB}$$

or $$X = 10\lg\left(\frac{V_2^2/R_2}{V_1^2/R_1}\right)\text{dB}$$

If $R_1 = R_2$,

then $$X = 10\lg\left(\frac{I_2^2}{I_1^2}\right)\text{dB}$$

or

$$X = 10 \lg\left(\frac{V_2^2}{V_1^2}\right) dB$$

i.e. $X = 20 \lg\left(\dfrac{I_2}{I_1}\right) dB$

or $X = 20 \lg\left(\dfrac{V_2}{V_1}\right) dB$

(from the laws of logarithms).

From equation (1), X decibels is a logarithmic ratio of two similar quantities and is not an absolute unit of measurement. It is therefore necessary to state a **reference level** to measure a number of decibels above or below that reference. The most widely used reference level for power is 1 mW, and when power levels are expressed in decibels, above or below the 1 mW reference level, the unit given to the new power level is dBm.

A voltmeter can be re-scaled to indicate the power level directly in decibels. The scale is generally calibrated by taking a reference level of 0 dB when a power of 1 mW is dissipated in a 600 Ω resistor (this being the natural impedance of a simple transmission line). The reference voltage V is then obtained from

$$P = \frac{V^2}{R},$$

i.e. $1 \times 10^{-3} = \dfrac{V^2}{600}$

from which, $V = 0.775$ volts. In general, the number of dBm,

$$X = 20 \lg\left(\frac{V}{0.775}\right)$$

Thus $V = 0.20$ V corresponds to $20 \lg\left(\dfrac{0.2}{0.775}\right)$

$$= -11.77 \, dBm \text{ and}$$

$V = 0.90$ V corresponds to $20 \lg\left(\dfrac{0.90}{0.775}\right)$

$$= +1.3 \, dBm, \text{ and so on.}$$

A typical **decibelmeter**, or **dB meter**, scale is shown in Fig. 10.30. Errors are introduced with dB meters when the circuit impedance is not 600 Ω.

Problem 12.   The ratio of two powers is (a) 3 (b) 20 (c) 4 (d) 1/20. Determine the decibel power ratio in each case.

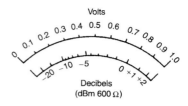

Figure 10.30

From above, the power ratio in decibels, X, is given by:
$X = 10 \lg(P_2/P_1)$

(a)   When $\dfrac{P_2}{P_1} = 3$,

$$X = 10 \lg(3) = 10(0.477)$$
$$= \mathbf{4.77 \, dB}$$

(b)   When $\dfrac{P_2}{P_1} = 20$,

$$X = 10 \lg(20) = 10(1.30)$$
$$= \mathbf{13.0 \, dB}$$

(c)   When $\dfrac{P_2}{P_1} = 400$,

$$X = 10 \lg(400) = 10(2.60)$$
$$= \mathbf{26.0 \, dB}$$

(d)   When $\dfrac{P_2}{P_1} = \dfrac{1}{20} = 0.05$,

$$X = 10 \lg(0.05) = 10(-1.30)$$
$$= \mathbf{-13.0 \, dB}$$

(a), (b) and (c) represent power gains and (d) represents a power loss or attenuation.

Problem 13.   The current input to a system is 5 mA and the current output is 20 mA. Find the decibel current ratio assuming the input and load resistances of the system are equal.

From above, the decibel current ratio is

$$20 \lg\left(\frac{I_2}{I_1}\right) = 20 \lg\left(\frac{20}{5}\right)$$
$$= 20 \lg 4 = 20(0.60)$$
$$= \mathbf{12 \, dB \ gain}$$

Problem 14.   6% of the power supplied to a cable appears at the output terminals. Determine the power loss in decibels.

If P_1 = input power and P_2 = output power then

$$\frac{P_2}{P_1} = \frac{6}{100} = 0.06$$

$$\text{Decibel power ratio} = 10\lg\left(\frac{P_2}{P_1}\right) = 10\lg(0.06)$$

$$= 10(-1.222) = -12.22\,\text{dB}$$

Hence the decibel power loss, or attenuation, is 12.22 dB.

Problem 15.   An amplifier has a gain of 14 dB and its input power is 8 mW. Find its output power.

Decibel power ratio $= 10\lg(P_2/P_1)$ where P_1 = input power = 8 mW, and P_2 = output power. Hence

$$14 = 10\lg\left(\frac{P_2}{P_1}\right)$$

from which

$$1.4 = \lg\left(\frac{P_2}{P_1}\right)$$

and $10^{1.4} = \dfrac{P_2}{P_1}$ from the definition of a logarithm

i.e. $25.12 = \dfrac{P_2}{P_1}$

Output power, $P_2 = 25.12\,P_1 = (25.12)(8)$

$$= \textbf{201 mW or 0.201 W}$$

Problem 16.   Determine, in decibels, the ratio of output power to input power of a 3 stage communications system, the stages having gains of 12 dB, 15 dB and −8 dB. Find also the overall power gain.

The decibel ratio may be used to find the overall power ratio of a chain simply by adding the decibel power ratios together. Hence the overall decibel

power ratio $= 12 + 15 - 8 = \textbf{19 dB gain}$.

Thus $19 = 10\lg\left(\dfrac{P_2}{P_1}\right)$

from which $1.9 = \lg\left(\dfrac{P_2}{P_1}\right)$

and $10^{1.9} = \dfrac{P_2}{P_1} = 79.4$

Thus the overall power gain, $\dfrac{P_2}{P_1} = 79.4$

[For the first stage,

$$12 = 10\lg\left(\frac{P_2}{P_1}\right)$$

from which

$$\frac{P_2}{P_1} = 10^{1.2} = 15.85$$

Similarly for the second stage,

$$\frac{P_2}{P_1} = 31.62$$

and for the third stage,

$$\frac{P_2}{P_1} = 0.1585$$

The overall power ratio is thus
$15.85 \times 31.62 \times 0.1585 = \textbf{79.4}$]

Problem 17.   The output voltage from an amplifier is 4 V. If the voltage gain is 27 dB, calculate the value of the input voltage assuming that the amplifier input resistance and load resistance are equal.

Voltage gain in decibels $= 27 = 20\lg(V_2/V_1) = 20\lg(4/V_1)$. Hence

$$\frac{27}{20} = \lg\left(\frac{4}{V_1}\right)$$

i.e. $1.35 = \lg\left(\dfrac{4}{V_1}\right)$

Thus $10^{1.35} = \dfrac{4}{V_1}$

from which $V_1 = \dfrac{4}{10^{1.35}}$

$$= \frac{4}{22.39}$$

$$= 0.179\,\text{V}$$

Hence the input voltage V_1 is 0.179 V

Now try the following exercise

Exercise 54   Further problems on logarithmic ratios

1. The ratio of two powers is (a) 3 (b) 10 (c) 20 (d) 10000. Determine the decibel power ratio for each.
   [(a) 4.77 dB (b) 10 dB (c) 13 dB (d) 40 dB]

2. The ratio of two powers is (a) $\frac{1}{10}$ (b) $\frac{1}{3}$ (c) $\frac{1}{40}$ (d) $\frac{1}{100}$. Determine the decibel power ratio for each.
   [(a) −10 dB (b) −4.77 dB (c) −16.02 dB (d) −20 dB]

3. The input and output currents of a system are 2 mA and 10 mA respectively. Determine the decibel current ratio of output to input current assuming input and output resistances of the system are equal.
   [13.98 dB]

4. 5% of the power supplied to a cable appears at the output terminals. Determine the power loss in decibels.
   [13 dB]

5. An amplifier has a gain of 24 dB and its input power is 10 mW. Find its output power.
   [2.51 W]

6. Determine, in decibels, the ratio of the output power to input power of a four stage system, the stages having gains of 10 dB, 8 dB, −5 dB and 7 dB. Find also the overall power gain.
   [20 dB, 100]

7. The output voltage from an amplifier is 7 mV. If the voltage gain is 25 dB calculate the value of the input voltage assuming that the amplifier input resistance and load resistance are equal.
   [0.39 mV]

8. The voltage gain of a number of cascaded amplifiers are 23 dB, −5.8 dB, −12.5 dB and 3.8 dB. Calculate the overall gain in decibels assuming that input and load resistances for each stage are equal. If a voltage of 15 mV is applied to the input of the system, determine the value of the output voltage.
   [8.5 dB, 39.91 mV]

9. The scale of a voltmeter has a decibel scale added to it, which is calibrated by taking a reference level of 0 dB when a power of 1 mW is dissipated in a 600 Ω resistor. Determine the voltage at (a) 0 dB (b) 1.5 dB (c) −15 dB (d) What decibel reading corresponds to 0.5 V?
   [(a) 0.775 V (b) 0.921 V (c) 0.138 V (d) −3.807 dB]

10.17   Null method of measurement

A **null method of measurement** is a simple, accurate and widely used method which depends on an instrument reading being adjusted to read zero current only. The method assumes:

(i)   if there is any deflection at all, then some current is flowing;

(ii)   if there is no deflection, then no current flows (i.e. a null condition).

Hence it is unnecessary for a meter sensing current flow to be calibrated when used in this way. A sensitive milliammeter or microammeter with centre zero position setting is called a **galvanometer**. Examples where the method is used are in the Wheatstone bridge (see Section 10.18), in the d.c. potentiometer (see Section 10.19) and with a.c. bridges (see Section 10.20).

10.18   Wheatstone bridge

Figure 10.31 shows a **Wheatstone bridge** circuit which compares an unknown resistance R_x with others of known values, i.e. R_1 and R_2, which have fixed values, and R_3, which is variable. R_3 is varied until zero deflection is obtained on the galvanometer G. No current then

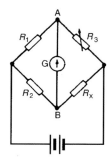

Figure 10.31

flows through the meter, $V_A = V_B$, and the bridge is said to be 'balanced'. At balance,

$$R_1 R_x = R_2 R_3 \text{ i.e. } R_x = \frac{R_2 R_3}{R_1} \text{ ohms}$$

Problem 18. In a Wheatstone bridge ABCD, a galvanometer is connected between A and C, and a battery between B and D. A resistor of unknown value is connected between A and B. When the bridge is balanced, the resistance between B and C is $100\,\Omega$, that between C and D is $10\,\Omega$ and that between D and A is $400\,\Omega$. Calculate the value of the unknown resistance.

The Wheatstone bridge is shown in Fig. 10.32 where R_x is the unknown resistance. At balance, equating the products of opposite ratio arms, gives:

$$(R_x)(10) = (100)(400)$$

and

$$R_x = \frac{(100)(400)}{10} = 4000\,\Omega$$

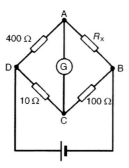

Figure 10.32

Hence, the unknown resistance, $R_x = 4\,\text{k}\Omega$.

10.19 D.C. potentiometer

The **d.c. potentiometer** is a null-balance instrument used for determining values of e.m.f.'s and p.d.s. by comparison with a known e.m.f. or p.d. In Fig. 10.33(a), using a standard cell of known e.m.f. E_1, the slider S is moved along the slide wire until balance is obtained

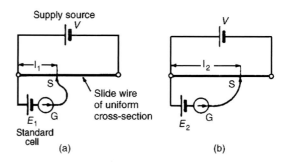

Figure 10.33

(i.e. the galvanometer deflection is zero), shown as length l_1.

The standard cell is now replaced by a cell of unknown e.m.f. E_2 (see Fig. 10.33(b)) and again balance is obtained (shown as l_2). Since $E_1 \propto l_1$ and $E_2 \propto l_2$ then

$$\frac{E_1}{E_2} = \frac{l_1}{l_2}$$

and

$$E_2 = E_1 \left(\frac{l_2}{l_1}\right) \text{volts}$$

A potentiometer may be arranged as a resistive two-element potential divider in which the division ratio is adjustable to give a simple variable d.c. supply. Such devices may be constructed in the form of a resistive element carrying a sliding contact which is adjusted by a rotary or linear movement of the control knob.

Problem 19. In a d.c. potentiometer, balance is obtained at a length of 400 mm when using a standard cell of 1.0186 volts. Determine the e.m.f. of a dry cell if balance is obtained with a length of 650 mm.

$E_1 = 1.0186\,\text{V}$, $l_1 = 400\,\text{mm}$ and $l_2 = 650\,\text{mm}$
With reference to Fig. 10.33,

$$\frac{E_1}{E_2} = \frac{l_1}{l_2}$$

from which,

$$\boldsymbol{E_2} = E_1 \left(\frac{l_2}{l_1}\right) = (1.0186)\left(\frac{650}{400}\right)$$

$$= \textbf{1.655 volts}$$

Now try the following exercise

Exercise 55 Further problems on the Wheatstone bridge and d.c. potentiometer

1. In a Wheatstone bridge PQRS, a galvanometer is connected between Q and S and a voltage source between P and R. An unknown resistor R_X is connected between P and Q. When the bridge is balanced, the resistance between Q and R is $200\,\Omega$, that between R and S is $10\,\Omega$ and that between S and P is $150\,\Omega$. Calculate the value of R_X. [$3\,k\Omega$]

2. Balance is obtained in a d.c. potentiometer at a length of 31.2 cm when using a standard cell of 1.0186 volts. Calculate the e.m.f. of a dry cell if balance is obtained with a length of 46.7 cm. [1.525 V]

10.20 A.C. bridges

A Wheatstone bridge type circuit, shown in Fig. 10.34, may be used in a.c. circuits to determine unknown values of inductance and capacitance, as well as resistance.

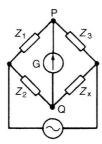

Figure 10.34

When the potential differences across Z_3 and Z_x (or across Z_1 and Z_2) are equal in magnitude and phase, then the current flowing through the galvanometer, G, is zero. At balance, $Z_1 Z_x = Z_2 Z_3$ from which

$$Z_x = \frac{Z_2 Z_3}{Z_1} \ \Omega$$

There are many forms of a.c. bridge, and these include: the Maxwell, Hay, Owen and Heaviside bridges for measuring inductance, and the De Sauty, Schering and Wien bridges for measuring capacitance. A **commercial or universal bridge** is one which can be used to measure resistance, inductance or capacitance. A.c. bridges require a knowledge of complex numbers (i.e. j notation, where $j = \sqrt{-1}$).

A Maxwell-Wien bridge for measuring the inductance L and resistance r of an inductor is shown in Fig. 10.35.

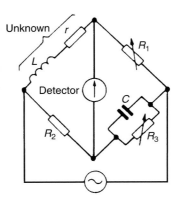

Figure 10.35

At balance the products of diagonally opposite impedances are equal. Thus

$$Z_1 Z_2 = Z_3 Z_4$$

Using complex quantities, $Z_1 = R_1$, $Z_2 = R_2$,

$$Z_3 = \frac{R_3(-jX_C)}{R_3 - jX_C} \left(\text{i.e. } \frac{\text{product}}{\text{sum}}\right)$$

and $Z_4 = r + jX_L$. Hence

$$R_1 R_2 = \frac{R_3(-jX_C)}{R_3 - jX_C}(r + jX_L)$$

i.e. $R_1 R_2 (R_3 - jX_C) = (-jR_3 X_C)(r + jX_L)$

$R_1 R_2 R_3 - jR_1 R_2 X_C = -jrR_3 X_C - j^2 R_3 X_C X_L$

i.e. $R_1 R_2 R_3 - jR_1 R_2 X_C = -jrR_3 X_C + R_3 X_C X_L$

(since $j^2 = -1$).

Equating the real parts gives:

$$R_1 R_2 R_3 = R_3 X_C X_L$$

from which, $\quad X_L = \dfrac{R_1 R_2}{X_C}$

i.e. $\quad 2\pi f L = \dfrac{R_1 R_2}{\dfrac{1}{2\pi f C}} = R_1 R_2 (2\pi f C)$

Hence inductance,

$$L = R_1 R_2 C \text{ henry} \qquad (2)$$

Equating the imaginary parts gives:

$$-R_1 R_2 X_C = -r R_3 X_C$$

from which, resistance,

$$r = \dfrac{R_1 R_2}{R_3} \text{ ohms} \qquad (3)$$

Problem 20. For the a.c. bridge shown in Fig. 10.35 determine the values of the inductance and resistance of the coil when $R_1 = R_2 = 400\,\Omega$, $R_3 = 5\,\text{k}\Omega$ and $C = 7.5\,\mu\text{F}$.

From equation (2) above, inductance

$$L = R_1 R_2 C = (400)(400)(7.5 \times 10^{-6})$$
$$= \textbf{1.2 H}$$

From equation (3) above, resistance,

$$r = \dfrac{R_1 R_2}{R_3} = \dfrac{(400)(400)}{5000} = \textbf{32}\,\boldsymbol{\Omega}$$

From equation (2),

$$R_2 = \dfrac{L}{R_1 C}$$

and from equation (3),

$$R_3 = \dfrac{R_1}{r} R_2$$

Hence $\quad R_3 = \dfrac{R_1}{r} \dfrac{L}{R_1 C} = \dfrac{L}{Cr}$

If the frequency is constant then $R_3 \propto L/r \propto \omega L/r \propto$ Q-factor (see Chapters 15 and 16). Thus the bridge

can be adjusted to give a direct indication of Q-factor. A Q-meter is described in Section 10.21 following.

Now try the following exercise

Exercise 56 Further problem on a.c. bridges

1. A Maxwell bridge circuit ABCD has the following arm impedances: AB, $250\,\Omega$ resistance; BC, $15\,\mu\text{F}$ capacitor in parallel with a $10\,\text{k}\Omega$ resistor; CD, $400\,\Omega$ resistor; DA, unknown inductor having inductance L and resistance R. Determine the values of L and R assuming the bridge is balanced.

[1.5 H, 10 Ω]

10.21 Q-meter

The **Q-factor** for a series L–C–R circuit is the voltage magnification at resonance, i.e.

$$\text{Q-factor} = \frac{\text{voltage across capacitor}}{\text{supply voltage}}$$

$$= \frac{V_c}{V} \quad \text{(see Chapter 15)}.$$

The simplified circuit of a **Q-meter**, used for measuring Q-factor, is shown in Fig. 10.36. Current from a variable frequency oscillator flowing through a very low resistance r develops a variable frequency voltage, V_r, which is applied to a series L–R–C circuit. The frequency is then varied until resonance causes voltage V_c to reach a maximum value. At resonance V_r and V_c are noted. Then

$$\text{Q-factor} = \frac{V_c}{V_r} = \frac{V_c}{Ir}$$

In a practical Q-meter, V_r is maintained constant and the electronic voltmeter can be calibrated to indicate the Q-factor directly. If a variable capacitor C is used and the oscillator is set to a given frequency, then C can be adjusted to give resonance. In this way inductance L may be calculated using

$$f_r = \frac{1}{2\pi \sqrt{LC}}$$

Since $\quad Q = \dfrac{2\pi f L}{R}$

then R may be calculated.

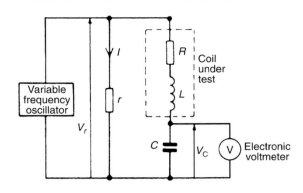

Figure 10.36

Q-meters operate at various frequencies and instruments exist with frequency ranges from 1 kHz to 50 MHz. Errors in measurement can exist with Q-meters since the coil has an effective parallel self capacitance due to capacitance between turns. The accuracy of a Q-meter is approximately ±5%.

Problem 21. When connected to a Q-meter an inductor is made to resonate at 400 kHz. The Q-factor of the circuit is found to be 100 and the capacitance of the Q-meter capacitor is set to 400 pF. Determine (a) the inductance, and (b) the resistance of the inductor.

Resonant frequency, $f_r = 400\,\text{kHz} = 400 \times 10^3\,\text{Hz}$, Q-factor $= 100$ and capacitance, $C = 400\,\text{pF} = 400 \times 10^{-12}\,\text{F}$. The circuit diagram of a Q-meter is shown in Fig. 10.36.

(a) At resonance,

$$f_r = \frac{1}{2\pi\sqrt{LC}}$$

for a series L–C–R circuit.

Hence $\qquad 2\pi f_r = \dfrac{1}{\sqrt{LC}}$

from which

$$(2\pi f_r)^2 = \frac{1}{LC}$$

and **inductance**,

$$L = \frac{1}{(2\pi f_r)^2 C}$$

$$= \frac{1}{(2\pi \times 400 \times 10^3)^2 (400 \times 10^{-12})}\,\text{H}$$

$$= \mathbf{396\,\mu H\ or\ 0.396\,mH}$$

(b) Q-factor at resonance $= 2\pi f_r L/R$ from which resistance

$$R = \frac{2\pi f_r L}{Q}$$

$$= \frac{2\pi (400 \times 10^3)(0.396 \times 10^{-3})}{100}$$

$$= \mathbf{9.95\,\Omega}$$

Now try the following exercise

Exercise 57   **Further problem on the Q-meter**

1. A Q-meter measures the Q-factor of a series L-C-R circuit to be 200 at a resonant frequency of 250 kHz. If the capacitance of the Q-meter capacitor is set to 300 pF determine (a) the inductance L, and (b) the resistance R of the inductor.   [(a) 1.351 mH (b) 10.61 Ω]

10.22   Measurement errors

Errors are always introduced when using instruments to measure electrical quantities. The errors most likely to occur in measurements are those due to:

(i) the limitations of the instrument;

(ii) the operator;

(iii) the instrument disturbing the circuit.

(i)   Errors in the limitations of the instrument

The **calibration accuracy** of an instrument depends on the precision with which it is constructed. Every instrument has a margin of error which is expressed as a percentage of the instruments full-scale deflection. For example, industrial grade instruments have an accuracy of ±2% of f.s.d. Thus if a voltmeter has a f.s.d. of 100 V and it indicates 40 V say, then the actual voltage may be anywhere between 40 ± (2% of 100), or 40 ± 2, i.e. between 38 V and 42 V.

When an instrument is calibrated, it is compared against a standard instrument and a graph is drawn of 'error' against 'meter deflection'. A typical graph is shown in Fig. 10.37 where it is seen that the accuracy varies over the scale length. Thus a meter with a ±2% f.s.d. accuracy would tend to have an accuracy which is much better than ±2% f.s.d. over much of the range.

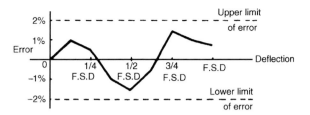

Figure 10.37

(ii) Errors by the operator

It is easy for an operator to misread an instrument. With linear scales the values of the sub-divisions are reasonably easy to determine; non-linear scale graduations are more difficult to estimate. Also, scales differ from instrument to instrument and some meters have more than one scale (as with multimeters) and mistakes in reading indications are easily made. When reading a meter scale it should be viewed from an angle perpendicular to the surface of the scale at the location of the pointer; a meter scale should not be viewed 'at an angle'. Errors by the operator are eliminated with digital instruments.

(iii) Errors due to the instrument disturbing the circuit

Any instrument connected into a circuit will affect that circuit to some extent. Meters require some power to operate, but provided this power is small compared with the power in the measured circuit, then little error will result. Incorrect positioning of instruments in a circuit can be a source of errors. For example, let a resistance be measured by the voltmeter-ammeter method as shown in Fig. 10.38. Assuming 'perfect' instruments, the resistance should be given by the voltmeter reading divided by the ammeter reading (i.e. $R = V/I$). However, in Fig. 10.38(a), $V/I = R + r_a$ and in Fig. 10.38(b) the current through the ammeter is that through the resistor plus that through the voltmeter. Hence the voltmeter reading divided by the ammeter reading will not give the true value of the resistance R for either method of connection.

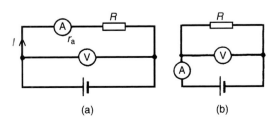

(a)   (b)

Figure 10.38

Problem 22. The current flowing through a resistor of $5\,k\Omega \pm 0.4\%$ is measured as $2.5\,mA$ with an accuracy of measurement of $\pm 0.5\%$. Determine the nominal value of the voltage across the resistor and its accuracy.

Voltage, $V = IR = (2.5 \times 10^{-3})(5 \times 10^3) = 12.5\,V$. The maximum possible error is $0.4\% + 0.5\% = 0.9\%$.
Hence the voltage, $V = 12.5\,V \pm 0.9\%$ of $12.5\,V$
0.9% of $12.5 = 0.9/100 \times 12.5 = 0.1125\,V = 0.11\,V$ correct to 2 significant figures.

Hence the voltage V may also be expressed as **12.5 ± 0.11 volts** (i.e. a voltage lying between $12.39\,V$ and $12.61\,V$).

Problem 23. The current I flowing in a resistor R is measured by a 0–10 A ammeter which gives an indication of 6.25 A. The voltage V across the resistor is measured by a 0–50 V voltmeter, which gives an indication of 36.5 V. Determine the resistance of the resistor, and its accuracy of measurement if both instruments have a limit of error of 2% of f.s.d. Neglect any loading effects of the instruments.

Resistance,

$$R = \frac{V}{I} = \frac{36.5}{6.25} = 5.84\,\Omega$$

Voltage error is $\pm 2\%$ of $50\,V = \pm 1.0\,V$ and expressed as a percentage of the voltmeter reading gives

$$\frac{\pm 1}{36.5} \times 100\% = \pm 2.74\%$$

Current error is $\pm 2\%$ of $10\,A = \pm 0.2\,A$ and expressed as a percentage of the ammeter reading gives

$$\frac{\pm 0.2}{6.25} \times 100\% = \pm 3.2\%$$

Maximum relative error = sum of errors = $2.74\% + 3.2\% = \pm 5.94\%$ and 5.94% of $5.84\,\Omega = 0.347\,\Omega$. Hence the resistance of the resistor may be expressed as:

$5.84\,\Omega \pm 5.94\%$ or $5.84 \pm 0.35\,\Omega$

(rounding off)

Problem 24. The arms of a Wheatstone bridge ABCD have the following resistances: AB: $R_1 = 1000\,\Omega \pm 1.0\%$; BC: $R_2 = 100\,\Omega \pm 0.5\%$; CD: unknown resistance R_x; DA: $R_3 = 432.5\,\Omega \pm 0.2\%$. Determine the value of the unknown resistance and its accuracy of measurement.

The Wheatstone bridge network is shown in Fig. 10.39 and at balance:

$$R_1 R_x = R_2 R_3,$$

i.e. $\quad R_x = \dfrac{R_2 R_3}{R_1} = \dfrac{(100)(432.5)}{1000} = 43.25\,\Omega$

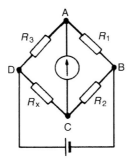

Figure 10.39

The maximum relative error of R_x is given by the sum of the three individual errors,
i.e. $1.0\% + 0.5\% + 0.2\% = 1.7\%$.

Hence $\qquad\qquad R_x = 43.25\,\Omega \pm 1.7\%$

1.7% of $43.25\,\Omega = 0.74\,\Omega$ (rounding off). Thus R_x may also be expressed as

$$R_x = 43.25 \pm 0.74\,\Omega$$

Now try the following exercises

Exercise 58   Further problems on measurement errors

1. The p.d. across a resistor is measured as 37.5 V with an accuracy of $\pm 0.5\%$. The value of the resistor is $6\,k\Omega \pm 0.8\%$. Determine the current flowing in the resistor and its accuracy of measurement.

    $[6.25\,mA \pm 1.3\%$ or $6.25 \pm 0.08\,mA]$

2. The voltage across a resistor is measured by a 75 V f.s.d. voltmeter which gives an indication of 52 V. The current flowing in the resistor is measured by a 20 A f.s.d. ammeter which gives an indication of 12.5 A. Determine the resistance of the resistor and its accuracy if both instruments have an accuracy of $\pm 2\%$ of f.s.d.

    $[4.16\,\Omega \pm 6.08\%$ or $4.16 \pm 0.25\,\Omega]$

3. A Wheatstone bridge PQRS has the following arm resistances: PQ, $1\,k\Omega \pm 2\%$; QR, $100\,\Omega \pm 0.5\%$; RS, unknown resistance; SP, $273.6\,\Omega \pm 0.1\%$. Determine the value of the unknown resistance, and its accuracy of measurement.

    $[27.36\,\Omega \pm 2.6\%$ or $27.36\,\Omega \pm 0.71\,\Omega]$

Exercise 59   Short answer questions on electrical measuring instruments and measurements

1. What is the main difference between an analogue and a digital type of measuring instrument?

2. Name the three essential devices for all analogue electrical indicating instruments

3. Complete the following statements:
    (a) An ammeter has a ...... resistance and is connected ...... with the circuit
    (b) A voltmeter has a ...... resistance and is connected ...... with the circuit

4. State two advantages and two disadvantages of a moving-coil instrument

5. What effect does the connection of (a) a shunt (b) a multiplier have on a milliammeter?

6. State two advantages and two disadvantages of a moving-coil instrument

7. Name two advantages of electronic measuring instruments compared with moving-coil or moving-iron instruments

8. Briefly explain the principle of operation of an ohmmeter

9. Name a type of ohmmeter used for measuring (a) low resistance values (b) high resistance values

10. What is a multimeter?

11. When may a rectifier instrument be used in preference to either a moving-coil or moving-iron instrument?

12. Name five quantities that a c.r.o. is capable of measuring

13. What is harmonic analysis?

14. What is a feature of waveforms containing the fundamental and odd harmonics?

15. Express the ratio of two powers P_1 and P_2 in decibel units

16. What does a power level unit of dBm indicate?

17. What is meant by a null method of measurement?

18. Sketch a Wheatstone bridge circuit used for measuring an unknown resistance in a d.c. circuit and state the balance condition

19. How may a d.c. potentiometer be used to measure p.d.'s

20. Name five types of a.c. bridge used for measuring unknown inductance, capacitance or resistance

21. What is a universal bridge?

22. State the name of an a.c. bridge used for measuring inductance

23. Briefly describe how the measurement of Q-factor may be achieved

24. Why do instrument errors occur when measuring complex waveforms?

25. Define 'calibration accuracy' as applied to a measuring instrument

26. State three main areas where errors are most likely to occur in measurements

Exercise 60   Multi-choice questions on electrical measuring instruments and measurements
(Answers on page 420)

1. Which of the following would apply to a moving coil instrument?
   (a) An uneven scale, measuring d.c.
   (b) An even scale, measuring a.c.
   (c) An uneven scale, measuring a.c.
   (d) An even scale, measuring d.c.

2. In question 1, which would refer to a moving iron instrument?

3. In question 1, which would refer to a moving coil rectifier instrument?

4. Which of the following is needed to extend the range of a milliammeter to read voltages of the order of 100 V?
   (a) a parallel high-value resistance
   (b) a series high-value resistance
   (c) a parallel low-value resistance
   (d) a series low-value resistance

5. Fig. 10.40 shows a scale of a multi-range ammeter. What is the current indicated when switched to a 25 A scale?
   (a) 84 A   (b) 5.6 A
   (c) 14 A   (d) 8.4 A

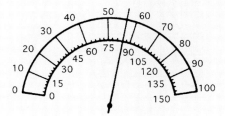

Figure 10.40

A sinusoidal waveform is displayed on a c.r.o. screen. The peak-to-peak distance is 5 cm and the distance between cycles is 4 cm. The 'variable' switch is on 100 μs/cm and the 'volts/cm' switch is on 10 V/cm. In questions 6 to 10, select the correct answer from the following:

(a) 25 V   (b) 5 V   (c) 0.4 ms
(d) 35.4 V   (e) 4 ms   (f) 50 V
(g) 250 Hz   (h) 2.5 V   (i) 2.5 kHz
(j) 17.7 V

6. Determine the peak-to-peak voltage

7. Determine the periodic time of the waveform

8. Determine the maximum value of the voltage

9. Determine the frequency of the waveform

10. Determine the r.m.s. value of the waveform

Figure 10.41 shows double-beam c.r.o. waveform traces. For the quantities stated in questions 11 to 17, select the correct answer from the following:

(a) 30 V   (b) 0.2 s   (c) 50 V

(d) $\dfrac{15}{\sqrt{2}}$ (e) 54° leading   (f) $\dfrac{250}{\sqrt{2}}$ V

(g) 15 V   (h) 100 μs   (i) $\dfrac{50}{\sqrt{2}}$ V

(j) 250 V   (k) 10 kHz   (l) 75 V

(m) 40 μs   (n) $\dfrac{3\pi}{10}$ rads lagging

(o) $\dfrac{25}{\sqrt{2}}$ V   (p) 5 Hz   (q) $\dfrac{30}{\sqrt{2}}$ V

(r) 25 kHz   (s) $\dfrac{75}{\sqrt{2}}$ V

(t) $\dfrac{3\pi}{10}$ rads leading

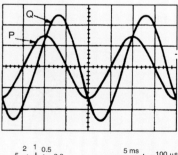

 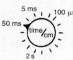

Figure 10.41

11. Amplitude of waveform P

12. Peak-to-peak value of waveform Q

13. Periodic time of both waveforms

14. Frequency of both waveforms

15. R.m.s. value of waveform P

16. R.m.s. value of waveform Q

17. Phase displacement of waveform Q relative to waveform P

18. The input and output powers of a system are 2 mW and 18 mW respectively. The decibel power ratio of output power to input power is:

(a) 9   (b) 9.54
(c) 1.9   (d) 19.08

19. The input and output voltages of a system are 500 μV and 500 mV respectively. The decibel voltage ratio of output to input voltage (assuming input resistance equals load resistance) is:

(a) 1000   (b) 30
(c) 0   (d) 60

20. The input and output currents of a system are 3 mA and 18 mA respectively. The decibel ratio of output to input current (assuming the input and load resistances are equal) is:

(a) 15.56   (b) 6
(c) 1.6   (d) 7.78

21. Which of the following statements is false?

(a) The Schering bridge is normally used for measuring unknown capacitances
(b) A.C. electronic measuring instruments can handle a much wider range of frequency than the moving coil instrument
(c) A complex waveform is one which is non-sinusoidal
(d) A square wave normally contains the fundamental and even harmonics

22. A voltmeter has a f.s.d. of 100 V, a sensitivity of 1 kΩ/V and an accuracy of ±2% of f.s.d. When the voltmeter is connected into a circuit it indicates 50 V. Which of the following statements is false?

(a) Voltage reading is 50±2 V
(b) Voltmeter resistance is 100 kΩ
(c) Voltage reading is 50 V±2%
(d) Voltage reading is 50 V±4%

23. A potentiometer is used to:
(a) compare voltages
(b) measure power factor
(c) compare currents
(d) measure phase sequence

Chapter 11

Semiconductor diodes

At the end of this chapter you should be able to:

- classify materials as conductors, semiconductors or insulators
- appreciate the importance of silicon and germanium
- understand n-type and p-type materials
- understand the p-n junction
- appreciate forward and reverse bias of p-n junctions
- recognise the symbols used to represent diodes in circuit diagrams
- understand the importance of diode characteristics and maximum ratings
- know the characteristics and applications of various types of diode – signal diodes, rectifiers, Zener diodes, silicon controlled rectifiers, light emitting diodes, varactor diodes and Schottky diodes.

11.1 Types of material

Materials may be classified as conductors, semiconductors or insulators. The classification depends on the value of resistivity of the material. Good conductors are usually metals and have resistivities in the order of 10^{-7} to $10^{-8}\,\Omega\text{m}$, semiconductors have resistivities in the order of 10^{-3} to $3 \times 10^3\,\Omega\text{m}$, and the resistivities of insulators are in the order of 10^4 to $10^{14}\,\Omega\text{m}$. Some typical approximate values at normal room temperatures are:

Conductors:

Aluminium	$2.7 \times 10^{-8}\,\Omega\text{m}$
Brass (70 Cu/30 Zn)	$8 \times 10^{-8}\,\Omega\text{m}$
Copper (pure annealed)	$1.7 \times 10^{-8}\,\Omega\text{m}$
Steel (mild)	$15 \times 10^{-8}\,\Omega\text{m}$

Semiconductors: (at 27°C)

Silicon	$2.3 \times 10^3\,\Omega\text{m}$
Germanium	$0.45\,\Omega\text{m}$

Insulators:

Glass	$\geq 10^{10}\,\Omega\text{m}$
Mica	$\geq 10^{11}\,\Omega\text{m}$
PVC	$\geq 10^{13}\,\Omega\text{m}$
Rubber (pure)	10^{12} to $10^{14}\,\Omega\text{m}$

In general, over a limited range of temperatures, the resistance of a conductor increases with temperature increase, the resistance of insulators remains approximately constant with variation of temperature and the resistance of semiconductor materials decreases as the temperature increases. For a specimen of each of these materials, having the same resistance (and thus completely different dimensions), at say, 15°C, the variation for a small increase in temperature to t°C is as shown in Fig. 11.1.

As the temperature of semiconductor materials is raised above room temperature, the resistivity is reduced and ultimately a point is reached where they effectively become conductors. For this reason, silicon should not operate at a working temperature in excess of 150°C to 200°C, depending on its purity, and germanium should not operate at a working temperature

DOI: 10.1016/B978-0-08-089056-2.00011-5

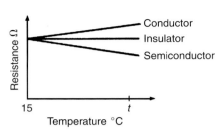

Figure 11.1

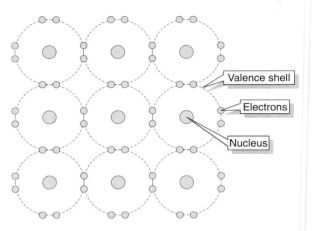

Figure 11.2

in excess of 75°C to 90°C, depending on its purity. As the temperature of a semiconductor is reduced below normal room temperature, the resistivity increases until, at very low temperatures the semiconductor becomes an insulator.

11.2   Semiconductor materials

From Chapter 2, it was stated that an atom contains both negative charge carriers (**electrons**) and positive charge carriers (**protons**). Electrons each carry a single unit of negative electric charge while protons each exhibit a single unit of positive charge. Since atoms normally contain an equal number of electrons and protons, the net charge present will be zero. For example, if an atom has eleven electrons, it will also contain eleven protons. The end result is that the negative charge of the electrons will be exactly balanced by the positive charge of the protons.

Electrons are in constant motion as they orbit around the nucleus of the atom. Electron orbits are organised into **shells**. The maximum number of electrons present in the first shell is two, in the second shell eight, and in the third, fourth and fifth shells it is 18, 32 and 50, respectively. In electronics, only the electron shell furthermost from the nucleus of an atom is important. It is important to note that the movement of electrons between atoms only involves those present in the outer **valence shell**.

If the valence shell contains the maximum number of electrons possible the electrons are rigidly bonded together and the material has the properties of an insulator (see Fig. 11.2). If, however, the valence shell does not have its full complement of electrons, the electrons can be easily detached from their orbital bonds, and the material has the properties associated with an electrical conductor.

In its pure state, silicon is an insulator because the covalent bonding rigidly holds all of the electrons leaving no free (easily loosened) electrons to conduct

current. If, however, an atom of a different element (i.e. an **impurity**) is introduced that has five electrons in its valence shell, a surplus electron will be present (see Fig. 11.3). These free electrons become available for use as charge carriers and they can be made to move through the lattice by applying an external potential difference to the material.

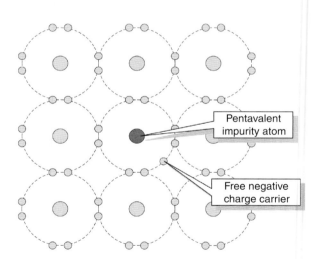

Figure 11.3

Similarly, if the impurity element introduced into the pure silicon lattice has three electrons in its valence shell, the absence of the fourth electron needed for proper covalent bonding will produce a number of spaces into which electrons can fit (see Fig. 11.4). These spaces are referred to as **holes**. Once again, current will flow when an external potential difference is applied to the material.

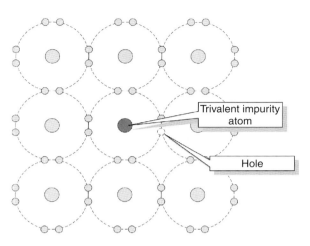

Figure 11.4

Regardless of whether the impurity element produces surplus electrons or holes, the material will no longer behave as an insulator, neither will it have the properties that we normally associate with a metallic conductor. Instead, we call the material a **semiconductor** – the term simply serves to indicate that the material is no longer a good insulator nor is it a good conductor but is somewhere in between. Examples of semiconductor materials include **silicon (Si)**, **germanium (Ge)**, **gallium arsenide (GaAs)**, and **indium arsenide (InAs)**.

Antimony, **arsenic** and **phosphorus** are **n-type impurities** and form an n-type material when any of these impurities are added to pure semiconductor material such as silicon or germanium. The amount of impurity added usually varies from 1 part impurity in 10^5 parts semiconductor material to 1 part impurity to 10^8 parts semiconductor material, depending on the resistivity required. **Indium, aluminium** and **boron** are all **p-type impurities** and form a p-type material when any of these impurities are added to a pure semiconductor.

The process of introducing an atom of another (impurity) element into the lattice of an otherwise pure material is called **doping**. When the pure material is doped with an impurity with five electrons in its valence shell (i.e. a **pentavalent impurity**) it will become an **n-type** (i.e. negative type) semiconductor material. If, however, the pure material is doped with an impurity having three electrons in its valence shell (i.e. a **trivalent impurity**) it will become a **p-type** (i.e. positive type) semiconductor material. Note that n-type semiconductor material contains an excess of negative charge carriers, and p-type material contains an excess of positive charge carriers.

In semiconductor materials, there are very few charge carriers per unit volume free to conduct. This is because the 'four electron structure' in the outer shell of the atoms (called **valency electrons**), form strong **covalent bonds** with neighbouring atoms, resulting in a tetrahedral (i.e. four-sided) structure with the electrons held fairly rigidly in place.

11.3 Conduction in semiconductor materials

Arsenic, antimony and phosphorus have five valency electrons and when a semiconductor is doped with one of these substances, some impurity atoms are incorporated in the tetrahedral structure. The 'fifth' valency electron is not rigidly bonded and is free to conduct, the impurity atom donating a charge carrier.

Indium, aluminium and boron have three valency electrons and when a semiconductor is doped with one of these substances, some of the semiconductor atoms are replaced by impurity atoms. One of the four bonds associated with the semiconductor material is deficient by one electron and this deficiency is called a **hole**. Holes give rise to conduction when a potential difference exists across the semiconductor material due to movement of electrons from one hole to another, as shown in Fig. 11.5. In this diagram, an electron moves from A to B, giving the appearance that the hole moves from B to A. Then electron C moves to A, giving the appearance that the hole moves to C, and so on.

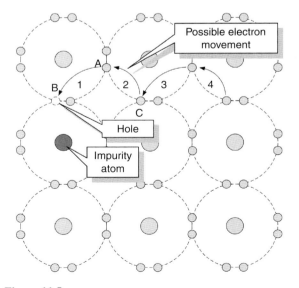

Figure 11.5

11.4   The p-n junction

A p-n junction is a piece of semiconductor material in which part of the material is p-type and part is n-type. In order to examine the charge situation, assume that separate blocks of p-type and n-type materials are pushed together. Also assume that a hole is a positive charge carrier and that an electron is a negative charge carrier.

At the junction, the donated electrons in the n-type material, called **majority carriers**, diffuse into the p-type material (diffusion is from an area of high density to an area of lower density) and the acceptor holes in the p-type material diffuse into the n-type material as shown by the arrows in Fig. 11.6. Because the n-type material has lost electrons, it acquires a positive potential with respect to the p-type material and thus tends to prevent further movement of electrons. The p-type material has gained electrons and becomes negatively charged with respect to the n-type material and hence tends to retain holes. Thus after a short while, the movement of electrons and holes stops due to the potential difference across the junction, called the **contact potential**. The area in the region of the junction becomes depleted of holes and electrons due to electron-hole recombination, and is called a **depletion layer**, as shown in Fig. 11.7.

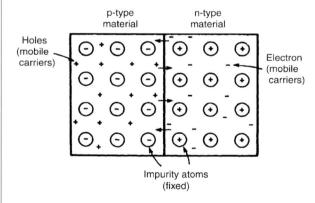

Figure 11.6

> **Problem 1.** Explain briefly the terms given below when they are associated with a p-n junction:
> (a) conduction in intrinsic semiconductors,
> (b) majority and minority carriers, and (c) diffusion.

(a)   Silicon or germanium with no doping atoms added are called **intrinsic semiconductors**. At room temperature, some of the electrons acquire sufficient energy for them to break the covalent bond between

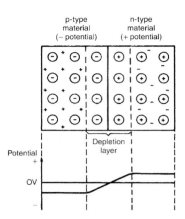

Figure 11.7

atoms and become free mobile electrons. This is called **thermal generation of electron-hole pairs**. Electrons generated thermally create a gap in the crystal structure called a hole, the atom associated with the hole being positively charged, since it has lost an electron. This positive charge may attract another electron released from another atom, creating a hole elsewhere. When a potential is applied across the semiconductor material, holes drift towards the negative terminal (unlike charges attract), and electrons towards the positive terminal, and hence a small current flows.

(b)   When additional mobile electrons are introduced by doping a semiconductor material with pentavalent atoms (atoms having five valency electrons), these mobile electrons are called **majority carriers**. The relatively few holes in the n-type material produced by intrinsic action are called **minority carriers**.

For p-type materials, the additional holes are introduced by doping with trivalent atoms (atoms having three valency electrons). The holes are apparently positive mobile charges and are majority carriers in the p-type material. The relatively few mobile electrons in the p-type material produced by intrinsic action are called minority carriers.

(c)   Mobile holes and electrons wander freely within the crystal lattice of a semiconductor material. There are more free electrons in n-type material than holes and more holes in p-type material than electrons. Thus, in their random wanderings, on average, holes pass into the n-type material and electrons into the p-type material. This process is called **diffusion**.

Intrinsic semiconductors have resistive properties, in that when an applied voltage across the material is reversed in polarity, a current of the same magnitude flows in the opposite direction. When a p-n junction is formed, the resistive property is replaced by a rectifying property, that is, current passes more easily in one direction than the other.

An n-type material can be considered to be a stationary crystal matrix of fixed positive charges together with a number of mobile negative charge carriers (electrons). The total number of positive and negative charges are equal. A p-type material can be considered to be a number of stationary negative charges together with mobile positive charge carriers (holes).

Again, the total number of positive and negative charges are equal and the material is neither positively nor negatively charged. When the materials are brought together, some of the mobile electrons in the n-type material diffuse into the p-type material. Also, some of the mobile holes in the p-type material diffuse into the n-type material.

Many of the majority carriers in the region of the junction combine with the opposite carriers to complete covalent bonds and create a region on either side of the junction with very few carriers. This region, called the **depletion layer**, acts as an insulator and is in the order of 0.5 μm thick. Since the n-type material has lost electrons, it becomes positively charged. Also, the p-type material has lost holes and becomes negatively charged, creating a potential across the junction, called the **barrier** or **contact potential**.

11.5   Forward and reverse bias

When an external voltage is applied to a p-n junction making the p-type material positive with respect to the n-type material, as shown in Fig. 11.8, the p-n junction is **forward biased**. The applied voltage opposes the contact potential, and, in effect, closes the depletion layer. Holes and electrons can now cross the junction and a current flows. An increase in the applied voltage above that required to narrow the depletion layer (about 0.2 V for germanium and 0.6 V for silicon), results in a rapid rise in the current flow.

When an external voltage is applied to a p-n junction making the p-type material negative with respect to the

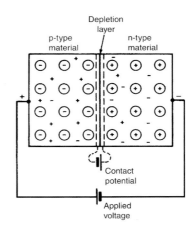

Figure 11.8

n-type material as is shown in Fig. 11.9, the p-n junction is **reverse biased**. The applied voltage is now in the same sense as the contact potential and opposes the movement of holes and electrons due to opening up the depletion layer. Thus, in theory, no current flows. However, at normal room temperature certain electrons in the covalent bond lattice acquire sufficient energy from the heat available to leave the lattice, generating mobile electrons and holes. This process is called **electron-hole generation by thermal excitation**.

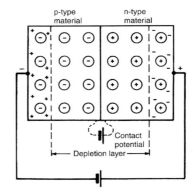

Figure 11.9

The electrons in the p-type material and holes in the n-type material caused by thermal excitation, are called minority carriers and these will be attracted by the applied voltage. Thus, in practice, a small current of a few microamperes for germanium and less than one microampere for silicon, at normal room temperature, flows under reverse bias conditions.

Graphs depicting the current-voltage relationship for forward and reverse biased p-n junctions, for both germanium and silicon, are shown in Fig. 11.10.

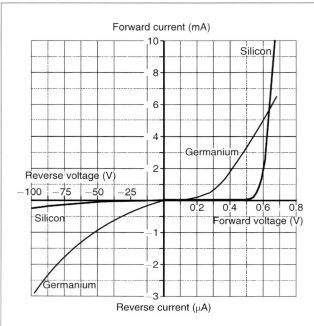

Figure 11.10

Problem 3. Sketch the forward and reverse characteristics of a silicon p-n junction diode and describe the shapes of the characteristics drawn.

A typical characteristic for a silicon p-n junction is shown in Fig. 11.10. When the positive terminal of the battery is connected to the p-type material and the negative terminal to the n-type material, the diode is forward biased. Due to like charges repelling, the holes in the p-type material drift towards the junction. Similarly the electrons in the n-type material are repelled by the negative bias voltage and also drift towards the junction. The width of the depletion layer and size of the contact potential are reduced. For applied voltages from 0 to about 0.6 V, very little current flows. At about 0.6 V, majority carriers begin to cross the junction in large numbers and current starts to flow. As the applied voltage is raised above 0.6 V, the current increases exponentially (see Fig. 11.10).

When the negative terminal of the battery is connected to the p-type material and the positive terminal to the n-type material the diode is reverse biased. The holes in the p-type material are attracted towards the negative terminal and the electrons in the n-type material are attracted towards the positive terminal (unlike charges attract). This drift increases the magnitude of both the contact potential and the thickness of the depletion layer, so that only very few majority carriers have sufficient energy to surmount the junction.

The thermally excited minority carriers, however, can cross the junction since it is, in effect, forward biased for these carriers. The movement of minority carriers results in a small constant current flowing. As the magnitude of the reverse voltage is increased a point will be reached where a large current suddenly starts to flow. The voltage at which this occurs is called the **breakdown voltage**. This current is due to two effects:

(i) the **Zener effect**, resulting from the applied voltage being sufficient to break some of the covalent bonds, and

(ii) the **avalanche effect**, resulting from the charge carriers moving at sufficient speed to break covalent bonds by collision.

Problem 4. The forward characteristic of a diode is shown in Fig. 11.11. Use the characteristic to determine (a) the current flowing in the diode when a forward voltage of 0.4 V is applied, (b) the voltage dropped across the diode when a forward current of 9 mA is flowing in it, (c) the resistance of the diode when the forward voltage is 0.6 V, and (d) whether the diode is a Ge or Si type.

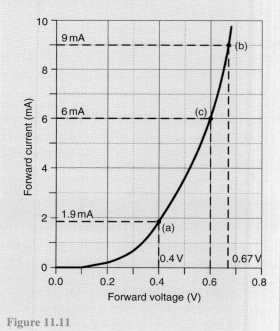

Figure 11.11

(a) From Fig. 11.11, when $V = 0.4$ V, **current flowing, $I = 1.9$ mA**

(b) When $I = 9$ mA, **the voltage dropped across the diode, $V = 0.67$ V**

(c) From the graph, when $V = 0.6\,\text{V}$, $I = 6\,\text{mA}$.

Thus, **resistance of the diode**,

$$\mathbf{R} = \frac{V}{I} = \frac{0.6}{6 \times 10^{-3}} = 0.1 \times 10^3 = \mathbf{100\,\Omega}$$

(d) The onset of conduction occurs at approximately 0.2 V. This suggests that the diode is a **Ge type**.

> **Problem 5.** Corresponding readings of current, I, and voltage, V, for a semiconductor device are given in the table:
>
> | V_f (V) | 0 | 0.1 | 0.2 | 0.3 | 0.4 | 0.5 | 0.6 | 0.7 | 0.8 |
> |---|---|---|---|---|---|---|---|---|---|
> | I_f (mA) | 0 | 0 | 0 | 0 | 0 | 1 | 9 | 24 | 50 |
>
> Plot the I/V characteristic for the device and identify the type of device.

The I/V characteristic is shown in Fig. 11.12. Since the device begins to conduct when a potential of approximately 0.6 V is applied to it we can infer that **the semiconductor material is silicon** rather than germanium.

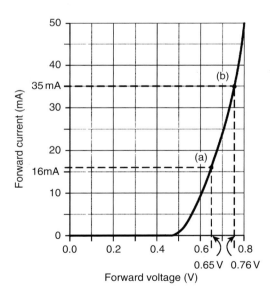

Figure 11.12

> **Problem 6.** For the characteristic of Fig. 11.12, determine for the device (a) the forward current when the forward voltage is 0.65 V, and (b) the forward voltage when the forward current is 35 mA.

(a) From Fig. 11.12, when the forward voltage is 0.65 V, **the forward current = 16 mA**

(b) When the forward current is 35 mA, **the forward voltage = 0.76 V**

Now try the following exercise

Exercise 61   Further problems on semiconductor materials and p-n junctions

1. Explain what you understand by the term intrinsic semiconductor and how an intrinsic semiconductor is turned into either a p-type or an n-type material.

2. Explain what is meant by minority and majority carriers in an n-type material and state whether the numbers of each of these carriers are affected by temperature.

3. A piece of pure silicon is doped with (a) pentavalent impurity and (b) trivalent impurity. Explain the effect these impurities have on the form of conduction in silicon.

4. With the aid of simple sketches, explain how pure germanium can be treated in such a way that conduction is predominantly due to (a) electrons and (b) holes.

5. Explain the terms given below when used in semiconductor terminology: (a) covalent bond, (b) trivalent impurity, (c) pentavalent impurity, (d) electron-hole pair generation.

6. Explain briefly why although both p-type and n-type materials have resistive properties when separate, they have rectifying properties when a junction between them exists.

7. The application of an external voltage to a junction diode can influence the drift of holes and electrons. With the aid of diagrams explain this statement and also how the direction and magnitude of the applied voltage affects the depletion layer.

8. State briefly what you understand by the terms: (a) reverse bias, (b) forward bias, (c) contact potential, (d) diffusion, (e) minority carrier conduction.

9. Explain briefly the action of a p-n junction diode: (a) on open-circuit, (b) when provided with a forward bias, and (c) when provided with a reverse bias. Sketch the characteristic curves for both forward and reverse bias conditions.

10. Draw a diagram illustrating the charge situation for an unbiased p-n junction. Explain the change in the charge situation when compared with that in isolated p-type and n-type materials. Mark on the diagram the depletion layer and the majority carriers in each region.

11. The graph shown in Fig. 11.13 was obtained during an experiment on a diode. (a) What type of diode is this? Give reasons. (b) Determine the forward current for a forward voltage of 0.5 V. (c) Determine the forward voltage for a forward current of 30 mA. (d) Determine the resistance of the diode when the forward voltage is 0.4 V.
[(a) Ge (b) 17 mA (c) 0.625 V (d) 50 Ω]

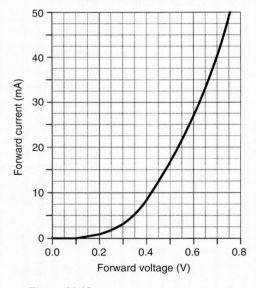

Figure 11.13

11.6 Semiconductor diodes

When a junction is formed between p-type and n-type semiconductor materials, the resulting device is called a **semiconductor diode**. This component offers an extremely low resistance to current flow in one

direction and an extremely high resistance to current flow in the other. This property allows diodes to be used in applications that require a circuit to behave differently according to the direction of current flowing in it. Note that an ideal diode would pass an infinite current in one direction and no current at all in the other direction.

A semiconductor diode is an encapsulated p-n junction fitted with connecting leads or tags for connection to external circuitry. Where an appreciable current is present (as is the case with many rectifier circuits) the diode may be mounted in a metal package designed to conduct heat away from the junction. The connection to the p-type material is referred to as the **anode** while that to the n-type material is called the **cathode**.

Various different types of diode are available for different applications. These include **rectifier diodes** for use in power supplies, **Zener diodes** for use as voltage reference sources, **light emitting diodes**, and **varactor diodes**. Figure 11.14 shows the symbols used to represent diodes in electronic circuit diagrams, where 'a' is the anode and 'k' the cathode.

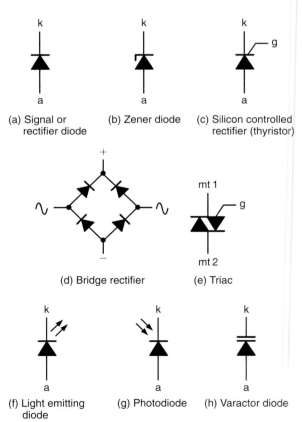

Figure 11.14

11.7   Characteristics and maximum ratings

Signal diodes require consistent forward characteristics with low forward voltage drop. Rectifier diodes need to be able to cope with high values of reverse voltage and large values of forward current, and consistency of characteristics is of secondary importance in such applications. Table 11.1 summarises the characteristics of some common semiconductor diodes. It is worth noting that diodes are limited by the amount of forward current and reverse voltage they can withstand. This limit is based on the physical size and construction of the diode.

A typical general-purpose diode may be specified as having a forward threshold voltage of 0.6 V and a reverse breakdown voltage of 200 V. If the latter is exceeded, the diode may suffer irreversible damage. Typical values of **maximum repetitive reverse voltage** (V_{RRM}) or **peak inverse voltage** (PIV) range from about 50 V to over 500 V. The reverse voltage may be increased until the maximum reverse voltage for which the diode is rated is reached. If this voltage is exceeded the junction may break down and the diode may suffer permanent damage.

11.8   Rectification

The process of obtaining unidirectional currents and voltages from alternating currents and voltages is called rectification. Semiconductor diodes are commonly used to convert alternating current (a.c.) to direct current (d.c.), in which case they are referred to as **rectifiers**. The simplest form of rectifier circuit makes use of a single diode and, since it operates on only either positive or negative half-cycles of the supply, it is known as a **half-wave rectifier**. Four diodes are connected as a **bridge rectifier** – see Fig. 11.14(d) – and are often used as a **full-wave rectifier**. Note that in both cases, automatic switching of the current is carried out by the diode(s). For methods of half-wave and full-wave rectification, see Section 14.7, page 221.

11.9   Zener diodes

Zener diodes are heavily doped silicon diodes that, unlike normal diodes, exhibit an abrupt reverse breakdown at relatively low voltages (typically less than 6 V). A similar effect, called **avalanche breakdown**, occurs in less heavily doped diodes. These avalanche diodes also exhibit a rapid breakdown with negligible current flowing below the avalanche voltage and a relatively large current flowing once the avalanche voltage has been reached. For avalanche diodes, this breakdown voltage usually occurs at voltages above 6 V. In practice, however, both types of diode are referred to as **Zener diodes**. The symbol for a Zener diode is shown in Fig. 11.14(b) whilst a typical Zener diode characteristic is shown in Fig. 11.15.

Table 11.1   Characteristics of some typical signal and rectifier diodes

Device code	Material	Max repetitive reverse voltage (V_{RRM})	Max forward current ($I_{F(max)}$)	Max reverse current ($I_{R(max)}$)	Application
1N4148	Silicon	100 V	75 mA	25 nA	General purpose
1N914	Silicon	100 V	75 mA	25 nA	General purpose
AA113	Germanium	60 V	10 mA	200 μA	RF detector
OA47	Germanium	25 V	110 mA	100 μA	Signal detector
OA91	Germanium	115 V	50 mA	275 μA	General purpose
1N4001	Silicon	50 V	1 A	10 μA	Low voltage rectifier
1N5404	Silicon	400 V	3 A	10 μA	High voltage rectifier
BY127	Silicon	1250 V	1 A	10 μA	High voltage rectifier

Section 1

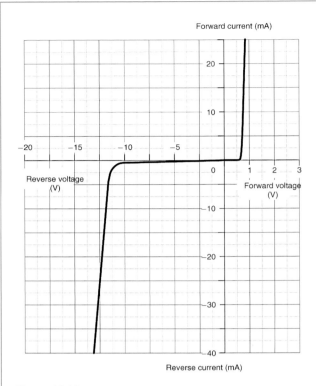

Figure 11.15

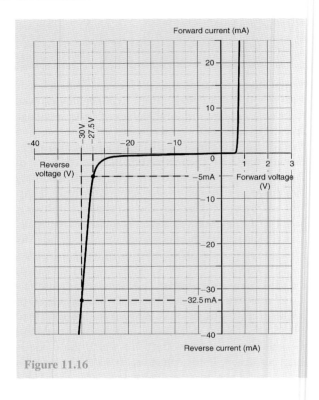

Figure 11.16

Whereas reverse breakdown is a highly undesirable effect in circuits that use conventional diodes, it can be extremely useful in the case of Zener diodes where the breakdown voltage is precisely known. When a diode is undergoing reverse breakdown and provided its maximum ratings are not exceeded, the voltage appearing across it will remain substantially constant (equal to the nominal Zener voltage) regardless of the current flowing. This property makes the Zener diode ideal for use as a **voltage regulator**.

Zener diodes are available in various families (according to their general characteristics, encapsulations and power ratings) with reverse breakdown (Zener) voltages in the range 2.4 V to 91 V.

Problem 7. The characteristic of a Zener diode is shown in Fig. 11.16. Use the characteristic to determine (a) the current flowing in the diode when a reverse voltage of 30 V is applied, (b) the voltage dropped across the diode when a reverse current of 5 mA is flowing in it, (c) the voltage rating for the Zener diode, and (d) the power dissipated in the Zener diode when a reverse voltage of 30 V appears across it.

(a) When $V = -30$ V, **the current flowing in the diode, $I = -32.5$ mA**

(b) When $I = -5$ mA, **the voltage dropped across the diode, $V = -27.5$ V**

(c) The characteristic shows the onset of Zener action at 27 V; this would suggest a **Zener voltage rating of 27 V**

(d) Power, $P = V \times I$, from which, **power dissipated when the reverse voltage is 30 V,**
$P = 30 \times (32.5 \times 10^{-3}) = 0.975$ W $=$ **975 mW**

11.10 Silicon controlled rectifiers

Silicon controlled rectifiers (or **thyristors**) are three-terminal devices which can be used for switching and a.c. power control. Silicon controlled rectifiers can switch very rapidly from conducting to a non-conducting state. In the off state, the silicon controlled rectifier exhibits negligible leakage current, while in the on state the device exhibits very low resistance. This results in very little power loss within the silicon controlled rectifier even when appreciable power levels are being controlled.

Once switched into the conducting state, the silicon controlled rectifier will remain conducting (i.e. it is latched in the on state) until the forward current is removed from the device. In d.c. applications this necessitates the interruption (or disconnection) of the supply before the device can be reset into its non-conducting state. Where the device is used with an alternating supply, the device will automatically become reset whenever the main supply reverses. The device can then be triggered on the next half-cycle having correct polarity to permit conduction.

Like their conventional silicon diode counterparts, silicon controlled rectifiers have anode and cathode connections; control is applied by means of a gate terminal, g. The symbol for a silicon controlled rectifier is shown in Fig. 11.14(c).

In normal use, a silicon controlled rectifier (SCR) is triggered into the conducting (on) state by means of the application of a current pulse to the gate terminal – see Fig. 11.17. The effective triggering of a silicon controlled rectifier requires a gate trigger pulse having a fast rise time derived from a low-resistance source. Triggering can become erratic when insufficient gate current is available or when the gate current changes slowly.

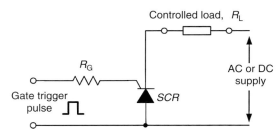

Figure 11.17

A typical silicon controlled rectifier for mains switching applications will require a gate trigger pulse of about 30 mA at 2.5 V to control a current of up to 5 A.

11.11 Light emitting diodes

Light emitting diodes (LED) can be used as general-purpose indicators and, compared with conventional filament lamps, operate from significantly smaller voltages and currents. LEDs are also very much more reliable than filament lamps. Most LEDs will provide a reasonable level of light output when a forward current of between 5 mA and 20 mA is applied.

Light emitting diodes are available in various formats with the round types being most popular. Round LEDs are commonly available in the 3 mm and 5 mm (0.2 inch)

diameter plastic packages and also in a 5 mm × 2 mm rectangular format. The viewing angle for round LEDs tends to be in the region of 20° to 40°, whereas for rectangular types this is increased to around 100°. The peak wavelength of emission depends on the type of semiconductor employed but usually lies in the range 630 to 690 nm. The symbol for an LED is shown in Fig. 11.14(f).

11.12 Varactor diodes

It was shown earlier that when a diode is operated in the reverse biased condition, the width of the depletion region increases as the applied voltage increases. Varying the width of the depletion region is equivalent to varying the plate separation of a very small capacitor such that the relationship between junction capacitance and applied reverse voltage will look something like that shown in Fig. 11.18. The typical variation of capacitance provided by a varactor is from about 50 pF to 10 pF as the reverse voltage is increased from 2 V to 20 V. The symbol for a varactor diode is shown in Fig. 11.14(h).

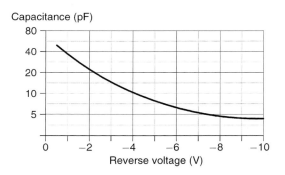

Figure 11.18

11.13 Schottky diodes

The conventional p-n junction diode explained in Section 11.4 operates well as a rectifier and switching device at relatively low frequencies (i.e. 50 Hz to 400 Hz) but its performance as a rectifier becomes seriously impaired at high frequencies due to the presence of stored charge carriers in the junction. These have the effect of momentarily allowing current to flow in the reverse direction when reverse voltage is applied. This problem becomes increasingly more problematic as the frequency of the a.c. supply is increased and the periodic time of the applied voltage becomes smaller.

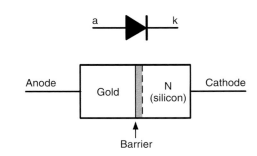

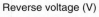

Figure 11.19

To avoid these problems a diode that uses a metal-semiconductor contact rather than a p-n junction (see Fig. 11.19) is employed. When compared with conventional silicon junction diodes, these **Schottky diodes** have a lower forward voltage (typically 0.35 V) and a slightly reduced maximum reverse voltage rating (typically 50 V to 200 V). Their main advantage, however, is that they operate with high efficiency in **switched-mode power supplies** (SMPS) at frequencies of up to 1 MHz. Schottky diodes are also extensively used in the construction of **integrated circuits** designed for high-speed digital logic applications.

Now try the following exercises

Exercise 62   Further problems on semiconductor diodes

1. Identify the types of diodes shown in Fig. 11.20.

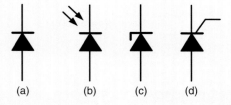

Figure 11.20

2. Sketch a circuit to show how a thyristor can be used as a controlled rectifier.

3. Sketch a graph showing how the capacitance of a varactor diode varies with applied reverse voltage.

4. State TWO advantages of light emitting diodes when compared with conventional filament indicating lamps.

5. State TWO applications for Schottky diodes.

6. The graph shown in Fig. 11.21 was obtained during an experiment on a Zener diode. (a) Estimate the Zener voltage for the diode. (b) Determine the reverse voltage for a reverse current of -20 mA. (c) Determine the reverse current for a reverse voltage of -5.5 V. (d) Determine the power dissipated by the diode when the reverse voltage is -6 V.
[(a) 5.6 (b) -5.8 V (c) -5 mA (d) 195 mW]

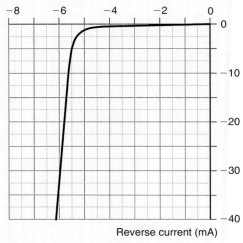

Figure 11.21

Exercise 63   Short answer problems on semiconductor diodes

1. A good conductor has a resistivity in the order of ...... to ...... Ωm

2. A semiconductor has a resistivity in the order of ...... to ...... Ωm

3. An insulator has a resistivity in the order of ...... to ...... Ωm

4. Over a limited range, the resistance of an insulator ...... with increase in temperature

5. Over a limited range, the resistance of a semiconductor ...... with increase in temperature

6. Over a limited range, the resistance of a conductor ...... with increase in temperature

7. The working temperature of germanium should not exceed ...... °C to ...... °C, depending on its ......

8. The working temperature of silicon should not exceed ...... °C to ...... °C, depending on its ......

9. Name four semiconductor materials used in the electronics industry

10. Name two n-type impurities

11. Name two p-type impurities

12. Antimony is called ...... impurity

13. Arsenic has ...... valency electrons

14. When phosphorus is introduced into a semiconductor material, mobile ...... result

15. Boron is called a ...... impurity

16. Indium has ...... valency electrons

17. When aluminium is introduced into a semiconductor material, mobile ...... result

18. When a p-n junction is formed, the n-type material acquires a ...... charge due to losing ......

19. When a p-n junction is formed, the p-type material acquires a ...... charge due to losing ......

20. What is meant by contact potential in a p-n junction?

21. With a diagram, briefly explain what a depletion layer is in a p-n junction

22. In a p-n junction, what is diffusion?

23. To forward bias a p-n junction, the ...... terminal of the battery is connected to the p-type material

24. To reverse bias a p-n junction, the positive terminal of the battery is connected to the ...... material

25. When a germanium p-n junction is forward biased, approximately ...... mV must be applied before an appreciable current starts to flow

26. When a silicon p-n junction is forward biased, approximately ...... mV must be applied before an appreciable current starts to flow

27. When a p-n junction is reversed biased, the thickness or width of the depletion layer ......

28. If the thickness or width of a depletion layer decreases, then the p-n junction is ...... biased

29. Name five types of diodes

30. What is meant by rectification?

31. What is a zener diode? State a typical practical application and sketch its circuit diagram symbol

32. What is a thyristor? State a typical practical application and sketch its circuit diagram symbol

33. What is an LED? Sketch its circuit diagram symbol

34. What is a varactor diode? Sketch its circuit diagram symbol

35. What is a Schottky diode? State a typical practical application and sketch its circuit diagram symbol

Exercise 64   Multi-choice questions on semiconductor diodes
(Answers on page 420)

In questions 1 to 5, select which statements are true.

1. In pure silicon:
    (a) the holes are the majority carriers
    (b) the electrons are the majority carriers
    (c) the holes and electrons exist in equal numbers

(d) conduction is due to there being more electrons than holes

2. Intrinsic semiconductor materials have:

(a) covalent bonds forming a tetrahedral structure

(b) pentavalent atoms added

(c) conduction by means of doping

(d) a resistance which increases with increase of temperature

3. Pentavalent impurities:

(a) have three valency electrons

(b) introduce holes when added to a semi-conductor material

(c) are introduced by adding aluminium atoms to a semiconductor material

(d) increase the conduction of a semicon-ductor material

4. Free electrons in a p-type material:

(a) are majority carriers

(b) take no part in conduction

(c) are minority carriers

(d) exist in the same numbers as holes

5. When an unbiased p-n junction is formed:

(a) the p-side is positive with respect to the n-side

(b) a contact potential exists

(c) electrons diffuse from the p-type material to the n-type material

(d) conduction is by means of majority carriers

In questions 6 to 10, select which statements are false.

6. (a) The resistance of an insulator remains approximately constant with increase of temperature

(b) The resistivity of a good conductor is about 10^7 to 10^8 ohm metres

(c) The resistivity of a conductor increases with increase of temperature

(d) The resistance of a semiconductor decreases with increase of tempera-ture

7. Trivalent impurities:

(a) have three valeney electrons

(b) introduce holes when added to a semi-conductor material

(c) can be introduced to a semiconductor material by adding antimony atoms to it

(d) increase the conductivity of a semi-conductor material when added to it

8. Free electrons in an n-type material:

(a) are majority carriers

(b) diffuse into the p-type material when a p-n junction is formed

(c) as a result of the diffusion process leave the n-type material positively charged

(d) exist in the same numbers as the holes in the n-type material

9. When a germanium p-n junction diode is forward biased:

(a) current starts to flow in an appreciable amount when the applied voltage is about 600 mV

(b) the thickness or width of the depletion layer is reduced

(c) the curve representing the current flow is exponential

(d) the positive terminal of the battery is connected to the p-type material

10. When a silicon p-n junction diode is reverse biased:

(a) a constant current flows over a large range of voltages

(b) current flow is due to electrons in the n-type material

(c) current type is due to minority carriers

(d) the magnitude of the reverse current flow is usually less than $1\,\mu A$

Chapter 12

Transistors

At the end of this chapter you should be able to:

- understand the structure of bipolar junction transistors (BJT) and junction gate field effect transistors (JFET)
- understand the action of BJT and JFET devices
- appreciate different classes and applications for BJT and JFET devices
- draw the circuit symbols for BJT and JFET devices
- appreciate common base, common emitter and common collector connections
- appreciate common gate, common source and common drain connections
- interpret characteristics for BJT and JFET devices
- appreciate how transistors are used as Class-A amplifiers
- use a load line to determine the performance of a transistor amplifier
- estimate quiescent operating conditions and gain from transistor characteristics and other data

12.1 Transistor classification

Transistors fall into **two main classes – bipolar** and **field effect**. They are also classified according to the semiconductor material employed – silicon or germanium, and to their field of application (for example, general purpose, switching, high frequency, and so on). Transistors are also classified according to the application that they are designed for, as shown in Table 12.1.

Table 12.1 Transistor classification

Low-frequency	Transistors designed specifically for audio low-frequency applications (below 100 kHz)
High-frequency	Transistors designed specifically for high radio-frequency applications (100 kHz and above)
Switching	Transistors designed for switching applications
Low-noise	Transistors that have low-noise characteristics and which are intended primarily for the amplification of low-amplitude signals
High-voltage	Transistors designed specifically to handle high voltages
Driver	Transistors that operate at medium power and voltage levels and which are often used to precede a final (power) stage which operates at an appreciable power level
Small-signal	Transistors designed for amplifying small voltages in amplifiers and radio receivers
Power	Transistor designed to handle high currents and voltages

DOI: 10.1016/B978-0-08-089056-2.00012-7

Note that these classifications can be combined so that it is possible, for example, to classify a transistor as a 'low-frequency power transistor' or as a 'low-noise high-frequency transistor'.

12.2 Bipolar junction transistors (BJT)

Bipolar transistors generally comprise n-p-n or p-n-p junctions of either silicon (Si) or germanium (Ge) material. The junctions are, in fact, produced in a single slice of silicon by diffusing impurities through a photographically reduced mask. Silicon transistors are superior when compared with germanium transistors in the vast majority of applications (particularly at high temperatures) and thus germanium devices are very rarely encountered in modern electronic equipment.

The construction of typical n-p-n and p-n-p transistors is shown in Figs 12.1 and 12.2. In order to conduct the heat away from the junction (important in medium- and high-power applications) the collector is connected to the metal case of the transistor.

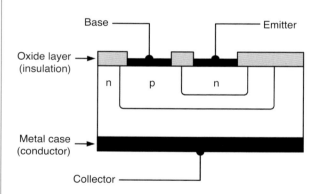

Figure 12.1

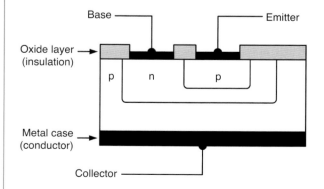

Figure 12.2

The **symbols** and simplified junction models for n-p-n and p-n-p transistors are shown in Fig. 12.3. It is important to note that the base region (p-type material in the case of an n-p-n transistor or n-type material in the case of a p-n-p transistor) is extremely narrow.

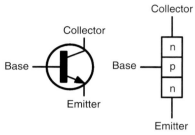

(a) n-p-n bipolar junction transistor (BJT)

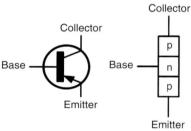

(b) p-n-p bipolar junction transistor (BJT)

Figure 12.3

12.3 Transistor action

In the **n-p-n transistor**, connected as shown in Fig. 12.4(a), transistor action is accounted for as follows:

(a) the majority carriers in the n-type emitter material are electrons

(b) the base-emitter junction is forward biased to these majority carriers and electrons cross the junction and appear in the base region

(c) the base region is very thin and only lightly doped with holes, so some recombination with holes occurs but many electrons are left in the base region

(d) the base-collector junction is reverse biased to holes in the base region and electrons in the collector region, but is forward biased to electrons in the base region; these electrons are attracted by the positive potential at the collector terminal

(e)   a large proportion of the electrons in the base region cross the base-collector junction into the collector region, creating a collector current

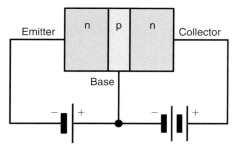

(a) n-p-n bipolar junction transistor

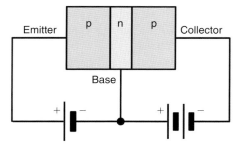

(b) p-n-p bipolar junction transistor

Figure 12.4

The **transistor action** for an n-p-n device is shown diagrammatically in Fig. 12.5(a). Conventional current

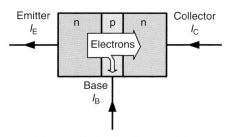

(a) n-p-n bipolar junction transistor

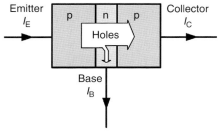

(b) p-n-p bipolar junction transistor

Figure 12.5

flow is taken to be in the direction of the motion of holes, that is, in the opposite direction to electron flow. Around 99.5% of the electrons leaving the emitter will cross the base-collector junction and only 0.5% of the electrons will recombine with holes in the narrow base region.

In the **p-n-p transistor**, connected as shown in Fig. 12.4(b), transistor action is accounted for as follows:

(a)   the majority carriers in the emitter p-type material are holes

(b)   the base-emitter junction is forward biased to the majority carriers and the holes cross the junction and appear in the base region

(c)   the base region is very thin and is only lightly doped with electrons so although some electron-hole pairs are formed, many holes are left in the base region

(d)   the base-collector junction is reverse biased to electrons in the base region and holes in the collector region, but forward biased to holes in the base region; these holes are attracted by the negative potential at the collector terminal

(e)   a large proportion of the holes in the base region cross the base-collector junction into the collector region, creating a collector current; conventional current flow is in the direction of hole movement

The **transistor action** for a p-n-p device is shown diagrammatically in Fig. 12.5(b). Around 99.5% of the holes leaving the emitter will cross the base-collector junction and only 0.5% of the holes will recombine with electrons in the narrow base region.

12.4   Leakage current

For an **n-p-n transistor**, the base-collector junction is reverse biased for majority carriers, but a small leakage current, I_{CBO}, flows from the collector to the base due to thermally generated minority carriers (holes in the collector and electrons in the base), being present. The base-collector junction is forward biased to these minority carriers.

Similarly, for a **p-n-p transistor**, the base-collector junction is reverse biased for majority carriers. However, a small leakage current, I_{CBO}, flows from the base to the collector due to thermally generated minority carriers (electrons in the collector and holes in the base), being present. Once again, the base-collector junction is forward biased to these minority carriers.

With modern transistors, leakage current is usually very small (typically less than 100 nA) and in most applications it can be ignored.

> **Problem 1.** With reference to a p-n-p transistor, explain briefly what is meant by the term 'transistor action' and why a bipolar junction transistor is so named.

For the transistor as depicted in Fig. 12.4(b), the emitter is relatively heavily doped with acceptor atoms (holes). When the emitter terminal is made sufficiently positive with respect to the base, the base-emitter junction is forward biased to the majority carriers. The majority carriers are holes in the emitter and these drift from the emitter to the base.

The base region is relatively lightly doped with donor atoms (electrons) and although some electron-hole recombinations take place, perhaps 0.5%, most of the holes entering the base, do not combine with electrons.

The base-collector junction is reverse biased to electrons in the base region, but forward biased to holes in the base region. Since the base is very thin and now is packed with holes, these holes pass the base-emitter junction towards the negative potential of the collector terminal. The control of current from emitter to collector is largely independent of the collector-base voltage and almost wholly governed by the emitter-base voltage.

The essence of transistor action is this current control by means of the base-emitter voltage. In a p-n-p transistor, holes in the emitter and collector regions are majority carriers, but are minority carriers when in the base region. Also thermally generated electrons in the emitter and collector regions are minority carriers as are holes in the base region. However, both majority and minority carriers contribute towards the total current flow (see Fig. 12.6). It is because a transistor makes use of both types of charge carriers (holes and electrons) that they are called **bipolar**. The transistor also comprises two p-n junctions and for this reason it is a **junction transistor**; hence the name – **bipolar junction transistor**.

12.5   Bias and current flow

In normal operation (i.e. for operation as a linear amplifier) the base-emitter junction of a transistor is forward biased and the collector-base junction is reverse biased. The base region is, however, made very narrow so that carriers are swept across it from emitter to collector so that only a relatively small current flows in the base. To put this into context, the current flowing in the emitter circuit is typically 100 times greater than that flowing in the base. The direction of conventional current flow is from emitter to collector in the case of a p-n-p transistor, and collector to emitter in the case of an n-p-n device, as shown in Fig. 12.7.

The equation that relates current flow in the collector, base, and emitter circuits (see Fig. 12.7) is:

$$I_E = I_B + I_C$$

where I_E is the emitter current, I_B is the base current, and I_C is the collector current (all expressed in the same units).

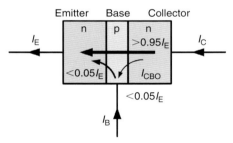

(a) n-p-n bipolar junction transistor

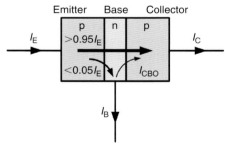

(b) p-n-p bipolar junction transistor

Figure 12.6

> **Problem 2.** A transistor operates with a collector current of 100 mA and an emitter current of 102 mA. Determine the value of base current.

Emitter current, $I_E = I_B + I_C$
from which, base current, $I_B = I_E - I_C$
Hence, **base current,** $I_B = 102 - 100 = \textbf{2 mA}$

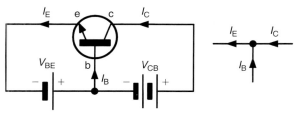

(a) n-p-n bipolar junction transistor (BJT)

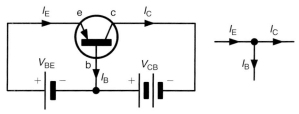

(b) p-n-p bipolar junction transistor (BJT)

Figure 12.7

12.6 Transistor operating configurations

Three basic circuit configurations are used for transistor amplifiers. These three circuit configurations depend upon which one of the three transistor connections is made common to both the input and the output. In the case of bipolar junction transistors, the configurations are known as **common-emitter**, **common-collector** (or **emitter-follower**), and **common-base**, as shown in Fig. 12.8.

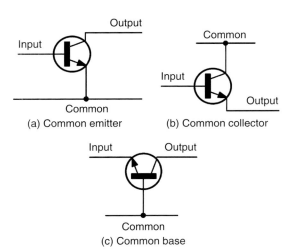

(a) Common emitter

(b) Common collector

(c) Common base

Figure 12.8

12.7 Bipolar transistor characteristics

The characteristics of a bipolar junction transistor are usually presented in the form of a set of graphs relating voltage and current present at the transistors terminals. Fig. 12.9 shows a typical **input characteristic** (I_B plotted against V_{BE}) for an n-p-n bipolar junction transistor operating in common-emitter mode. In this mode, the input current is applied to the base and the output current appears in the collector (the emitter is effectively **common** to both the input and output circuits as shown in Fig. 12.8(a)).

The input characteristic shows that very little base current flows until the base-emitter voltage V_{BE} exceeds 0.6 V. Thereafter, the base current increases rapidly – this characteristic bears a close resemblance to the forward part of the characteristic for a silicon diode.

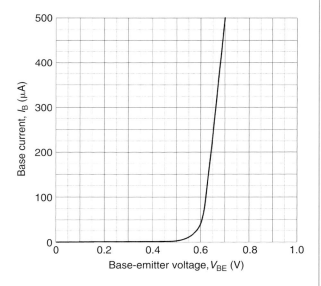

Figure 12.9

Figure 12.10 shows a typical set of **output (collector) characteristics** (I_C plotted against V_{CE}) for an n-p-n bipolar transistor. Each curve corresponds to a different value of base current. Note the 'knee' in the characteristic below $V_{CE} = 2$ V. Also note that the curves are quite flat. For this reason (i.e. since the collector current does not change very much as the collector-emitter voltage changes) we often refer to this as a **constant current characteristic**.

Figure 12.11 shows a typical **transfer characteristic** for an n-p-n bipolar junction transistor. Here I_C is plotted against I_B for a small-signal general-purpose transistor.

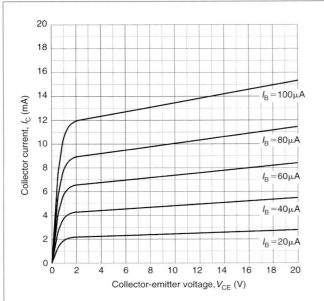

Figure 12.10

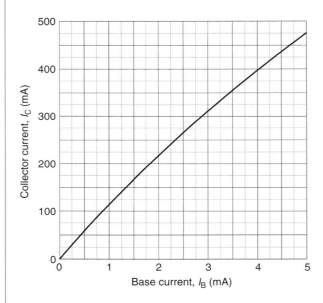

Figure 12.11

The slope of this curve (i.e. the ratio of I_C to I_B) is the common-emitter current gain of the transistor which is explored further in Section 12.9.

A circuit that can be used for obtaining the common-emitter characteristics of an n-p-n BJT is shown in Fig. 12.12. For the input characteristic, VR1 is set at a particular value and the corresponding values of V_{BE} and I_B are noted. This is repeated for various settings of VR1 and plotting the values gives the typical input characteristic of Fig. 12.9.

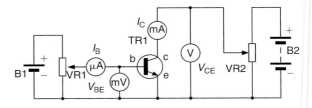

Figure 12.12

For the output characteristics, VR1 is varied so that I_B is, say, $20\,\mu A$. Then VR2 is set at various values and corresponding values of V_{CE} and I_C are noted. The graph of V_{CE}/I_C is then plotted for $I_B = 20\,\mu A$. This is repeated for, say, $I_B = 40\,\mu A$, $I_B = 60\,\mu A$, and so on. Plotting the values gives the typical output characteristics of Fig. 12.10.

12.8 Transistor parameters

The transistor characteristics met in the previous section provide us with some useful information that can help us to model the behaviour of a transistor. In particular, the three characteristic graphs can be used to determine the following parameters for operation in common-emitter mode:

Input resistance (from the input characteristic, Fig. 12.9)

$$\text{Static (or d.c.) input resistance} = \frac{V_{BE}}{I_B}$$

(from corresponding points on the graph)

$$\text{Dynamic (or a.c.) input resistance} = \frac{\Delta V_{BE}}{\Delta I_B}$$

(from the slope of the graph)

(Note that ΔV_{BE} means 'change of V_{BE}' and ΔI_B means 'change of I_B')

Output resistance (from the output characteristic, Fig. 12.10)

$$\text{Static (or d.c.) output resistance} = \frac{V_{CE}}{I_C}$$

(from corresponding points on the graph)

$$\text{Dynamic (or a.c.) output resistance} = \frac{\Delta V_{CE}}{\Delta I_C}$$

(from the slope of the graph)

(Note that ΔV_{CE} means 'change of V_{CE}' and ΔI_C means 'change of I_C')

Current gain (from the transfer characteristic, Fig. 12.11)

Static (or d.c.) current gain $= \dfrac{I_C}{I_B}$

(from corresponding points on the graph)

Dynamic (or a.c.) current gain $= \dfrac{\Delta I_C}{\Delta I_B}$

(from the slope of the graph)

(Note that ΔI_C means 'change of I_C' and ΔI_B means 'change of I_B')

The method for determining these parameters from the relevant characteristic is illustrated in the following worked problems.

Problem 3. Figure 12.13 shows the input characteristic for an n-p-n silicon transistor. When the base-emitter voltage is 0.65 V, determine (a) the value of base current, (b) the static value of input resistance, and (c) the dynamic value of input resistance.

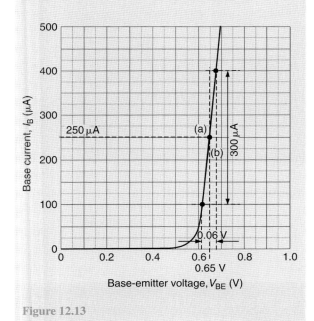

Figure 12.13

(a) From Fig. 12.13, when $V_{BE} = 0.65$ V, **base current, $I_B = 250\,\mu A$** (shown as (a) on the graph)

(b) When $V_{BE} = 0.65$ V, $I_B = 250\,\mu A$, hence, **the static value of input resistance**

$$= \frac{V_{BE}}{I_B} = \frac{0.65}{250 \times 10^{-6}} = \mathbf{2.6\,k\Omega}$$

(c) From Fig. 12.13, V_{BE} changes by 0.06 V when I_B changes by $300\,\mu A$ (as shown by (b) on the graph). Hence,

dynamic value of input resistance

$$= \frac{\Delta V_{BE}}{\Delta I_B} = \frac{0.06}{300 \times 10^{-6}} = \mathbf{200\,\Omega}$$

Problem 4. Figure 12.14 shows the output characteristic for an n-p-n silicon transistor. When the collector-emitter voltage is 10 V and the base current is $80\,\mu A$, determine (a) the value of collector current, (b) the static value of output resistance, and (c) the dynamic value of output resistance.

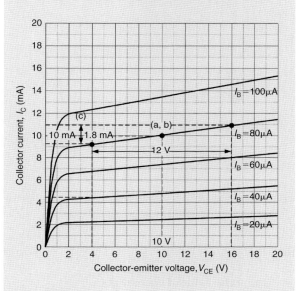

Figure 12.14

(a) From Fig. 12.14, when $V_{CE} = 10$ V and $I_B = 80\,\mu A$, (i.e. point (a, b) on the graph), the **collector current, $I_C = 10\,mA$**

(b) When $V_{CE} = 10$ V and $I_B = 80\,\mu A$ then $I_C = 10\,mA$ from part (a).

Hence,

the static value of output resistance

$$= \frac{V_{CE}}{I_C} = \frac{10}{10 \times 10^{-3}} = \mathbf{1\,k\Omega}$$

(c) When the change in V_{CE} is 12 V, the change in I_C is 1.8 mA (shown as point (c) on the graph)

Hence,

the dynamic value of output resistance

$$= \frac{\Delta V_{CE}}{\Delta I_C} = \frac{12}{1.8 \times 10^{-3}} = \mathbf{6.67\,k\Omega}$$

Problem 5. Figure 12.15 shows the transfer characteristic for an n-p-n silicon transistor. When the base current is 2.5 mA, determine (a) the value of collector current, (b) the static value of current gain, and (c) the dynamic value of current gain.

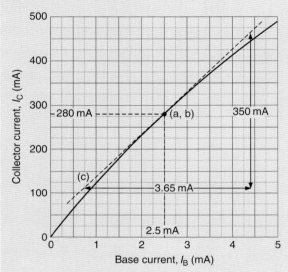

Figure 12.15

(a) From Fig. 12.15, when $I_B = 2.5$ mA, **collector current, $I_C = 280$ mA** (see point (a, b) on the graph)

(b) From part (a), when $I_B = 2.5$ mA, $I_C = 280$ mA hence,
the static value of current gain

$$= \frac{I_C}{I_B} = \frac{280 \times 10^{-3}}{2.5 \times 10^{-3}} = \mathbf{112}$$

(c) In Fig. 12.15, the tangent through the point (a, b) is shown by the broken straight line (c).
Hence,
the dynamic value of current gain

$$= \frac{\Delta I_C}{\Delta I_B} = \frac{(460 - 110) \times 10^{-3}}{(4.4 - 0.75) \times 10^{-3}} = \frac{350}{3.65} = \mathbf{96}$$

12.9 Current gain

As stated earlier, the common-emitter current gain is given by the ratio of collector current, I_C, to base current, I_B. We use the symbol h_{FE} to represent the static value of common-emitter current gain, thus:

$$h_{FE} = \frac{I_C}{I_B}$$

Similarly, we use h_{fe} to represent the dynamic value of common emitter current gain, thus:

$$h_{fe} = \frac{\Delta I_C}{\Delta I_B}$$

As we showed earlier, values of h_{FE} and h_{fe} can be obtained from the transfer characteristic (I_C plotted against I_B). Note that h_{FE} is found from corresponding static values while h_{fe} is found by measuring the slope of the graph. Also note that, if the transfer characteristic is linear, there is little (if any) difference between h_{FE} and h_{fe}.

It is worth noting that current gain (h_{fe}) varies with collector current. For most small-signal transistors, h_{fe} is a maximum at a collector current in the range 1 mA and 10 mA. Current gain also falls to very low values for power transistors when operating at very high values of collector current. Furthermore, most transistor parameters (particularly common-emitter current gain, h_{fe}) are liable to wide variation from one device to the next. It is, therefore, important to design circuits on the basis of the minimum value for h_{fe} in order to ensure successful operation with a variety of different devices.

Problem 6. A bipolar transistor has a common-emitter current gain of 125. If the transistor operates with a collector current of 50 mA, determine the value of base current.

Common-emitter current gain, $h_{FE} = \dfrac{I_C}{I_B}$

from which, **base current,**

$$I_B = \frac{I_C}{h_{FE}} = \frac{50 \times 10^{-3}}{125} = \mathbf{400\,\mu A}$$

12.10 Typical BJT characteristics and maximum ratings

Table 12.2 summarises the characteristics of some typical bipolar junction transistors for different applications, where I_C max is the maximum collector current, V_{CE} max is the maximum collector-emitter voltage, P_{TOT} max is the maximum device power dissipation, and h_{fe} is the typical value of common-emitter current gain.

Table 12.2 Transistor characteristics and maximum ratings

Device	Type	I_C max.	V_{CE} max.	P_{TOT} max.	h_{FE} typical	Application
BC108	n-p-n	100 mA	20 V	300 mW	125	General-purpose small-signal amplifier
BCY70	n-p-n	200 mA	−40 V	360 mW	150	General-purpose small-signal amplifier
2N3904	n-p-n	200 mA	40 V	310 mW	150	Switching
BF180	n-p-n	20 mA	20 V	150 mW	100	RF amplifier
2N3053	n-p-n	700 mA	40 V	800 mW	150	Low-frequency amplifier/driver
2N3055	n-p-n	15 A	60 V	115 W	50	Low-frequency power

Problem 7. Which of the bipolar transistors listed in Table 12.2 would be most suitable for each of the following applications: (a) the input stage of a radio receiver, (b) the output stage of an audio amplifier, and (c) generating a 5 V square wave pulse.

(a) **BF180**, since this transistor is designed for use in radio frequency (RF) applications

(b) **2N3055**, since this is the only device in the list that can operate at a sufficiently high power level

(c) **2N3904**, since switching transistors are designed for use in pulse and square wave applications

---

Now try the following exercise

Exercise 65   Further problems on bipolar junction transistors

1. Explain, with the aid of sketches, the operation of an n-p-n transistor and also explain why the collector current is very nearly equal to the emitter current.

2. Describe the basic principle of operation of a bipolar junction transistor, including why majority carriers crossing into the base from the emitter pass to the collector and why the collector current is almost unaffected by the collector potential.

3. Explain what is meant by 'leakage current' in a bipolar junction transistor and why this can usually be ignored.

4. For a transistor connected in common-emitter configuration, sketch the typical output characteristics relating collector current and the collector-emitter voltage, for various values of base current. Explain the shape of the characteristics.

5. Sketch the typical input characteristic relating base current and the base-emitter voltage for a transistor connected in common-emitter configuration and explain its shape.

6. With the aid of a circuit diagram, explain how the input and output characteristic of a common-emitter n-p-n transistor may be produced.

7. Define the term 'current gain' for a bipolar junction transistor operating in common-emitter mode.

8. A bipolar junction transistor operates with a collector current of 1.2 A and a base current

of 50 mA. What will the value of emitter current be? [1.25 A]

9. What is the value of common-emitter current gain for the transistor in problem 8? [24]

10. Corresponding readings of base current, I_B, and base-emitter voltage, V_{BE}, for a bipolar junction transistor are given in the table below:

V_{BE} (V)	0	0.1	0.2	0.3	0.4	0.5	0.6	0.7	0.8
I_B (μA)	0	0	0	0	1	3	19	57	130

Plot the I_B/V_{BE} characteristic for the device and use it to determine (a) the value of I_B when $V_{BE} = 0.65$ V, (b) the static value of input resistance when $V_{BE} = 0.65$ V, and (c) the dynamic value of input resistance when $V_{BE} = 0.65$ V.
[(a) 32.5 μA (b) 20 kΩ (c) 3 kΩ]

11. Corresponding readings of base current, I_B, and collector current, I_C, for a bipolar junction transistor are given in the table below:

I_B (μA)	0	10	20	30	40	50	60	70	80
I_C (mA)	0	1.1	2.1	3.1	4.0	4.9	5.8	6.7	7.6

Plot the I_C/I_B characteristic for the device and use it to determine the static value of common-emitter current gain when $I_B = 45$ μA. [98]

12.11 Field effect transistors

Field effect transistors are available in two basic forms; junction gate and insulated gate. The gate-source junction of a **junction gate field effect transistor (JFET)** is effectively a reverse-biased p-n junction. The gate connection of an **insulated gate field effect transistor (IGFET)**, on the other hand, is insulated from the channel and charge is capacitively coupled to the channel. To keep things simple, we will consider only JFET devices. Figure 12.16 shows the basic construction of an n-channel JFET.

JFET transistors comprise a channel of p-type or n-type material surrounded by material of the opposite polarity. The ends of the channel (in which conduction takes place) form electrodes known as the source

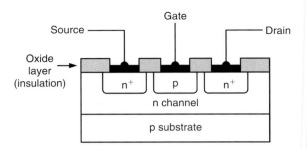

Figure 12.16

and drain. The effective width of the channel (in which conduction takes place) is controlled by a charge placed on the third (gate) electrode. The effective resistance between the source and drain is thus determined by the voltage present at the gate. (The + signs in Fig. 12.16 is used to indicate a region of heavy doping thus n^+ simply indicates a heavily doped n-type region.)

JFETs offer a very much higher input resistance when compared with bipolar transistors. For example, the input resistance of a bipolar transistor operating in common-emitter mode is usually around 2.5 kΩ. A JFET transistor operating in equivalent common-source mode would typically exhibit an input resistance of 100 MΩ! This feature makes JFET devices ideal for use in applications where a very high input resistance is desirable.

As with bipolar transistors, the characteristics of a FET are often presented in the form of a set of graphs relating voltage and current present at the transistors, terminals.

12.12 Field effect transistor characteristics

A typical **mutual characteristic** (I_D plotted against V_{GS}) for a small-signal general-purpose n-channel field effect transistor operating in common-source mode is shown in Fig. 12.17. This characteristic shows that the drain current is progressively reduced as the gate-source voltage is made more negative. At a certain value of V_{GS} the drain current falls to zero and the device is said to be cut-off.

Figure 12.18 shows a typical family of **output characteristics** (I_D plotted against V_{DS}) for a small-signal general-purpose n-channel FET operating in common-source mode. This characteristic comprises a family of curves, each relating to a different value of gate-source voltage V_{GS}. You might also like to compare this characteristic with the output characteristic for a transistor

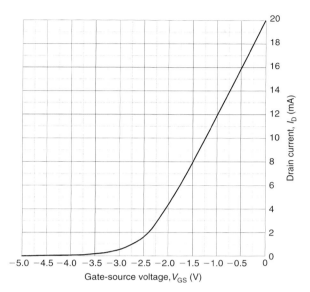

Figure 12.17

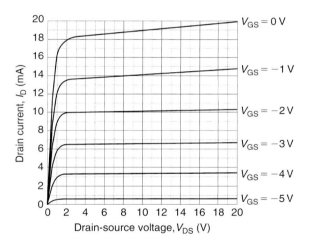

Figure 12.18

operating in common-emitter mode that you met earlier in Fig. 12.10.

As in the case of the bipolar junction transistor, the output characteristic curves for an n-channel FET have a 'knee' that occurs at low values of V_{DS}. Also, note how the curves become flattened above this value with the drain current I_D not changing very significantly for a comparatively large change in drain-source voltage V_{DS}. These characteristics are, in fact, even flatter than those for a bipolar transistor. Because of their flatness, they are often said to represent a constant current characteristic.

The gain offered by a field effect transistor is normally expressed in terms of its **forward transconductance**

(g_{fs} or Y_{fs}) in common-source mode. In this mode, the input voltage is applied to the gate and the output current appears in the drain (the source is effectively common to both the input and output circuits).

In common-source mode, **the static (or d.c.) forward transfer conductance** is given by:

$$g_{FS} = \frac{I_D}{V_{GS}}$$

(from corresponding points on the graph)

whilst **the dynamic (or a.c.) forward transfer conductance** is given by:

$$g_{fs} = \frac{\Delta I_D}{\Delta V_{GS}}$$

(from the slope of the graph)

(Note that ΔI_D means 'change of I_D' and ΔV_{GS} means 'change of V_{GS}')

The method for determining these parameters from the relevant characteristic is illustrated in worked problem 8 below.

Forward transfer conductance (g_{fs}) varies with drain current. For most small-signal devices, g_{fs}, is quoted for values of drain current between 1 mA and 10 mA. Most FET parameters (particularly forward transfer conductance) are liable to wide variation from one device to the next. It is, therefore, important to design circuits on the basis of the minimum value for g_{fs}, in order to ensure successful operation with a variety of different devices. The experimental circuit for obtaining the common-source characteristics of an n-channel JFET transistor is shown in Fig. 12.19.

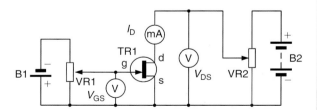

Figure 12.19

Problem 8.   Figure 12.20 shows the mutual characteristic for a junction gate field effect transistor. When the gate-source voltage is −2.5 V, determine (a) the value of drain current, (b) the dynamic value of forward transconductance.

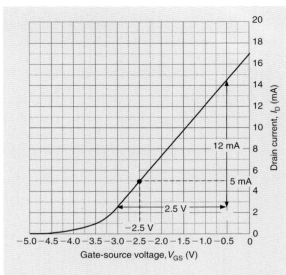

Figure 12.20

(a) From Fig. 12.20, when $V_{GS} = -2.5\,V$, the **drain current, $I_D = 5\,mA$**

(b) From Fig. 12.20

$$g_{fs} = \frac{\Delta I_D}{\Delta V_{GS}} = \frac{(14.5 - 2.5) \times 10^{-3}}{2.5}$$

i.e. **the dynamic value of forward transconductance** $= \dfrac{12 \times 10^{-3}}{2.5} = \mathbf{4.8\,mS}$

(note the unit – **siemens, S**)

Problem 9. A field effect transistor operates with a drain current of 100 mA and a gate source bias of $-1\,V$. The device has a g_{fs} value of 0.25. If the bias voltage decreases to $-1.1\,V$, determine (a) the change in drain current, and (b) the new value of drain current.

(a) The change in gate-source voltage (V_{GS}) is $-0.1\,V$ and the resulting change in drain current can be determined from:

$$g_{fs} = \frac{\Delta I_D}{\Delta V_{GS}}$$

Hence, **the change in drain current,**

$$\Delta I_D = g_{fs} \times \Delta V_{GS}$$

$$= 0.25 \times -0.1$$

$$= -0.025\,A = \mathbf{-25\,mA}$$

(b) The **new value of drain current** $= (100 - 25)$

$$= \mathbf{75\,mA}$$

12.13 Typical FET characteristics and maximum ratings

Table 12.3 summarises the characteristics of some typical field effect transistors for different applications, where I_D max is the maximum drain current, V_{DS} max is the maximum drain-source voltage, P_D max is the maximum drain power dissipation, and g_{fs} typ is the typical value of forward transconductance for the transistor. The list includes both depletion and enhancement types as well as junction and insulated gate types.

Problem 10. Which of the field effect transistors listed in Table 12.3 would be most suitable for each of the following applications: (a) the input stage of a radio receiver, (b) the output stage of a transmitter, and (c) switching a load connected to a high-voltage supply.

(a) **BF244A**, since this transistor is designed for use in radio frequency (RF) applications

(b) **MRF171A**, since this device is designed for RF power applications

(c) **IRF830**, since this device is intended for switching applications and can operate at up to 500 V

12.14 Transistor amplifiers

Three basic circuit arrangements are used for transistor amplifiers and these are based on the three circuit configurations that we met earlier (i.e. they depend upon which one of the three transistor connections is made common to both the input and the output). In the case of **bipolar transistors**, the configurations are known as **common emitter, common collector** (or emitter follower) and **common base**.

Where **field effect transistors** are used, the corresponding configurations are **common source, common drain** (or source follower) and **common gate**.

These basic circuit configurations depicted in Figs 12.21 and 12.22 exhibit quite different performance characteristics, as shown in Tables 12.4 and 12.5 respectively.

Table 12.3 FET characteristics and maximum ratings

Device	Type	I_D max.	V_{DS} max.	P_D max.	g_{fs} typ.	Application
2N2819	n-chan.	10 mA	25 V	200 mW	4.5 mS	General purpose
2N5457	n-chan.	10 mA	25 V	310 mW	1.2 mS	General purpose
2N7000	n-chan.	200 mA	60 V	400 mW	0.32 S	Low-power switching
BF244A	n-chan.	100 mA	30 V	360 mW	3.3 mS	RF amplifier
BSS84	p-chan.	−130 mA	−50 V	360 mW	0.27 S	Low-power switching
IRF830	n-chan.	4.5 A	500 V	75 W	3.0 S	Power switching
MRF171A	n-chan.	4.5 A	65 V	115 W	1.8 S	RF power amplifier

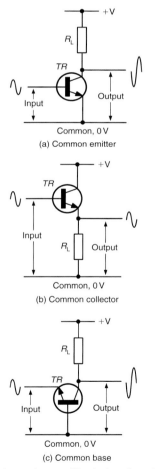

+V
RL
TR
Input
Output
Common, 0 V
(a) Common emitter
+V
TR
Input
RL
Output
Common, 0 V
(b) Common collector
+V
RL
TR
Input
Output
Common, 0 V
(c) Common base

Bipolar transistor amplifier circuit configurations

Figure 12.21

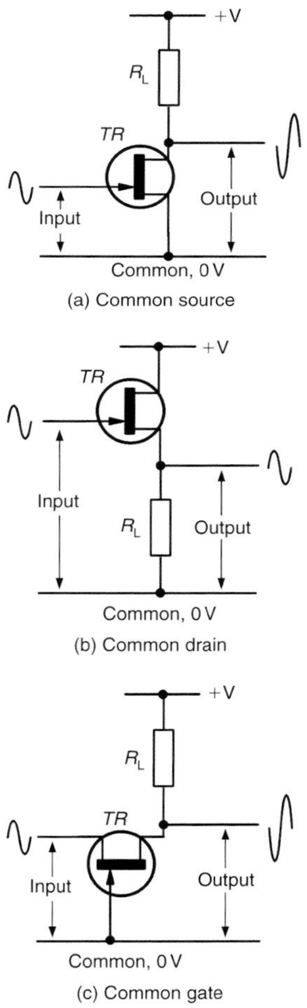

+V
RL
TR
Input
Output
Common, 0 V
(a) Common source
+V
TR
Input
RL
Output
Common, 0 V
(b) Common drain
+V
RL
TR
Input
Output
Common, 0 V
(c) Common gate

Field effect transistor amplifier circuit configurations

Figure 12.22

Table 12.4 Characteristics of BJT amplifiers

	Bipolar transistor amplifiers (see Figure 12.21)		
Parameter	Common emitter	Common collector	Common base
Voltage gain	medium/high (40)	unity (1)	high (200)
Current gain	high (200)	high (200)	unity (1)
Power gain	very high (8000)	high (200)	high (200)
Input resistance	medium (2.5 kΩ)	high (100 kΩ)	low (200 Ω)
Output resistance	medium/high (20 kΩ)	low (100 Ω)	high (100 kΩ)
Phase shift	180°	0°	0°
Typical applications	General purpose, AF and RF amplifiers	Impedance matching, input and output stages	RF and VHF amplifiers

Table 12.5 Characteristics of FET amplifiers

	Field effect transistor amplifiers (see Figure 12.22)		
Parameter	Common source	Common drain	Common gate
Voltage gain	medium/high (40)	unity (1)	high (250)
Current gain	very high (200 000)	very high (200 000)	unity (1)
Power gain	very high (8 000 000)	very high (200 000)	high (250)
Input resistance	very high (1 MΩ)	very high (1 MΩ)	low (500 Ω)
Output resistance	medium/high (50 kΩ)	low (200 Ω)	high (150 kΩ)
Phase shift	180°	0°	0°
Typical applications	General purpose, AF and RF amplifiers	Impedance matching stages	RF and VHF amplifiers

A requirement of most amplifiers is that the output signal should be a faithful copy of the input signal or be somewhat larger in amplitude. Other types of amplifier are 'non-linear', in which case their input and output waveforms will not necessarily be similar. In practice, the degree of linearity provided by an amplifier can be affected by a number of factors including the amount of bias applied and the amplitude of the input signal. It is also worth noting that a linear amplifier will become non-linear when the applied input signal exceeds a threshold value. Beyond this value the amplifier is said to be overdriven and the output will become increasingly distorted if the input signal is further increased.

The optimum value of bias for **linear (Class A) amplifiers** is that value which ensures that the active devices are operated at the mid-point of their characteristics. In practice, this means that a static value of collector current will flow even when there is no signal present. Furthermore, the collector current will flow throughout the complete cycle of an input signal (i.e. conduction will take place over an angle of $360°$). At no stage should the transistor be **saturated** ($V_{CE} \approx 0$ V or $V_{DS} \approx 0$ V) nor should it be **cut-off** ($V_{CE} \approx V_{CC}$ or $V_{DS} \approx V_{DD}$).

In order to ensure that a static value of collector current flows in a transistor, a small current must be applied to the base of the transistor. This current can be derived from the same voltage rail that supplies the collector circuit (via the **collector load**). Figure 12.23 shows a simple Class-A common-emitter circuit in which the **base bias resistor**, R1, and **collector load**

resistor, R2, are connected to a common positive supply rail.

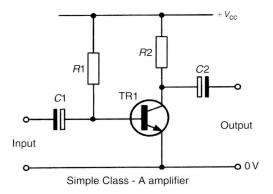

Figure 12.23

The a.c. signal is applied to the base terminal of the transistor via a coupling capacitor, C1. This capacitor removes the d.c. component of any signal applied to the input terminals and ensures that the base bias current delivered by R1 is unaffected by any device connected to the input. C2 couples the signal out of the stage and also prevents d.c. current flow appearing at the output terminals.

12.15 Load lines

The a.c. performance of a transistor amplifier stage can be predicted using a **load line** superimposed on the relevant set of output characteristics. For a bipolar transistor operating in common-emitter mode the required characteristics are I_C plotted against V_{CE}. One end of the load line corresponds to the supply voltage (V_{CC}) while the other end corresponds to the value of collector or drain current that would flow with the device totally saturated ($V_{CE} = 0\,V$). In this condition:

$$I_C = \frac{V_{CC}}{R_L}$$

where R_L is the value of collector or drain load resistance.

Figure 12.24 shows a load line superimposed on a set of output characteristics for a bipolar transistor operating in common-emitter mode. The quiescent point (or operating point) is the point on the load line that corresponds to the conditions that exist when no-signal is applied to the stage. In Fig. 12.24, the base bias current is set at $20\,\mu A$ so that the **quiescent point** effectively sits roughly halfway along the load line. This position

ensures that the collector voltage can swing both positively (above) and negatively (below) its quiescent value (V_{CQ}).

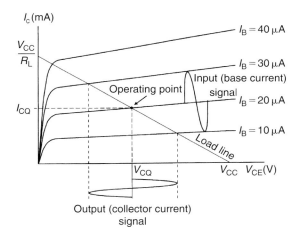

Figure 12.24

The effect of superimposing an alternating base current (of $20\,\mu A$ peak-peak) to the d.c. bias current (of $20\,\mu A$) can be clearly seen. The corresponding collector current signal can be determined by simply moving up and down the load line.

> **Problem 11.** The characteristic curves shown in Fig. 12.25 relate to a transistor operating in common-emitter mode. If the transistor is operated with $I_B = 30\,\mu A$, a load resistor of $1.2\,k\Omega$ and an 18 V supply, determine (a) the quiescent values of collector voltage and current (V_{CQ} and I_{CQ}), and (b) the peak-peak output voltage that would be produced by an input signal of $40\,\mu A$ peak-peak.

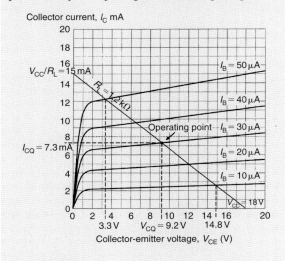

Figure 12.25

(a) First we need to construct the load line on Fig. 12.25. The two ends of the load line will correspond to V_{CC}, the 18 V supply, on the collector-emitter voltage axis and $18\,V/1.2\,k\Omega$ or 15 mA on the collector current axis.

Next we locate the **operating point** (or **quiescent point**) from the point of intersection of the $I_B = 30\,\mu A$ characteristic and the load line. Having located the operating point we can read off the **quiescent values**, i.e. the no-signal values, of collector-emitter voltage (V_{CQ}) and collector current (I_{CQ}). Hence, $V_{CQ} = 9.2\,V$ and $I_{CQ} = 7.3\,mA$

(b) Next we can determine the maximum and minimum values of collector-emitter voltage by locating the appropriate intercept points on Fig. 12.25. Note that the maximum and minimum values of base current will be $(30\,\mu A + 20\,\mu A) = 50\,\mu A$ on positive peaks of the signal and $(30\,\mu A - 20\,\mu A) = 10\,\mu A$ on negative peaks of the signal. The maximum and minimum values of V_{CE} are, respectively, 14.8 V and 3.3 V. Hence,

the output voltage swing $= (14.8\,V - 3.3\,V)$

$$= 11.5\,V\ \textbf{peak-peak}$$

Problem 12. An n-p-n transistor has the following characteristics, which may be assumed to be linear between the values of collector voltage stated.

Base current (µA)	Collector current (mA) for collector voltages of:	
	1 V	5 V
30	1.4	1.6
50	3.0	3.5
70	4.6	5.2

The transistor is used as a common-emitter amplifier with load resistor $R_L = 1.2\,k\Omega$ and a collector supply of 7 V. The signal input resistance is $1\,k\Omega$. If an input current of $20\,\mu A$ peak varies sinusoidally about a mean bias of $50\,\mu A$, estimate (a) the quiescent values of collector voltage and current, (b) the output voltage swing, (c) the voltage gain, (d) the dynamic current gain, and (e) the power gain.

The characteristics are drawn as shown in Fig. 12.26.

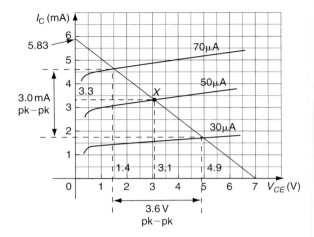

Figure 12.26

The two ends of the load line will correspond to V_{CC}, the 7 V supply, on the collector-emitter voltage axis and $7\,V/1.2\,k\Omega = 5.83\,mA$ on the collector current axis.

(a) The operating point (or quiescent point), X, is located from the point of intersection of the $I_B = 50\,\mu A$ characteristic and the load line. Having located the operating point we can read off the **quiescent values**, i.e. the no-signal values, of collector-emitter voltage (V_{CQ}) and collector current (I_{CQ}). Hence, $V_{CQ} = 3.1\,V$ and $I_{CQ} = 3.3\,mA$

(b) The maximum and minimum values of collector-emitter voltage may be determined by locating the appropriate intercept points on Fig. 12.26. Note that the maximum and minimum values of base current will be $(50\,\mu A + 20\,\mu A) = 70\,\mu A$ on positive peaks of the signal and $(50\,\mu A - 20\,\mu A) = 30\,\mu A$ on negative peaks of the signal. The maximum and minimum values of V_{CE} are, respectively, 4.9 V and 1.4 V. Hence,

the output voltage swing $= (4.9\,V - 1.4\,V)$

$$= 3.5\,V\ \textbf{peak-peak}$$

(c) Voltage gain $= \dfrac{\text{change in collector voltage}}{\text{change in base voltage}}$

The change in collector voltage $= 3.5\,V$ from part (b).

The input voltage swing is given by: $i_b R_i$,

where i_b is the base current swing $= (70 - 30) = 40\,\mu A$ and R_i is the input resistance $= 1\,k\Omega$.

Hence,
input voltage swing $= 40 \times 10^{-6} \times 1 \times 10^{3}$
$$= 40\,\text{mV}$$
$$= \text{change in base voltage.}$$

Thus,

voltage gain $= \dfrac{\text{change in collector voltage}}{\text{change in base voltage}}$

$$= \frac{\Delta V_C}{\Delta V_B} = \frac{3.5}{40 \times 10^{-3}} = \mathbf{87.5}$$

(d) Dynamic current gain, $h_{\text{fe}} = \dfrac{\Delta I_C}{\Delta I_B}$

From Figure 12.26, the output current swing, i.e. the change in collector current, $\Delta I_C = 3.0\,\text{mA}$ peak to peak. The input base current swing, the change in base current, $\Delta I_B = 40\,\mu\text{A}$.

Hence, **the dynamic current gain**,

$$h_{\text{fe}} = \frac{\Delta I_C}{\Delta I_B} = \frac{3.0 \times 10^{-3}}{40 \times 10^{-6}} = \mathbf{75}$$

(e) For a resistive load, the power gain is given by:

$$\textbf{power gain} = \text{voltage gain} \times \text{current gain}$$
$$= 87.5 \times 75 = \mathbf{6562.5}$$

Now try the following exercises

Exercise 66   Further problems on transistors

1. State whether the following statements are true or false:

    (a) The purpose of a transistor amplifier is to increase the frequency of the input signal.

    (b) The gain of an amplifier is the ratio of the output signal amplitude to the input signal amplitude.

    (c) The output characteristics of a transistor relate the collector current to the base current.

    (d) If the load resistor value is increased the load line gradient is reduced.

    (e) In a common-emitter amplifier, the output voltage is shifted through 180° with reference to the input voltage.

    (f) In a common-emitter amplifier, the input and output currents are in phase.

(g) The dynamic current gain of a transistor is always greater than the static current gain.
[(a) false (b) true (c) false (d) true
(e) true (f) true (g) true]

2. In relation to a simple transistor amplifier stage, explain what is meant by the terms: (a) Class-A (b) saturation (c) cut-off (d) quiescent point.

3. Sketch the circuit of a simple Class-A BJT amplifier and explain the function of the components.

4. Explain, with the aid of a labelled sketch, how a load line can be used to determine the operating point of a simple Class-A transistor amplifier.

5. Sketch circuits showing how a JFET can be connected as an amplifier in: (a) common source configuration, (b) common drain configuration, (c) common gate configuration. State typical values of voltage gain and input resistance for each circuit.

6. The output characteristics for a BJT are shown in Fig. 12.27. If this device is used in a common-emitter amplifier circuit operating from a 12 V supply with a base bias of $60\,\mu\text{A}$ and a load resistor of $1\,\text{k}\Omega$, determine (a) the quiescent values of collector-emitter voltage and collector current, and (b) the peak-peak collector voltage when an $80\,\mu\text{A}$ peak-peak signal current is applied.
[(a) 5 V, 7 mA (b) 8.5 V]

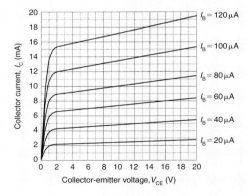

Figure 12.27

7. The output characteristics of a JFET are shown in Fig. 12.28. If this device is used in an

amplifier circuit operating from an 18 V supply with a gate-source bias voltage of −3 V and a load resistance of 900 Ω, determine (a) the quiescent values of drain-source voltage and drain current, (b) the peak-peak output voltage when an input voltage of 2 V peak-peak is applied, and (c) the voltage gain of the stage.

[(a) 12.2 V, 6.1 mA (b) 5.5 V (c) 2.75]

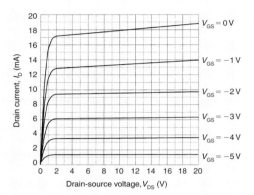

Figure 12.28

8. An amplifier has a current gain of 40 and a voltage gain of 30. Determine the power gain.

[1200]

9. The output characteristics of a transistor in common-emitter mode configuration can be regarded as straight lines connecting the following points.

	$I_B = 20\,\mu A$		$50\,\mu A$		$80\,\mu A$	
V_{CE} (v)	1.0	8.0	1.0	8.0	1.0	8.0
I_C (mA)	1.2	1.4	3.4	4.2	6.1	8.1

Plot the characteristics and superimpose the load line for a 1 kΩ load, given that the supply voltage is 9 V and the d.c. base bias is 50 μA. The signal input resistance is 800 Ω. When a peak input current of 30 μA varies sinusoidally about a mean bias of 50 μA, determine (a) the quiescent values of collector voltage and current, V_{CQ} and I_{CQ}, (b) the output voltage swing, (c) the voltage gain, (d) the dynamic current gain, and (e) the power gain.

[(a) 5.2 V, 3.7 mA (b) 5.1 V (c) 106
(d) 87 (e) 9222]

Exercise 67   Short answer questions on transistors

1. In a p-n-p transistor the p-type material regions are called the ...... and ...... , and the n-type material region is called the ......

2. In an n-p-n transistor, the p-type material region is called the ...... and the n-type material regions are called the ...... and the ......

3. In a p-n-p transistor, the base-emitter junction is ......biased and the base-collector junction is ...... biased

4. In an n-p-n transistor, the base-collector junction is ...... biased and the base-emitter junction is ...... biased

5. Majority charge carriers in the emitter of a transistor pass into the base region. Most of them do not recombine because the base is ...... doped

6. Majority carriers in the emitter region of a transistor pass the base-collector junction because for these carriers it is ...... biased

7. Conventional current flow is in the direction of ...... flow

8. Leakage current flows from ...... to ...... in an n-p-n transistor

9. The input characteristic of I_B against V_{BE} for a transistor in common-emitter configuration is similar in shape to that of a ....

10. From a transistor input characteristic,

$$\text{static input resistance} = \frac{......}{......} \text{ and}$$

$$\text{dynamic input resistance} = \frac{......}{......}$$

11. From a transistor output characteristic,

$$\text{static output resistance} = \frac{......}{......} \text{ and}$$

$$\text{dynamic output resistance} = \frac{......}{......}$$

12. From a transistor transfer characteristic,

$$\text{static current gain} = \frac{......}{......} \text{and dynamic}$$

$$\text{current gain} = \frac{......}{......}$$

13. Complete the following statements that refer to a transistor amplifier:

   (a) An increase in base current causes collector current to ......

   (b) When base current increases, the voltage drop across the load resistor ......

   (c) Under no-signal conditions the power supplied by the battery to an amplifier equals the power dissipated in the load plus the power dissipated in the ......

   (d) The load line has a ...... gradient

   (e) The gradient of the load line depends upon the value of ......

   (f) The position of the load line depends upon ......

   (g) The current gain of a common-emitter amplifier is always greater than ......

   (h) The operating point is generally positioned at the ...... of the load line

14. Explain, with a diagram, the construction of a junction gate field effect transistor. State the advantage of a JFET over a bipolar transistor

15. Sketch typical mutual and output characteristics for a small-signal general-purpose FET operating in common-source mode

16. Name and sketch three possible circuit arrangements used for transistor amplifiers

17. Name and sketch three possible circuit arrangements used for FETs

18. Draw a circuit diagram showing how a transistor can be used as a common-emitter amplifier. Explain briefly the purpose of all the components you show in your diagram

19. Explain how a load line is used to predict a.c. performance of a transistor amplifier

20. What is the quiescent point on a load line?

Exercise 68   Multi-choice problems on transistors
(Answers on page 420)

In Problems 1 to 10 select the correct answer from those given.

1. In normal operation, the junctions of a p-n-p transistor are:

   (a) both forward biased

   (b) base-emitter forward biased and base-collector reverse biased

   (c) both reverse biased

   (d) base-collector forward biased and base-emitter reverse biased

2. In normal operation, the junctions of an n-p-n transistor are:

   (a) both forward biased

   (b) base-emitter forward biased and base-collector reverse biased

   (c) both reverse biased

   (d) base-collector forward biased and base-emitter reverse biased

3. The current flow across the base-emitter junction of a p-n-p transistor

   (a) mainly electrons

   (b) equal numbers of holes and electrons

   (c) mainly holes

   (d) the leakage current

4. The current flow across the base-emitter junction of an n-p-n transistor consists of

   (a) mainly electrons

   (b) equal numbers of holes and electrons

   (c) mainly holes

   (d) the leakage current

5. In normal operation an n-p-n transistor connected in common-base configuration has

   (a) the emitter at a lower potential than the base

   (b) the collector at a lower potential than the base

   (c) the base at a lower potential than the emitter

   (d) the collector at a lower potential than the emitter

6. In normal operation, a p-n-p transistor connected in common-base configuration has

   (a) the emitter at a lower potential than the base

   (b) the collector at a higher potential than the base

   (c) the base at a higher potential than the emitter

   (d) the collector at a lower potential than the emitter

7. If the per unit value of electrons which leave the emitter and pass to the collector is 0.9 in an n-p-n transistor and the emitter current is 4 mA, then
   (a) the base current is approximately 4.4 mA
   (b) the collector current is approximately 3.6 mA
   (c) the collector current is approximately 4.4 mA
   (d) the base current is approximately 3.6 mA

8. The base region of a p-n-p transistor is
   (a) very thin and heavily doped with holes
   (b) very thin and heavily doped with electrons
   (c) very thin and lightly doped with holes
   (d) very thin and lightly doped with electrons

9. The voltage drop across the base-emitter junction of a p-n-p silicon transistor in normal operation is about
   (a) 200 mV (b) 600 mV (c) zero
   (d) 4.4 V

10. For a p-n-p transistor,
    (a) the number of majority carriers crossing the base-emitter junction largely depends on the collector voltage
    (b) in common-base configuration, the collector current is proportional to the collector-base voltage
    (c) in common-emitter configuration, the base current is less than the base current in common-base configuration
    (d) the collector current flow is independent of the emitter current flow for a given value of collector-base voltage

In questions 11 to 15, which refer to the amplifier shown in Fig. 12.29, select the correct answer from those given.

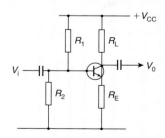

Figure 12.29

11. If R_L short-circuited:
    (a) the amplifier signal output would fall to zero
    (b) the collector current would fall to zero
    (c) the transistor would overload

12. If R_2 open-circuited:
    (a) the amplifier signal output would fall to zero
    (b) the operating point would be affected and the signal would distort
    (c) the input signal would not be applied to the base

13. A voltmeter connected across R_E reads zero. Most probably
    (a) the transistor base-emitter junction has short-circuited
    (b) R_L has open-circuited
    (c) R_2 has short-circuited

14. A voltmeter connected across R_L reads zero. Most probably
    (a) the V_{CC} supply battery is flat
    (b) the base collector junction of the transistor has gone open circuit
    (c) R_L has open-circuited

15. If R_E short-circuited:
    (a) the load line would be unaffected
    (b) the load line would be affected

In questions 16 to 20, which refer to the output characteristics shown in Fig. 12.30, select the correct answer from those given.

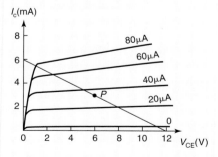

Figure 12.30

16. The load line represents a load resistor of
    (a) 1 kΩ   (b) 2 kΩ
    (c) 3 kΩ   (d) 0.5 kΩ

17. The no-signal collector dissipation for the operating point marked P is
    (a) 12 mW   (b) 15 mW
    (c) 18 mW   (d) 21 mW

18. The greatest permissible peak input current would be about
    (a) 30 μA   (b) 35 μA
    (c) 60 μA   (d) 80 μA

19. The greatest possible peak output voltage would then be about
    (a) 5.2 V   (b) 6.5 V
    (c) 8.8 V   (d) 13 V

20. The power dissipated in the load resistor under no-signal conditions is:
    (a) 16 mW   (b) 18 mW
    (c) 20 mW   (d) 22 mW

Revision Test 3

This revision test covers the material contained in Chapters 8 to 12. *The marks for each question are shown in brackets at the end of each question.*

1. A conductor, 25 cm long is situated at right-angles to a magnetic field. Determine the strength of the magnetic field if a current of 12 A in the conductor produces a force on it of 4.5 N. (3)

2. An electron in a television tube has a charge of 1.5×10^{-19} C and travels at 3×10^7 m/s perpendicular to a field of flux density $20\,\mu$T. Calculate the force exerted on the electron in the field. (3)

3. A lorry is travelling at 100 km/h. Assuming the vertical component of the earth's magnetic field is $40\,\mu$T and the back axle of the lorry is 1.98 m, find the e.m.f. generated in the axle due to motion. (4)

4. An e.m.f. of 2.5 kV is induced in a coil when a current of 2 A collapses to zero in 5 ms. Calculate the inductance of the coil. (4)

5. Two coils, P and Q, have a mutual inductance of 100 mH. If a current of 3 A in coil P is reversed in 20 ms, determine (a) the average e.m.f. induced in coil Q, and (b) the flux change linked with coil Q if it is wound with 200 turns. (5)

6. A moving coil instrument gives a f.s.d. when the current is 50 mA and has a resistance of $40\,\Omega$. Determine the value of resistance required to enable the instrument to be used (a) as a 0–5 A ammeter, and (b) as a 0–200 V voltmeter. State the mode of connection in each case. (8)

7. An amplifier has a gain of 20 dB. Its input power is 5 mW. Calculate its output power. (3)

8. A sinusoidal voltage trace displayed on an asciloscope is shown in Fig. RT3.1; the 'time/cm' switch is on 50 ms and the 'volts/cm' switch is on 2 V/cm. Determine for the waveform (a) the frequency (b) the peak-to-peak voltage (c) the amplitude (d) the r.m.s. value. (7)

9. With reference to a p-n junction, briefly explain the following terms: (a) majority carriers (b) contact potential (c) depletion layer (d) forward bias (e) reverse bias. (10)

10. Briefly describe each of the following, drawing their circuit diagram symbol and stating typical applications: (a) zenor diode (b) silicon controlled rectifier (c) light emitting diode (d) varactor diode (e) Schottky diode. (20)

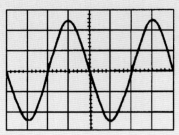

Figure RT3.1

11. The following values were obtained during an experiment on a varactor diode.

Voltage, V	5	10	15	20	25
Capacitance, pF	42	28	18	12	8

Plot a graph showing the variation of capacitance with voltage for the varactor. Label your axes clearly and use your graph to determine (a) the capacitance when the reverse voltage is -17.5 V, (b) the reverse voltage for a capacitance of 35 pF, and (c) the change in capacitance when the voltage changes from -2.5 V to -22.5 V. (8)

12. Briefly describe, with diagrams, the action of an n-p-n transistor. (7)

13. The output characteristics of a common-emitter transistor amplifier are given below. Assume that the characteristics are linear between the values of collector voltage stated.

	$I_B = 10\,\mu$A		$40\,\mu$A		$70\,\mu$A	
V_{CE} (V)	1.0	7.0	1.0	7.0	1.0	7.0
I_C (mA)	0.6	0.7	2.5	2.9	4.6	5.35

Plot the characteristics and superimpose the load line for a 1.5 kΩ load and collector supply voltage of 8 V. The signal input resistance is 1.2 kΩ. When a peak input current of $30\,\mu$A varies sinusoidally about a mean bias of $40\,\mu$A, determine (a) the quiescent values of collector voltage and current, (b) the output voltage swing, (c) the voltage gain, (d) the dynamic current gain, and (e) the power gain. (18)

General:

Charge $Q = It$ Force $F = ma$

Work $W = Fs$ Power $P = \dfrac{W}{t}$

Energy $W = Pt$

Ohm's law $V = IR$ or $I = \dfrac{V}{R}$ or $R = \dfrac{V}{I}$

Conductance $G = \dfrac{1}{R}$ Resistance $R = \dfrac{\rho l}{a}$

Power $P = VI = I^2R = \dfrac{V^2}{R}$

Resistance at $\theta°C$, $R_\theta = R_0(1 + \alpha_0\theta)$

Terminal p.d. of source, $V = E - Ir$

Series circuit $R = R_1 + R_2 + R_3 + \cdots$

Parallel network $\dfrac{1}{R} = \dfrac{1}{R_1} + \dfrac{1}{R_2} + \dfrac{1}{R_3} + \cdots$

Capacitors and Capacitance:

$E = \dfrac{V}{d}$ $C = \dfrac{Q}{V}$ $Q = It$ $D = \dfrac{Q}{A}$

$\dfrac{D}{E} = \varepsilon_0\varepsilon_r$ $C = \dfrac{\varepsilon_0\varepsilon_r A(n-1)}{d}$ $W = \dfrac{1}{2}CV^2$

Capacitors in parallel $C = C_1 + C_2 + C_3 + \cdots$

Capacitors in series $\dfrac{1}{C} = \dfrac{1}{C_1} + \dfrac{1}{C_2} + \dfrac{1}{C_3} + \cdots$

Magnetic Circuits:

$B = \dfrac{\Phi}{A}$ $F_m = NI$ $H = \dfrac{NI}{l}$ $\dfrac{B}{H} = \mu_0\mu_r$

$S = \dfrac{mmf}{\Phi} = \dfrac{l}{\mu_0\mu_r A}$

Electromagnetism:

$F = BIl\sin\theta$ $F = QvB$

Electromagnetic Induction:

$E = Blv\sin\theta$ $E = -N\dfrac{d\Phi}{dt} = -L\dfrac{dI}{dt}$

$W = \dfrac{1}{2}LI^2$ $L = \dfrac{N\Phi}{I} = \dfrac{N^2}{S}$ $E_2 = -M\dfrac{dI_1}{dt}$

$M = \dfrac{N_1 N_2}{S}$

Measurements:

Shunt $R_s = \dfrac{I_a r_a}{I_s}$ Multiplier $R_M = \dfrac{V - Ir_a}{I}$

Power in decibels $= 10\log\dfrac{P_2}{P_1}$

$= 20\log\dfrac{I_2}{I_1}$

$= 20\log\dfrac{V_2}{V_1}$

Wheatstone bridge $R_X = \dfrac{R_2 R_3}{R_1}$

Potentiometer $E_2 = E_1\left(\dfrac{l_2}{l_1}\right)$

Further Electrical and Electronic Principles

Chapter 13

D.C. circuit theory

At the end of this chapter you should be able to:

- state and use Kirchhoff's laws to determine unknown currents and voltages in d.c. circuits

- understand the superposition theorem and apply it to find currents in d.c. circuits

- understand general d.c. circuit theory

- understand Thévenin's theorem and apply a procedure to determine unknown currents in d.c. circuits

- recognize the circuit diagram symbols for ideal voltage and current sources

- understand Norton's theorem and apply a procedure to determine unknown currents in d.c. circuits

- appreciate and use the equivalence of the Thévenin and Norton equivalent networks

- state the maximum power transfer theorem and use it to determine maximum power in a d.c. circuit

13.1 Introduction

The laws which determine the currents and voltage drops in d.c. networks are: (a) Ohm's law (see Chapter 2), (b) the laws for resistors in series and in parallel (see Chapter 5), and (c) Kirchhoff's laws (see Section 13.2 following). In addition, there are a number of circuit theorems which have been developed for solving problems in electrical networks. These include:

  (i)   the superposition theorem (see Section 13.3),

 (ii)   Thévenin's theorem (see Section 13.5),

(iii)   Norton's theorem (see Section 13.7), and

(iv)   the maximum power transfer theorem (see Section 13.8)

13.2 Kirchhoff's laws

Kirchhoff's laws state:

(a) **Current Law.** *At any junction in an electric circuit the total current flowing towards that junction is*

equal to the total current flowing away from the junction, i.e. $\Sigma I = 0$

Thus, referring to Fig. 13.1:

$$I_1 + I_2 = I_3 + I_4 + I_5$$

or $I_1 + I_2 - I_3 - I_4 - I_5 = 0$

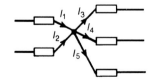

Figure 13.1

(b) **Voltage Law.** *In any closed loop in a network, the algebraic sum of the voltage drops (i.e. products of current and resistance) taken around the loop is equal to the resultant e.m.f. acting in that loop.*

Thus, referring to Fig. 13.2:

$$E_1 - E_2 = IR_1 + IR_2 + IR_3$$

DOI: 10.1016/B978-0-08-089056-2.00013-9

(Note that if current flows away from the positive terminal of a source, that source is considered by convention to be positive. Thus moving anticlockwise around the loop of Fig. 13.2, E_1 is positive and E_2 is negative.)

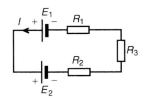

Figure 13.2

Problem 1. (a) Find the unknown currents marked in Fig. 13.3(a). (b) Determine the value of e.m.f. E in Fig. 13.3(b).

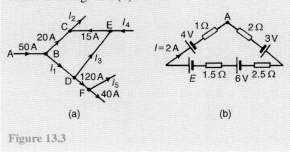

(a)   (b)

Figure 13.3

(a) Applying Kirchhoff's current law:

For junction B: $50 = 20 + I_1$

Hence $I_1 = 30\,A$

For junction C: $20 + 15 = I_2$

Hence $I_2 = 35\,A$

For junction D: $I_1 = I_3 + 120$

i.e. $30 = I_3 + 120$

Hence $I_3 = -90\,A$

(i.e. in the opposite direction to that shown in Fig. 13.3(a))

For junction E: $I_4 + I_3 = 15$

i.e. $I_4 = 15 - (-90)$

Hence $I_4 = 105\,A$

For junction F: $120 = I_5 + 40$

Hence $I_5 = 80\,A$

(b) Applying Kirchhoff's voltage law and moving clockwise around the loop of Fig. 13.3(b) starting at point A:

$$3 + 6 + E - 4 = (I)(2) + (I)(2.5)$$
$$+ (I)(1.5) + (I)(1)$$
$$= I(2 + 2.5 + 1.5 + 1)$$

i.e. $5 + E = 2(7)$, since $I = 2\,A$

Hence $E = 14 - 5 = 9\,V$

Problem 2. Use Kirchhoff's laws to determine the currents flowing in each branch of the network shown in Fig. 13.4.

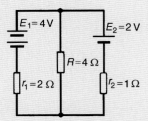

Figure 13.4

Procedure

1. Use Kirchhoff's current law and label current directions on the original circuit diagram. The directions chosen are arbitrary, but it is usual, as a starting point, to assume that current flows from the positive terminals of the batteries. This is shown in Fig. 13.5 where the three branch currents are expressed in terms of I_1 and I_2 only, since the current through R is $(I_1 + I_2)$

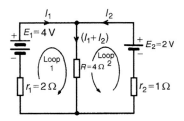

Figure 13.5

2. Divide the circuit into two loops and apply Kirchhoff's voltage law to each. From loop 1 of Fig. 13.5, and moving in a clockwise direction as indicated (the direction chosen does not matter), gives

$$E_1 = I_1 r_1 + (I_1 + I_2)R$$

i.e. $4 = 2I_1 + 4(I_1 + I_2)$,

i.e. $6I_1 + 4I_2 = 4$ (1)

From loop 2 of Fig. 13.5, and moving in an anticlockwise direction as indicated (once again, the choice of direction does not matter; it does not have to be in the same direction as that chosen for the first loop), gives:

$$E_2 = I_2 r_2 + (I_1 + I_2)R$$

i.e. $2 = I_2 + 4(I_1 + I_2)$

i.e. $4I_1 + 5I_2 = 2$ (2)

3. Solve Equations (1) and (2) for I_1 and I_2

$2 \times$ (1) gives: $12I_1 + 8I_2 = 8$ (3)

$3 \times$ (2) gives: $12I_1 + 15I_2 = 6$ (4)

(3) − (4) gives: $-7I_2 = 2$

hence $I_2 = -2/7 = \mathbf{-0.286\,A}$

(i.e. I_2 is flowing in the opposite direction to that shown in Fig. 13.5)

From (1) $6I_1 + 4(-0.286) = 4$

$$6I_1 = 4 + 1.144$$

Hence $I_1 = \dfrac{5.144}{6} = \mathbf{0.857\,A}$

Current flowing through resistance R is

$$(I_1 + I_2) = 0.857 + (-0.286)$$

$$= \mathbf{0.571\,A}$$

Note that a third loop is possible, as shown in Fig. 13.6, giving a third equation which can be used as a check:

$$E_1 - E_2 = I_1 r_1 - I_2 r_2$$

$$4 - 2 = 2I_1 - I_2$$

$$2 = 2I_1 - I_2$$

[Check: $2I_1 - I_2 = 2(0.857) - (-0.286) = 2$]

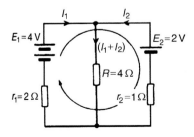

Figure 13.6

Problem 3.   Determine, using Kirchhoff's laws, each branch current for the network shown in Fig. 13.7.

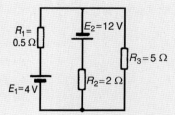

Figure 13.7

1. Currents, and their directions are shown labelled in Fig. 13.8 following Kirchhoff's current law. It is usual, although not essential, to follow conventional current flow with current flowing from the positive terminal of the source

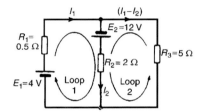

Figure 13.8

2. The network is divided into two loops as shown in Fig. 13.8. Applying Kirchhoff's voltage law gives: For loop 1:

$$E_1 + E_2 = I_1 R_1 + I_2 R_2$$

i.e. $16 = 0.5I_1 + 2I_2$ (1)

For loop 2:

$$E_2 = I_2 R_2 - (I_1 - I_2)R_3$$

Note that since loop 2 is in the opposite direction to current $(I_1 - I_2)$, the volt drop across R_3 (i.e. $(I_1 - I_2)(R_3)$) is by convention negative.

Thus $12 = 2I_2 - 5(I_1 - I_2)$

i.e. $12 = -5I_1 + 7I_2$ (2)

3. Solving Equations (1) and (2) to find I_1 and I_2:

$10 \times$ (1) gives: $160 = 5I_1 + 20I_2$ (3)

(2) + (3) gives: $172 = 27I_2$

hence $I_2 = \dfrac{172}{27} = \mathbf{6.37\,A}$

From (1): $16 = 0.5I_1 + 2(6.37)$

$$I_1 = \frac{16 - 2(6.37)}{0.5} = \mathbf{6.52\,A}$$

Current flowing in $R_3 = (I_1 - I_2)$

$$= 6.52 - 6.37 = \mathbf{0.15\,A}$$

Problem 4. For the bridge network shown in Fig. 13.9 determine the currents in each of the resistors.

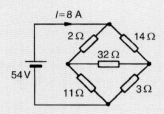

Figure 13.9

Let the current in the $2\,\Omega$ resistor be I_1, then by Kirchhoff's current law, the current in the $14\,\Omega$ resistor is $(I - I_1)$. Let the current in the $32\,\Omega$ resistor be I_2 as shown in Fig. 13.10. Then the current in the $11\,\Omega$ resistor is $(I_1 - I_2)$ and that in the $3\,\Omega$ resistor is $(I - I_1 + I_2)$. Applying Kirchhoff's voltage law to loop 1 and moving in a clockwise direction as shown in Fig. 13.10 gives:

$$54 = 2I_1 + 11(I_1 - I_2)$$

i.e. $13I_1 - 11I_2 = 54 \qquad (1)$

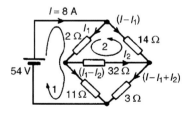

Figure 13.10

Applying Kirchhoff's voltage law to loop 2 and moving in a anticlockwise direction as shown in Fig. 13.10 gives:

$$0 = 2I_1 + 32I_2 - 14(I - I_1)$$

However $\qquad I = 8\,A$

Hence $\qquad 0 = 2I_1 + 32I_2 - 14(8 - I_1)$

i.e. $\qquad 16I_1 + 32I_2 = 112 \qquad (2)$

Equations (1) and (2) are simultaneous equations with two unknowns, I_1 and I_2.

$16 \times (1)$ gives: $\qquad 208I_1 - 176I_2 = 864 \qquad (3)$

$13 \times (2)$ gives: $\qquad 208I_1 + 416I_2 = 1456 \qquad (4)$

$(4) - (3)$ gives: $\qquad 592I_2 = 592$

$$I_2 = 1\,A$$

Substituting for I_2 in (1) gives:

$$13I_1 - 11 = 54$$

$$I_1 = \frac{65}{13} = 5\,A$$

Hence, the current flowing in the $2\,\Omega$ resistor

$$= I_1 = \mathbf{5\,A}$$

the current flowing in the $14\,\Omega$ resistor

$$= (I - I_1) = 8 - 5 = \mathbf{3\,A}$$

the current flowing in the $32\,\Omega$ resistor

$$= I_2 = \mathbf{1\,A}$$

the current flowing in the $11\,\Omega$ resistor

$$= (I_1 - I_2) = 5 - 1 = \mathbf{4\,A}$$

and the current flowing in the $3\,\Omega$ resistor

$$= I - I_1 + I_2 = 8 - 5 + 1 = \mathbf{4\,A}$$

Now try the following exercise

Exercise 69 Further problems on Kirchhoff's laws

1. Find currents I_3, I_4 and I_6 in Fig. 13.11
   $$[I_3 = 2\,A,\ I_4 = -1\,A,\ I_6 = 3\,A]$$

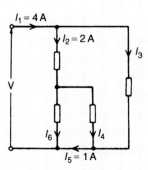

Figure 13.11

2. For the networks shown in Fig. 13.12, find the values of the currents marked.

$$[(a)\ I_1 = 4\,\text{A},\ I_2 = -1\,\text{A},\ I_3 = 13\,\text{A}$$
$$(b)\ I_1 = 40\,\text{A},\ I_2 = 60\,\text{A},\ I_3 = 120\,\text{A}$$
$$I_4 = 100\,\text{A},\ I_5 = -80\,\text{A}]$$

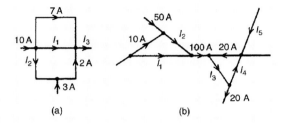

(a)   (b)

Figure 13.12

3. Calculate the currents I_1 and I_2 in Fig. 13.13.

$$[I_1 = 0.8\,\text{A},\ I_2 = 0.5\,\text{A}]$$

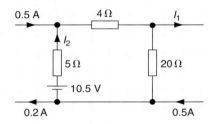

Figure 13.13

4. Use Kirchhoff's laws to find the current flowing in the $6\,\Omega$ resistor of Fig. 13.14 and the power dissipated in the $4\,\Omega$ resistor.

$$[2.162\,\text{A},\ 42.07\,\text{W}]$$

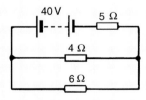

Figure 13.14

5. Find the current flowing in the $3\,\Omega$ resistor for the network shown in Fig. 13.15(a). Find also the p.d. across the $10\,\Omega$ and $2\,\Omega$ resistors.

$$[2.715\,\text{A},\ 7.410\,\text{V},\ 3.948\,\text{V}]$$

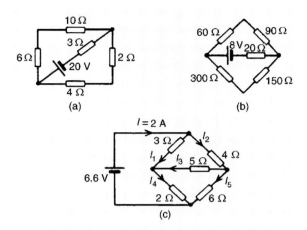

(a)   (b)

(c)

Figure 13.15

6. For the network shown in Fig. 13.15(b) find: (a) the current in the battery, (b) the current in the $300\,\Omega$ resistor, (c) the current in the $90\,\Omega$ resistor, and (d) the power dissipated in the $150\,\Omega$ resistor.

$$[(a)\ 60.38\,\text{mA}\ (b)\ 15.10\,\text{mA}$$
$$(c)\ 45.28\,\text{mA}\ (d)\ 34.20\,\text{mW}]$$

7. For the bridge network shown in Fig. 13.15(c), find the currents I_1 to I_5

$$[I_1 = 1.26\,\text{A},\ I_2 = 0.74\,\text{A},\ I_3 = 0.16\,\text{A},$$
$$I_4 = 1.42\,\text{A},\ I_5 = 0.58\,\text{A}]$$

13.3   The superposition theorem

The superposition theorem **states:**

In any network made up of linear resistances and containing more than one source of e.m.f., the resultant current flowing in any branch is the algebraic sum of the currents that would flow in that branch if each source was considered separately, all other sources being replaced at that time by their respective internal resistances.

The superposition theorem is demonstrated in the following worked problems

Problem 5.   Figure 13.16 shows a circuit containing two sources of e.m.f., each with their internal resistance. Determine the current in each branch of the network by using the superposition theorem.

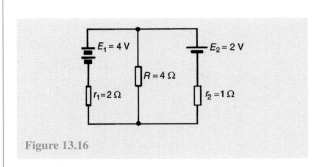

Figure 13.16

Procedure:

1. Redraw the original circuit with source E_2 removed, being replaced by r_2 only, as shown in Fig. 13.17(a)

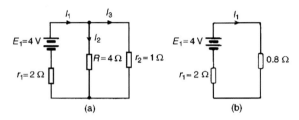

Figure 13.17

2. Label the currents in each branch and their directions as shown in Fig. 13.17(a) and determine their values. (Note that the choice of current directions depends on the battery polarity, which, by convention is taken as flowing from the positive battery terminal as shown)
   R in parallel with r_2 gives an equivalent resistance of $(4 \times 1)/(4+1)=0.8\,\Omega$
   From the equivalent circuit of Fig. 13.17(b),

$$I_1 = \frac{E_1}{r_1+0.8} = \frac{4}{2+0.8}$$
$$= 1.429\,\text{A}$$

From Fig. 13.17(a),

$$I_2 = \left(\frac{1}{4+1}\right)I_1 = \frac{1}{5}(1.429) = 0.286\,\text{A}$$

and $I_3 = \left(\frac{4}{4+1}\right)I_1 = \frac{4}{5}(1.429) = 1.143\,\text{A}$

by current division

3. Redraw the original circuit with source E_1 removed, being replaced by r_1 only, as shown in Fig. 13.18(a)

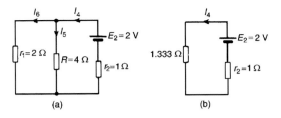

Figure 13.18

4. Label the currents in each branch and their directions as shown in Fig. 13.18(a) and determine their values.
   r_1 in parallel with R gives an equivalent resistance of $(2 \times 4)/(2+4)=8/6=1.333\,\Omega$
   From the equivalent circuit of Fig. 13.18(b)

$$I_4 = \frac{E_2}{1.333+r_2} = \frac{2}{1.333+1} = 0.857\,\text{A}$$

From Fig. 13.18(a),

$$I_5 = \left(\frac{2}{2+4}\right)I_4 = \frac{2}{6}(0.857) = 0.286\,\text{A}$$

$$I_6 = \left(\frac{4}{2+4}\right)I_4 = \frac{4}{6}(0.857) = 0.571\,\text{A}$$

5. Superimpose Fig. 13.18(a) on to Fig. 13.17(a) as shown in Fig. 13.19

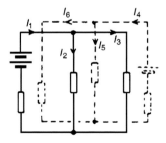

Figure 13.19

6. Determine the algebraic sum of the currents flowing in each branch.
   Resultant current flowing through source 1, i.e.

$$I_1 - I_6 = 1.429 - 0.571$$
$$= \mathbf{0.858\,A}\ \textbf{(discharging)}$$

Resultant current flowing through source 2, i.e.

$$I_4 - I_3 = 0.857 - 1.143$$
$$= \mathbf{-0.286\,A}\ \textbf{(charging)}$$

Resultant current flowing through resistor R, i.e.

$$I_2 + I_5 = 0.286 + 0.286$$

$$= \mathbf{0.572\,A}$$

The resultant currents with their directions are shown in Fig. 13.20

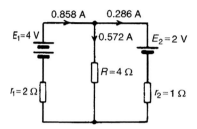

Figure 13.20

Problem 6.   For the circuit shown in Fig. 13.21, find, using the superposition theorem, (a) the current flowing in and the p.d. across the $18\,\Omega$ resistor, (b) the current in the 8 V battery and (c) the current in the 3 V battery.

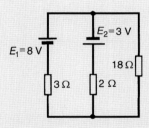

Figure 13.21

1. Removing source E_2 gives the circuit of Fig. 13.22(a)

2. The current directions are labelled as shown in Fig. 13.22(a), I_1 flowing from the positive terminal of E_1

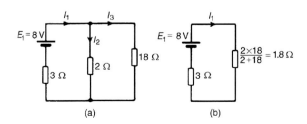

Figure 13.22

From Fig. 13.22(b),

$$I_1 = \frac{E_1}{3 + 1.8} = \frac{8}{4.8} = 1.667\,A$$

From Fig. 13.22(a),

$$I_2 = \left(\frac{18}{2 + 18}\right) I_1 = \frac{18}{20}(1.667) = 1.500\,A$$

and $$I_3 = \left(\frac{2}{2 + 18}\right) I_1 = \frac{2}{20}(1.667) = 0.167\,A$$

3. Removing source E_1 gives the circuit of Fig. 13.23(a) (which is the same as Fig. 13.23(b))

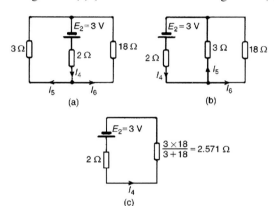

Figure 13.23

4. The current directions are labelled as shown in Figures 13.23(a) and 13.23(b), I_4 flowing from the positive terminal of E_2
   From Fig. 13.23(c),

$$I_4 = \frac{E_2}{2 + 2.571} = \frac{3}{4.571} = 0.656\,A$$

   From Fig. 13.23(b),

$$I_5 = \left(\frac{18}{3 + 18}\right) I_4 = \frac{18}{21}(0.656) = 0.562\,A$$

$$I_6 = \left(\frac{3}{3 + 18}\right) I_4 = \frac{3}{21}(0.656) = 0.094\,A$$

5. Superimposing Fig. 13.23(a) on to Fig. 13.22(a) gives the circuit in Fig. 13.24

6. (a) Resultant current in the $18\,\Omega$ resistor

$$= I_3 - I_6$$

$$= 0.167 - 0.094 = \mathbf{0.073\,A}$$

   P.d. across the $18\,\Omega$ resistor

$$= 0.073 \times 18 = \mathbf{1.314\,V}$$

Section 2

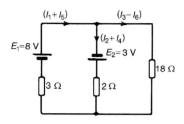

Figure 13.24

(b) Resultant current in the 8 V battery
$$= I_1 + I_5 = 1.667 + 0.562$$
$$= \textbf{2.229 A (discharging)}$$

(c) Resultant current in the 3 V battery
$$= I_2 + I_4 = 1.500 + 0.656$$
$$= \textbf{2.156 A (discharging)}$$

For a practical laboratory experiment on the superposition theorem, see Chapter 24, page 408.

Now try the following exercise

Exercise 70   Further problems on the superposition theorem

1. Use the superposition theorem to find currents I_1, I_2 and I_3 of Fig. 13.25.
$$[I_1 = 2\,A, I_2 = 3\,A, I_3 = 5\,A]$$

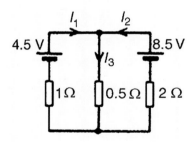

Figure 13.25

2. Use the superposition theorem to find the current in the $8\,\Omega$ resistor of Fig. 13.26.
[0.385 A]

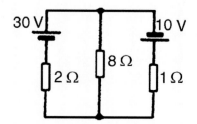

Figure 13.26

3. Use the superposition theorem to find the current in each branch of the network shown in Fig. 13.27.
[10 V battery discharges at 1.429 A
4 V battery charges at 0.857 A
Current through $10\,\Omega$ resistor is 0.571 A]

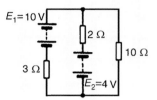

Figure 13.27

4. Use the superposition theorem to determine the current in each branch of the arrangement shown in Fig. 13.28.
[24 V battery charges at 1.664 A
52 V battery discharges at 3.280 A
Current in $20\,\Omega$ resistor is 1.616 A]

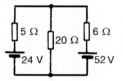

Figure 13.28

13.4   General d.c. circuit theory

The following points involving d.c. circuit analysis need to be appreciated before proceeding with problems using Thévenin's and Norton's theorems:

(i)   The open-circuit voltage, E, across terminals AB in Fig. 13.29 is equal to 10 V, since no current flows through the $2\,\Omega$ resistor and hence no voltage drop occurs.

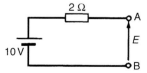

Figure 13.29

(ii) The open-circuit voltage, E, across terminals AB in Fig. 13.30(a) is the same as the voltage across the 6 Ω resistor. The circuit may be redrawn as shown in Fig. 13.30(b)

$$E = \left(\frac{6}{6+4}\right)(50)$$

by voltage division in a series circuit, i.e. $E = 30\,\text{V}$

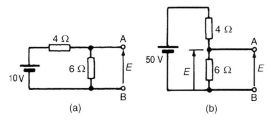

Figure 13.30

(iii) For the circuit shown in Fig. 13.31(a) representing a practical source supplying energy, $V = E - Ir$, where E is the battery e.m.f., V is the battery terminal voltage and r is the internal resistance of the battery (as shown in Section 4.6). For the circuit shown in Fig. 13.31(b),

$$V = E - (-I)r, \text{ i.e. } V = E + Ir$$

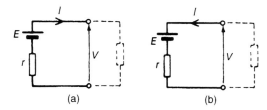

Figure 13.31

(iv) The resistance 'looking-in' at terminals AB in Fig. 13.32(a) is obtained by reducing the circuit in stages as shown in Figures 13.32(b) to (d). Hence the equivalent resistance across AB is 7 Ω.

(v) For the circuit shown in Fig. 13.33(a), the 3 Ω resistor carries no current and the p.d. across the 20 Ω resistor is 10 V. Redrawing the circuit gives Fig. 13.33(b), from which

$$E = \left(\frac{4}{4+6}\right) \times 10 = 4\,\text{V}$$

(vi) If the 10 V battery in Fig. 13.33(a) is removed and replaced by a short-circuit, as shown in Fig. 13.33(c), then the 20 Ω resistor may be

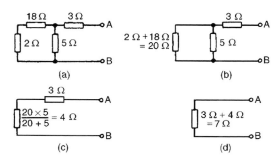

Figure 13.32

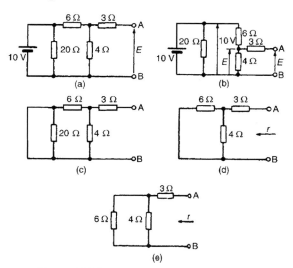

Figure 13.33

removed. The reason for this is that a short-circuit has zero resistance, and 20 Ω in parallel with zero ohms gives an equivalent resistance of $(20 \times 0)/(20 + 0)$ i.e. 0 Ω. The circuit is then as shown in Fig. 13.33(d), which is redrawn in Fig. 13.33(e). From Fig. 13.33(e), the equivalent resistance across AB,

$$r = \frac{6 \times 4}{6+4} + 3 = 2.4 + 3 = 5.4\,\Omega$$

(vii) To find the voltage across AB in Fig. 13.34: Since the 20 V supply is across the 5 Ω and 15 Ω resistors in series then, by voltage division, the voltage drop across AC,

$$V_{AC} = \left(\frac{5}{5+15}\right)(20) = 5\,\text{V}$$

Similarly,

$$V_{CB} = \left(\frac{12}{12+3}\right)(20) = 16\,\text{V}.$$

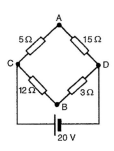

Figure 13.34

V_C is at a potential of $+20$ V.
$$V_A = V_C - V_{AC} = +20 - 5 = 15 \text{ V}$$
and $\quad V_B = V_C - V_{BC} = +20 - 16 = 4 \text{ V}$.
Hence the voltage between AB is $V_A - V_B = 15 - 4 = 11$ V and current would flow from A to B since A has a higher potential than B.

(viii) In Fig. 13.35(a), to find the equivalent resistance across AB the circuit may be redrawn as in Figs 13.35(b) and (c). From Fig. 13.27(c), the equivalent resistance across AB
$$= \frac{5 \times 15}{5 + 15} + \frac{12 \times 3}{12 + 3}$$
$$= 3.75 + 2.4 = \mathbf{6.15 \, \Omega}$$

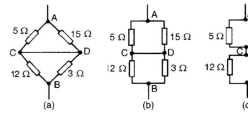

Figure 13.35

(ix) In the worked problems in Sections 13.5 and 13.7 following, it may be considered that Thévenin's and Norton's theorems have no obvious advantages compared with, say, Kirchhoff's laws. However, these theorems can be used to analyse part of a circuit and in much more complicated networks the principle of replacing the supply by a constant voltage source in series with a resistance (or impedance) is very useful.

13.5 Thévenin's theorem

Thévenin's theorem **states:**

The current in any branch of a network is that which would result if an e.m.f. equal to the p.d. across a break

made in the branch, were introduced into the branch, all other e.m.f.'s being removed and represented by the internal resistances of the sources.

The procedure adopted when using Thévenin's theorem is summarised below. To determine the current in any branch of an active network (i.e. one containing a source of e.m.f.):

(i) remove the resistance R from that branch,

(ii) determine the open-circuit voltage, E, across the break,

(iii) remove each source of e.m.f. and replace them by their internal resistances and then determine the resistance, r, 'looking-in' at the break,

(iv) determine the value of the current from the equivalent circuit shown in Fig. 13.36, i.e.

$$I = \frac{E}{R + r}$$

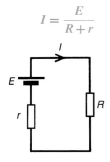

Figure 13.36

Problem 7. Use Thévenin's theorem to find the current flowing in the $10\,\Omega$ resistor for the circuit shown in Fig. 13.37.

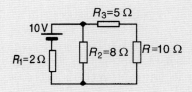

Figure 13.37

Following the above procedure:

(i) The $10\,\Omega$ resistance is removed from the circuit as shown in Fig. 13.38(a)

(ii) There is no current flowing in the $5\,\Omega$ resistor and current I_1 is given by

$$I_1 = \frac{10}{R_1 + R_2} = \frac{10}{2 + 8} = 1 \text{ A}$$

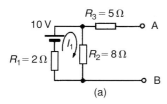

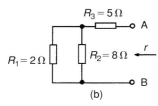

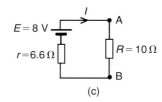

Figure 13.38

P.d. across $R_2 = I_1R_2 = 1 \times 8 = 8$ V. Hence p.d. across AB, i.e. the open-circuit voltage across the break, $E = 8$ V

(iii) Removing the source of e.m.f. gives the circuit of Fig. 13.38(b). Resistance,

$$r = R_3 + \frac{R_1R_2}{R_1 + R_2} = 5 + \frac{2 \times 8}{2 + 8}$$
$$= 5 + 1.6 = 6.6\,\Omega$$

(iv) The equivalent Thévenin's circuit is shown in Fig. 13.38(c)

$$\text{Current } I = \frac{E}{R + r} = \frac{8}{10 + 6.6} = \frac{8}{16.6}$$
$$= 0.482\,\text{A}$$

Hence the current flowing in the 10 Ω resistor of Fig. 13.37 is **0.482 A**.

Problem 8. For the network shown in Fig. 13.39 determine the current in the 0.8 Ω resistor using Thévenin's theorem.

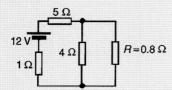

Figure 13.39

Following the procedure:

(i) The 0.8 Ω resistor is removed from the circuit as shown in Fig. 13.40(a).

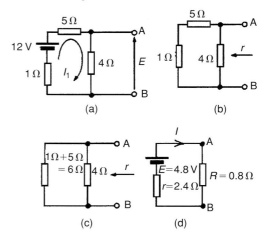

Figure 13.40

(ii) Current $I_1 = \dfrac{12}{1 + 5 + 4} = \dfrac{12}{10} = 1.2$ A

P.d. across 4 Ω resistor $= 4I_1 = (4)(1.2) = 4.8$ V. Hence p.d. across AB, i.e. the open-circuit voltage across AB, $E = 4.8$ V

(iii) Removing the source of e.m.f. gives the circuit shown in Fig. 13.40(b). The equivalent circuit of Fig. 13.40(b) is shown in Fig. 13.40(c), from which, resistance

$$r = \frac{4 \times 6}{4 + 6} = \frac{24}{10} = 2.4\,\Omega$$

(iv) The equivalent Thévenin's circuit is shown in Fig. 13.40(d), from which, current

$$I = \frac{E}{r + R} = \frac{4.8}{2.4 + 0.8} = \frac{4.8}{3.2}$$

$$= \mathbf{1.5\,A = current\ in\ the\ 0.8\,\Omega\ resistor}$$

Problem 9. Use Thévenin's theorem to determine the current I flowing in the 4 Ω resistor shown in Fig. 13.41. Find also the power dissipated in the 4 Ω resistor.

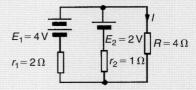

Figure 13.41

Following the procedure:

(i) The $4\,\Omega$ resistor is removed from the circuit as shown in Fig. 13.42(a)

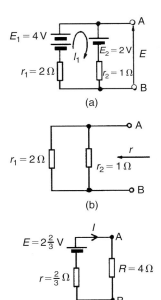

(a)

(b)

(c)

Figure 13.42

(ii) Current $I_1 = \dfrac{E_1 - E_2}{r_1 + r_2} = \dfrac{4-2}{2+1} = \dfrac{2}{3}\,\text{A}$

P.d. across AB,

$$E = E_1 - I_1 r_1 = 4 - \frac{2}{3}(2) = 2\frac{2}{3}\,\text{V}$$

(see Section 13.4(iii)). (Alternatively, p.d. across AB, $E = E_2 + I_1 r_2 = 2 + \frac{2}{3}(1) = 2\frac{2}{3}\,\text{V}$)

(iii) Removing the sources of e.m.f. gives the circuit shown in Fig. 13.42(b), from which, resistance

$$r = \frac{2 \times 1}{2+1} = \frac{2}{3}\,\Omega$$

(iv) The equivalent Thévenin's circuit is shown in Fig. 13.42(c), from which, current,

$$I = \frac{E}{r+R} = \frac{2\frac{2}{3}}{\frac{2}{3}+4} = \frac{8/3}{14/3} = \frac{8}{14}$$

$$= \mathbf{0.571\,A}$$

$$= \textbf{current in the } 4\,\Omega \textbf{ resistor}$$

Power dissipated in the $4\,\Omega$ resistor,
$P = I^2 R = (0.571)^2 (4) = \mathbf{1.304\,W}$

Problem 10. Determine the current in the $5\,\Omega$ resistance of the network shown in Fig. 13.43 using Thévenin's theorem. Hence find the currents flowing in the other two branches.

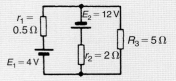

Figure 13.43

Following the procedure:

(i) The $5\,\Omega$ resistance is removed from the circuit as shown in Fig. 13.44(a)

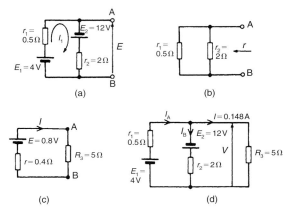

(a)

(b)

(c)

(d)

Figure 13.44

(ii) Current $I_1 = \dfrac{12+4}{0.5+2} = \dfrac{16}{2.5} = 6.4\,\text{A}$

P.d. across AB,

$$E = E_1 - I_1 r_1 = 4 - (6.4)(0.5) = 0.8\,\text{V}$$

(see Section 13.4(iii)). (Alternatively, $E = -E_2 + I_1 r_1 = -12 + (6.4)(2) = 0.8\,\text{V}$)

(iii) Removing the sources of e.m.f. gives the circuit shown in Fig. 13.44(b), from which resistance

$$r = \frac{0.5 \times 2}{0.5+2} = \frac{1}{2.5} = 0.4\,\Omega$$

(iv) The equivalent Thévenin's circuit is shown in Fig. 13.44(c), from which, current

$$I = \frac{E}{r+R} = \frac{0.8}{0.4+5} = \frac{0.8}{5.4} = \mathbf{0.148\,A}$$

$$= \textbf{current in the } 5\,\Omega \textbf{ resistor}$$

From Fig. 13.44(d),

$$\text{voltage } V = IR_3 = (0.148)(5) = 0.74\,\text{V}$$

From Section 13.4(iii),

$$V = E_1 - I_A r_1$$

i.e. $$0.74 = 4 - (I_A)(0.5)$$

Hence current, $I_A = \dfrac{4-0.74}{0.5} = \dfrac{3.26}{0.5} = \mathbf{6.52\,A}$

Also from Fig. 13.44(d),

$$V = -E_2 + I_B r_2$$

i.e. $$0.74 = -12 + (I_B)(2)$$

Hence current $I_B = \dfrac{12+0.74}{2} = \dfrac{12.74}{2} = \mathbf{6.37\,A}$

[Check, from Fig. 13.44(d), $I_A = I_B + I$, correct to 2 significant figures by Kirchhoff's current law]

Problem 11. Use Thévenin's theorem to determine the current flowing in the $3\,\Omega$ resistance of the network shown in Fig. 13.45. The voltage source has negligible internal resistance.

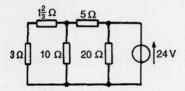

Figure 13.45

(Note the symbol for an ideal voltage source in Fig. 13.45 – from BS EN 60617-2: 1996, which superseded BS 3939-2: 1985 – and may be used as an alternative to the battery symbol.)

Following the procedure

(i) The $3\,\Omega$ resistance is removed from the circuit as shown in Fig. 13.46(a).

(ii) The $1\frac{2}{3}\,\Omega$ resistance now carries no current. P.d. across $10\,\Omega$ resistor

$$= \left(\frac{10}{10+5}\right)(24) = \mathbf{16\,V}$$

(see Section 13.4(v)). Hence p.d. across AB, $E = 16\,\text{V}$.

(iii) Removing the source of e.m.f. and replacing it by its internal resistance means that the $20\,\Omega$ resistance is short-circuited as shown in Fig. 13.46(b)

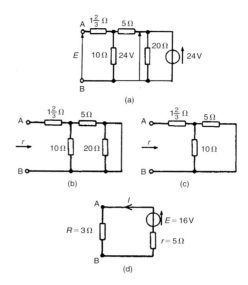

Figure 13.46

since its internal resistance is zero. The $20\,\Omega$ resistance may thus be removed as shown in Fig. 13.46(c) (see Section 13.4 (vi)).

From Fig. 13.46(c), resistance,

$$r = 1\frac{2}{3} + \frac{10 \times 5}{10+5} = 1\frac{2}{3} + \frac{50}{15} = 5\,\Omega$$

(iv) The equivalent Thévenin's circuit is shown in Fig. 13.46(d), from which, current,

$$I = \frac{E}{r+R} = \frac{16}{3+5} = \frac{16}{8} = \mathbf{2\,A}$$

$$= \textbf{current in the } 3\,\Omega \textbf{ resistance}$$

Problem 12. A Wheatstone Bridge network is shown in Fig. 13.47. Calculate the current flowing in the $32\,\Omega$ resistor, and its direction, using Thévenin's theorem. Assume the source of e.m.f. to have negligible resistance.

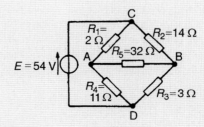

Figure 13.47

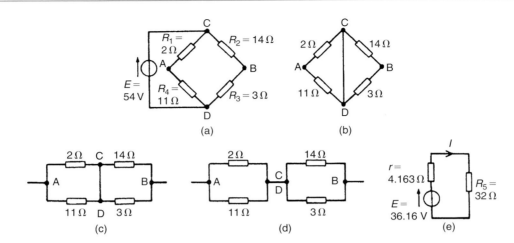

Figure 13.48

Following the procedure:

(i)   The $32\,\Omega$ resistor is removed from the circuit as shown in Fig. 13.48(a)

(ii) The p.d. between A and C,

$$V_{AC} = \left(\frac{R_1}{R_1 + R_4}\right)(E) = \left(\frac{2}{2 + 11}\right)(54)$$
$$= 8.31\,\text{V}$$

The p.d. between B and C,

$$V_{BC} = \left(\frac{R_2}{R_2 + R_3}\right)(E) = \left(\frac{14}{14 + 3}\right)(54)$$
$$= 44.47\,\text{V}$$

Hence the p.d. between A and B$=44.47-8.31=$**36.16 V**

Point C is at a potential of $+54$ V. Between C and A is a voltage drop of 8.31 V. Hence the voltage at point A is $54-8.31=45.69$ V. Between C and B is a voltage drop of 44.47 V. Hence the voltage at point B is $54-44.47=9.53$ V. Since the voltage at A is greater than at B, current must flow in the direction A to B. (See Section 13.4 (vii))

(iii) Replacing the source of e.m.f. with a short-circuit (i.e. zero internal resistance) gives the circuit shown in Fig. 13.48(b). The circuit is redrawn and simplified as shown in Fig. 13.48(c) and (d), from which the resistance between terminals A and B,

$$r = \frac{2 \times 11}{2 + 11} + \frac{14 \times 3}{14 + 3}$$
$$= \frac{22}{13} + \frac{42}{17}$$

$$= 1.692 + 2.471$$
$$= \mathbf{4.163\,\Omega}$$

(iv) The equivalent Thévenin's circuit is shown in Fig. 13.48(e), from which, current

$$I = \frac{E}{r + R_5}$$
$$= \frac{36.16}{4.163 + 32} = 1\,\text{A}$$

Hence the current in the $32\,\Omega$ resistor of Fig. 13.47 is 1A, flowing from A to B
For a practical laboratory experiment on Thévenin's theorem, see Chapter 24, page 410.

Now try the following exercise

Exercise 71   Further problems on Thévenin's theorem

1. Use Thévenin's theorem to find the current flowing in the $14\,\Omega$ resistor of the network shown in Fig. 13.49. Find also the power dissipated in the $14\,\Omega$ resistor.

    [0.434 A, 2.64 W]

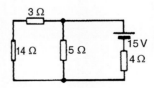

Figure 13.49

2. Use Thévenin's theorem to find the current flowing in the 6 Ω resistor shown in Fig. 13.50 and the power dissipated in the 4 Ω resistor.

[2.162 A, 42.07 W]

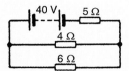

Figure 13.50

3. Repeat problems 1 to 4 of Exercise 70, page 190, using Thévenin's theorem.

4. In the network shown in Fig. 13.51, the battery has negligible internal resistance. Find, using Thévenin's theorem, the current flowing in the 4 Ω resistor.   [0.918 A]

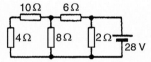

Figure 13.51

5. For the bridge network shown in Fig. 13.52, find the current in the 5 Ω resistor, and its direction, by using Thévenin's theorem.

[0.153 A from B to A]

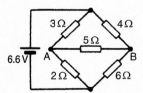

Figure 13.52

13.6   Constant-current source

A source of electrical energy can be represented by a source of e.m.f. in series with a resistance. In Section 13.5, the Thévenin constant-voltage source consisted of a constant e.m.f. E in series with an internal resistance r. However this is not the only form of representation. A source of electrical energy can also be represented by a constant-current source in parallel with a resistance. It may be shown that the two forms are equivalent. An **ideal constant-voltage generator** is one with zero internal resistance so that it supplies the same voltage to all loads. An **ideal constant-current generator** is one with infinite internal resistance so that it supplies the same current to all loads.

Note the symbol for an ideal current source (from BS EN 60617-2: 1996, which superseded BS 3939-2: 1985), shown in Fig. 13.53.

13.7   Norton's theorem

Norton's theorem **states:**

The current that flows in any branch of a network is the same as that which would flow in the branch if it were connected across a source of electrical energy, the short-circuit current of which is equal to the current that would flow in a short-circuit across the branch, and the internal resistance of which is equal to the resistance which appears across the open-circuited branch terminals.

The procedure adopted when using Norton's theorem is summarised below. To determine the current flowing in a resistance R of a branch AB of an active network:

(i)   short-circuit branch AB

(ii)   determine the short-circuit current I_{SC} flowing in the branch

(iii)   remove all sources of e.m.f. and replace them by their internal resistance (or, if a current source exists, replace with an open-circuit), then determine the resistance r, 'looking-in' at a break made between A and B

(iv)   determine the current I flowing in resistance R from the Norton equivalent network shown in Fig. 13.53, i.e.

$$I = \left(\frac{r}{r+R}\right) I_{SC}$$

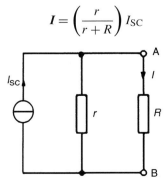

Figure 13.53

Problem 13. Use Norton's theorem to determine the current flowing in the $10\,\Omega$ resistance for the circuit shown in Fig. 13.54.

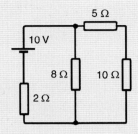

Figure 13.54

Following the above procedure:

(i)   The branch containing the $10\,\Omega$ resistance is short-circuited as shown in Fig. 13.55(a)

(ii) Fig. 13.55(b) is equivalent to Fig. 13.55(a).

Hence $I_{SC} = \dfrac{10}{2} = 5\,A$

(iii) If the $10\,V$ source of e.m.f. is removed from Fig. 13.55(a) the resistance 'looking-in' at a break made between A and B is given by:

$$r = \frac{2 \times 8}{2 + 8} = 1.6\,\Omega$$

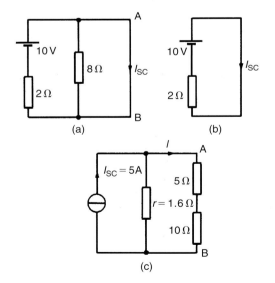

Figure 13.55

(iv) From the Norton equivalent network shown in Fig. 13.55(c) the current in the $10\,\Omega$ resistance,

by current division, is given by:

$$I = \left(\frac{1.6}{1.6 + 5 + 10}\right)(5) = \mathbf{0.482\,A}$$

as obtained previously in Problem 7 using Thévenin's theorem.

Problem 14. Use Norton's theorem to determine the current I flowing in the $4\,\Omega$ resistance shown in Fig. 13.56.

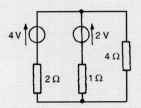

Figure 13.56

Following the procedure:

(i)   The $4\,\Omega$ branch is short-circuited as shown in Fig. 13.57(a)

(ii) From Fig. 13.57(a),

$$I_{SC} = I_1 + I_2 = \frac{4}{2} + \frac{2}{1} = 4\,A$$

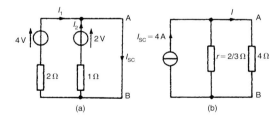

Figure 13.57

(iii) If the sources of e.m.f. are removed the resistance 'looking-in' at a break made between A and B is given by:

$$r = \frac{2 \times 1}{2 + 1} = \frac{2}{3}\,\Omega$$

(iv) From the Norton equivalent network shown in Fig. 13.57(b) the current in the $4\,\Omega$ resistance is given by:

$$I = \left(\frac{\frac{2}{3}}{\frac{2}{3} + 4}\right)(4) = \mathbf{0.571\,A},$$

as obtained previously in problems 2, 5 and 9 using Kirchhoff's laws and the theorems of superposition and Thévenin

Problem 15.   Determine the current in the $5\,\Omega$ resistance of the network shown in Fig. 13.58 using Norton's theorem. Hence find the currents flowing in the other two branches.

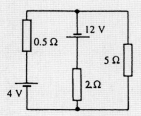

Figure 13.58

Following the procedure:

(i)   The $5\,\Omega$ branch is short-circuited as shown in Fig. 13.59(a)

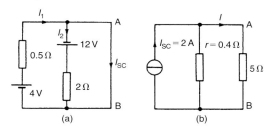

(a)   (b)

Figure 13.59

(ii)   From Fig. 13.59(a),

$$I_{SC} = I_1 - I_2 = \frac{4}{0.5} - \frac{12}{2} = 8 - 6 = \mathbf{2\,A}$$

(iii)   If each source of e.m.f. is removed the resistance 'looking-in' at a break made between A and B is given by:

$$r = \frac{0.5 \times 2}{0.5 + 2} = 0.4\,\Omega$$

(iv)   From the Norton equivalent network shown in Fig. 13.59(b) the current in the $5\,\Omega$ resistance is given by:

$$I = \left(\frac{0.4}{0.4 + 5}\right)(2) = \mathbf{0.148\,A},$$

as obtained previously in Problem 10 using Thévenin's theorem.

The currents flowing in the other two branches are obtained in the same way as in Problem 10. Hence the current flowing from the 4 V source is **6.52 A** and the current flowing from the 12 V source is **6.37 A**.

Problem 16.   Use Norton's theorem to determine the current flowing in the $3\,\Omega$ resistance of the network shown in Fig. 13.60. The voltage source has negligible internal resistance.

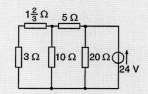

Figure 13.60

Following the procedure:

(i)   The branch containing the $3\,\Omega$ resistance is short-circuited as shown in Fig. 13.61(a)

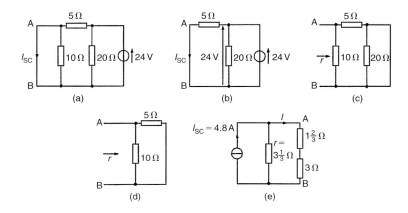

(a)   (b)   (c)

(d)   (e)

Figure 13.61

(ii) From the equivalent circuit shown in Fig. 13.61(b),

$$I_{SC} = \frac{24}{5} = 4.8\,\text{A}$$

(iii) If the 24 V source of e.m.f. is removed the resistance 'looking-in' at a break made between A and B is obtained from Fig. 13.61(c) and its equivalent circuit shown in Fig. 13.61(d) and is given by:

$$r = \frac{10 \times 5}{10 + 5} = \frac{50}{15} = 3\frac{1}{3}\,\Omega$$

(iv) From the Norton equivalent network shown in Fig. 13.61(e) the current in the 3 Ω resistance is given by:

$$I = \left(\frac{3\frac{1}{3}}{3\frac{1}{3} + 1\frac{2}{3} + 3}\right)(4.8) = 2\,\text{A},$$

as obtained previously in Problem 11 using Thévenin's theorem.

Problem 17. Determine the current flowing in the 2 Ω resistance in the network shown in Fig. 13.62.

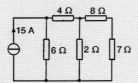

Figure 13.62

Following the procedure:

(i) The 2 Ω resistance branch is short-circuited as shown in Fig. 13.63(a)

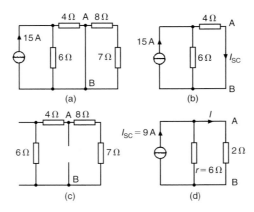

Figure 13.63

(ii) Fig. 13.63(b) is equivalent to Fig. 13.63(a). Hence

$$I_{SC} = \frac{6}{6+4}(15) = \textbf{9 A} \text{ by current division.}$$

(iii) If the 15 A current source is replaced by an open-circuit then from Fig. 13.63(c) the resistance 'looking-in' at a break made between A and B is given by $(6+4)\,\Omega$ in parallel with $(8+7)\,\Omega$, i.e.

$$r = \frac{(10)(15)}{10+15} = \frac{150}{25} = 6\,\Omega$$

(iv) From the Norton equivalent network shown in Fig. 13.63(d) the current in the 2 Ω resistance is given by:

$$I = \left(\frac{6}{6+2}\right)(9) = \textbf{6.75 A}$$

Now try the following exercise

Exercise 72   Further problems on Norton's theorem

1. Repeat Problems 1–4 of Exercise 70, page 186, by using Norton's theorem.

2. Repeat Problems 1, 2, 4 and 5 of Exercise 71, page 196, by using Norton's theorem.

3. Determine the current flowing in the 6 Ω resistance of the network shown in Fig. 13.64 by using Norton's theorem.   [2.5 mA]

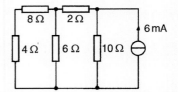

Figure 13.64

13.8 Thévenin and Norton equivalent networks

The Thévenin and Norton networks shown in Fig. 13.65 are equivalent to each other. The resistance 'looking-in' at terminals AB is the same in each of the networks, i.e. r.

If terminals AB in Fig. 13.65(a) are short-circuited, the short-circuit current is given by E/r. If terminals

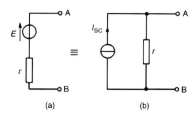

Figure 13.65

AB in Fig. 13.65(b) are short-circuited, the short-circuit current is I_{SC}. For the circuit shown in Fig. 13.65(a) to be equivalent to the circuit in Fig. 13.65(b) the same short-circuit current must flow. Thus $I_{SC} = E/r$.

Figure 13.66 shows a source of e.m.f. E in series with a resistance r feeding a load resistance R

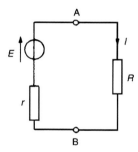

Figure 13.66

From Fig. 13.66,

$$I = \frac{E}{r+R} = \frac{E/r}{(r+R)/r} = \left(\frac{r}{r+R}\right)\frac{E}{r}$$

i.e. $$I = \left(\frac{r}{r+R}\right)I_{SC}$$

From Fig. 13.67 it can be seen that, when viewed from the load, the source appears as a source of current I_{SC} which is divided between r and R connected in parallel.

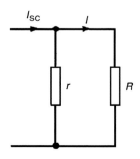

Figure 13.67

Thus the two representations shown in Fig. 13.65 are equivalent.

Problem 18.   Convert the circuit shown in Fig. 13.68 to an equivalent Norton network.

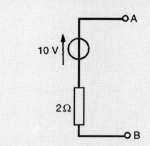

Figure 13.68

If terminals AB in Fig. 13.68 are short-circuited, the short-circuit current $I_{SC} = 10/2 = 5$ A.

The resistance 'looking-in' at terminals AB is $2\,\Omega$. Hence the equivalent Norton network is as shown in Fig. 13.69

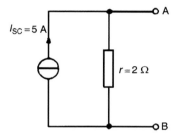

Figure 13.69

Problem 19.   Convert the network shown in Fig. 13.70 to an equivalent Thévenin circuit.

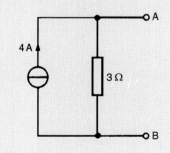

Figure 13.70

The open-circuit voltage E across terminals AB in Fig. 13.70 is given by:

$$E = (I_{SC})(r) = (4)(3) = 12\,\text{V}.$$

The resistance 'looking-in' at terminals AB is $3\,\Omega$. Hence the equivalent Thévenin circuit is as shown in Fig. 13.71

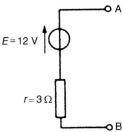

Figure 13.71

Problem 20. (a) Convert the circuit to the left of terminals AB in Fig. 13.72 to an equivalent Thévenin circuit by initially converting to a Norton equivalent circuit. (b) Determine the current flowing in the $1.8\,\Omega$ resistor.

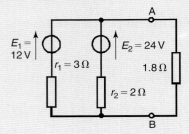

Figure 13.72

(a) For the branch containing the 12 V source, converting to a Norton equivalent circuit gives $I_{SC} = 12/3 = 4\,A$ and $r_1 = 3\,\Omega$. For the branch containing the 24 V source, converting to a Norton equivalent circuit gives $I_{SC2} = 24/2 = 12\,A$ and $r_2 = 2\,\Omega$. Thus Fig. 13.73(a) shows a network equivalent to Fig. 13.72

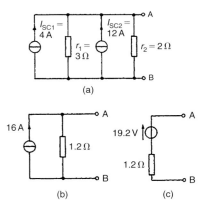

Figure 13.73

From Fig. 13.73(a) the total short-circuit current is $4 + 12 = 16\,A$ and the total resistance is given by $(3 \times 2)/(3 + 2) = \mathbf{1.2\,\Omega}$. Thus Fig. 13.73(a) simplifies to Fig. 13.73(b). The open-circuit voltage across AB of Fig. 13.73(b), $E = (16)(1.2) = \mathbf{19.2\,V}$, and the resistance 'looking-in' at AB is $1.2\,\Omega$. Hence the Thévenin equivalent circuit is as shown in Fig. 13.73(c).

(b) When the $1.8\,\Omega$ resistance is connected between terminals A and B of Fig. 13.73(c) the current I flowing is given by

$$I = \left(\frac{19.2}{1.2 + 1.8}\right) = \mathbf{6.4\,A}$$

Problem 21. Determine by successive conversions between Thévenin and Norton equivalent networks a Thévenin equivalent circuit for terminals AB of Fig. 13.74. Hence determine the current flowing in the $200\,\Omega$ resistance.

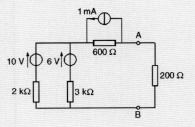

Figure 13.74

For the branch containing the 10 V source, converting to a Norton equivalent network gives $I_{SC} = 10/2000 = 5\,mA$ and $r_1 = 2\,k\Omega$
For the branch containing the 6 V source, converting to a Norton equivalent network gives $I_{SC} = 6/3000 = 2\,mA$ and $r_2 = 3\,k\Omega$
Thus the network of Fig. 13.74 converts to Fig. 13.75(a). Combining the 5 mA and 2 mA current sources gives the equivalent network of Fig. 13.75(b) where the short-circuit current for the original two branches considered is 7 mA and the resistance is $(2 \times 3)/(2 + 3) = 1.2\,k\Omega$

Both of the Norton equivalent networks shown in Fig. 13.75(b) may be converted to Thévenin equivalent circuits. The open-circuit voltage across CD is $(7 \times 10^{-3})(1.2 \times 10^3) = 8.4\,V$ and the resistance 'looking-in' at CD is $1.2\,k\Omega$. The open-circuit voltage across EF is $(1 \times 10^{-3})(600) = 0.6\,V$ and the resistance 'looking-in' at EF is $0.6\,k\Omega$. Thus Fig. 13.75(b)

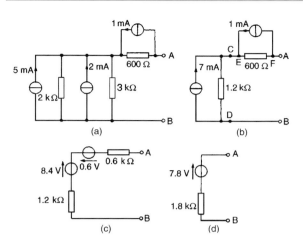

Figure 13.75

converts to Fig. 13.75(c). Combining the two Thévenin circuits gives $E = 8.4 - 0.6 = 7.8$ V and the resistance $r = (1.2 + 0.6)$ k$\Omega = \mathbf{1.8\,k\Omega}$

Thus the Thévenin equivalent circuit for terminals AB of Fig. 13.74 is as shown in Fig. 13.75(d)

Hence the current I flowing in a 200 Ω resistance connected between A and B is given by

$$I = \frac{7.8}{1800 + 200}$$

$$= \frac{7.8}{2000} = \mathbf{3.9\,mA}$$

Now try the following exercise

Exercise 73   Further problems on Thévenin and Norton equivalent networks

1. Convert the circuits shown in Fig. 13.76 to Norton equivalent networks.
   $$[(a)\ I_{SC} = 25\,A,\ r = 2\,\Omega$$
   $$(b)\ I_{SC} = 2\,mA,\ r = 5\,\Omega]$$

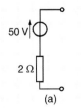
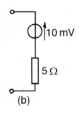

Figure 13.76

2. Convert the networks shown in Fig. 13.77 to Thévenin equivalent circuits.
   $$[(a)\ E = 20\,V,\ r = 4\,\Omega$$
   $$(b)\ E = 12\,mV,\ r = 3\,\Omega]$$

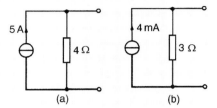

Figure 13.77

3. (a) Convert the network to the left of terminals AB in Fig. 13.78 to an equivalent Thévenin circuit by initially converting to a Norton equivalent network.

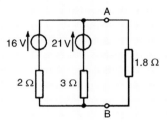

Figure 13.78

   (b) Determine the current flowing in the 1.8 Ω resistance connected between A and B in Fig. 13.78.
   $$[(a)\ E = 18\,V,\ r = 1.2\,\Omega\ (b)\ 6\,A]$$

4. Determine, by successive conversions between Thévenin and Norton equivalent networks, a Thévenin equivalent circuit for terminals AB of Fig. 13.79. Hence determine the current flowing in a 6 Ω resistor connected between A and B.
   $$[E = 9\tfrac{1}{3}\,V,\ r = 1\,\Omega,\ 1\tfrac{1}{3}\,A]$$

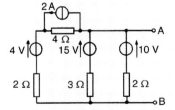

Figure 13.79

5. For the network shown in Fig. 13.80, convert each branch containing a voltage source to its

Norton equivalent and hence determine the current flowing in the 5 Ω resistance.

[1.22 A]

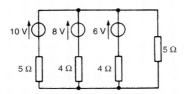

Figure 13.80

13.9 Maximum power transfer theorem

The maximum power transfer theorem states:
The power transferred from a supply source to a load is at its maximum when the resistance of the load is equal to the internal resistance of the source.

Hence, in Fig. 13.81, when $R = r$ the power transferred from the source to the load is a maximum.

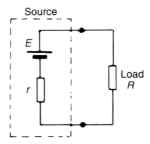

Figure 13.81

Typical practical applications of the maximum power transfer theorem are found in stereo amplifier design, seeking to maximise power delivered to speakers, and in electric vehicle design, seeking to maximise power delivered to drive a motor.

Problem 22. The circuit diagram of Fig. 13.82 shows dry cells of source e.m.f. 6 V, and internal resistance 2.5 Ω. If the load resistance R_L is varied from 0 to 5 Ω in 0.5 Ω steps, calculate the power dissipated by the load in each case. Plot a graph of R_L (horizontally) against power (vertically) and determine the maximum power dissipated.

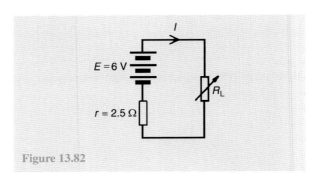

Figure 13.82

When $R_L = 0$, current $I = E/(r + R_L) = 6/2.5 = 2.4$ A and power dissipated in R_L, $P = I^2 R_L$ i.e.
$P = (2.4)^2(0) = 0$ W.
When $R_L = 0.5$ Ω,
current $I = E/(r + R_L) = 6/(2.5 + 0.5) = 2$ A and
$P = I^2 R_L = (2)^2(0.5) = 2.00$ W.
When $R_L = 1.0$ Ω, current $I = 6/(2.5 + 1.0) = 1.714$ A and $P = (1.714)^2(1.0) = 2.94$ W.

With similar calculations the following table is produced:

$R_L(\Omega)$	0	0.5	1.0	1.5	2.0	2.5
$I = \dfrac{E}{r + R_L}$	2.4	2.0	1.714	1.5	1.333	1.2
$P = I^2 R_L$ (W)	0	2.00	2.94	3.38	3.56	3.60
$R_L(\Omega)$	3.0	3.5	4.0	4.5	5.0	
$I = \dfrac{E}{r + R_L}$	1.091	1.0	0.923	0.857	0.8	
$P = I^2 R_L$ (W)	3.57	3.50	3.41	3.31	3.20	

A graph of R_L against P is shown in Fig. 13.83. **The maximum value of power is 3.60 W** which occurs when R_L is 2.5 Ω, i.e. **maximum power occurs when $R_L = r$**, which is what the maximum power transfer theorem states.

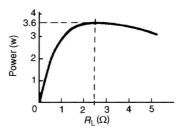

Figure 13.83

Problem 23. A d.c. source has an open-circuit voltage of 30 V and an internal resistance of 1.5 Ω. State the value of load resistance that gives maximum power dissipation and determine the value of this power.

The circuit diagram is shown in Fig. 13.84. From the maximum power transfer theorem, for maximum power dissipation, $R_L = r = \mathbf{1.5\,\Omega}$

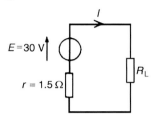

Figure 13.84

From Fig. 13.84, current $I = E/(r + R_L)$

$$= 30/(1.5 + 1.5) = 10\,\text{A}$$

Power $P = I^2 R_L = (10)^2(1.5) = \mathbf{150\,W} = $ maximum power dissipated

Problem 24. Find the value of the load resistor R_L shown in Fig. 13.85 that gives maximum power dissipation and determine the value of this power.

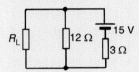

Figure 13.85

Using the procedure for Thévenin's theorem:

(i) Resistance R_L is removed from the circuit as shown in Fig. 13.86(a)

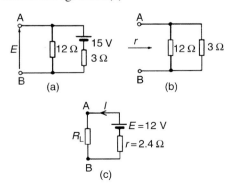

Figure 13.86

(ii) The p.d. across AB is the same as the p.d. across the 12 Ω resistor. Hence

$$E = \left(\frac{12}{12 + 3}\right)(15) = 12\,\text{V}$$

(iii) Removing the source of e.m.f. gives the circuit of Fig. 13.86(b), from which, resistance,

$$r = \frac{12 \times 3}{12 + 3} = \frac{36}{15} = 2.4\,\Omega$$

(iv) The equivalent Thévenin's circuit supplying terminals AB is shown in Fig. 13.86(c), from which,

$$\text{current, } I = \frac{E}{r + R_L}$$

For maximum power, $R_L = r = \mathbf{2.4\,\Omega}$

Thus current, $I = \dfrac{12}{2.4 + 2.4} = 2.5\,\text{A}$

Power, P, dissipated in load R_L,
$P = I^2 R_L = (2.5)^2(2.4) = \mathbf{15\,W}$.

Now try the following exercises

Exercise 74 Further problems on the maximum power transfer theorem

1. A d.c. source has an open-circuit voltage of 20 V and an internal resistance of 2 Ω. Determine the value of the load resistance that gives maximum power dissipation. Find the value of this power. [2 Ω, 50 W]

2. Determine the value of the load resistance R_L shown in Fig. 13.87 that gives maximum power dissipation and find the value of the power.
   $[R_L = 1.6\,\Omega,\ P = 57.6\,\text{W}]$

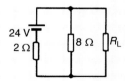

Figure 13.87

3. A d.c. source having an open-circuit voltage of 42 V and an internal resistance of 3 Ω is connected to a load of resistance R_L. Determine the maximum power dissipated by the load. [147 W]

4. A voltage source comprising six 2 V cells, each having an internal resistance of $0.2\,\Omega$, is connected to a load resistance R. Determine the maximum power transferred to the load.
[30 W]

5. The maximum power dissipated in a $4\,\Omega$ load is 100 W when connected to a d.c. voltage V and internal resistance r. Calculate (a) the current in the load, (b) internal resistance r, and (c) voltage V. [(a) 5 A (b) $4\,\Omega$ (c) 40 V]

Exercise 75   Short answer questions on d.c. circuit theory

1. Name two laws and three theorems which may be used to find unknown currents and p.d.'s in electrical circuits

2. State Kirchhoff's current law

3. State Kirchhoff's voltage law

4. State, in your own words, the superposition theorem

5. State, in your own words, Thévenin's theorem

6. State, in your own words, Norton's theorem

7. State the maximum power transfer theorem for a d.c. circuit

Exercise 76   Multi-choice questions on d.c. circuit theory
(Answers on page 420)

1. Which of the following statements is true:
   For the junction in the network shown in Fig. 13.88:
   (a) $I_5 - I_4 = I_3 - I_2 + I_1$
   (b) $I_1 + I_2 + I_3 = I_4 + I_5$
   (c) $I_2 + I_3 + I_5 = I_1 + I_4$
   (d) $I_1 - I_2 - I_3 - I_4 + I_5 = 0$

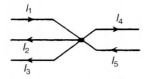

Figure 13.88

2. Which of the following statements is true?
   For the circuit shown in Fig. 13.89:
   (a) $E_1 + E_2 + E_3 = Ir_1 + Ir_2 + I_3r_3$
   (b) $E_2 + E_3 - E_1 - I(r_1 + r_2 + r_3) = 0$
   (c) $I(r_1 + r_2 + r_3) = E_1 - E_2 - E_3$
   (d) $E_2 + E_3 - E_1 = Ir_1 + Ir_2 + Ir_3$

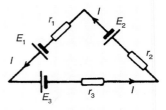

Figure 13.89

3. For the circuit shown in Fig. 13.90, the internal resistance r is given by:
   (a) $\dfrac{I}{V - E}$ (b) $\dfrac{V - E}{I}$
   (c) $\dfrac{I}{E - V}$ (d) $\dfrac{E - V}{I}$

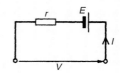

Figure 13.90

4. For the circuit shown in Fig. 13.91, voltage V is:
   (a) 12 V (b) 2 V (c) 10 V (d) 0 V

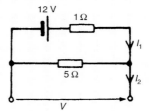

Figure 13.91

5. For the circuit shown in Fig. 13.91, current I_1 is:
   (a) 2 A   (b) 14.4 A
   (c) 0.5 A   (d) 0 A

6. For the circuit shown in Fig. 13.91, current I_2 is:
   (a) 2 A   (b) 14.4 A
   (c) 0.5 A   (d) 0 A

7. The equivalent resistance across terminals AB of Fig. 13.92 is:
   (a) 9.31 Ω   (b) 7.24 Ω
   (c) 10.0 Ω   (d) 6.75 Ω

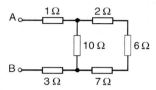

Figure 13.92

8. With reference to Fig. 13.93, which of the following statements is correct?
   (a) $V_{PQ} = 2\,V$
   (b) $V_{PQ} = 15\,V$
   (c) When a load is connected between P and Q, current would flow from Q to P
   (d) $V_{PQ} = 20\,V$

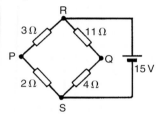

Figure 13.93

9. In Fig. 13.93, if the 15 V battery is replaced by a short-circuit, the equivalent resistance across terminals PQ is:
   (a) 20 Ω   (b) 4.20 Ω
   (c) 4.13 Ω   (d) 4.29 Ω

10. For the circuit shown in Fig. 13.94, maximum power transfer from the source is required. For this to be so, which of the following statements is true?
    (a) $R_2 = 10\,\Omega$ (b) $R_2 = 30\,\Omega$
    (c) $R_2 = 7.5\,\Omega$ (d) $R_2 = 15\,\Omega$

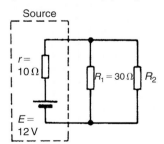

Figure 13.94

11. The open-circuit voltage E across terminals XY of Fig. 13.95 is:
    (a) 0 V   (b) 20 V
    (c) 4 V   (d) 16 V

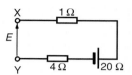

Figure 13.95

12. The maximum power transferred by the source in Fig. 13.96 is:
    (a) 5 W   (b) 200 W
    (c) 40 W   (d) 50 W

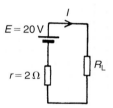

Figure 13.96

13. For the circuit shown in Fig. 13.97, voltage V is:
    (a) 0 V   (b) 20 V
    (c) 4 V   (d) 16 V

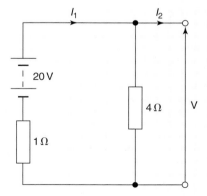

Figure 13.97

14. For the circuit shown in Fig. 13.97, current I_1 is:

(a) 25 A   (b) 4 A
(c) 0 A   (d) 20 A

15. For the circuit shown in Fig. 13.97, current I_2 is:
    (a) 25 A   (b) 4 A
    (c) 0 A   (d) 20 A

16. The current flowing in the branches of a d.c. circuit may be determined using:
    (a) Kirchhoff's laws
    (b) Lenz's law
    (c) Faraday's laws
    (d) Fleming's left-hand rule

Chapter 14

Alternating voltages and currents

At the end of this chapter you should be able to:

- appreciate why a.c. is used in preference to d.c.
- describe the principle of operation of an a.c. generator
- distinguish between unidirectional and alternating waveforms
- define cycle, period or periodic time T and frequency f of a waveform
- perform calculations involving $T = 1/f$
- define instantaneous, peak, mean and r.m.s. values, and form and peak factors for a sine wave
- calculate mean and r.m.s. values and form and peak factors for given waveforms
- understand and perform calculations on the general sinusoidal equation $v = V_m \sin(\omega t \pm \phi)$
- understand lagging and leading angles
- combine two sinusoidal waveforms (a) by plotting graphically, (b) by drawing phasors to scale and (c) by calculation
- understand rectification, and describe methods of obtaining half-wave and full-wave rectification
- appreciate methods of smoothing a rectified output waveform

14.1 Introduction

Electricity is produced by generators at power stations and then distributed by a vast network of transmission lines (called the National Grid system) to industry and for domestic use. It is easier and cheaper to generate alternating current (a.c.) than direct current (d.c.) and a.c. is more conveniently distributed than d.c. since its voltage can be readily altered using transformers. Whenever d.c. is needed in preference to a.c., devices called rectifiers are used for conversion (see Section 14.7).

14.2 The a.c. generator

Let a single turn coil be free to rotate at constant angular velocity symmetrically between the poles of a magnet system as shown in Fig. 14.1.

An e.m.f. is generated in the coil (from Faraday's laws) which varies in magnitude and reverses its direction at regular intervals. The reason for this is shown in Fig. 14.2. In positions (a), (e) and (i) the conductors of the loop are effectively moving along the magnetic field, no flux is cut and hence no e.m.f. is induced. In position (c) maximum flux is cut and hence maximum e.m.f. is induced. In position (g), maximum flux is cut

DOI: 10.1016/B978-0-08-089056-2.00014-0

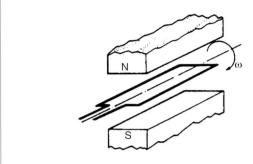

Figure 14.1

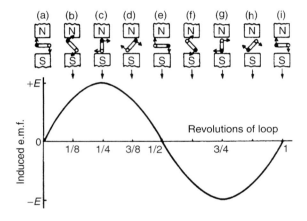

Figure 14.2

and hence maximum e.m.f. is again induced. However, using Fleming's right-hand rule, the induced e.m.f. is in the opposite direction to that in position (c) and is thus shown as $-E$. In positions (b), (d), (f) and (h) some flux is cut and hence some e.m.f. is induced. If all such

positions of the coil are considered, in one revolution of the coil, one cycle of alternating e.m.f. is produced as shown. This is the principle of operation of the a.c. generator (i.e. the alternator).

14.3 Waveforms

If values of quantities which vary with time t are plotted to a base of time, the resulting graph is called a **waveform**. Some typical waveforms are shown in Fig. 14.3. Waveforms (a) and (b) are **unidirectional waveforms**, for, although they vary considerably with time, they flow in one direction only (i.e. they do not cross the time axis and become negative). Waveforms (c) to (g) are called **alternating waveforms** since their quantities are continually changing in direction (i.e. alternately positive and negative).

A waveform of the type shown in Fig. 14.3(g) is called a **sine wave**. It is the shape of the waveform of e.m.f. produced by an alternator and thus the mains electricity supply is of 'sinusoidal' form.

One complete series of values is called a **cycle** (i.e. from O to P in Fig. 14.3(g)).

The time taken for an alternating quantity to complete one cycle is called the **period** or the **periodic time, T,** of the waveform.

The number of cycles completed in one second is called the **frequency, f,** of the supply and is measured in **hertz, Hz**. The standard frequency of the electricity supply in Great Britain is 50 Hz

$$T = \frac{1}{f} \quad \text{or} \quad f = \frac{1}{T}$$

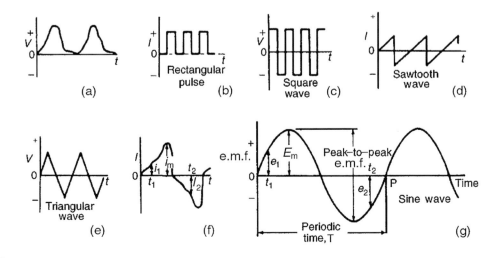

Figure 14.3

Problem 1. Determine the periodic time for frequencies of (a) 50 Hz and (b) 20 kHz.

(a) Periodic time $T = \dfrac{1}{f} = \dfrac{1}{50} = 0.02\,\text{s}$ or **20 ms**

(b) Periodic time $T = \dfrac{1}{f} = \dfrac{1}{20\,000}$

$$= 0.00005\,\text{s or } 50\,\mu\text{s}$$

Problem 2. Determine the frequencies for periodic times of (a) 4 ms (b) 4 μs.

(a) Frequency $f = \dfrac{1}{T} = \dfrac{1}{4 \times 10^{-3}}$

$$= \dfrac{1000}{4} = 250\,\text{Hz}$$

(b) Frequency $f = \dfrac{1}{T} = \dfrac{1}{4 \times 10^{-6}} = \dfrac{1\,000\,000}{4}$

$$= 250\,000\,\text{Hz}$$

$$\text{or } 250\,\text{kHz or } 0.25\,\text{MHz}$$

Problem 3. An alternating current completes 5 cycles in 8 ms. What is its frequency?

Time for 1 cycle $= (8/5)\,\text{ms} = 1.6\,\text{ms} = $ periodic time T.

$$\text{Frequency } f = \dfrac{1}{T} = \dfrac{1}{1.6 \times 10^{-3}} = \dfrac{1000}{1.6}$$

$$= \dfrac{10\,000}{16} = 625\,\text{Hz}$$

Now try the following exercise

Exercise 77   Further problems on frequency and periodic time

1. Determine the periodic time for the following frequencies:
    (a) 2.5 Hz   (b) 100 Hz   (c) 40 kHz
    [(a) 0.4 s (b) 10 ms (c) 25 μs]

2. Calculate the frequency for the following periodic times:
    (a) 5 ms   (b) 50 μs   (c) 0.2 s
    [(a) 200 Hz (b) 20 kHz (c) 5 Hz]

3. An alternating current completes 4 cycles in 5 ms. What is its frequency?   [800 Hz]

14.4   A.C. values

Instantaneous values are the values of the alternating quantities at any instant of time. They are represented by small letters, i, v, e, etc., (see Fig. 14.3(f) and (g)).

The largest value reached in a half-cycle is called the **peak value** or the **maximum value** or the **amplitude** of the waveform. Such values are represented by V_m, I_m, E_m, etc. (see Fig. 14.3(f) and (g)). A **peak-to-peak** value of e.m.f. is shown in Fig. 14.3(g) and is the difference between the maximum and minimum values in a cycle.

The **average** or **mean value** of a symmetrical alternating quantity, (such as a sine wave), is the average value measured over a half-cycle, (since over a complete cycle the average value is zero).

$$\text{Average or mean value} = \frac{\text{area under the curve}}{\text{length of base}}$$

The area under the curve is found by approximate methods such as the trapezoidal rule, the mid-ordinate rule or Simpson's rule. Average values are represented by V_{AV}, I_{AV}, E_{AV}, etc.

For a sine wave:

$$\text{average value} = 0.637 \times \text{maximum value}$$

$$(\text{i.e. } 2/\pi \times \text{maximum value})$$

The **effective value** of an alternating current is that current which will produce the same heating effect as an equivalent direct current. The effective value is called the **root mean square (r.m.s.) value** and whenever an alternating quantity is given, it is assumed to be the r.m.s. value. For example, the domestic mains supply in Great Britain is 240 V and is assumed to mean '240 V r.m.s.'. The symbols used for r.m.s. values are I, V, E, etc. For a non-sinusoidal waveform as shown in Fig. 14.4 the r.m.s. value is given by:

$$I = \sqrt{\frac{i_1^2 + i_2^2 + \cdots + i_n^2}{n}}$$

where n is the number of intervals used.

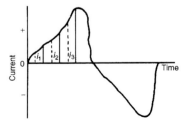

Figure 14.4

For a sine wave:

r.m.s. value = 0.707 × maximum value

(i.e.$1/\sqrt{2}$ × maximum value)

$$\text{Form factor} = \frac{\text{r.m.s. value}}{\text{average value}}$$

For a sine wave, form factor = 1.11

$$\text{Peak factor} = \frac{\text{maximum value}}{\text{r.m.s. value}}$$

For a sine wave, peak factor = 1.41.
   The values of form and peak factors give an indication of the shape of waveforms.

Problem 4. For the periodic waveforms shown in Fig. 14.5 determine for each: (i) frequency (ii) average value over half a cycle (iii) r.m.s. value (iv) form factor and (v) peak factor.

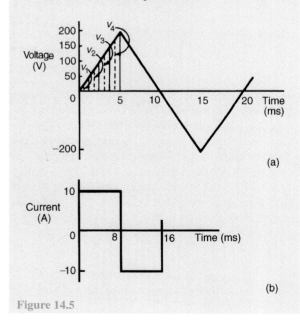

Figure 14.5

(a) **Triangular waveform** (Fig. 14.5(a)).

   (i) Time for 1 complete cycle = 20 ms = periodic time, T. Hence

$$\text{frequency } f = \frac{1}{T} = \frac{1}{20 \times 10^{-3}}$$
$$= \frac{1000}{20} = \mathbf{50\,Hz}$$

(ii) Area under the triangular waveform for a half-cycle = $\frac{1}{2}$ × base × height

$$= \tfrac{1}{2} \times (10 \times 10^{-3}) \times 200 = 1 \text{ volt second}$$

$$\left.\begin{array}{r}\text{Average value} \\ \text{of waveform}\end{array}\right\} = \frac{\text{area under curve}}{\text{length of base}}$$

$$= \frac{1 \text{ volt second}}{10 \times 10^{-3}\text{second}}$$

$$= \frac{1000}{10} = \mathbf{100\,V}$$

(iii) In Fig. 14.5(a), the first 1/4 cycle is divided into 4 intervals. Thus

$$\text{r.m.s. value} = \sqrt{\frac{v_1^2 + v_2^2 + v_3^2 + v_4^2}{4}}$$

$$= \sqrt{\frac{25^2 + 75^2 + 125^2 + 175^2}{4}}$$

$$= \mathbf{114.6\,V}$$

(Note that the greater the number of intervals chosen, the greater the accuracy of the result. For example, if twice the number of ordinates as that chosen above are used, the r.m.s. value is found to be 115.6 V)

(iv) Form factor = $\dfrac{\text{r.m.s. value}}{\text{average value}}$

$$= \frac{114.6}{100} = \mathbf{1.15}$$

(v) Peak factor = $\dfrac{\text{maximum value}}{\text{r.m.s. value}}$

$$= \frac{200}{114.6} = \mathbf{1.75}$$

(b) **Rectangular waveform** (Fig. 14.5(b)).

   (i) Time for 1 complete cycle = 16 ms = periodic time, T. Hence

$$\text{frequency, } f = \frac{1}{T} = \frac{1}{16 \times 10^{-3}} = \frac{1000}{16}$$

$$= \mathbf{62.5\,Hz}$$

(ii) $\left.\begin{array}{r}\text{Average value over} \\ \text{half a cycle}\end{array}\right\} = \dfrac{\text{area under curve}}{\text{length of base}}$

$$= \frac{10 \times (8 \times 10^{-3})}{8 \times 10^{-3}}$$

$$= \mathbf{10\,A}$$

(iii)   The r.m.s. value $= \sqrt{\dfrac{i_1^2 + i_2^2 + i_3^2 + i_4^2}{4}} = \mathbf{10\,A}$, however many intervals are chosen, since the waveform is rectangular.

(iv)   Form factor $= \dfrac{\text{r.m.s. value}}{\text{average value}} = \dfrac{10}{10} = \mathbf{1}$

(v)   Peak factor $= \dfrac{\text{maximum value}}{\text{r.m.s. value}} = \dfrac{10}{10} = \mathbf{1}$

Problem 5.   The following table gives the corresponding values of current and time for a half-cycle of alternating current.

time t (ms)	0	0.5	1.0	1.5	2.0	2.5
current i (A)	0	7	14	23	40	56

time t (ms)	3.0	3.5	4.0	4.5	5.0
current i (A)	68	76	60	5	0

Assuming the negative half-cycle is identical in shape to the positive half-cycle, plot the waveform and find (a) the frequency of the supply, (b) the instantaneous values of current after 1.25 ms and 3.8 ms, (c) the peak or maximum value, (d) the mean or average value, and (e) the r.m.s. value of the waveform.

The half-cycle of alternating current is shown plotted in Fig. 14.6

(a)   Time for a half-cycle $= 5$ ms; hence the time for 1 cycle, i.e. the periodic time, $T = 10$ ms or 0.01 s

$$\text{Frequency, } f = \frac{1}{T} = \frac{1}{0.01} = \mathbf{100\,Hz}$$

(b)   Instantaneous value of current after 1.25 ms is **19 A**, from Fig. 14.6. Instantaneous value of current after 3.8 ms is **70 A**, from Fig. 14.6

(c)   Peak or maximum value $= \mathbf{76\,A}$

(d)   Mean or average value $= \dfrac{\text{area under curve}}{\text{length of base}}$

Using the mid-ordinate rule with 10 intervals, each of width 0.5 ms gives:

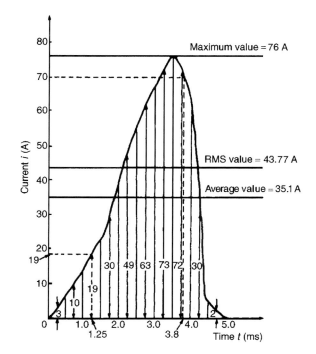

Figure 14.6

$$\left.\begin{array}{c}\text{area under}\\\text{curve}\end{array}\right\} = (0.5 \times 10^{-3})[3 + 10 + 19 + 30$$
$$+ 49 + 63 + 73$$
$$+ 72 + 30 + 2]$$
$$(\text{see Fig. 14.6})$$
$$= (0.5 \times 10^{-3})(351)$$

$$\left.\begin{array}{c}\text{Hence mean or}\\\text{average value}\end{array}\right\} = \frac{(0.5 \times 10^{-3})(351)}{5 \times 10^{-3}}$$
$$= \mathbf{35.1\,A}$$

(e)   R.m.s. value $= \sqrt{\dfrac{\begin{array}{c}3^2 + 10^2 + 19^2 + 30^2 + 49^2\\ + 63^2 + 73^2 + 72^2 + 30^2 + 2^2\end{array}}{10}}$

$$= \sqrt{\frac{19\,157}{10}} = \mathbf{43.8\,A}$$

Problem 6.   Calculate the r.m.s. value of a sinusoidal current of maximum value 20 A.

For a sine wave,

$$\text{r.m.s. value} = 0.707 \times \text{maximum value}$$
$$= 0.707 \times 20 = \mathbf{14.14\,A}$$

Problem 7.   Determine the peak and mean values for a 240 V mains supply.

For a sine wave, r.m.s. value of voltage $V = 0.707 \times V_m$. A 240 V mains supply means that 240 V is the r.m.s. value, hence

$$V_m = \frac{V}{0.707} = \frac{240}{0.707} = \textbf{339.5 V}$$
$$= \textbf{peak value}$$

Mean value

$$V_{AV} = 0.637 V_m = 0.637 \times 339.5 = \textbf{216.3 V}$$

Problem 8. A supply voltage has a mean value of 150 V. Determine its maximum value and its r.m.s. value.

For a sine wave, mean value $= 0.637 \times$ maximum value. Hence

$$\textbf{maximum value} = \frac{\text{mean value}}{0.637} = \frac{150}{0.637}$$
$$= \textbf{235.5 V}$$

R.m.s. value $= 0.707 \times$ maximum value
$$= 0.707 \times 235.5 = \textbf{166.5 V}$$

Now try the following exercise

Exercise 78   Further problems on a.c. values of waveforms

1. An alternating current varies with time over half a cycle as follows:

Current (A)	0	0.7	2.0	4.2	8.4
time (ms)	0	1	2	3	4

Current (A)	8.2	2.5	1.0	0.4	0.2	0
time (ms)	5	6	7	8	9	10

The negative half-cycle is similar. Plot the curve and determine:
(a) the frequency (b) the instantaneous values at 3.4 ms and 5.8 ms (c) its mean value and (d) its r.m.s. value.
[(a) 50 Hz (b) 5.5 A, 3.1 A
(c) 2.8 A (d) 4.0 A]

2. For the waveforms shown in Fig. 14.7 determine for each (i) the frequency (ii) the average value over half a cycle (iii) the r.m.s. value (iv) the form factor (v) the peak factor.

[(a) (i) 100 Hz (ii) 2.50 A (iii) 2.87 A
     (iv) 1.15   (v) 1.74
 (b) (i) 250 Hz (ii) 20 V   (iii) 20 V
     (iv) 1.0   (v) 1.0
 (c) (i) 125 Hz (ii) 18 A   (iii) 19.56 A
     (iv) 1.09   (v) 1.23
 (d) (i) 250 Hz (ii) 25 V   (iii) 50 V
     (iv) 2.0   (v) 2.0]

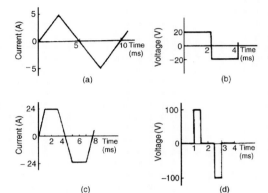

Figure 14.7

3. An alternating voltage is triangular in shape, rising at a constant rate to a maximum of 300 V in 8 ms and then falling to zero at a constant rate in 4 ms. The negative half-cycle is identical in shape to the positive half-cycle. Calculate (a) the mean voltage over half a cycle, and (b) the r.m.s. voltage.
[(a) 150 V (b) 170 V]

4. An alternating e.m.f. varies with time over half a cycle as follows:

E.m.f. (V)	0	45	80	155	215
time (ms)	0	1.5	3.0	4.5	6.0

E.m.f. (V)	320	210	95	0
time (ms)	7.5	9.0	10.5	12.0

The negative half-cycle is identical in shape to the positive half-cycle. Plot the waveform and determine (a) the periodic time and frequency (b) the instantaneous value of voltage at 3.75 ms (c) the times when the voltage is 125 V (d) the mean value, and (e) the r.m.s. value

[(a) 24 ms, 41.67 Hz   (b) 115 V
(c) 4 ms and 10.1 ms   (d) 142 V
(e) 171 V]

5. Calculate the r.m.s. value of a sinusoidal curve of maximum value 300 V   [212.1 V]

6. Find the peak and mean values for a 200 V mains supply   [282.9 V, 180.2 V]

7. Plot a sine wave of peak value 10.0 A. Show that the average value of the waveform is 6.37 A over half a cycle, and that the r.m.s. value is 7.07 A

8. A sinusoidal voltage has a maximum value of 120 V. Calculate its r.m.s. and average values.   [84.8 V, 76.4 V]

9. A sinusoidal current has a mean value of 15.0 A. Determine its maximum and r.m.s. values.   [23.55 A, 16.65 A]

14.5 Electrical safety – insulation and fuses

Insulation is used to prevent 'leakage', and when determining what type of insulation should be used, the maximum voltage present must be taken into account. For this reason, **peak values are always considered when choosing insulation materials**.

Fuses are the weak link in a circuit and are used to break the circuit if excessive current is drawn. Excessive current could lead to a fire. Fuses rely on the heating effect of the current, and for this reason, **r.m.s. values must always be used when calculating the appropriate fuse size**.

14.6 The equation of a sinusoidal waveform

In Fig. 14.8, 0A represents a vector that is free to rotate anticlockwise about 0 at an angular velocity of ω rad/s. A rotating vector is known as a **phasor**.

After time t seconds the vector 0A has turned through an angle ωt. If the line BC is constructed perpendicular to 0A as shown, then

$$\sin \omega t = \frac{BC}{0B} \quad \text{i.e. } BC = 0B \sin \omega t$$

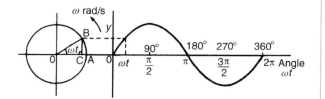

Figure 14.8

If all such vertical components are projected on to a graph of y against angle ωt (in radians), a sine curve results of maximum value 0A. Any quantity which varies sinusoidally can thus be represented as a phasor.

A sine curve may not always start at 0°. To show this a periodic function is represented by $y = \sin(\omega t \pm \phi)$, where ϕ is the phase (or angle) difference compared with $y = \sin \omega t$. In Fig. 14.9(a), $y_2 = \sin(\omega t + \phi)$ starts ϕ radians earlier than $y_1 = \sin \omega t$ and is thus said to **lead** y_1 by ϕ radians. Phasors y_1 and y_2 are shown in Fig. 14.9(b) at the time when $t = 0$.

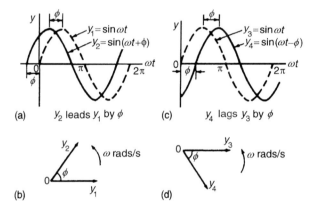

Figure 14.9

In Fig. 14.9(c), $y_4 = \sin(\omega t - \phi)$ starts ϕ radians later than $y_3 = \sin \omega t$ and is thus said to **lag** y_3 by ϕ radians. Phasors y_3 and y_4 are shown in Fig. 14.9(d) at the time when $t = 0$.

Given the general sinusoidal voltage, $v = V_m \sin(\omega t \pm \phi)$, then

(i) Amplitude or maximum value $= V_m$

(ii) Peak to peak value $= 2V_m$

(iii) Angular velocity $= \omega$ rad/s

(iv) Periodic time, $T = 2\pi/\omega$ seconds

(v) Frequency, $f = \omega/2\pi$ Hz (since $\omega = 2\pi f$)

(vi) $\phi =$ angle of lag or lead (compared with $v = V_m \sin \omega t$)

Problem 9. An alternating voltage is given by $v = 282.8 \sin 314t$ volts. Find (a) the r.m.s. voltage, (b) the frequency, and (c) the instantaneous value of voltage when $t = 4$ ms.

(a) The general expression for an alternating voltage is $v = V_m \sin(\omega t \pm \phi)$. Comparing $v = 282.8 \sin 314t$ with this general expression gives the peak voltage as 282.8 V. Hence the r.m.s. voltage $= 0.707 \times$ maximum value
$$= 0.707 \times 282.8 = \textbf{200 V}$$

(b) Angular velocity, $\omega = 314$ rad/s, i.e. $2\pi f = 314$. Hence frequency,
$$f = \frac{314}{2\pi} = \textbf{50 Hz}$$

(c) When $t = 4$ ms,
$$v = 282.8 \sin(314 \times 4 \times 10^{-3})$$
$$= 282.8 \sin(1.256) = \textbf{268.9 V}$$

Note that 1.256 radians $= \left[1.256 \times \dfrac{180°}{\pi} \right]$
$$= 71.96°$$

Hence $v = 282.8 \sin 71.96° = \textbf{268.9 V}$, as above.

Problem 10. An alternating voltage is given by $v = 75 \sin(200\pi t - 0.25)$ volts. Find (a) the amplitude, (b) the peak-to-peak value, (c) the r.m.s. value, (d) the periodic time, (e) the frequency, and (f) the phase angle (in degrees and minutes) relative to $75 \sin 200\pi t$.

Comparing $v = 75 \sin(200\pi t - 0.25)$ with the general expression $v = V_m \sin(\omega t \pm \phi)$ gives:

(a) Amplitude, or peak value $= \textbf{75 V}$

(b) Peak-to-peak value $= 2 \times 75 = \textbf{150 V}$

(c) The r.m.s. value $= 0.707 \times$ maximum value
$$= 0.707 \times 75 = \textbf{53 V}$$

(d) Angular velocity, $\omega = 200\pi$ rad/s. Hence periodic time,
$$T = \frac{2\pi}{\omega} = \frac{2\pi}{200\pi} = \frac{1}{100} = \textbf{0.01 s or 10 ms}$$

(e) Frequency, $f = \dfrac{1}{T} = \dfrac{1}{0.01} = \textbf{100 Hz}$

(f) Phase angle, $\phi = 0.25$ radians lagging $75 \sin 200\pi t$
$$0.25 \text{ rads} = 0.25 \times \frac{180°}{\pi} = 14.32°$$

Hence phase angle $= \textbf{14.32° lagging}$

Problem 11. An alternating voltage, v, has a periodic time of 0.01 s and a peak value of 40 V. When time t is zero, $v = -20$ V. Express the instantaneous voltage in the form $v = V_m \sin(\omega t \pm \phi)$.

Amplitude, $V_m = 40$ V.

Periodic time $T = \dfrac{2\pi}{\omega}$ hence angular velocity,
$$\omega = \frac{2\pi}{T} = \frac{2\pi}{0.01} = 200\pi \text{ rad/s}.$$
$v = V_m \sin(\omega t + \phi)$ thus becomes
$$v = 40 \sin(200\pi t + \phi) \text{ volts}.$$

When time $t = 0$, $v = -20$ V

i.e. $-20 = 40 \sin \phi$

so that $\sin \phi = -20/40 = -0.5$

Hence $\phi = \sin^{-1}(-0.5) = -30°$
$$= \left(-30 \times \frac{\pi}{180}\right) \text{ rads} = -\frac{\pi}{6} \text{ rads}$$

Thus $v = \textbf{40} \sin\left(\textbf{200}\pi\textbf{t} - \dfrac{\pi}{\textbf{6}}\right) \textbf{V}$

Problem 12. The current in an a.c. circuit at any time t seconds is given by: $i = 120 \sin(100\pi t + 0.36)$ amperes. Find (a) the peak value, the periodic time, the frequency and phase angle relative to $120 \sin 100\pi t$, (b) the value of the current when $t = 0$, (c) the value of the current when $t = 8$ ms, (d) the time when the current first reaches 60 A, and (e) the time when the current is first a maximum.

(a) Peak value $= \textbf{120 A}$

Periodic time $T = \dfrac{2\pi}{\omega}$
$$= \frac{2\pi}{100\pi} \quad (\text{since } \omega = 100\pi)$$
$$= \frac{1}{50} = \textbf{0.02 s or 20 ms}$$

Frequency, $f = \dfrac{1}{T} = \dfrac{1}{0.02} = \textbf{50 Hz}$

Phase angle $= 0.36$ rads

$$= 0.36 \times \frac{180°}{\pi} = \textbf{20.63° leading}$$

(b) When $t = 0$,

$$i = 120\sin(0 + 0.36)$$

$$= 120\sin 20.63° = \textbf{42.3 A}$$

(c) When $t = 8$ ms,

$$i = 120\sin\left[100\pi\left(\frac{8}{10^3}\right) + 0.36\right]$$

$$= 120\sin 2.8733$$

$$= \textbf{31.8 A}$$

(d) When $i = 60$ A, $60 = 120\sin(100\pi t + 0.36)$ thus $(60/120) = \sin(100\pi t + 0.36)$ so that $(100\pi t + 0.36) = \sin^{-1} 0.5 = 30°$ $= \pi/6$ rads $= 0.5236$ rads. Hence time,

$$t = \frac{0.5236 - 0.36}{100\pi} = \textbf{0.521 ms}$$

(e) When the current is a maximum, $i = 120$ A.

Thus $120 = 120\sin(100\pi t + 0.36)$

$$1 = \sin(100\pi t + 0.36)$$

$$(100\pi t + 0.36) = \sin^{-1} 1 = 90°$$

$$= (\pi/2)\,\text{rads}$$

$$= 1.5708\,\text{rads}.$$

Hence time, $t = \dfrac{1.5708 - 0.36}{100\pi} = \textbf{3.85 ms}$

For a practical laboratory experiment on the use of the CRO to measure voltage, frequency and phase, see Chapter 24, page 412.

Now try the following exercise

Exercise 79   Further problems on
$$v = V_m\sin(\omega t \pm \phi)$$

1. An alternating voltage is represented by $v = 20\sin 157.1\,t$ volts. Find (a) the maximum value (b) the frequency (c) the periodic time. (d) What is the angular velocity of the phasor representing this waveform?
    [(a) 20 V (b) 25 Hz (c) 0.04 s (d) 157.1 rads/s]

2. Find the peak value, the r.m.s. value, the frequency, the periodic time and the phase angle (in degrees) of the following alternating quantities:
    (a) $v = 90\sin 400\pi t$ volts
    [90 V, 63.63 V, 200 Hz, 5 ms, 0°]
    (b) $i = 50\sin(100\pi t + 0.30)$ amperes
    [50 A, 35.35 A, 50 Hz, 0.02 s, 17.19° lead]
    (c) $e = 200\sin(628.4\,t - 0.41)$ volts
    [200 V, 141.4 V, 100 Hz, 0.01 s, 23.49° lag]

3. A sinusoidal current has a peak value of 30 A and a frequency of 60 Hz. At time $t = 0$, the current is zero. Express the instantaneous current i in the form $i = I_m\sin\omega t$.
    [$i = 30\sin 120\pi t$ A]

4. An alternating voltage v has a periodic time of 20 ms and a maximum value of 200 V. When time $t = 0$, $v = -75$ volts. Deduce a sinusoidal expression for v and sketch one cycle of the voltage showing important points.
    [$v = 200\sin(100\pi t - 0.384)$ V]

5. The voltage in an alternating current circuit at any time t seconds is given by $v = 60\sin 40\,t$ volts. Find the first time when the voltage is (a) 20 V (b) -30 V.
    [(a) 8.496 ms (b) 91.63 ms]

6. The instantaneous value of voltage in an a.c. circuit at any time t seconds is given by $v = 100\sin(50\pi t - 0.523)$ V. Find:
    (a) the peak-to-peak voltage, the frequency, the periodic time and the phase angle
    (b) the voltage when $t = 0$
    (c) the voltage when $t = 8$ ms
    (d) the times in the first cycle when the voltage is 60 V
    (e) the times in the first cycle when the voltage is -40 V
    (f) the first time when the voltage is a maximum.
    Sketch the curve for one cycle showing relevant points.
    [(a) 200 V, 25 Hz, 0.04 s, 29.97° lagging (b) -49.95 V (c) 66.96 V (d) 7.426 ms, 19.23 ms (e) 25.95 ms, 40.71 ms (f) 13.33 ms]

14.7 Combination of waveforms

The resultant of the addition (or subtraction) of two sinusoidal quantities may be determined either:

(a) by plotting the periodic functions graphically (see worked Problems 13 and 16), or

(b) by resolution of phasors by drawing or calculation (see worked Problems 14 and 15)

> **Problem 13.** The instantaneous values of two alternating currents are given by $i_1 = 20\sin\omega t$ amperes and $i_2 = 10\sin(\omega t + \pi/3)$ amperes. By plotting i_1 and i_2 on the same axes, using the same scale, over one cycle, and adding ordinates at intervals, obtain a sinusoidal expression for $i_1 + i_2$

$i_1 = 20\sin\omega t$ and $i_2 = 10\sin(\omega t + \pi/3)$ are shown plotted in Fig. 14.10. Ordinates of i_1 and i_2 are added at, say, $15°$ intervals (a pair of dividers are useful for this). For example,

at $30°$, $i_1 + i_2 = 10 + 10 = 20\,\text{A}$

at $60°$, $i_1 + i_2 = 17.3 + 8.7 = 26\,\text{A}$

at $150°$, $i_1 + i_2 = 10 + (-5) = 5\,\text{A}$, and so on.

ωt (degrees)	0	30	60	90
$\sin\omega t$	0	0.5	0.866	1
$i_1 = 20\sin\omega t$	0	10	17.32	20

$(\omega t + 60)$	60	90	120	150
$\sin(\omega t + \frac{\pi}{3})$	0.866	1	0.866	0.5
$i_2 = 10\sin(\omega t + \frac{\pi}{3})$	8.66	10	8.66	5

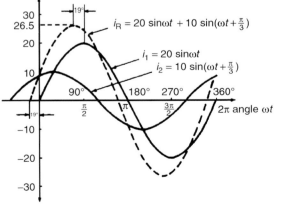

Figure 14.10

The resultant waveform for $i_1 + i_2$ is shown by the broken line in Fig. 14.10. It has the same period, and hence frequency, as i_1 and i_2. The amplitude or peak value is $26.5\,\text{A}$

The resultant waveform leads the curve $i_1 = 20\sin\omega t$ by $19°$ i.e. $(19 \times \pi/180)\,\text{rads} = 0.332\,\text{rads}$

Hence the sinusoidal expression for the resultant $i_1 + i_2$ is given by:

$$i_R = i_1 + i_2 = 26.5\sin(\omega t + 0.332)\,\text{A}$$

> **Problem 14.** Two alternating voltages are represented by $v_1 = 50\sin\omega t$ volts and $v_2 = 100\sin(\omega t - \pi/6)\,\text{V}$. Draw the phasor diagram and find, by calculation, a sinusoidal expression to represent $v_1 + v_2$

Phasors are usually drawn at the instant when time $t = 0$. Thus v_1 is drawn horizontally 50 units long and v_2 is drawn 100 units long lagging v_1 by $\pi/6$ rads, i.e. $30°$. This is shown in Fig. 14.11(a) where 0 is the point of rotation of the phasors.

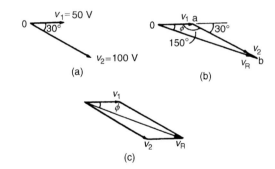

Figure 14.11

Procedure to draw phasor diagram to represent $v_1 + v_2$:

(i) Draw v_1 horizontal 50 units long, i.e. oa of Fig. 14.11(b)

(ii) Join v_2 to the end of v_1 at the appropriate angle, i.e. ab of Fig. 14.11(b)

(iii) The resultant $v_R = v_1 + v_2$ is given by the length ob and its phase angle may be measured with respect to v_1

Alternatively, when two phasors are being added the resultant is always the diagonal of the parallelogram, as shown in Fig. 14.11(c).

From the drawing, by measurement, $v_R = 145\,\text{V}$ and angle $\phi = 20°$ lagging v_1.

A more accurate solution is obtained by calculation, using the cosine and sine rules. Using the cosine rule on triangle 0ab of Fig. 14.11(b) gives:

$$v_R^2 = v_1^2 + v_2^2 - 2v_1v_2\cos 150°$$
$$= 50^2 + 100^2 - 2(50)(100)\cos 150°$$
$$= 2500 + 10000 - (-8660)$$
$$v_R = \sqrt{21\,160} = 145.5\,\text{V}$$

Using the sine rule,

$$\frac{100}{\sin\phi} = \frac{145.5}{\sin 150°}$$

from which
$$\sin\phi = \frac{100\sin 150°}{145.5}$$
$$= 0.3436$$

and $\phi = \sin^{-1}0.3436 = 0.35$ radians, and lags v_1. Hence

$$\boldsymbol{v_R = v_1 + v_2 = 145.5\sin(\omega t - 0.35)\,\text{V}}$$

Problem 15. Find a sinusoidal expression for $(i_1 + i_2)$ of Problem 13, (a) by drawing phasors, (b) by calculation.

(a) The relative positions of i_1 and i_2 at time $t = 0$ are shown as phasors in Fig. 14.12(a). The phasor diagram in Fig. 14.12(b) shows the resultant i_R, and i_R is measured as 26 A and angle ϕ as 19° or 0.33 rads leading i_1.

Hence, by drawing, $i_R = 26\sin(\omega t + 0.33)\,\text{A}$

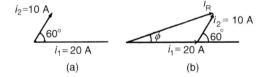

Figure 14.12

(b) From Fig. 14.12(b), by the cosine rule:

$$i_R^2 = 20^2 + 10^2 - 2(20)(10)(\cos 120°)$$

from which $i_R = \boldsymbol{26.46\,\text{A}}$

By the sine rule:
$$\frac{10}{\sin\phi} = \frac{26.46}{\sin 120°}$$

from which $\phi = 19.10°$ (i.e. 0.333 rads)

Hence, by calculation,

$$\boldsymbol{i_R = 26.46\sin(\omega t + 0.333)\,\text{A}}$$

An alternative method of calculation is to use **complex numbers** (see '*Engineering Mathematics*').

Then $i_1 + i_2 = 20\sin\omega t + 10\sin\left(\omega t + \dfrac{\pi}{3}\right)$

$$\equiv 20\angle 0 + 10\angle\frac{\pi}{3}\text{rad or}$$
$$20\angle 0° + 10\angle 60°$$
$$= (20 + j0) + (5 + j8.66)$$
$$= (25 + j8.66)$$
$$= 26.46\angle 19.106° \text{ or } 26.46\angle 0.333\,\text{rad}$$
$$\equiv \boldsymbol{26.46\sin(\omega t + 0.333)\,\text{A}}$$

Problem 16. Two alternating voltages are given by $v_1 = 120\sin\omega t$ volts and $v_2 = 200\sin(\omega t - \pi/4)$ volts. Obtain sinusoidal expressions for $v_1 - v_2$ (a) by plotting waveforms, and (b) by resolution of phasors.

(a) $v_1 = 120\sin\omega t$ and $v_2 = 200\sin(\omega t - \pi/4)$ are shown plotted in Fig. 14.13. Care must be taken when subtracting values of ordinates especially when at least one of the ordinates is negative. For example

at 30°, $v_1 - v_2 = 60 - (-52) = 112\,\text{V}$
at 60°, $v_1 - v_2 = 104 - 52 = 52\,\text{V}$
at 150°, $v_1 - v_2 = 60 - 193 = -133\,\text{V}$ and so on.

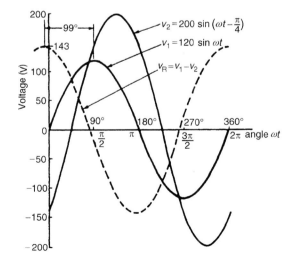

Figure 14.13

The resultant waveform, $v_R = v_1 - v_2$, is shown by the broken line in Fig. 14.13 The maximum value of v_R is 143 V and the waveform is seen to lead v_1 by 99° (i.e. 1.73 radians)

Hence, by drawing,

$v_R = v_1 - v_2 = 143 \sin(\omega t + 1.73)$ volts

(b) The relative positions of v_1 and v_2 are shown at time $t = 0$ as phasors in Fig. 14.14(a). Since the resultant of $v_1 - v_2$ is required, $-v_2$ is drawn in the opposite direction to $+v_2$ and is shown by the broken line in Fig. 14.14(a). The phasor diagram with the resultant is shown in Fig. 14.14(b) where $-v_2$ is added phasorially to v_1.

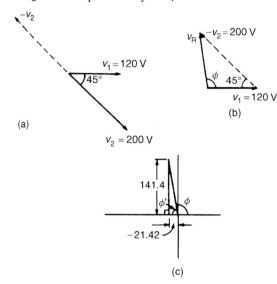

Figure 14.14

By resolution:

Sum of horizontal components of v_1 and $v_2 = 120 \cos 0° - 200 \cos 45° = -21.42$

Sum of vertical components of v_1 and $v_2 = 120 \sin 0° + 200 \sin 45° = 141.4$

From Fig. 14.14(c), resultant

$$v_R = \sqrt{(-21.42)^2 + (141.4)^2}$$

$$= 143.0$$

and $\tan \phi' = \dfrac{141.4}{21.42}$

$$= \tan 6.6013$$

from which, $\phi' = \tan^{-1} 6.6013$

$$= 81.39°$$

and $\phi = 98.61°$ or 1.721 radians

Hence, by resolution of phasors,

$v_R = v_1 - v_2 = 143.0 \sin(\omega t + 1.721)$ volts

(By complex numbers:

$$v_R = v_1 - v_2 = 120\angle 0 - 200\angle - \frac{\pi}{4}$$

$$= (120 + j0) - (141.42 - j141.42)$$

$$= -21.42 + j141.42$$

$$= 143.0\angle 98.61° \quad \text{or} \quad 143.9\angle 1.721 \text{ rad}$$

Hence, $v_R = v_1 - v_2 = 143.0 \sin(\omega t + 1.721)$ **volts)**

Now try the following exercise

1. The instantaneous values of two alternating voltages are given by $v_1 = 5 \sin \omega t$ and $v_2 = 8 \sin(\omega t - \pi/6)$. By plotting v_1 and v_2 on the same axes, using the same scale, over one cycle, obtain expressions for (a) $v_1 + v_2$ and (b) $v_1 - v_2$

   [(a) $v_1 + v_2 = 12.6 \sin(\omega t - 0.32)$ V
   (b) $v_1 - v_2 = 4.4 \sin(\omega t + 2)$ V]

2. Repeat Problem 1 using calculation
   [(a) $12.58 \sin(\omega t - 0.324)$
   (b) $4.44 \sin(\omega t + 2.02)$]

3. Construct a phasor diagram to represent $i_1 + i_2$ where $i_1 = 12 \sin \omega t$ and $i_2 = 15 \sin(\omega t + \pi/3)$. By measurement, or by calculation, find a sinusoidal expression to represent $i_1 + i_2$

   [$23.43 \sin(\omega t + 0.588)$]

Determine, either by plotting graphs and adding ordinates at intervals, or by calculation, the following periodic functions in the form $v = V_m \sin(\omega t \pm \phi)$

4. $10 \sin \omega t + 4 \sin(\omega t + \pi/4)$
   [$13.14 \sin(\omega t + 0.217)$]

5. $80 \sin(\omega t + \pi/3) + 50 \sin(\omega t - \pi/6)$
   [$94.34 \sin(\omega t + 0.489)$]

6. $100 \sin \omega t - 70 \sin(\omega t - \pi/3)$
   [$88.88 \sin(\omega t + 0.751)$]

7. The voltage drops across two components when connected in series across

an a.c. supply are $v_1 = 150 \sin 314.2t$ and $v_2 = 90 \sin (314.2t - \pi/5)$ volts respectively. Determine (a) the voltage of the supply, in trigonometric form, (b) the r.m.s. value of the supply voltage, and (c) the frequency of the supply.

$$[(a) \; 229 \sin(314.2t - 0.233)\,V$$
$$(b) \; 161.9\,V \; (c) \; 50\,Hz]$$

8. If the supply to a circuit is $25 \sin 628.3t$ volts and the voltage drop across one of the components is $18 \sin (628.3t - 0.52)$ volts, calculate (a) the voltage drop across the remainder of the circuit, (b) the supply frequency, and (c) the periodic time of the supply.

$$[(a) \; 12.96 \sin(628.3t + 0.762)\,V$$
$$(b) \; 100\,Hz \; (c) \; 10\,ms]$$

9. The voltages across three components in a series circuit when connected across an a.c. supply are:

$$v_1 = 30 \sin \left(300\pi t - \frac{\pi}{6} \right) \text{ volts,}$$

$$v_2 = 40 \sin \left(300\pi t + \frac{\pi}{4} \right) \text{ volts and}$$

$$v_3 = 50 \sin \left(300\pi t + \frac{\pi}{3} \right) \text{ volts.}$$

Calculate (a) the supply voltage, in sinusoidal form, (b) the frequency of the supply, (c) the periodic time, and (d) the r.m.s. value of the supply.

$$[(a) \; 97.39 \sin(300\pi t + 0.620)\,V$$
$$(b) \; 150\,Hz \; (c) \; 6.67\,ms \; (d) \; 68.85\,V]$$

14.8   Rectification

The process of obtaining unidirectional currents and voltages from alternating currents and voltages is called rectification. Automatic switching in circuits is achieved using diodes (see Chapter 11).

Half-wave rectification

Using a single diode, D, as shown in Fig. 14.15, **half-wave rectification** is obtained. When P is sufficiently positive with respect to Q, diode D is switched on and current i flows. When P is negative with respect to Q, diode D is switched off. Transformer T isolates the equipment from direct connection with the mains supply and enables the mains voltage to be changed.

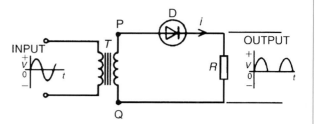

Figure 14.15

Thus, an alternating, sinusoidal waveform applied to the transformer primary is rectified into a unidirectional waveform. Unfortunately, the output waveform shown in Fig. 14.15 is not constant (i.e. steady), and as such, would be unsuitable as a d.c. power supply for electronic equipment. It would, however, be satisfactory as a battery charger. In section 14.8, methods of smoothing the output waveform are discussed.

Full-wave rectification using a centre-tapped transformer

Two diodes may be used as shown in Fig. 14.16 to obtain **full-wave rectification** where a centre-tapped transformer T is used. When P is sufficiently positive with respect to Q, diode D_1 conducts and current flows (shown by the broken line in Fig. 14.16). When S is positive with respect to Q, diode D_2 conducts and current flows (shown by the continuous line in Fig. 14.16).

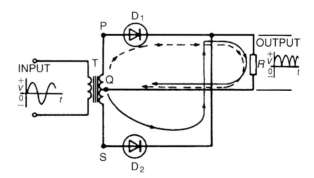

Figure 14.16

The current flowing in the load R is in the same direction for both half-cycles of the input. The output waveform is thus as shown in Fig. 14.16. The output is unidirectional, but is not constant; however, it is better than the output waveform produced with a half-wave rectifier. Section 14.8 explains how the waveform may be improved so as to be of more use.

A **disadvantage** of this type of rectifier is that centre-tapped transformers are expensive.

Full-wave bridge rectification

Four diodes may be used in a **bridge rectifier** circuit, as shown in Fig. 14.17 to obtain **full-wave rectification**. (Note, the term 'bridge' means a network of four elements connected to form a square, the input being applied to two opposite corners and the output being taken from the remaining two corners.) As for the rectifier shown in Fig. 14.16, the current flowing in load R is in the same direction for both half-cycles of the input giving the output waveform shown.

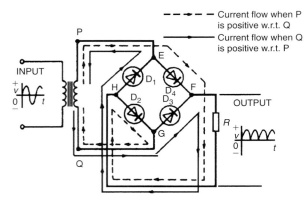

Figure 14.17

Following the broken line in Fig. 14.17:
When P is positive with respect to Q, current flows from the transformer to point E, through diode D_4 to point F, then through load R to point H, through D_2 to point G, and back to the transformer.

Following the full line in Fig. 14.17:
When Q is positive with respect to P, current flows from the transformer to point G, through diode D_3 to point F, then through load R to point H, through D_1 to point E, and back to the transformer. The output waveform is not steady and needs improving; a method of smoothing is explained in the next section.

14.9   Smoothing of the rectified output waveform

The pulsating outputs obtained from the half- and full-wave rectifier circuits are not suitable for the operation of equipment that requires a steady d.c. output, such as would be obtained from batteries. For example, for applications such as audio equipment, a supply with a large variation is unacceptable since it produces 'hum' in the output. **Smoothing** is the process of removing the worst of the output waveform variations.

To smooth out the pulsations a large capacitor, C, is connected across the output of the rectifier, as shown in Fig. 14.18; the effect of this is to maintain the output voltage at a level which is very near to the peak of the output waveform. The improved waveforms for half-wave and full-wave rectifiers are shown in more detail in Fig. 14.19.

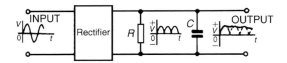

Figure 14.18

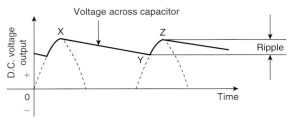

(a) Half-wave rectifier

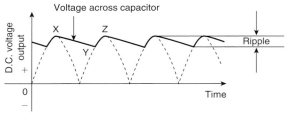

(b) Full-wave rectifier

Figure 14.19

During each pulse of output voltage, the capacitor C charges to the same potential as the peak of the waveform, as shown as point X in Fig. 14.19. As the waveform dies away, the capacitor discharges across the load, as shown by XY. The output voltage is then restored to the peak value the next time the rectifier conducts, as shown by YZ. This process continues as shown in Fig. 14.19.

Capacitor C is called a **reservoir capacitor** since it stores and releases charge between the peaks of the rectified waveform.

The variation in potential between points X and Y is called **ripple**, as shown in Fig. 14.19; the object is to reduce ripple to a minimum. Ripple may be reduced even further by the addition of inductance and another

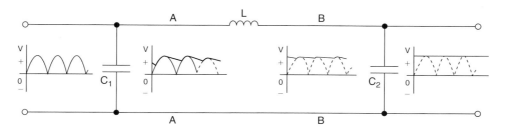

Figure 14.20

capacitor in a '**filter**' circuit arrangement, as shown in Fig. 14.20.

The output voltage from the rectifier is applied to capacitor C_1 and the voltage across points AA is shown in Fig. 14.20, similar to the waveforms of Fig. 14.19. The load current flows through the inductance L; when current is changing, e.m.f.'s are induced, as explained in Chapter 9. By Lenz's law, the induced voltages will oppose those causing the current changes.

As the ripple voltage increases and the load current increases, the induced e.m.f. in the inductor will oppose the increase. As the ripple voltage falls and the load current falls, the induced e.m.f. will try to maintain the current flow.

The voltage across points BB in Fig. 14.20 and the current in the inductance are almost ripple-free. A further capacitor, C_2, completes the process.

For a practical laboratory experiment on the use of the CRO with a bridge rectifier circuit, see Chapter 24, page 413.

Now try the following exercises

Exercise 81   Short answer questions on alternating voltages and currents

1. Briefly explain the principle of operation of the simple alternator

2. What is meant by (a) waveform (b) cycle

3. What is the difference between an alternating and a unidirectional waveform?

4. The time to complete one cycle of a waveform is called the ......

5. What is frequency? Name its unit

6. The mains supply voltage has a special shape of waveform called a ......

7. Define peak value

8. What is meant by the r.m.s. value?

9. The domestic mains electricity voltage in Great Britain is ......

10. What is the mean value of a sinusoidal alternating e.m.f. which has a maximum value of 100 V?

11. The effective value of a sinusoidal waveform is ...... × maximum value

12. What is a phasor quantity?

13. Complete the statement:
    Form factor = ... ÷ ......, and for a sine wave, form factor = ...

14. Complete the statement:
    Peak factor = ... ÷ ......, and for a sine wave, peak factor = ...

15. A sinusoidal current is given by $i = I_m \sin(\omega t \pm \alpha)$. What do the symbols I_m, ω and α represent?

16. How is switching obtained when converting a.c. to d.c.?

17. Draw an appropriate circuit diagram suitable for half-wave rectifications and explain its operation

18. Explain, with a diagram, how full-wave rectification is obtained using a centre-tapped transformer

19. Explain, with a diagram, how full-wave rectification is obtained using a bridge rectifier circuit

20. Explain a simple method of smoothing the output of a rectifier

Exercise 82 **Multi-choice questions on alternating voltages and currents**

(Answers on page 420)

1. The value of an alternating current at any given instant is:
   (a) a maximum value
   (b) a peak value
   (c) an instantaneous value
   (d) an r.m.s. value

2. An alternating current completes 100 cycles in 0.1 s. Its frequency is:
   (a) 20 Hz   (b) 100 Hz
   (c) 0.002 Hz   (d) 1 kHz

3. In Fig. 14.21, at the instant shown, the generated e.m.f. will be:
   (a) zero
   (b) an r.m.s. value
   (c) an average value
   (d) a maximum value

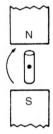

Figure 14.21

4. The supply of electrical energy for a consumer is usually by a.c. because:
   (a) transmission and distribution are more easily effected
   (b) it is most suitable for variable speed motors
   (c) the volt drop in cables is minimal
   (d) cable power losses are negligible

5. Which of the following statements is false?
   (a) It is cheaper to use a.c. than d.c.
   (b) Distribution of a.c. is more convenient than with d.c. since voltages may be readily altered using transformers
   (c) An alternator is an a.c. generator
   (d) A rectifier changes d.c. to a.c.

6. An alternating voltage of maximum value 100 V is applied to a lamp. Which of the following direct voltages, if applied to the lamp, would cause the lamp to light with the same brilliance?
   (a) 100 V   (b) 63.7 V
   (c) 70.7 V   (d) 141.4 V

7. The value normally stated when referring to alternating currents and voltages is the:
   (a) instantaneous value
   (b) r.m.s. value
   (c) average value
   (d) peak value

8. State which of the following is false. For a sine wave:
   (a) the peak factor is 1.414
   (b) the r.m.s. value is 0.707 × peak value
   (c) the average value is 0.637 × r.m.s. value
   (d) the form factor is 1.11

9. An a.c. supply is 70.7 V, 50 Hz. Which of the following statements is false?
   (a) The periodic time is 20 ms
   (b) The peak value of the voltage is 70.7 V
   (c) The r.m.s. value of the voltage is 70.7 V
   (d) The peak value of the voltage is 100 V

10. An alternating voltage is given by $v = 100\sin(50\pi t - 0.30)$ V.
    Which of the following statements is true?
    (a) The r.m.s. voltage is 100 V
    (b) The periodic time is 20 ms
    (c) The frequency is 25 Hz
    (d) The voltage is leading $v = 100\sin 50\pi t$ by 0.30 radians

11. The number of complete cycles of an alternating current occurring in one second is known as:
    (a) the maximum value of the alternating current
    (b) the frequency of the alternating current
    (c) the peak value of the alternating current
    (d) the r.m.s. or effective value

12. A rectifier conducts:
    (a) direct currents in one direction
    (b) alternating currents in one direction
    (c) direct currents in both directions
    (d) alternating currents in both directions

This revision test covers the material contained in Chapter 13 to 14. *The marks for each question are shown in brackets at the end of each question.*

1. Find the current flowing in the 5 Ω resistor of the circuit shown in Fig. RT4.1 using (a) Kirchhoff's laws, (b) the superposition theorem, (c) Thévenin's theorem, (d) Norton's theorem.

   Demonstrate that the same answer results from each method.

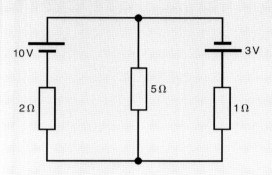

   Figure RT4.1

   Find also the current flowing in each of the other two branches of the circuit. (27)

2. A d.c. voltage source has an internal resistance of 2 Ω and an open-circuit voltage of 24 V. State the value of load resistance that gives maximum power dissipation and determine the value of this power. (5)

3. A sinusoidal voltage has a mean value of 3.0 A. Determine it's maximum and r.m.s. values. (4)

4. The instantaneous value of current in an a.c. circuit at any time t seconds is given by: $i = 50\sin(100\pi t - 0.45)$ mA. Determine
   (a) the peak to peak current, the frequency, the periodic time and the phase angle (in degrees)
   (b) the current when $t = 0$
   (c) the current when $t = 8$ ms
   (d) the first time when the voltage is a maximum.
   Sketch the current for one cycle showing relevant points. (14)

Chapter 15

Single-phase series a.c. circuits

At the end of this chapter you should be able to:

- draw phasor diagrams and current and voltage waveforms for (a) purely resistive (b) purely inductive and (c) purely capacitive a.c. circuits
- perform calculations involving $X_L = 2\pi fL$ and $X_C = 1/(2\pi fC)$
- draw circuit diagrams, phasor diagrams and voltage and impedance triangles for R–L, R–C and R–L–C series a.c. circuits and perform calculations using Pythagoras' theorem, trigonometric ratios and $Z = V/I$
- understand resonance
- derive the formula for resonant frequency and use it in calculations
- understand Q-factor and perform calculations using

$$\frac{V_L (\text{or } V_C)}{V} \quad \text{or} \quad \frac{\omega_r L}{R} \quad \text{or} \quad \frac{1}{\omega_r CR} \quad \text{or} \quad \frac{1}{R}\sqrt{\frac{L}{C}}$$

- understand bandwidth and half-power points
- perform calculations involving $(f_2 - f_1) = f_r/Q$
- understand selectivity and typical values of Q-factor
- appreciate that power P in an a.c. circuit is given by $P = VI\cos\phi$ or $I_R^2 R$ and perform calculations using these formulae
- understand true, apparent and reactive power and power factor and perform calculations involving these quantities

15.1 Purely resistive a.c. circuit

In a purely resistive a.c. circuit, the current I_R and applied voltage V_R are in phase. See Fig. 15.1

15.2 Purely inductive a.c. circuit

In a purely inductive a.c. circuit, the current I_L **lags** the applied voltage V_L by $90°$ (i.e. $\pi/2$ rads). See Fig. 15.2

In a purely inductive circuit the opposition to the flow of alternating current is called the **inductive reactance**, X_L

$$X_L = \frac{V_L}{I_L} = 2\pi fL \; \Omega$$

where f is the supply frequency, in hertz, and L is the inductance, in henry's. X_L is proportional to f as shown in Fig. 15.3

DOI: 10.1016/B978-0-08-089056-2.00015-2

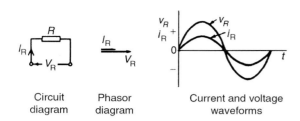

Figure 15.1

Circuit diagram   Phasor diagram   Current and voltage waveforms

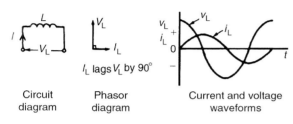

I_L lags V_L by 90°

Circuit diagram   Phasor diagram   Current and voltage waveforms

Figure 15.2

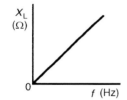

Figure 15.3

Problem 1. (a) Calculate the reactance of a coil of inductance 0.32 H when it is connected to a 50 Hz supply. (b) A coil has a reactance of 124 Ω in a circuit with a supply of frequency 5 kHz. Determine the inductance of the coil.

(a) Inductive reactance,

$$X_L = 2\pi fL = 2\pi (50)(0.32) = \mathbf{100.5\,\Omega}$$

(b) Since $X_L = 2\pi fL$, inductance

$$L = \frac{X_L}{2\pi f} = \frac{124}{2\pi (5000)} \text{H} = \mathbf{3.95\,mH}$$

Problem 2. A coil has an inductance of 40 mH and negligible resistance. Calculate its inductive reactance and the resulting current if connected to (a) a 240 V, 50 Hz supply, and (b) a 100 V, 1 kHz supply.

(a) Inductive reactance,

$$X_L = 2\pi fL$$
$$= 2\pi (50)(40 \times 10^{-3}) = \mathbf{12.57\,\Omega}$$

$$\text{Current, } I = \frac{V}{X_L} = \frac{240}{12.57} = \mathbf{19.09\,A}$$

(b) Inductive reactance,

$$X_L = 2\pi (1000)(40 \times 10^{-3}) = \mathbf{251.3\,\Omega}$$

$$\text{Current, } I = \frac{V}{X_L} = \frac{100}{251.3} = \mathbf{0.398\,A}$$

15.3 Purely capacitive a.c. circuit

In a purely capacitive a.c. circuit, the current I_C **leads** the applied voltage V_C by 90° (i.e. $\pi/2$ rads). See Fig. 15.4

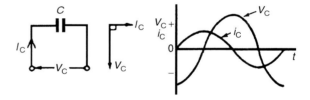

Figure 15.4

In a purely capacitive circuit the opposition to the flow of alternating current is called the **capacitive reactance**, X_C

$$X_C = \frac{V_C}{I_C} = \frac{1}{2\pi fC}\;\Omega$$

where C is the capacitance in farads.
X_C varies with frequency f as shown in Fig. 15.5

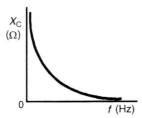

Figure 15.5

Problem 3.   Determine the capacitive reactance of a capacitor of $10\,\mu\text{F}$ when connected to a circuit of frequency (a) 50 Hz (b) 20 kHz

(a)   Capacitive reactance

$$X_C = \frac{1}{2\pi fC}$$

$$= \frac{1}{2\pi(50)(10 \times 10^{-6})}$$

$$= \frac{10^6}{2\pi(50)(10)} = \mathbf{318.3\,\Omega}$$

(b) $X_C = \dfrac{1}{2\pi fC}$

$$= \frac{1}{2\pi(20 \times 10^3)(10 \times 10^{-6})}$$

$$= \frac{10^6}{2\pi(20 \times 10^3)(10)}$$

$$= \mathbf{0.796\,\Omega}$$

Hence as the frequency is increased from 50 Hz to 20 kHz, X_C decreases from $318.3\,\Omega$ to $0.796\,\Omega$ (see Fig. 15.5)

Problem 4.   A capacitor has a reactance of $40\,\Omega$ when operated on a 50 Hz supply. Determine the value of its capacitance.

Since

$$X_C = \frac{1}{2\pi fC}$$

capacitance $C = \dfrac{1}{2\pi fX_C}$

$$= \frac{1}{2\pi(50)(40)}\,\text{F}$$

$$= \frac{10^6}{2\pi(50)(40)}\,\mu\text{F}$$

$$= \mathbf{79.58\,\mu F}$$

Problem 5.   Calculate the current taken by a $23\,\mu\text{F}$ capacitor when connected to a 240 V, 50 Hz supply.

$$\text{Current}\quad I = \frac{V}{X_C}$$

$$= \frac{V}{\left(\dfrac{1}{2\pi fC}\right)}$$

$$= 2\pi fCV$$

$$= 2\pi(50)(23 \times 10^{-6})(240)$$

$$= \mathbf{1.73\,A}$$

CIVIL

The relationship between voltage and current for the inductive and capacitive circuits can be summarised using the word 'CIVIL', which represents the following: **In a capacitor (C) the current (I) is ahead of the voltage (V), and the voltage (V) is ahead of the current (I) for the inductor (L).**

Now try the following exercise

Exercise 83   Further problems on purely inductive and capacitive a.c. circuits

1.   Calculate the reactance of a coil of inductance 0.2 H when it is connected to (a) a 50 Hz, (b) a 600 Hz, and (c) a 40 kHz supply.
[(a) $62.83\,\Omega$ (b) $754\,\Omega$ (c) $50.27\,\text{k}\Omega$]

2.   A coil has a reactance of $120\,\Omega$ in a circuit with a supply frequency of 4 kHz. Calculate the inductance of the coil.   [4.77 mH]

3.   A supply of 240 V, 50 Hz is connected across a pure inductance and the resulting current is 1.2 A. Calculate the inductance of the coil.
[0.637 H]

4.   An e.m.f. of 200 V at a frequency of 2 kHz is applied to a coil of pure inductance 50 mH. Determine (a) the reactance of the coil, and (b) the current flowing in the coil.
[(a) $628\,\Omega$ (b) 0.318 A]

5.   A 120 mH inductor has a 50 mA, 1 kHz alternating current flowing through it. Find the p.d. across the inductor.   [37.7 V]

6.   Calculate the capacitive reactance of a capacitor of $20\,\mu\text{F}$ when connected to an a.c. circuit of frequency (a) 20 Hz, (b) 500 Hz, (c) 4 kHz
[(a) $397.9\,\Omega$ (b) $15.92\,\Omega$ (c) $1.989\,\Omega$]

7.   A capacitor has a reactance of $80\,\Omega$ when connected to a 50 Hz supply. Calculate the value of its capacitance.   [$39.79\,\mu\text{F}$]

8. Calculate the current taken by a $10\,\mu\text{F}$ capacitor when connected to a 200 V, 100 Hz supply.
    [1.257 A]

9. A capacitor has a capacitive reactance of $400\,\Omega$ when connected to a 100 V, 25 Hz supply. Determine its capacitance and the current taken from the supply.   [15.92 µF, 0.25 A]

10. Two similar capacitors are connected in parallel to a 200 V, 1 kHz supply. Find the value of each capacitor if the circuit current is 0.628 A.   [0.25 µF]

15.4   R–L series a.c. circuit

In an a.c. circuit containing inductance L and resistance R, the applied voltage V is the phasor sum of V_R and V_L (see Fig. 15.6), and thus the current I lags the applied voltage V by an angle lying between $0°$ and $90°$ (depending on the values of V_R and V_L), shown as angle ϕ. In any a.c. series circuit the current is common to each component and is thus taken as the reference phasor.

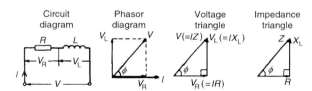

Figure 15.6

From the phasor diagram of Fig. 15.6, the 'voltage triangle' is derived.
For the R–L circuit:

$$V = \sqrt{V_R^2 + V_L^2} \quad \text{(by Pythagoras' theorem)}$$

and

$$\tan\phi = \frac{V_L}{V_R} \quad \text{(by trigonometric ratios)}$$

In an a.c. circuit, the ratio applied voltage V to current I is called the impedance, Z, i.e.

$$Z = \frac{V}{I}\ \Omega$$

If each side of the voltage triangle in Fig. 15.6 is divided by current I then the 'impedance triangle' is derived.

For the R–L circuit: $Z = \sqrt{R^2 + X_L^2}$

$$\tan\phi = \frac{X_L}{R}$$

$$\sin\phi = \frac{X_L}{Z}$$

and
$$\cos\phi = \frac{R}{Z}$$

Problem 6.   In a series R–L circuit the p.d. across the resistance R is 12 V and the p.d. across the inductance L is 5 V. Find the supply voltage and the phase angle between current and voltage.

From the voltage triangle of Fig. 15.6, supply voltage

$$V = \sqrt{12^2 + 5^2}$$

i.e.
$$V = \textbf{13 V}$$

(Note that in a.c. circuits, the supply voltage is **not** the arithmetic sum of the p.d.'s across components. It is, in fact, the **phasor sum**)

$$\tan\phi = \frac{V_L}{V_R} = \frac{5}{12}$$

from which, circuit phase angle

$$\phi = \tan^{-1}\left(\frac{5}{12}\right) = \textbf{22.62° lagging}$$

('Lagging' infers that the current is 'behind' the voltage, since phasors revolve anticlockwise)

Problem 7.   A coil has a resistance of $4\,\Omega$ and an inductance of 9.55 mH. Calculate (a) the reactance, (b) the impedance, and (c) the current taken from a 240 V, 50 Hz supply. Determine also the phase angle between the supply voltage and current.

$R=4\,\Omega$, $L=9.55\,\text{mH}=9.55\times10^{-3}\,\text{H}$, $f=50\,\text{Hz}$ and $V=240\,\text{V}$

(a) Inductive reactance,

$$X_L = 2\pi f L$$
$$= 2\pi(50)(9.55\times10^{-3})$$
$$= \textbf{3}\,\boldsymbol{\Omega}$$

(b)   Impedance,

$$Z = \sqrt{R^2 + X_L^2} = \sqrt{4^2 + 3^2} = \mathbf{5\,\Omega}$$

(c)   Current,

$$I = \frac{V}{Z} = \frac{240}{5} = \mathbf{48\,A}$$

The circuit and phasor diagrams and the voltage and impedance triangles are as shown in Fig. 15.6

Since $\tan\phi = \dfrac{X_L}{R}$

$$\phi = \tan^{-1}\frac{X_L}{R}$$

$$= \tan^{-1}\frac{3}{4}$$

$$= \mathbf{36.87°\ lagging}$$

Problem 8.   A coil takes a current of 2 A from a 12 V d.c. supply. When connected to a 240 V, 50 Hz supply the current is 20 A. Calculate the resistance, impedance, inductive reactance and inductance of the coil.

Resistance

$$R = \frac{\text{d.c. voltage}}{\text{d.c. current}} = \frac{12}{2} = 6\,\Omega$$

Impedance

$$Z = \frac{\text{a.c. voltage}}{\text{a.c. current}} = \frac{240}{20} = 12\,\Omega$$

Since

$$Z = \sqrt{R^2 + X_L^2}$$

inductive reactance,

$$X_L = \sqrt{Z^2 - R^2} = \sqrt{12^2 - 6^2} = 10.39\,\Omega$$

Since $X_L = 2\pi fL$, inductance,

$$L = \frac{X_L}{2\pi f} = \frac{10.39}{2\pi(50)} = \mathbf{33.1\,mH}$$

This problem indicates a simple method for finding the inductance of a coil, i.e. firstly to measure the current when the coil is connected to a d.c. supply of known voltage, and then to repeat the process with an a.c. supply.

For a practical laboratory experiment on the measurement of inductance of a coil, see Chapter 24, page 414.

Problem 9.   A coil of inductance 318.3 mH and negligible resistance is connected in series with a 200 Ω resistor to a 240 V, 50 Hz supply. Calculate (a) the inductive reactance of the coil, (b) the impedance of the circuit, (c) the current in the circuit, (d) the p.d. across each component, and (e) the circuit phase angle.

$L = 318.3\,\text{mH} = 0.3183\,\text{H}$, $R = 200\,\Omega$,
$V = 240\,\text{V}$ and $f = 50\,\text{Hz}$.
The circuit diagram is as shown in Fig. 15.6

(a)   Inductive reactance

$$X_L = 2\pi fL = 2\pi(50)(0.3183) = \mathbf{100\,\Omega}$$

(b)   Impedance

$$Z = \sqrt{R^2 + X_L^2}$$

$$= \sqrt{200^2 + 100^2} = \mathbf{223.6\,\Omega}$$

(c)   Current

$$I = \frac{V}{Z} = \frac{240}{223.6} = \mathbf{1.073\,A}$$

(d)   The p.d. across the coil,

$$V_L = IX_L = 1.073 \times 100 = \mathbf{107.3\,V}$$

The p.d. across the resistor,

$$V_R = IR = 1.073 \times 200 = \mathbf{214.6\,V}$$

[Check: $\sqrt{V_R^2 + V_L^2} = \sqrt{214.6^2 + 107.3^2} = 240\,\text{V}$, the supply voltage]

(e)   From the impedance triangle, angle

$$\phi = \tan^{-1}\frac{X_L}{R} = \tan^{-1}\left(\frac{100}{200}\right)$$

Hence the phase angle $\phi = \mathbf{26.57°\ lagging}$.

Problem 10.   A coil consists of a resistance of 100 Ω and an inductance of 200 mH. If an alternating voltage, v, given by $v = 200\sin 500t$ volts is applied across the coil, calculate (a) the circuit impedance, (b) the current flowing, (c) the p.d. across the resistance, (d) the p.d. across the inductance, and (e) the phase angle between voltage and current.

Since $v = 200 \sin 500t$ volts then $V_m = 200\,\text{V}$ and $\omega = 2\pi f = 500\,\text{rad/s}$

Hence r.m.s. voltage

$$V = 0.707 \times 200 = 141.4\,\text{V}$$

Inductive reactance,

$$X_L = 2\pi fL$$
$$= \omega L = 500 \times 200 \times 10^{-3} = 100\,\Omega$$

(a) Impedance

$$Z = \sqrt{R^2 + X_L^2}$$
$$= \sqrt{100^2 + 100^2} = \mathbf{141.4\,\Omega}$$

(b) Current

$$I = \frac{V}{Z} = \frac{141.4}{141.4} = \mathbf{1\,A}$$

(c) P.d. across the resistance

$$V_R = IR = 1 \times 100 = \mathbf{100\,V}$$

P.d. across the inductance

$$V_L = IX_L = 1 \times 100 = \mathbf{100\,V}$$

(d) Phase angle between voltage and current is given by:

$$\tan\phi = \frac{X_L}{R}$$

from which,

$$\phi = \tan^{-1}\left(\frac{100}{100}\right)$$

hence $\qquad \boldsymbol{\phi = 45°}$ or $\dfrac{\pi}{4}$ **rads**

Problem 11. A pure inductance of 1.273 mH is connected in series with a pure resistance of $30\,\Omega$. If the frequency of the sinusoidal supply is 5 kHz and the p.d. across the $30\,\Omega$ resistor is 6 V, determine the value of the supply voltage and the voltage across the 1.273 mH inductance. Draw the phasor diagram.

The circuit is shown in Fig. 15.7(a)

Supply voltage, $V = IZ$

Current $I = \dfrac{V_R}{R} = \dfrac{6}{30} = 0.20\,\text{A}$

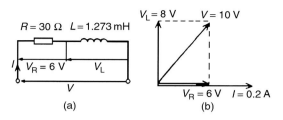

Figure 15.7

Inductive reactance

$$X_L = 2\pi fL$$
$$= 2\pi(5 \times 10^3)(1.273 \times 10^{-3})$$
$$= 40\,\Omega$$

Impedance,

$$Z = \sqrt{R^2 + X_L^2} = \sqrt{30^2 + 40^2} = 50\,\Omega$$

Supply voltage

$$V = IZ = (0.20)(50) = \mathbf{10\,V}$$

Voltage across the 1.273 mH inductance,

$$V_L = IX_L = (0.2)(40) = \mathbf{8\,V}$$

The phasor diagram is shown in Fig. 15.7(b)

(Note that in a.c. circuits, the supply voltage is **not** the arithmetic sum of the p.d.'s across components but the **phasor sum**)

Problem 12. A coil of inductance 159.2 mH and resistance $20\,\Omega$ is connected in series with a $60\,\Omega$ resistor to a 240 V, 50 Hz supply. Determine (a) the impedance of the circuit, (b) the current in the circuit, (c) the circuit phase angle, (d) the p.d. across the $60\,\Omega$ resistor, and (e) the p.d. across the coil. (f) Draw the circuit phasor diagram showing all voltages.

The circuit diagram is shown in Fig. 15.8(a). When impedances are connected in series the individual resistances may be added to give the total circuit resistance. The equivalent circuit is thus shown in Fig. 15.8(b). Inductive reactance $X_L = 2\pi fL$

$$= 2\pi(50)(159.2 \times 10^{-3}) = 50\,\Omega$$

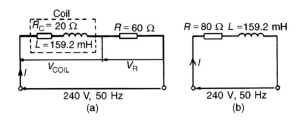

Figure 15.8

(a)   Circuit impedance,

$$Z = \sqrt{R^2 + X_L^2} = \sqrt{80^2 + 50^2} = \textbf{94.34}\,\boldsymbol{\Omega}$$

(b)   Circuit current, $I = \dfrac{V}{Z} = \dfrac{240}{94.34} = \textbf{2.544 A}$.

(c)   Circuit phase angle $\phi = \tan^{-1} X_L/R$
$$= \tan^{-1}(50/80)$$
$$= \textbf{32° lagging}$$

From Fig. 15.8(a):

(d) $V_R = IR = (2.544)(60) = \textbf{152.6 V}$

(e) $V_{COIL} = IZ_{COIL}$, where

$$Z_{COIL} = \sqrt{R_C^2 + X_L^2} = \sqrt{20^2 + 50^2} = 53.85\,\Omega.$$

Hence $V_{COIL} = (2.544)\,(53.85) = \textbf{137.0 V}$

(f)   For the phasor diagram, shown in Fig. 15.9,
$V_L = IX_L = (2.544)(50) = 127.2$ V.
$V_{RCOIL} = IR_C = (2.544)(20) = 50.88$ V

The 240 V supply voltage is the phasor sum of V_{COIL} and V_R as shown in the phasor diagram in Fig. 15.9

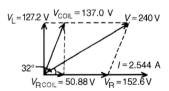

Figure 15.9

Now try the following exercise

Exercise 84   Further problems on R–L a.c. series circuits

1.   Determine the impedance of a coil which has a resistance of $12\,\Omega$ and a reactance of $16\,\Omega$.
[$20\,\Omega$]

2.   A coil of inductance 80 mH and resistance $60\,\Omega$ is connected to a 200 V, 100 Hz supply. Calculate the circuit impedance and the current taken from the supply. Find also the phase angle between the current and the supply voltage.
[$78.27\,\Omega$, 2.555 A, 39.95° lagging]

3.   An alternating voltage given by $v = 100 \sin 240t$ volts is applied across a coil of resistance $32\,\Omega$ and inductance 100 mH. Determine (a) the circuit impedance, (b) the current flowing, (c) the p.d. across the resistance, and (d) the p.d. across the inductance.
[(a) $40\,\Omega$ (b) 1.77 A (c) 56.64 V (d) 42.48 V]

4.   A coil takes a current of 5 A from a 20 V d.c. supply. When connected to a 200 V, 50 Hz a.c. supply the current is 25 A. Calculate the (a) resistance, (b) impedance, and (c) inductance of the coil.
[(a) $4\,\Omega$ (b) $8\,\Omega$ (c) 22.05 mH]

5.   A resistor and an inductor of negligible resistance are connected in series to an a.c. supply. The p.d. across the resistor is 18 V and the p.d. across the inductor is 24 V. Calculate the supply voltage and the phase angle between voltage and current.   [30 V, 53.13° lagging]

6.   A coil of inductance 636.6 mH and negligible resistance is connected in series with a $100\,\Omega$ resistor to a 250 V, 50 Hz supply. Calculate (a) the inductive reactance of the coil, (b) the impedance of the circuit, (c) the current in the circuit, (d) the p.d. across each component, and (e) the circuit phase angle.
[(a) $200\,\Omega$ (b) $223.6\,\Omega$ (c) 1.118 A (d) 223.6 V, 111.8 V (e) 63.43° lagging]

15.5   R–C series a.c. circuit

In an a.c. series circuit containing capacitance C and resistance R, the applied voltage V is the phasor sum of V_R and V_C (see Fig. 15.10) and thus the current I leads the applied voltage V by an angle lying between 0° and 90° (depending on the values of V_R and V_C), shown as angle α.

From the phasor diagram of Fig. 15.10, the **'voltage triangle'** is derived.

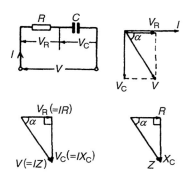

Figure 15.10

For the $R - C$ circuit:

$$V = \sqrt{V_R^2 + V_C^2} \quad \text{(by Pythagoras' theorem)}$$

and

$$\tan\alpha = \frac{V_C}{V_R} \quad \text{(by trigonometric ratios)}$$

As stated in Section 15.4, in an a.c. circuit, the ratio applied voltage V to current I is called the **impedance** Z, i.e. $Z = V/I \ \Omega$

If each side of the voltage triangle in Fig. 15.10 is divided by current I then the **'impedance triangle'** is derived.

For the $R - C$ circuit: $Z = \sqrt{R^2 + X_C^2}$

$$\tan\alpha = \frac{X_C}{R} \quad \sin\alpha = \frac{X_C}{Z} \quad \text{and} \quad \cos\alpha = \frac{R}{Z}$$

Problem 13. A resistor of 25 Ω is connected in series with a capacitor of 45 μF. Calculate (a) the impedance, and (b) the current taken from a 240 V, 50 Hz supply. Find also the phase angle between the supply voltage and the current.

$R = 25\,\Omega$, $C = 45\,\mu\text{F} = 45 \times 10^{-6}\,\text{F}$, $V = 240\,\text{V}$ and $f = 50\,\text{Hz}$. The circuit diagram is as shown in Fig. 15.10

Capacitive reactance,

$$X_C = \frac{1}{2\pi fC}$$

$$= \frac{1}{2\pi(50)(45 \times 10^{-6})} = 70.74\,\Omega$$

(a)   Impedance $Z = \sqrt{R^2 + X_C^2} = \sqrt{25^2 + 70.74^2}$

$$= \mathbf{75.03\,\Omega}$$

(b)   Current $I = V/Z = 240/75.03 = \mathbf{3.20\,A}$

Phase angle between the supply voltage and current, $\alpha = \tan^{-1}(X_C/R)$ hence

$$\alpha = \tan^{-1}\left(\frac{70.74}{25}\right) = \mathbf{70.54°\ leading}$$

('Leading' infers that the current is 'ahead' of the voltage, since phasors revolve anticlockwise)

Problem 14. A capacitor C is connected in series with a 40 Ω resistor across a supply of frequency 60 Hz. A current of 3 A flows and the circuit impedance is 50 Ω. Calculate (a) the value of capacitance, C, (b) the supply voltage, (c) the phase angle between the supply voltage and current, (d) the p.d. across the resistor, and (e) the p.d. across the capacitor. Draw the phasor diagram.

(a)   Impedance $Z = \sqrt{R^2 + X_C^2}$

Hence $X_C = \sqrt{Z^2 - R^2} = \sqrt{50^2 - 40^2} = 30\,\Omega$

$X_C = \dfrac{1}{2\pi fC}$ hence,

$$C = \frac{1}{2\pi fX_C} = \frac{1}{2\pi(60)(30)}\,F = \mathbf{88.42\,\mu F}$$

(b)   Since $Z = V/I$ then $V = IZ = (3)(50) = \mathbf{150\,V}$

(c)   Phase angle, $\alpha = \tan^{-1}X_C/R = \tan^{-1}(30/40) = \mathbf{36.87°\ leading}$.

(d)   P.d. across resistor, $V_R = IR = (3)(40) = \mathbf{120\,V}$

(e)   P.d. across capacitor, $V_C = IX_C = (3)(30) = \mathbf{90\,V}$

The phasor diagram is shown in Fig. 15.11, where the supply voltage V is the phasor sum of V_R and V_C.

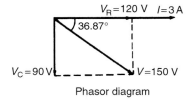

Phasor diagram

Figure 15.11

Now try the following exercise

Exercise 85 **Further problems on R–C a.c. circuits**

1. A voltage of 35 V is applied across a $C-R$ series circuit. If the voltage across the resistor is 21 V, find the voltage across the capacitor.
[28 V]

2. A resistance of 50 Ω is connected in series with a capacitance of 20 μF. If a supply of 200 V, 100 Hz is connected across the arrangement find (a) the circuit impedance, (b) the current flowing, and (c) the phase angle between voltage and current.
[(a) 93.98 Ω (b) 2.128 A (c) 57.86° leading]

3. A 24.87 μF capacitor and a 30 Ω resistor are connected in series across a 150 V supply. If the current flowing is 3 A find (a) the frequency of the supply, (b) the p.d. across the resistor and (c) the p.d. across the capacitor.
[(a) 160 Hz (b) 90 V (c) 120 V]

4. An alternating voltage $v = 250 \sin 800t$ volts is applied across a series circuit containing a 30 Ω resistor and 50 μF capacitor. Calculate (a) the circuit impedance, (b) the current flowing, (c) the p.d. across the resistor, (d) the p.d. across the capacitor, and (e) the phase angle between voltage and current.
[(a) 39.05 Ω (b) 4.526 A (c) 135.8 V (d) 113.2 V (e) 39.81° leading]

5. A 400 Ω resistor is connected in series with a 2358 pF capacitor across a 12 V a.c. supply. Determine the supply frequency if the current flowing in the circuit is 24 mA [225 kHz]

15.6 R–L–C series a.c. circuit

In an a.c. series circuit containing resistance R, inductance L and capacitance C, the applied voltage V is the phasor sum of V_R, V_L and V_C (see Fig. 15.12). V_L and V_C are anti-phase, i.e. displaced by 180°, and there are three phasor diagrams possible – each depending on the relative values of V_L and V_C.

When $X_L > X_C$ (Fig. 15.12(b)):

$$Z = \sqrt{R^2 + (X_L - X_C)^2}$$

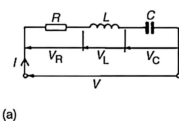

(a)

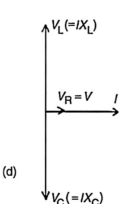

(d)

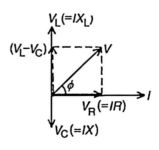

(b)

IMPEDANCE TRIANGLE

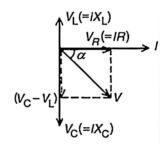

(c)

IMPEDANCE TRIANGLE

Figure 15.12

and $\qquad \tan \phi = \dfrac{X_L - X_C}{R}$

When $X_C > X_L$ (Fig. 15.12(c)):

$$Z = \sqrt{R^2 + (X_C - X_L)^2}$$

and $\qquad \tan \alpha = \dfrac{X_C - X_L}{R}$

When $X_L = X_C$ (Fig. 15.12(d)), the applied voltage V and the current I are in phase. This effect is called **series resonance** (see Section 15.7).

> **Problem 15.** A coil of resistance $5\,\Omega$ and inductance $120\,mH$ in series with a $100\,\mu F$ capacitor, is connected to a $300\,V$, $50\,Hz$ supply. Calculate (a) the current flowing, (b) the phase difference between the supply voltage and current, (c) the voltage across the coil, and (d) the voltage across the capacitor.

The circuit diagram is shown in Fig. 15.13

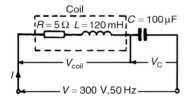

Figure 15.13

$$X_L = 2\pi f L = 2\pi(50)(120 \times 10^{-3}) = \textbf{37.70}\,\boldsymbol{\Omega}$$

$$X_C = \frac{1}{2\pi f C} = \frac{1}{2\pi(50)(100 \times 10^{-6})} = \textbf{31.83}\,\boldsymbol{\Omega}$$

Since X_L is greater than X_C the circuit is inductive.

$$X_L - X_C = 37.70 - 31.83 = 5.87\,\Omega$$

Impedance

$$Z = \sqrt{R^2 + (X_L - X_C)^2}$$
$$= \sqrt{5^2 + 5.87^2} = 7.71\,\Omega$$

(a) Current $I = \dfrac{V}{Z} = \dfrac{300}{7.71} = \textbf{38.91 A}$

(b) Phase angle

$$\phi = \tan^{-1}\left(\frac{X_L - X_C}{R}\right)$$
$$= \tan^{-1}\left(\frac{5.87}{5}\right) = \textbf{49.58}^\circ$$

(c) Impedance of coil

$$Z_{COIL} = \sqrt{R^2 + X_L^2}$$
$$= \sqrt{5^2 + 37.7^2} = 38.03\,\Omega$$

Voltage across coil

$$V_{COIL} = I Z_{COIL}$$
$$= (38.91)(38.03) = \textbf{1480 V}$$

Phase angle of coil

$$= \tan^{-1}\frac{X_L}{R}$$
$$= \tan^{-1}\left(\frac{37.7}{5}\right) = \textbf{82.45}^\circ \textbf{ lagging}$$

(d) Voltage across capacitor

$$V_C = I X_C = (38.91)(31.83) = \textbf{1239 V}$$

The phasor diagram is shown in Fig. 15.14. The supply voltage V is the phasor sum of V_{COIL} and V_C.

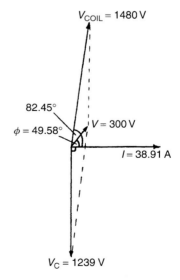

Figure 15.14

Series-connected impedances

For series-connected impedances the total circuit impedance can be represented as a single L–C–R circuit by combining all values of resistance together, all values of inductance together and all values of capacitance together, (remembering that for series connected capacitors

$$\frac{1}{C} = \frac{1}{C_1} + \frac{1}{C_2} + \cdots \Big)$$

For example, the circuit of Fig. 15.15(a) showing three impedances has an equivalent circuit of Fig. 15.15(b).

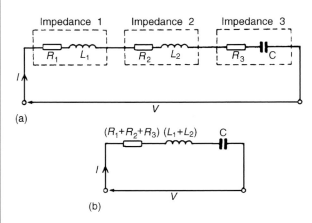

Figure 15.15

> **Problem 16.** The following three impedances are connected in series across a 40 V, 20 kHz supply: (i) a resistance of 8 Ω, (ii) a coil of inductance 130 μH and 5 Ω resistance, and (iii) a 10 Ω resistor in series with a 0.25 μF capacitor. Calculate (a) the circuit current, (b) the circuit phase angle, and (c) the voltage drop across each impedance.

The circuit diagram is shown in Fig. 15.16(a). Since the total circuit resistance is $8+5+10$, i.e. 23 Ω, an equivalent circuit diagram may be drawn as shown in Fig. 15.16(b).
Inductive reactance,

$$X_L = 2\pi fL = 2\pi(20 \times 10^3)(130 \times 10^{-6}) = 16.34\,\Omega$$

Capacitive reactance,

$$X_C = \frac{1}{2\pi fC} = \frac{1}{2\pi(20 \times 10^3)(0.25 \times 10^{-6})}$$

$$= 31.83\,\Omega$$

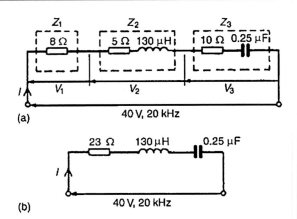

Figure 15.16

Since $X_C > X_L$, the circuit is capacitive (see phasor diagram in Fig. 15.12(c)).

$$X_C - X_L = 31.83 - 16.34 = 15.49\,\Omega$$

(a) Circuit impedance, $Z = \sqrt{R^2 + (X_C - X_L)^2}$

$$= \sqrt{23^2 + 15.49^2} = 27.73\,\Omega$$

Circuit current, $I = V/Z = 40/27.73 = \textbf{1.442 A}$

From Fig. 15.12(c), circuit phase angle

$$\phi = \tan^{-1}\left(\frac{X_C - X_L}{R}\right)$$

i.e.

$$\phi = \tan^{-1}\left(\frac{15.49}{23}\right) = \textbf{33.96° leading}$$

(b) From Fig. 15.16(a),

$$V_1 = IR_1 = (1.442)(8) = \textbf{11.54 V}$$
$$V_2 = IZ_2 = I\sqrt{5^2 + 16.34^2}$$

$$= (1.442)(17.09) = \textbf{24.64 V}$$
$$V_3 = IZ_3 = I\sqrt{10^2 + 31.83^2}$$

$$= (1.442)(33.36) = \textbf{48.11 V}$$

The 40 V supply voltage is the phasor sum of V_1, V_2 and V_3

> **Problem 17.** Determine the p.d.'s V_1 and V_2 for the circuit shown in Fig. 15.17 if the frequency of the supply is 5 kHz. Draw the phasor diagram and hence determine the supply voltage V and the circuit phase angle.

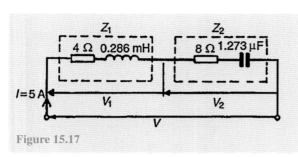

Figure 15.17

For impedance Z_1: $R_1 = 4\,\Omega$ and

$$X_L = 2\pi f L$$
$$= 2\pi(5 \times 10^3)(0.286 \times 10^{-3})$$
$$= 8.985\,\Omega$$

$$V_1 = IZ_1 = I\sqrt{R^2 + X_L^2}$$
$$= 5\sqrt{4^2 + 8.985^2} = 49.18\,\text{V}$$

Phase angle $\phi_1 = \tan^{-1}\left(\dfrac{X_L}{R}\right) = \tan^{-1}\left(\dfrac{8.985}{4}\right)$

$$= \mathbf{66.0°\ lagging}$$

For impedance Z_2: $R_2 = 8\,\Omega$ and

$$X_C = \frac{1}{2\pi f C} = \frac{1}{2\pi(5 \times 10^3)(1.273 \times 10^{-6})}$$
$$= 25.0\,\Omega$$

$$V_2 = IZ_2 = I\sqrt{R^2 + X_C^2} = 5\sqrt{8^2 + 25.0^2}$$
$$= 131.2\,\text{V}.$$

Phase angle $\phi_2 = \tan^{-1}\left(\dfrac{X_C}{R}\right) = \tan^{-1}\left(\dfrac{25.0}{8}\right)$

$$= 72.26°\ \text{leading}$$

The phasor diagram is shown in Fig. 15.18

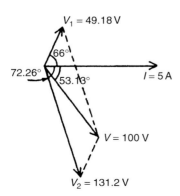

Figure 15.18

The phasor sum of V_1 and V_2 gives the supply voltage V of 100 V at a phase angle of **53.13° leading**. These values may be determined by drawing or by calculation – either by resolving into horizontal and vertical components or by the cosine and sine rules.

Now try the following exercise

Exercise 86   Further problems on $R-L-C$ a.c. circuits

1. A $40\,\mu\text{F}$ capacitor in series with a coil of resistance $8\,\Omega$ and inductance 80 mH is connected to a 200 V, 100 Hz supply. Calculate (a) the circuit impedance, (b) the current flowing, (c) the phase angle between voltage and current, (d) the voltage across the coil, and (e) the voltage across the capacitor.
   [(a) $13.18\,\Omega$ (b) 15.17 A (c) 52.63° lagging (d) 772.1 V (e) 603.6 V]

2. Find the values of resistance R and inductance L in the circuit of Fig. 15.19.
   [$R = 131\,\Omega$, $L = 0.545$ H]

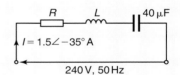

Figure 15.19

3. Three impedances are connected in series across a 100 V, 2 kHz supply. The impedances comprise:
   (i) an inductance of 0.45 mH and $2\,\Omega$ resistance,
   (ii) an inductance of $570\,\mu\text{H}$ and $5\,\Omega$ resistance, and
   (iii) a capacitor of capacitance $10\,\mu\text{F}$ and resistance $3\,\Omega$.

   Assuming no mutual inductive effects between the two inductances calculate (a) the circuit impedance, (b) the circuit current, (c) the circuit phase angle, and (d) the voltage across each impedance. Draw the phasor diagram.
   [(a) $11.12\,\Omega$ (b) 8.99 A (c) 25.92° lagging (d) 53.92 V, 78.53 V, 76.46 V]

4. For the circuit shown in Fig. 15.20 determine the voltages V_1 and V_2 if the supply frequency

is 1 kHz. Draw the phasor diagram and hence determine the supply voltage V and the circuit phase angle.

$$[V_1 = 26.0\,\text{V}, V_2 = 67.05\,\text{V},$$
$$V = 50\,\text{V}, 53.14° \text{ leading}]$$

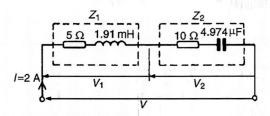

$I=2\,\text{A}$

Figure 15.20

15.7 Series resonance

As stated in Section 15.6, for an $R{-}L{-}C$ series circuit, when $X_L = X_C$ (Fig. 15.12(d)), the applied voltage V and the current I are in phase. This effect is called **series resonance**. At resonance:

(i) $V_L = V_C$

(ii) $Z = R$ (i.e. the minimum circuit impedance possible in an $L{-}C{-}R$ circuit)

(iii) $I = V/R$ (i.e. the maximum current possible in an $L{-}C{-}R$ circuit)

(iv) Since $X_L = X_C$, then $2\pi f_r L = 1/2\pi f_r C$ from which,

$$f_r^2 = \frac{1}{(2\pi)^2 LC}$$

and

$$f_r = \frac{1}{2\pi\sqrt{LC}}\,\text{Hz}$$

where f_r is the resonant frequency.

(v) The series resonant circuit is often described as an **acceptor circuit** since it has its minimum impedance, and thus maximum current, at the resonant frequency.

(vi) Typical graphs of current I and impedance Z against frequency are shown in Fig. 15.21

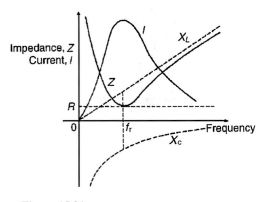

Figure 15.21

> **Problem 18.** A coil having a resistance of $10\,\Omega$ and an inductance of 125 mH is connected in series with a $60\,\mu\text{F}$ capacitor across a 120 V supply. At what frequency does resonance occur? Find the current flowing at the resonant frequency.

Resonant frequency,

$$f_r = \frac{1}{2\pi\sqrt{LC}}\,\text{Hz} = \frac{1}{2\pi\sqrt{\left[\left(\dfrac{125}{10^3}\right)\left(\dfrac{60}{10^6}\right)\right]}}$$

$$= \frac{1}{2\pi\sqrt{\left(\dfrac{125\times 6}{10^8}\right)}} = \frac{1}{2\pi\left(\dfrac{\sqrt{(125)(6)}}{10^4}\right)}$$

$$= \frac{10^4}{2\pi\sqrt{(125)(6)}} = \mathbf{58.12\,Hz}$$

At resonance, $X_L = X_C$ and impedance $Z = R$. Hence current, $I = V/R = 120/10 = \mathbf{12\,A}$

> **Problem 19.** The current at resonance in a series $L{-}C{-}R$ circuit is $100\,\mu\text{A}$. If the applied voltage is 2 mV at a frequency of 200 kHz, and the circuit inductance is $50\,\mu\text{H}$, find (a) the circuit resistance, and (b) the circuit capacitance.

(a) $I = 100\,\mu\text{A} = 100 \times 10^{-6}\,\text{A}$ and $V = 2\,\text{mV} = 2 \times 10^{-3}\,\text{V}$.

At resonance, impedance $Z =$ resistance R. Hence

$$R = \frac{V}{I} = \frac{2 \times 10^{-3}}{100 \times 10^{-6}} = \frac{2 \times 10^6}{100 \times 10^3} = \mathbf{20\,\Omega}$$

(b) At resonance $X_L = X_C$ i.e.

$$2\pi f L = \frac{1}{2\pi f C}$$

Hence capacitance

$$C = \frac{1}{(2\pi f)^2 L}$$

$$= \frac{1}{(2\pi \times 200 \times 10^3)^2 (50 \times 10^{-6})} \text{ F}$$

$$= \frac{(10^6)(10^6)}{(4\pi)^2 (10^{10})(50)} \mu\text{F}$$

$$= \mathbf{0.0127\,\mu F} \text{ or } \mathbf{12.7\,nF}$$

15.8 Q-factor

At resonance, if R is small compared with X_L and X_C, it is possible for V_L and V_C to have voltages many times greater than the supply voltage (see Fig. 15.12(d), page 234)

$$\text{Voltage magnification at resonance}$$

$$= \frac{\text{voltage across } L \text{ (or } C)}{\text{supply voltage } V}$$

This ratio is a measure of the quality of a circuit (as a resonator or tuning device) and is called the **Q-factor**. Hence

$$\text{Q-factor} = \frac{V_L}{V} = \frac{IX_L}{IR} = \frac{X_L}{R} = \frac{2\pi f_r L}{R}$$

Alternatively,

$$\text{Q-factor} = \frac{V_C}{V} = \frac{IX_C}{IR} = \frac{X_C}{R} = \frac{1}{2\pi f_r C R}$$

At resonance

$$f_r = \frac{1}{2\pi \sqrt{LC}}$$

i.e. $$2\pi f_r = \frac{1}{\sqrt{LC}}$$

Hence

$$\text{Q-factor} = \frac{2\pi f_r L}{R} = \frac{1}{\sqrt{LC}}\left(\frac{L}{R}\right) = \frac{1}{R}\sqrt{\frac{L}{C}}$$

Problem 20. A coil of inductance 80 mH and negligible resistance is connected in series with a capacitance of 0.25 μF and a resistor of resistance 12.5 Ω across a 100 V, variable frequency supply. Determine (a) the resonant frequency, and (b) the current at resonance. How many times greater than the supply voltage is the voltage across the reactances at resonance?

(a) Resonant frequency

$$f_r = \frac{1}{2\pi \sqrt{\left(\frac{80}{10^3}\right)\left(\frac{0.25}{10^6}\right)}}$$

$$= \frac{1}{2\pi \sqrt{\frac{(8)(0.25)}{10^8}}} = \frac{10^4}{2\pi \sqrt{2}}$$

$$= \mathbf{1125.4\,Hz} \text{ or } \mathbf{1.1254\,kHz}$$

(b) Current at resonance $I = V/R = 100/12.5 = \mathbf{8\,A}$
Voltage across inductance, at resonance,

$$V_L = IX_L = (I)(2\pi f L)$$

$$= (8)(2\pi)(1125.4)(80 \times 10^{-3})$$

$$= 4525.5 \text{ V}$$

(Also, voltage across capacitor,

$$V_C = IX_C = \frac{I}{2\pi f C}$$

$$= \frac{8}{2\pi(1125.4)(0.25 \times 10^{-6})}$$

$$= 4525.5 \text{ V)}$$

Voltage magnification at resonance $= V_L/V$ or $V_C/V = 4525.5/100 = \mathbf{45.255}$ i.e. at resonance, the voltage across the reactances are 45.255 times greater than the supply voltage. Hence **the Q-factor of the circuit is 45.255**

Problem 21. A series circuit comprises a coil of resistance 2 Ω and inductance 60 mH, and a 30 μF capacitor. Determine the Q-factor of the circuit at resonance.

At resonance,

$$Q\text{-factor} = \frac{1}{R}\sqrt{\frac{L}{C}} = \frac{1}{2}\sqrt{\frac{60 \times 10^{-3}}{30 \times 10^{-6}}}$$

$$= \frac{1}{2}\sqrt{\frac{60 \times 10^{6}}{30 \times 10^{3}}}$$

$$= \frac{1}{2}\sqrt{2000} = \mathbf{22.36}$$

Problem 22. A coil of negligible resistance and inductance 100 mH is connected in series with a capacitance of 2 μF and a resistance of 10 Ω across a 50 V, variable frequency supply. Determine (a) the resonant frequency, (b) the current at resonance, (c) the voltages across the coil and the capacitor at resonance, and (d) the Q-factor of the circuit.

(a)   Resonant frequency,

$$f_r = \frac{1}{2\pi \sqrt{LC}} = \frac{1}{2\pi\sqrt{\left(\frac{100}{10^3}\right)\left(\frac{2}{10^6}\right)}}$$

$$= \frac{1}{2\pi\sqrt{\frac{20}{10^8}}} = \frac{1}{\frac{2\pi\sqrt{20}}{10^4}}$$

$$= \frac{10^4}{2\pi\sqrt{20}} = \mathbf{355.9\,Hz}$$

(b)   Current at resonance $I = V/R = 50/10 = \mathbf{5\,A}$

(c)   Voltage across coil at resonance,

$$V_L = IX_L = I(2\pi f_r L)$$

$$= (5)(2\pi \times 355.9 \times 100 \times 10^{-3}) = \mathbf{1118\,V}$$

Voltage across capacitance at resonance,

$$V_C = IX_C = \frac{I}{2\pi f_r C}$$

$$= \frac{5}{2\pi(355.9)(2 \times 10^{-6})} = \mathbf{1118\,V}$$

(d)   Q-factor (i.e. voltage magnification at resonance)

$$= \frac{V_L}{V} \text{ or } \frac{V_C}{V} = \frac{1118}{50} = \mathbf{22.36}$$

Q-factor may also have been determined by

$$\frac{2\pi f_r L}{R} \quad \text{or} \quad \frac{1}{2\pi f_r CR} \quad \text{or} \quad \frac{1}{R}\sqrt{\frac{L}{C}}$$

Now try the following exercise

Exercise 87   Further problems on series resonance and Q-factor

1.   Find the resonant frequency of a series a.c. circuit consisting of a coil of resistance 10 Ω and inductance 50 mH and capacitance 0.05 μF. Find also the current flowing at resonance if the supply voltage is 100 V.

[3.183 kHz, 10 A]

2.   The current at resonance in a series L–C–R circuit is 0.2 mA. If the applied voltage is 250 mV at a frequency of 100 kHz and the circuit capacitance is 0.04 μF, find the circuit resistance and inductance.

[1.25 kΩ, 63.3 μH]

3.   A coil of resistance 25 Ω and inductance 100 mH is connected in series with a capacitance of 0.12 μF across a 200 V, variable frequency supply. Calculate (a) the resonant frequency, (b) the current at resonance, and (c) the factor by which the voltage across the reactance is greater than the supply voltage.

[(a) 1.453 kHz (b) 8 A (c) 36.51]

4.   A coil of 0.5 H inductance and 8 Ω resistance is connected in series with a capacitor across a 200 V, 50 Hz supply. If the current is in phase with the supply voltage, determine the capacitance of the capacitor and the p.d. across its terminals.   [20.26 μF, 3.928 kV]

5.   Calculate the inductance which must be connected in series with a 1000 pF capacitor to give a resonant frequency of 400 kHz.

[0.158 mH]

6.   A series circuit comprises a coil of resistance 20 Ω and inductance 2 mH and a 500 pF capacitor. Determine the Q-factor of the circuit at resonance. If the supply voltage is 1.5 V, what is the voltage across the capacitor?

[100, 150 V]

15.9 Bandwidth and selectivity

Figure 15.22 shows how current I varies with frequency in an $R-L-C$ series circuit. At the resonant frequency f_r, current is a maximum value, shown as I_r. Also shown are the points A and B where the current is 0.707 of the maximum value at frequencies f_1 and f_2. The power delivered to the circuit is I^2R. At $I = 0.707 \, I_r$, the power is $(0.707 \, I_r)^2 R = 0.5 \, I_r^2 R$, i.e. half the power that occurs at frequency f_r. The points corresponding to f_1 and f_2 are called the **half-power points**. The distance between these points, i.e. $(f_2 - f_1)$, is called the **bandwidth**.

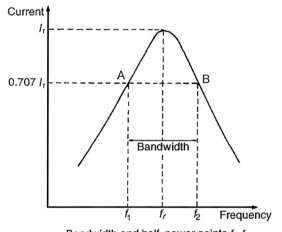

Bandwidth and half-power points f_1, f_2

Figure 15.22

It may be shown that

$$Q = \frac{f_r}{(f_2 - f_1)}$$

or

$$(f_2 - f_1) = \frac{f_r}{Q}$$

Problem 23. A filter in the form of a series $L-R-C$ circuit is designed to operate at a resonant frequency of 5 kHz. Included within the filter is a 20 mH inductance and 10 Ω resistance. Determine the bandwidth of the filter.

Q-factor at resonance is given by:

$$Q_r = \frac{\omega_r L}{R} = \frac{(2\pi \times 5000)(20 \times 10^{-3})}{10}$$

$$= 62.83$$

Since $Q_r = f_r / (f_2 - f_1)$, **bandwidth**,

$$(f_2 - f_1) = \frac{f_r}{Q} = \frac{5000}{62.83} = \textbf{79.6 Hz}$$

Selectivity is the ability of a circuit to respond more readily to signals of a particular frequency to which it is tuned than to signals of other frequencies. The response becomes progressively weaker as the frequency departs from the resonant frequency. The higher the Q-factor, the narrower the bandwidth and the more selective is the circuit. Circuits having high Q-factors (say, in the order of 100 to 300) are therefore useful in communications engineering. A high Q-factor in a series power circuit has disadvantages in that it can lead to dangerously high voltages across the insulation and may result in electrical breakdown.

For a practical laboratory experiment on series a.c. circuits and resonance, see Chapter 24, page 415.

15.10 Power in a.c. circuits

In Figs 15.23(a)–(c), the value of power at any instant is given by the product of the voltage and current at that instant, i.e. the instantaneous power, $p = vi$, as shown by the broken lines.

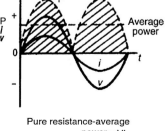

Pure resistance-average power = VI

(a)

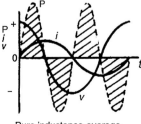

Pure inductance-average power = 0

(b)

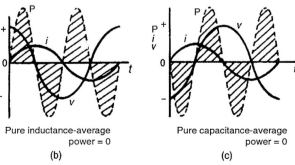

Pure capacitance-average power = 0

(c)

Figure 15.23

Section 2

(a) For a purely resistive a.c. circuit, the average power dissipated, P, is given by: $P = VI = I^2R = V^2/R$ **watts** (V and I being r.m.s. values) See Fig. 15.23(a)

(b) For a purely inductive a.c. circuit, the average power is zero. See Fig. 15.23(b)

(c) For a purely capacitive a.c. circuit, the average power is zero. See Fig. 15.23(c)

Figure 15.24 shows current and voltage waveforms for an R–L circuit where the current lags the voltage by angle ϕ. The waveform for power (where $p = vi$) is shown by the broken line, and its shape, and hence average power, depends on the value of angle ϕ.

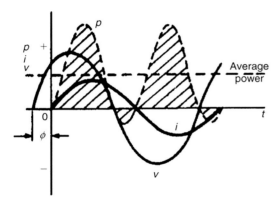

Figure 15.24

For an R–L, R–C or R–L–C series a.c. circuit, the average power P is given by:

$$P = VI\cos\phi \text{ watts}$$

or $\qquad\qquad P = I^2R \text{ watts}$

(V and I being r.m.s. values)

> **Problem 24.** An instantaneous current, $i = 250\sin\omega t$ mA flows through a pure resistance of $5\,\text{k}\Omega$. Find the power dissipated in the resistor.

Power dissipated, $P = I^2R$ where I is the r.m.s. value of current. If $i = 250\sin\omega t$ mA, then $I_m = 0.250$ A and r.m.s. current, $I = (0.707 \times 0.250)$ A. Hence **power** $P = (0.707 \times 0.250)^2(5000) = \textbf{156.2 watts}$.

> **Problem 25.** A series circuit of resistance $60\,\Omega$ and inductance 75 mH is connected to a 110 V, 60 Hz supply. Calculate the power dissipated.

Inductive reactance, $X_L = 2\pi fL$
$$= 2\pi(60)(75 \times 10^{-3})$$
$$= 28.27\,\Omega$$

Impedance, $Z = \sqrt{R^2 + X_L^2}$
$$= \sqrt{60^2 + 28.27^2}$$
$$= 66.33\,\Omega$$

Current, $I = V/Z = 110/66.33 = 1.658$ A.

To calculate power dissipation in an a.c. circuit two formulae may be used:

(i) $P = I^2R = (1.658)^2(60) = \textbf{165 W}$

or

(ii) $P = VI\cos\phi$ where $\cos\phi = \dfrac{R}{Z} = \dfrac{60}{66.33}$
$$= 0.9046$$

Hence $P = (110)(1.658)(0.9046) = \textbf{165 W}$

15.11 Power triangle and power factor

Figure 15.25(a) shows a phasor diagram in which the current I lags the applied voltage V by angle ϕ. The horizontal component of V is $V\cos\phi$ and the vertical component of V is $V\sin\phi$. If each of the voltage phasors is multiplied by I, Fig. 15.25(b) is obtained and is known as the **'power triangle'**.

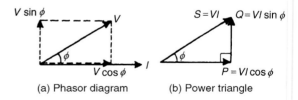

(a) Phasor diagram   (b) Power triangle

Figure 15.25

Apparent power,
$$S = VI \text{ voltamperes (VA)}$$

True or active power,
$$P = VI\cos\phi \text{ watts (W)}$$

Reactive power,
$$Q = VI\sin\phi \text{ reactive}$$
$$\text{voltamperes (var)}$$

$$\text{Power factor} = \frac{\text{True power } P}{\text{Apparent power } S}$$

For sinusoidal voltages and currents,

$$\text{power factor} = \frac{P}{S} = \frac{VI\cos\phi}{VI}$$

i.e. p.f. $= \cos\phi = \dfrac{R}{Z}$ (from Fig. 15.6)

The relationships stated above are also true when current I leads voltage V.

Problem 26. A pure inductance is connected to a 150 V, 50 Hz supply, and the apparent power of the circuit is 300 VA. Find the value of the inductance.

Apparent power $S = VI$.
Hence current $I = S/V = 300/150 = 2$ A.
Inductive reactance $X_L = V/I = 150/2 = 75\,\Omega$.
Since $X_L = 2\pi fL$,

$$\text{inductance } L = \frac{X_L}{2\pi f} = \frac{75}{2\pi(50)} = \mathbf{0.239\,H}$$

Problem 27. A transformer has a rated output of 200 kVA at a power factor of 0.8. Determine the rated power output and the corresponding reactive power.

$VI = 200\,\text{kVA} = 200 \times 10^3$ and p.f. $= 0.8 = \cos\phi$.
Power output, $P = VI\cos\phi = (200 \times 10^3)(0.8)$
$$= \mathbf{160\,kW}.$$
Reactive power, $Q = VI\sin\phi$. If $\cos\phi = 0.8$, then $\phi = \cos^{-1}0.8 = 36.87°$.
Hence $\sin\phi = \sin 36.87° = 0.6$
Hence **reactive power,** $Q = (200 \times 10^3)(0.6)$
$$= \mathbf{120\,kvar}.$$

Problem 28. A load takes 90 kW at a power factor of 0.5 lagging. Calculate the apparent power and the reactive power.

True power $P = 90\,\text{kW} = VI\cos\phi$ and
power factor $= 0.5 = \cos\phi$.

$$\textbf{Apparent power}, S = VI = \frac{P}{\cos\phi} = \frac{90}{0.5} = \mathbf{180\,kVA}$$

Angle $\phi = \cos^{-1}0.5 = 60°$
hence $\sin\phi = \sin 60° = 0.866$
Hence **reactive power,**
$Q = VI\sin\phi = 180 \times 10^3 \times 0.866 = \mathbf{156\,kvar}$.

Problem 29. The power taken by an inductive circuit when connected to a 120 V, 50 Hz supply is 400 W and the current is 8 A. Calculate (a) the resistance, (b) the impedance, (c) the reactance, (d) the power factor, and (e) the phase angle between voltage and current.

(a) Power $P = I^2R$ hence $R = \dfrac{P}{I^2} = \dfrac{400}{8^2} = \mathbf{6.25\,\Omega}$.

(b) Impedance $Z = \dfrac{V}{I} = \dfrac{120}{8} = \mathbf{15\,\Omega}$.

(c) Since $Z = \sqrt{R^2 + X_L^2}$, then
$X_L = \sqrt{Z^2 - R^2} = \sqrt{15^2 - 6.25^2} = \mathbf{13.64\,\Omega}$.

(d) **Power factor** $= \dfrac{\text{true power}}{\text{apparent power}} = \dfrac{VI\cos\phi}{VI}$
$$= \frac{400}{(120)(8)} = \mathbf{0.4167}$$

(e) p.f. $= \cos\phi = 0.4167$ hence
phase angle, $\phi = \cos^{-1}0.4167 = \mathbf{65.37°\ lagging}$.

Problem 30. A circuit consisting of a resistor in series with a capacitor takes 100 watts at a power factor of 0.5 from a 100 V, 60 Hz supply. Find (a) the current flowing, (b) the phase angle, (c) the resistance, (d) the impedance, and (e) the capacitance.

(a) Power factor $= \dfrac{\text{true power}}{\text{apparent power}}$, i.e. $0.5 = \dfrac{100}{100 \times I}$
hence current,

$$I = \frac{100}{(0.5)(100)} = \mathbf{2\,A}$$

(b) Power factor $= 0.5 = \cos\phi$ hence phase angle,
$\phi = \cos^{-1}0.5 = \mathbf{60°\ leading}$

(c) Power $P = I^2R$ hence resistance,

$$R = \frac{P}{I^2} = \frac{100}{2^2} = \mathbf{25\,\Omega}$$

(d) Impedance $Z = \dfrac{V}{I} = \dfrac{100}{2} = \mathbf{50\,\Omega}$

(e) Capacitive reactance, $X_C = \sqrt{Z^2 - R^2}$
$$= \sqrt{50^2 - 25^2} = 43.30\,\Omega.$$

$$X_C = 1/2\pi fC.$$

Hence capacitance $C = \dfrac{1}{2\pi f X_C} = \dfrac{1}{2\pi (60)(43.30)}$ F

$= \mathbf{61.26\,\mu F}$

Now try the following exercises

Exercise 88   Further problems on power in a.c. circuits

1. A voltage $v = 200\sin\omega t$ volts is applied across a pure resistance of $1.5\,\text{k}\Omega$. Find the power dissipated in the resistor.
   [13.33 W]

2. A $50\,\mu\text{F}$ capacitor is connected to a 100 V, 200 Hz supply. Determine the true power and the apparent power.   [0, 628.3 VA]

3. A motor takes a current of 10 A when supplied from a 250 V a.c. supply. Assuming a power factor of 0.75 lagging find the power consumed. Find also the cost of running the motor for 1 week continuously if 1 kWh of electricity costs 12.20 p.
   [1875 W, £38.43]

4. A motor takes a current of 12 A when supplied from a 240 V a.c. supply. Assuming a power factor of 0.70 lagging, find the power consumed.   [2.016 kW]

5. A transformer has a rated output of 100 kVA at a power factor of 0.6. Determine the rated power output and the corresponding reactive power.   [60 kW, 80 kvar]

6. A substation is supplying 200 kVA and 150 kvar. Calculate the corresponding power and power factor.   [132 kW, 0.66]

7. A load takes 50 kW at a power factor of 0.8 lagging. Calculate the apparent power and the reactive power.   [62.5 kVA, 37.5 kvar]

8. A coil of resistance $400\,\Omega$ and inductance 0.20 H is connected to a 75 V, 400 Hz supply. Calculate the power dissipated in the coil.
   [5.452 W]

9. An $80\,\Omega$ resistor and a $6\,\mu\text{F}$ capacitor are connected in series across a 150 V, 200 Hz supply. Calculate (a) the circuit impedance, (b) the current flowing, and (c) the power dissipated in the circuit.
   [(a) $154.9\,\Omega$ (b) 0.968 A (c) 75 W]

10. The power taken by a series circuit containing resistance and inductance is 240 W when connected to a 200 V, 50 Hz supply. If the current flowing is 2 A find the values of the resistance and inductance.   [$60\,\Omega$, 255 mH]

11. The power taken by a C–R series circuit, when connected to a 105 V, 2.5 kHz supply, is 0.9 kW and the current is 15 A. Calculate (a) the resistance, (b) the impedance, (c) the reactance, (d) the capacitance, (e) the power factor, and (f) the phase angle between voltage and current.
    [(a) $4\,\Omega$ (b) $7\,\Omega$ (c) $5.745\,\Omega$ (d) $11.08\,\mu\text{F}$ (e) 0.571 (f) 55.18° leading]

12. A circuit consisting of a resistor in series with an inductance takes 210 W at a power factor of 0.6 from a 50 V, 100 Hz supply. Find (a) the current flowing, (b) the circuit phase angle, (c) the resistance, (d) the impedance, and (e) the inductance.
    [(a) 7 A (b) 53.13° lagging (c) $4.286\,\Omega$ (d) $7.143\,\Omega$ (e) 9.095 mH]

13. A 200 V, 60 Hz supply is applied to a capacitive circuit. The current flowing is 2 A and the power dissipated is 150 W. Calculate the values of the resistance and capacitance.
    [$37.5\,\Omega$, $28.61\,\mu\text{F}$]

Exercise 89   Short answer questions on single-phase a.c. circuits

1. Complete the following statements:
   (a) In a purely resistive a.c. circuit the current is …… with the voltage
   (b) In a purely inductive a.c. circuit the current …… the voltage by …… degrees
   (c) In a purely capacitive a.c. circuit the current …… the voltage by …… degrees

2. Draw phasor diagrams to represent (a) a purely resistive a.c. circuit (b) a purely inductive a.c. circuit (c) a purely capacitive a.c. circuit

3. What is inductive reactance? State the symbol and formula for determining inductive reactance

4. What is capacitive reactance? State the symbol and formula for determining capacitive reactance

5. Draw phasor diagrams to represent (a) a coil (having both inductance and resistance), and (b) a series capacitive circuit containing resistance

6. What does 'impedance' mean when referring to an a.c. circuit?

7. Draw an impedance triangle for an R–L circuit. Derive from the triangle an expression for (a) impedance, and (b) phase angle

8. Draw an impedance triangle for an R–C circuit. From the triangle derive an expression for (a) impedance, and (b) phase angle

9. What is series resonance?

10. Derive a formula for resonant frequency f_r in terms of L and C

11. What does the Q-factor in a series circuit mean?

12. State three formulae used to calculate the Q-factor of a series circuit at resonance

13. State an advantage of a high Q-factor in a series high-frequency circuit

14. State a disadvantage of a high Q-factor in a series power circuit

15. State two formulae which may be used to calculate power in an a.c. circuit

16. Show graphically that for a purely inductive or purely capacitive a.c. circuit the average power is zero

17. Define 'power factor'

18. Define (a) apparent power (b) reactive power

19. Define (a) bandwidth (b) selectivity

Exercise 90   Multi-choice questions on single-phase a.c. circuits
(Answers on page 420)

1. An inductance of 10 mH connected across a 100 V, 50 Hz supply has an inductive reactance of
   (a) $10\pi\ \Omega$ (b) $1000\pi\ \Omega$
   (c) $\pi\ \Omega$ (d) $\pi\ H$

2. When the frequency of an a.c. circuit containing resistance and inductance is increased, the current
   (a) decreases   (b) increases
   (c) stays the same

3. In question 2, the phase angle of the circuit
   (a) decreases   (b) increases
   (c) stays the same

4. When the frequency of an a.c. circuit containing resistance and capacitance is decreased, the current
   (a) decreases   (b) increases
   (c) stays the same

5. In question 4, the phase angle of the circuit
   (a) decreases   (b) increases
   (c) stays the same

6. A capacitor of $1\,\mu F$ is connected to a 50 Hz supply. The capacitive reactance is
   (a) $50\,M\Omega$ (b) $\dfrac{10}{\pi}\,k\Omega$
   (c) $\dfrac{\pi}{10^4}\,\Omega$ (d) $\dfrac{10}{\pi}\,\Omega$

7. In a series a.c. circuit the voltage across a pure inductance is 12 V and the voltage across a pure resistance is 5 V. The supply voltage is
   (a) 13 V   (b) 17 V
   (c) 7 V   (d) 2.4 V

8. Inductive reactance results in a current that
   (a) leads the voltage by 90°
   (b) is in phase with the voltage
   (c) leads the voltage by π rad
   (d) lags the voltage by $\pi/2$ rad

9. Which of the following statements is false?
   (a) Impedance is at a minimum at resonance in an a.c. circuit
   (b) The product of r.m.s. current and voltage gives the apparent power in an a.c. circuit
   (c) Current is at a maximum at resonance in an a.c. circuit
   (d) $\dfrac{\text{Apparent power}}{\text{True power}}$ gives power factor

10. The impedance of a coil, which has a resistance of X ohms and an inductance of Y henrys, connected across a supply of frequency K Hz, is

(a) $2\pi KY$ (b) $X+Y$

(c) $\sqrt{X^2+Y^2}$ (d) $\sqrt{X^2+(2\pi KY)^2}$

11. In question 10, the phase angle between the current and the applied voltage is given by

    (a) $\tan^{-1}\dfrac{Y}{X}$ (b) $\tan^{-1}\dfrac{2\pi KY}{X}$

    (c) $\tan^{-1}\dfrac{X}{2\pi KY}$ (d) $\tan\left(\dfrac{2\pi KY}{X}\right)$

12. When a capacitor is connected to an a.c. supply the current
    (a) leads the voltage by $180°$
    (b) is in phase with the voltage
    (c) leads the voltage by $\pi/2$ rad
    (d) lags the voltage by $90°$

13. When the frequency of an a.c. circuit containing resistance and capacitance is increased the impedance
    (a) increases   (b) decreases
    (c) stays the same

14. In an $R–L–C$ series a.c. circuit a current of $5\,A$ flows when the supply voltage is $100\,V$. The phase angle between current and voltage is $60°$ lagging. Which of the following statements is false?
    (a) The circuit is effectively inductive
    (b) The apparent power is $500\,VA$
    (c) The equivalent circuit reactance is $20\,\Omega$
    (d) The true power is $250\,W$

15. A series a.c. circuit comprising a coil of inductance $100\,mH$ and resistance $1\,\Omega$ and a $10\,\mu F$ capacitor is connected across a $10\,V$ supply. At resonance the p.d. across the capacitor is
    (a) $10\,kV$ (b) $1\,kV$
    (c) $100\,V$ (d) $10\,V$

16. The amplitude of the current I flowing in the circuit of Fig. 15.26 is:
    (a) $21\,A$ (b) $16.8\,A$
    (c) $28\,A$ (d) $12\,A$

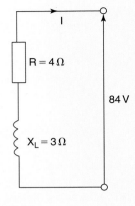

Figure 15.26

17. If the supply frequency is increased at resonance in a series $R–L–C$ circuit and the values of L, C and R are constant, the circuit will become:
    (a) capacitive   (b) resistive
    (c) inductive   (d) resonant

18. For the circuit shown in Fig. 15.27, the value of Q-factor is:
    (a) 50 (b) 100
    (c) 5×10^{-4} (d) 40

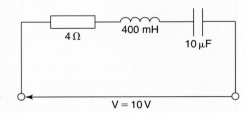

Figure 15.27

19. A series $R–L–C$ circuit has a resistance of $8\,\Omega$, an inductance of $100\,mH$ and a capacitance of $5\,\mu F$. If the current flowing is $2\,A$, the impedance at resonance is:
    (a) $160\,\Omega$ (b) $16\,\Omega$
    (c) $8\,m\Omega$ (d) $8\,\Omega$

Chapter 16

Single-phase parallel a.c. circuits

At the end of this chapter you should be able to:

- calculate unknown currents, impedances and circuit phase angle from phasor diagrams for (a) R–L (b) R–C (c) L–C (d) LR–C parallel a.c. circuits
- state the condition for parallel resonance in an LR–C circuit
- derive the resonant frequency equation for an LR–C parallel a.c. circuit
- determine the current and dynamic resistance at resonance in an LR–C parallel circuit
- understand and calculate Q-factor in an LR–C parallel circuit
- understand how power factor may be improved

16.1 Introduction

In parallel circuits, such as those shown in Figs 16.1 and 16.2, the voltage is common to each branch of the network and is thus taken as the reference phasor when drawing phasor diagrams.

For any parallel a.c. circuit:

True or active power, $P = VI \cos\phi$ watts (W)

or $P = I_R^2 R$ watts

Apparent power, $S = VI$ voltamperes (VA)

Reactive power, $Q = VI \sin\phi$ reactive voltamperes (var)

$$\text{Power factor} = \frac{\text{true power}}{\text{apparent power}} = \frac{P}{S} = \cos\phi$$

(These formulae are the same as for series a.c. circuits as used in Chapter 15.)

16.2 R–L parallel a.c. circuit

In the two branch parallel circuit containing resistance R and inductance L shown in Fig. 16.1, the current flowing in the resistance, I_R, is in-phase with the supply voltage V and the current flowing in the inductance, I_L, lags the supply voltage by 90°. The supply current I is the phasor sum of I_R and I_L and thus the current I lags the applied voltage V by an angle lying between 0° and 90° (depending on the values of I_R and I_L), shown as angle ϕ in the phasor diagram.

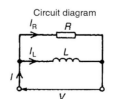
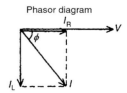

Figure 16.1

DOI: 10.1016/B978-0-08-089056-2.00016-4

From the phasor diagram: $I = \sqrt{I_R^2 + I_L^2}$ (by Pythagoras' theorem) where

$$I_R = \frac{V}{R} \quad \text{and} \quad I_L = \frac{V}{X_L}$$

$$\tan\phi = \frac{I_L}{I_R} \quad \sin\phi = \frac{I_L}{I} \quad \text{and} \quad \cos\phi = \frac{I_R}{I}$$

(by trigonometric ratios)

$$\text{Circuit impedance, } Z = \frac{V}{I}$$

Problem 1. A 20 Ω resistor is connected in parallel with an inductance of 2.387 mH across a 60 V, 1 kHz supply. Calculate (a) the current in each branch, (b) the supply current, (c) the circuit phase angle, (d) the circuit impedance, and (e) the power consumed.

The circuit and phasor diagrams are as shown in Fig. 16.1

(a) Current flowing in the resistor,

$$I_R = \frac{V}{R} = \frac{60}{20} = 3\,\text{A}$$

Current flowing in the inductance,

$$I_L = \frac{V}{X_L} = \frac{V}{2\pi f L}$$

$$= \frac{60}{2\pi(1000)(2.387 \times 10^{-3})} = 4\,\text{A}$$

(b) From the phasor diagram, supply current,

$$I = \sqrt{I_R^2 + I_L^2} = \sqrt{3^2 + 4^2} = 5\,\text{A}$$

(c) Circuit phase angle,

$$\phi = \tan^{-1}\frac{I_L}{I_R} = \tan^{-1}\frac{4}{3} = 53.13°\,\text{lagging}$$

(d) Circuit impedance,

$$Z = \frac{V}{I} = \frac{60}{5} = 12\,\Omega$$

(e) Power consumed

$$P = VI\cos\phi = (60)(5)(\cos 53.13°)$$

$$= 180\,\text{W}$$

(Alternatively, power consumed, $P = I_R^2 R = (3)^2(20) = 180\,\text{W}$)

Now try the following exercise

Exercise 91 Further problems on R–L parallel a.c. circuits

1. A 30 Ω resistor is connected in parallel with a pure inductance of 3 mH across a 110 V, 2 kHz supply. Calculate (a) the current in each branch, (b) the circuit current, (c) the circuit phase angle, (d) the circuit impedance, (e) the power consumed, and (f) the circuit power factor.

   [(a) $I_R = 3.67$ A, $I_L = 2.92$ A (b) 4.69 A
   (c) 38.51° lagging (d) 23.45 Ω
   (e) 404 W (f) 0.782 lagging]

2. A 40 Ω resistance is connected in parallel with a coil of inductance L and negligible resistance across a 200 V, 50 Hz supply and the supply current is found to be 8 A. Sketch the phasor diagram and determine the inductance of the coil.   [102 mH]

16.3 R–C parallel a.c. circuit

In the two branch parallel circuit containing resistance R and capacitance C shown in Fig. 16.2, I_R is in-phase with the supply voltage V and the current flowing in the capacitor, I_C, leads V by 90°. The supply current I is the phasor sum of I_R and I_C and thus the current I leads the applied voltage V by an angle lying between 0° and 90° (depending on the values of I_R and I_C), shown as angle α in the phasor diagram.

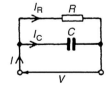 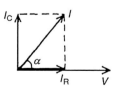

Figure 16.2

From the phasor diagram: $I = \sqrt{I_R^2 + I_C^2}$ (by Pythagoras' theorem) where

$$I_R = \frac{V}{R} \quad \text{and} \quad I_C = \frac{V}{X_C}$$

$$\tan\alpha = \frac{I_C}{I_R} \quad \sin\alpha = \frac{I_C}{I} \quad \text{and} \quad \cos\alpha = \frac{I_R}{I}$$

(by trigonometric ratios)

$$\text{Circuit impedance, } Z = \frac{V}{I}$$

Problem 2. A 30 μF capacitor is connected in parallel with an 80 Ω resistor across a 240 V, 50 Hz supply. Calculate (a) the current in each branch, (b) the supply current, (c) the circuit phase angle, (d) the circuit impedance, (e) the power dissipated, and (f) the apparent power.

The circuit and phasor diagrams are as shown in Fig. 16.2

(a) Current in resistor,

$$I_R = \frac{V}{R} = \frac{240}{80} = 3\,\text{A}$$

Current in capacitor,

$$I_C = \frac{V}{X_C} = \frac{V}{\left(\dfrac{1}{2\pi f C}\right)} = 2\pi f C V$$

$$= 2\pi(50)(30 \times 10^6)(240) = \mathbf{2.262\,A}$$

(b) Supply current,

$$I = \sqrt{I_R^2 + I_C^2} = \sqrt{3^2 + 2.262^2}$$

$$= \mathbf{3.757\,A}$$

(c) Circuit phase angle,

$$\alpha = \tan^{-1}\frac{I_C}{I_R} = \tan^{-1}\frac{2.262}{3}$$

$$= \mathbf{37.02°\ leading}$$

(d) Circuit impedance,

$$Z = \frac{V}{I} = \frac{240}{3.757} = \mathbf{63.88\,\Omega}$$

(e) True or active power dissipated,

$$P = VI\cos\alpha = (240)(3.757)\cos 37.02°$$

$$= \mathbf{720\,W}$$

(Alternatively, true power

$$P = I_R^2 R = (3)^2(80) = 720\,\text{W})$$

(f) Apparent power,

$$S = VI = (240)(3.757) = \mathbf{901.7\,VA}$$

Problem 3. A capacitor C is connected in parallel with a resistor R across a 120 V, 200 Hz supply. The supply current is 2 A at a power factor of 0.6 leading. Determine the values of C and R.

The circuit diagram is shown in Fig. 16.3(a).

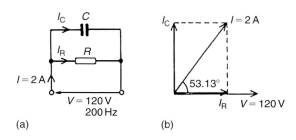

(a)   (b)

Figure 16.3

Power factor $= \cos\phi = 0.6$ leading, hence

$$\phi = \cos^{-1}0.6 = 53.13°\ \text{leading}.$$

From the phasor diagram shown in Fig. 16.3(b),

$$I_R = I\cos 53.13° = (2)(0.6)$$

$$= \mathbf{1.2\,A}$$

and $\quad I_C = I\sin 53.13° = (2)(0.8)$

$$= \mathbf{1.6\,A}$$

(Alternatively, I_R and I_C can be measured from the scaled phasor diagram.)
From the circuit diagram,

$$I_R = \frac{V}{R} \text{ from which}$$

$$R = \frac{V}{I_R}$$

$$= \frac{120}{1.2} = \mathbf{100\,\Omega}$$

and $\quad I_C = \dfrac{V}{X_C}$

$$= 2\pi f C V \text{ from which}$$

$$C = \frac{I_C}{2\pi f V}$$

$$= \frac{1.6}{2\pi(200)(120)}$$

$$= \mathbf{10.61\,\mu F}$$

Now try the following exercise

Exercise 92   Further problems on R–C parallel a.c. circuits

1. A 1500 nF capacitor is connected in parallel with a 16 Ω resistor across a 10 V, 10 kHz supply. Calculate (a) the current in each branch, (b) the supply current, (c) the circuit phase angle, (d) the circuit impedance, (e) the power consumed, (f) the apparent power, and (g) the circuit power factor. Sketch the phasor diagram.
    [(a) $I_R = 0.625$ A, $I_C = 0.943$ A (b) 1.131 A
    (c) 56.46° leading (d) 8.84 Ω (e) 6.25 W
    (f) 11.31 VA (g) 0.553 leading]

2. A capacitor C is connected in parallel with a resistance R across a 60 V, 100 Hz supply. The supply current is 0.6 A at a power factor of 0.8 leading. Calculate the value of R and C.
    [$R = 125$ Ω, $C = 9.55$ μF]

16.4 L–C parallel circuit

In the two branch parallel circuit containing inductance L and capacitance C shown in Fig. 16.4, I_L lags V by 90° and I_C leads V by 90°

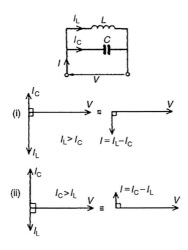

Figure 16.4

Theoretically there are three phasor diagrams possible – each depending on the relative values of I_L and I_C:

(i) $I_L > I_C$ (giving a supply current, $I = I_L - I_C$ lagging V by 90°)

(ii) $I_C > I_L$ (giving a supply current, $I = I_C - I_L$ leading V by 90°)

(iii) $I_L = I_C$ (giving a supply current, $I = 0$).

The latter condition is not possible in practice due to circuit resistance inevitably being present (as in the circuit described in Section 16.5).

For the L–C parallel circuit,

$$I_L = \frac{V}{X_L} \quad I_C = \frac{V}{X_C}$$

$I =$ **phasor difference between I_L and I_C, and**

$$Z = \frac{V}{I}$$

Problem 4.   A pure inductance of 120 mH is connected in parallel with a 25 μF capacitor and the network is connected to a 100 V, 50 Hz supply. Determine (a) the branch currents, (b) the supply current and its phase angle, (c) the circuit impedance, and (d) the power consumed.

The circuit and phasor diagrams are as shown in Fig. 16.4

(a)   Inductive reactance,

$$X_L = 2\pi fL = 2\pi(50)(120 \times 10^{-3})$$

$$= 37.70 \, \Omega$$

Capacitive reactance,

$$X_C = \frac{1}{2\pi fC} = \frac{1}{2\pi(50)(25 \times 10^{-6})}$$

$$= 127.3 \, \Omega$$

Current flowing in inductance,

$$I_L = \frac{V}{X_L} = \frac{100}{37.70} = \mathbf{2.653 \, A}$$

Current flowing in capacitor,

$$I_C = \frac{V}{X_C} = \frac{100}{127.3} = \mathbf{0.786 \, A}$$

(b) I_L and I_C are anti-phase, hence supply current,

$$I = I_L - I_C = 2.653 - 0.786 = \mathbf{1.867 \, A}$$

and **the current lags the supply voltage V by 90°** (see Fig. 16.4(i))

(c)   Circuit impedance,

$$Z = \frac{V}{I} = \frac{100}{1.867} = \mathbf{53.56\,\Omega}$$

(d)   Power consumed,

$$P = VI\cos\phi = (100)(1.867)\cos 90° = \mathbf{0\,W}$$

Problem 5.   Repeat Problem 4 for the condition when the frequency is changed to 150 Hz.

(a)   Inductive reactance,

$$X_L = 2\pi(150)(120 \times 10^{-3}) = 113.1\,\Omega$$

Capacitive reactance,

$$X_C = \frac{1}{2\pi(150)(25 \times 10^{-6})} = 42.44\,\Omega$$

Current flowing in inductance,

$$I_L = \frac{V}{X_L} = \frac{100}{113.1} = \mathbf{0.884\,A}$$

Current flowing in capacitor,

$$I_C = \frac{V}{X_C} = \frac{100}{42.44} = \mathbf{2.356\,A}$$

(b)   Supply current,

$$I = I_C - I_L = 2.356 - 0.884 = \mathbf{1.472\,A}$$

leading V by 90° (see Fig. 16.4(ii))

(c)   Circuit impedance,

$$Z = \frac{V}{I} = \frac{100}{1.472} = \mathbf{67.93\,\Omega}$$

(d)   Power consumed,

$$P = VI\cos\phi = \mathbf{0\,W} \text{ (since } \phi = 90°)$$

From problems 4 and 5:

(i)   When $X_L < X_C$ then $I_L > I_C$ and I lags V by 90°

(ii)   When $X_L > X_C$ then $I_L < I_C$ and I leads V by 90°

(iii)   In a parallel circuit containing no resistance the power consumed is zero

Now try the following exercise

1.   An inductance of 80 mH is connected in parallel with a capacitance of 10 μF across a 60 V, 100 Hz supply. Determine (a) the branch currents, (b) the supply current, (c) the circuit phase angle, (d) the circuit impedance, and (e) the power consumed.
   [(a) $I_C = 0.377$ A, $I_L = 1.194$ A (b) 0.817 A (c) 90° lagging (d) 73.44 Ω (e) 0 W]

2.   Repeat Problem 1 for a supply frequency of 200 Hz.
   [(a) $I_C = 0.754$ A, $I_L = 0.597$ A (b) 0.157 A (c) 90° leading (d) 382.2 Ω (e) 0 W]

16.5   *LR–C* parallel a.c. circuit

In the two branch circuit containing capacitance C in parallel with inductance L and resistance R in series (such as a coil) shown in Fig. 16.5(a), the phasor diagram for the LR branch alone is shown in Fig. 16.5(b) and the phasor diagram for the C branch is shown alone in Fig. 16.5(c). Rotating each and superimposing on one another gives the complete phasor diagram shown in Fig. 16.5(d).

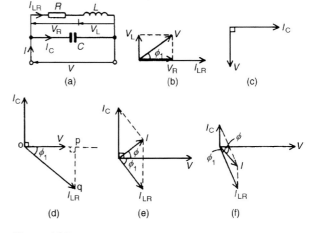

Figure 16.5

The current I_{LR} of Fig. 16.5(d) may be resolved into horizontal and vertical components. The horizontal component, shown as op is $I_{LR}\cos\phi_1$ and the vertical component, shown as pq is $I_{LR} \sin\phi_1$. There are three possible conditions for this circuit:

(i) $I_C > I_{LR} \sin\phi_1$ (giving a supply current I leading V by angle ϕ – as shown in Fig. 16.5(e))

(ii) $I_{LR} \sin\phi > I_C$ (giving I lagging V by angle ϕ – as shown in Fig. 16.5(f))

(iii) $I_C = I_{LR} \sin\phi_1$ (this is called **parallel resonance**, see Section 16.6)

There are two methods of finding the phasor sum of currents I_{LR} and I_C in Fig. 16.5(e) and (f). These are: (i) by a scaled phasor diagram, or (ii) by resolving each current into their 'in-phase' (i.e. horizontal) and 'quadrature' (i.e. vertical) **components**, as demonstrated in problems 6 and 7. With reference to the phasor diagrams of Fig. 16.5:

Impedance of LR branch, $Z_{LR} = \sqrt{R^2 + X_L^2}$

Current, $I_{LR} = \dfrac{V}{Z_{LR}}$ and $I_C = \dfrac{V}{X_C}$

Supply current

$I =$ **phasor sum of I_{LR} and I_C (by drawing)**

$$= \sqrt{(I_{LR}\cos\phi_1)^2 + (I_{LR}\sin\phi_1 \sim I_C)^2}$$

(by calculation)

where $\sim$ means 'the difference between'.

$$\text{Circuit impedance } Z = \frac{V}{I}$$

$$\tan\phi_1 = \frac{V_L}{V_R} = \frac{X_L}{R}$$

$$\sin\phi_1 = \frac{X_L}{Z_{LR}} \quad \text{and} \quad \cos\phi_1 = \frac{R}{Z_{LR}}$$

$$\tan\phi = \frac{I_{LR}\sin\phi_1 \sim I_C}{I_{LR}\cos\phi_1} \quad \text{and} \quad \cos\phi = \frac{I_{LR}\cos\phi_1}{I}$$

Problem 6. A coil of inductance 159.2 mH and resistance $40\,\Omega$ is connected in parallel with a $30\,\mu$F capacitor across a 240 V, 50 Hz supply. Calculate (a) the current in the coil and its phase angle, (b) the current in the capacitor and its phase angle, (c) the supply current and its phase angle, (d) the circuit impedance, (e) the power consumed, (f) the apparent power, and (g) the reactive power. Draw the phasor diagram.

The circuit diagram is shown in Fig. 16.6(a).

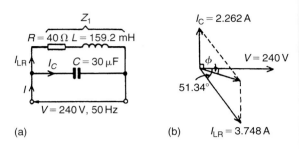

(a)   (b)

Figure 16.6

(a) For the coil, inductive reactance $X_L = 2\pi f L = 2\pi(50)(159.2 \times 10^{-3}) = 50\,\Omega$.

$$\text{Impedance } Z_1 = \sqrt{R^2 + X_L^2}$$
$$= \sqrt{40^2 + 50^2}$$
$$= 64.03\,\Omega$$

Current in coil

$$I_{LR} = \frac{V}{Z_1} = \frac{240}{64.03} = \textbf{3.748\,A}$$

Branch phase angle

$$\phi_1 = \tan^{-1}\frac{X_L}{R} = \tan^{-1}\frac{50}{40}$$
$$= \tan^{-1}1.25 = \textbf{51.34}° \textbf{ lagging}$$

(see phasor diagram in Fig. 16.6(b))

(b) Capacitive reactance,

$$X_C = \frac{1}{2\pi f C} = \frac{1}{2\pi(50)(30 \times 10^{-6})}$$
$$= 106.1\,\Omega$$

Current in capacitor,

$$I_C = \frac{V}{X_C} = \frac{240}{106.1}$$
$$= \textbf{2.262\,A leading the supply}$$
$$\textbf{voltage by 90}°$$

(see phasor diagram of Fig. 16.6(b)).

(c) The supply current I is the phasor sum of I_{LR} and I_C. This may be obtained by drawing the phasor diagram to scale and measuring the current I and its phase angle relative to V. (Current I will always be the diagonal of the parallelogram formed as in Fig. 16.6(b).)

Alternatively the current I_{LR} and I_C may be resolved into their horizontal (or 'in-phase') and vertical (or 'quadrature') components.

The horizontal component of I_{LR} is:

$$I_{LR}\cos 51.34° = 3.748\cos 51.34° = 2.341\,A.$$

The horizontal component of I_C is

$$I_C\cos 90° = 0$$

Thus the total horizontal component,

$$I_H = \mathbf{2.341\,A}$$

The vertical component of I_{LR}

$$= -I_{LR}\sin 51.34° = -3.748\sin 51.34°$$
$$= -2.927\,A$$

The vertical component of I_C

$$= I_C\sin 90° = 2.262\sin 90° = 2.262\,A$$

Thus the total vertical component,

$$I_V = -2.927 + 2.262 = \mathbf{-0.665\,A}$$

I_H and I_V are shown in Fig. 16.7, from which,

$$I = \sqrt{2.341^2 + (-0.665)^2} = 2.434\,A$$

$$\text{Angle } \phi = \tan^{-1}\frac{0.665}{2.341} = 15.86° \text{ lagging}$$

Hence **the supply current $I = 2.434\,A$ lagging V by 15.86°**

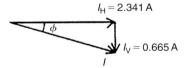

Figure 16.7

(d) Circuit impedance,

$$Z = \frac{V}{I} = \frac{240}{2.434} = \mathbf{98.60\,\Omega}$$

(e) Power consumed,

$$P = VI\cos\phi = (240)(2.434)\cos 15.86°$$
$$= \mathbf{562\,W}$$

(Alternatively, $P = I_R^2 R = I_{LR}^2 R$ (in this case)

$$= (3.748)^2(40) = \mathbf{562\,W})$$

(f) Apparent power,

$$S = VI = (240)(2.434) = \mathbf{584.2\,VA}$$

(g) Reactive power,

$$Q = VI\sin\phi = (240)(2.434)(\sin 15.86°)$$
$$= \mathbf{159.6\,var}$$

Problem 7. A coil of inductance 0.12 H and resistance 3 kΩ is connected in parallel with a 0.02 μF capacitor and is supplied at 40 V at a frequency of 5 kHz. Determine (a) the current in the coil, and (b) the current in the capacitor. (c) Draw to scale the phasor diagram and measure the supply current and its phase angle; check the answer by calculation. Determine (d) the circuit impedance and (e) the power consumed.

The circuit diagram is shown in Fig. 16.8(a).

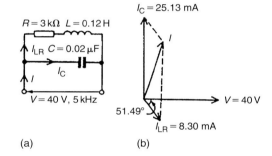

Figure 16.8

(a) Inductive reactance,

$$X_L = 2\pi f L = 2\pi(5000)(0.12) = 3770\,\Omega$$

Impedance of coil,

$$Z_1 = \sqrt{R^2 + X_L} = \sqrt{3000^2 + 3770^2}$$
$$= 4818\,\Omega$$

Current in coil,

$$I_{LR} = \frac{V}{Z_1} = \frac{40}{4818} = \mathbf{8.30\,mA}$$

Branch phase angle

$$\phi = \tan^{-1}\frac{X_L}{R} = \tan^{-1}\frac{3770}{3000}$$
$$= \mathbf{51.49° \text{ lagging}}$$

(b) Capacitive reactance,

$$X_C = \frac{1}{2\pi f C} = \frac{1}{2\pi(5000)(0.02 \times 10^{-6})}$$

$$= 1592\,\Omega$$

Capacitor current,

$$I_C = \frac{V}{X_C} = \frac{40}{1592}$$

$$= 25.13\,\text{mA leading } V \text{ by } 90°$$

(c) Currents I_{LR} and I_C are shown in the phasor diagram of Fig. 16.8(b). The parallelogram is completed as shown and the supply current is given by the diagonal of the parallelogram. The current I is measured as **19.3 mA** leading voltage V by **74.5°**. By calculation,

$$I = \sqrt{(I_{LR}\cos 51.49°)^2 + (I_C - I_{LR}\sin 51.49°)^2}$$

$$= 19.34\,\text{mA}$$

and

$$\phi = \tan^{-1}\left(\frac{I_C - I_{LR}\sin 51.5°}{I_{LR}\cos 51.5°}\right) = 74.50°$$

(d) Circuit impedance,

$$Z = \frac{V}{I} = \frac{40}{19.34 \times 10^{-3}} = 2.068\,\text{k}\Omega$$

(e) Power consumed,

$$P = VI\cos\phi$$

$$= (40)(19.34 \times 10^{-3})\cos 74.50°$$

$$= 206.7\,\text{mW}$$

(Alternatively, $P = I_R^2 R$

$$= I_{LR}^2 R$$

$$= (8.30 \times 10^{-3})^2 (3000)$$

$$= 206.7\,\text{mW})$$

Now try the following exercise

Exercise 94 Further problems on *LR–C* parallel a.c. circuit

1. A coil of resistance $60\,\Omega$ and inductance $318.4\,\text{mH}$ is connected in parallel with a $15\,\mu\text{F}$ capacitor across a $200\,\text{V}$, $50\,\text{Hz}$ supply. Calculate (a) the current in the coil, (b) the current in the capacitor, (c) the supply current and its phase angle, (d) the circuit impedance, (e) the power consumed, (f) the apparent power, and (g) the reactive power. Sketch the phasor diagram.
   [(a) 1.715 A (b) 0.943 A (c) 1.028 A at 30.88° lagging (d) 194.6 Ω (e) 176.5 W (f) 205.6 VA (g) 105.5 var]

2. A 25 nF capacitor is connected in parallel with a coil of resistance $2\,\text{k}\Omega$ and inductance $0.20\,\text{H}$ across a $100\,\text{V}$, $4\,\text{kHz}$ supply. Determine (a) the current in the coil, (b) the current in the capacitor, (c) the supply current and its phase angle (by drawing a phasor diagram to scale, and also by calculation), (d) the circuit impedance, and (e) the power consumed.
   [(a) 18.48 mA (b) 62.83 mA (c) 46.17 mA at 81.49° leading (d) 2.166 kΩ (e) 0.683 W]

16.6 Parallel resonance and Q-factor

Parallel resonance

Resonance occurs in the two branch network containing capacitance C in parallel with inductance L and resistance R in series (see Fig. 16.5(a)) when the quadrature (i.e. vertical) component of current I_{LR} is equal to I_C. At this condition the supply current I is in-phase with the supply voltage V.

Resonant frequency

When the quadrature component of I_{LR} is equal to I_C then: $I_C = I_{LR}\sin\phi_1$ (see Fig. 16.9). Hence

$$\frac{V}{X_C} = \left(\frac{V}{Z_{LR}}\right)\left(\frac{X_L}{Z_{LR}}\right) \quad \text{(from Section 16.5)}$$

from which,

$$Z_{LR}^2 = X_L X_C = (2\pi f_r L)\left(\frac{1}{2\pi f_r C}\right) = \frac{L}{C} \quad (1)$$

Hence

$$\left[\sqrt{R^2 + X_L^2}\right]^2 = \frac{L}{C} \quad \text{and} \quad R^2 + X_L^2 = \frac{L}{C}$$

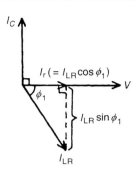

Figure 16.9

Thus $\quad (2\pi f_r L)^2 = \dfrac{L}{C} - R^2$ and

$$2\pi f_r L = \sqrt{\dfrac{L}{C} - R^2}$$

and $\qquad f_r = \dfrac{1}{2\pi L}\sqrt{\dfrac{L}{C} - R^2}$

$$= \dfrac{1}{2\pi}\sqrt{\dfrac{L}{L^2 C} - \dfrac{R^2}{L^2}}$$

i.e. parallel resonant frequency,

$$f_r = \dfrac{1}{2\pi}\sqrt{\dfrac{1}{LC} - \dfrac{R^2}{L^2}}$$

(When R is negligible, then $f_r = \dfrac{1}{2\pi\sqrt{LC}}$, which is the same as for series resonance)

Current at resonance

Current at resonance,

$$I_r = I_{LR}\cos\phi_1 \quad \text{(from Fig. 16.9)}$$

$$= \left(\dfrac{V}{Z_{LR}}\right)\left(\dfrac{R}{Z_{LR}}\right) \quad \text{(from Section 16.5)}$$

$$= \dfrac{V R}{Z_{LR}^2}$$

However, from equation (1), $Z_{LR}^2 = L/C$ hence

$$I_r = \dfrac{VR}{(L/C)} = \dfrac{VRC}{L} \qquad (2)$$

The current is at a **minimum** at resonance.

Dynamic resistance

Since the current at resonance is in-phase with the voltage the impedance of the circuit acts as a resistance. This resistance is known as the **dynamic resistance**, R_D (or sometimes, the dynamic impedance).

From equation (2), impedance at resonance

$$= \dfrac{V}{I_r} = \dfrac{V}{\left(\dfrac{VRC}{L}\right)}$$

$$= \dfrac{L}{RC}$$

i.e. dynamic resistance,

$$R_D = \dfrac{L}{RC}\ \text{ohms}$$

Graphs of current and impedance against frequency near to resonance for a parallel circuit are shown in Fig. 16.10, and are seen to be the reverse of those in a series circuit (from page 238).

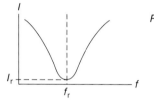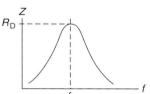

Figure 16.10

Rejector circuit

The parallel resonant circuit is often described as a **rejector** circuit since it presents its maximum impedance at the resonant frequency and the resultant current is a minimum.

Mechanical analogy

Electrical resonance for the parallel circuit can be likened to a mass hanging on a spring which, if pulled down and released, will oscillate up and down but due to friction the oscillations will slowly die. To maintain the oscillation the mass would require a small force applied each time it reaches its point of maximum travel and this is exactly what happens with the electrical circuit. A small current is required to overcome the losses and maintain the oscillations of current. Figure 16.11 shows the two cases.

Section 2

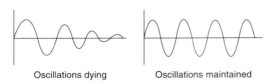

Oscillations dying   Oscillations maintained

Figure 16.11

Applications of resonance

One use for resonance is to establish a condition of **stable frequency** in circuits designed to produce a.c. signals. Usually, a parallel circuit is used for this purpose, with the capacitor and inductor directly connected together, exchanging energy between each other. Just as a pendulum can be used to stabilise the frequency of a clock mechanism's oscillations, so can a parallel circuit be used to stabilise the electrical frequency of an a.c. oscillator circuit.

Another use for resonance is in applications where the effects of greatly increased or decreased impedance at a particular frequency is desired. A resonant circuit can be used to 'block' (i.e. present high impedance toward) a frequency or range of frequencies, thus acting as a sort of frequency **'filter'** to strain certain frequencies out of a mix of others. In fact, these particular circuits are called filters, and their design is considered in Chapter 17. In essence, this is how analogue radio receiver tuner circuits work to filter, or select, one station frequency out of the mix of different radio station frequency signals intercepted by the antenna.

Q-factor

Currents higher than the supply current can circulate within the parallel branches of a parallel resonant circuit, the current leaving the capacitor and establishing the magnetic field of the inductor, this then collapsing and recharging the capacitor, and so on. The **Q-factor** of a parallel resonant circuit is the ratio of the current circulating in the parallel branches of the circuit to the supply current, i.e. the current magnification.

Q-factor at resonance = current magnification

$$= \frac{\text{circulating current}}{\text{supply current}}$$

$$= \frac{I_C}{I_r} = \frac{I_{LR}\sin\phi_1}{I_r}$$

$$= \frac{I_{LR}\sin\phi_1}{I_{LR}\cos\phi_1}$$

$$= \frac{\sin\phi_1}{\cos\phi_1} = \tan\phi_1$$

$$= \frac{X_L}{R}$$

i.e. Q-factor at resonance $= \dfrac{2\pi f_r L}{R}$

(which is the same as for a series circuit).
Note that in a **parallel** circuit the Q-factor is a measure of **current magnification**, whereas in a **series** circuit it is a measure of **voltage magnification**.
At mains frequencies the Q-factor of a parallel circuit is usually low, typically less than 10, but in radio-frequency circuits the Q-factor can be very high.

Problem 8. A pure inductance of 150 mH is connected in parallel with a 40 μF capacitor across a 50 V, variable frequency supply. Determine (a) the resonant frequency of the circuit and (b) the current circulating in the capacitor and inductance at resonance.

The circuit diagram is shown in Fig. 16.12.

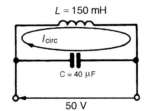

$L = 150$ mH

I_{circ}

$C = 40$ μF

50 V

Figure 16.12

(a) Parallel resonant frequency,

$$f_r = \frac{1}{2\pi}\sqrt{\frac{1}{LC} - \frac{R^2}{L^2}}$$

However, resistance $R = 0$, hence,

$$f_r = \frac{1}{2\pi}\sqrt{\frac{1}{LC}}$$

$$= \frac{1}{2\pi}\sqrt{\frac{1}{(150 \times 10^{-3})(40 \times 10^{-6})}}$$

$$= \frac{1}{2\pi}\sqrt{\frac{10^7}{(15)(4)}} = \frac{10^3}{2\pi}\sqrt{\frac{1}{6}}$$

$$= \mathbf{64.97\,Hz}$$

(b)   Current circulating in L and C at resonance,

$$I_{CIRC} = \frac{V}{X_C} = \frac{V}{\left(\dfrac{1}{2\pi f_r C}\right)} = 2\pi f_r C V$$

Hence

$$I_{CIRC} = 2\pi(64.97)(40 \times 10^{-6})(50)$$
$$= \mathbf{0.816\,A}$$

(Alternatively,

$$I_{CIRC} = \frac{V}{X_L} = \frac{V}{2\pi f_r L} = \frac{50}{2\pi(64.97)(0.15)}$$
$$= \mathbf{0.817\,A})$$

Problem 9. A coil of inductance 0.20 H and resistance 60 Ω is connected in parallel with a 20 μF capacitor across a 20 V, variable frequency supply. Calculate (a) the resonant frequency, (b) the dynamic resistance, (c) the current at resonance and (d) the circuit Q-factor at resonance.

(a)   Parallel resonant frequency,

$$f_r = \frac{1}{2\pi}\sqrt{\frac{1}{LC} - \frac{R^2}{L^2}}$$

$$= \frac{1}{2\pi}\sqrt{\frac{1}{(0.20)(20 \times 10^{-6})} - \frac{(60)^2}{(0.20)^2}}$$

$$= \frac{1}{2\pi}\sqrt{2\,50\,000 - 90\,000} = \frac{1}{2\pi}\sqrt{1\,60\,000}$$

$$= \frac{1}{2\pi}(400) = \mathbf{63.66\,Hz}$$

(b)   Dynamic resistance,

$$R_D = \frac{L}{RC} = \frac{0.20}{(60)(20 \times 10^{-6})} = \mathbf{166.7\,\Omega}$$

(c)   Current at resonance,

$$I_r = \frac{V}{R_D} = \frac{20}{166.7} = \mathbf{0.12\,A}$$

(d)   Circuit Q-factor at resonance

$$= \frac{2\pi f_r L}{R} = \frac{2\pi(63.66)(0.20)}{60} = \mathbf{1.33}$$

Alternatively, Q-factor at resonance

$$= \text{current magnification (for a parallel circuit)}$$

$$= \frac{I_C}{I_r}$$

$$I_c = \frac{V}{X_C} = \frac{V}{\left(\dfrac{1}{2\pi f_r C}\right)} = 2\pi f_r C V$$

$$= 2\pi(63.66)(20 \times 10^{-6})(20) = 0.16\,A$$

Hence Q-factor $= I_C/I_r = 0.16/0.12 = \mathbf{1.33}$,   as obtained above.

Problem 10. A coil of inductance 100 mH and resistance 800 Ω is connected in parallel with a variable capacitor across a 12 V, 5 kHz supply. Determine for the condition when the supply current is a minimum: (a) the capacitance of the capacitor, (b) the dynamic resistance, (c) the supply current, and (d) the Q-factor.

(a)   The supply current is a minimum when the parallel circuit is at resonance and resonant frequency,

$$f_r = \frac{1}{2\pi}\sqrt{\frac{1}{LC} - \frac{R^2}{L^2}}$$

Transposing for C gives:

$$(2\pi f_r)^2 = \frac{1}{LC} - \frac{R^2}{L^2}$$

$$(2\pi f_r)^2 + \frac{R^2}{L^2} = \frac{1}{LC}$$

$$\text{and } C = \frac{1}{L\left\{(2\pi f_r)^2 + \dfrac{R^2}{L^2}\right\}}$$

When $L = 100$ mH, $R = 800\,\Omega$ and $f_r = 5000$ Hz,

$$C = \frac{1}{100 \times 10^{-3}\left\{(2\pi(5000))^2 + \dfrac{800^2}{(100 \times 10^{-3})^2}\right\}}$$

$$= \frac{1}{0.1\{\pi^2 10^8 + (0.64)(10^8)\}}\,F$$

$$= \frac{10^6}{0.1(10.51 \times 10^8)}\,\mu F$$

$$= \mathbf{0.009515\,\mu F} \text{ or } \mathbf{9.515\,nF}$$

(b) Dynamic resistance,

$$R_D = \frac{L}{CR} = \frac{100 \times 10^{-3}}{(9.515 \times 10^{-9})(800)}$$

$$= \mathbf{13.14\,k\Omega}$$

(c) Supply current at resonance,

$$I_r = \frac{V}{R_D} = \frac{12}{13.14 \times 10^3} = \mathbf{0.913\,mA}$$

(d) Q-factor at resonance

$$= \frac{2\pi f_r L}{R} = \frac{2\pi(5000)(100 \times 10^{-3})}{800} = \mathbf{3.93}$$

Alternatively, Q-factor at resonance

$$= \frac{I_C}{I_r} = \frac{(V/X_C)}{I_r} = \frac{2\pi f_r C V}{I_r}$$

$$= \frac{2\pi(5000)(9.515 \times 10^{-9})(12)}{0.913 \times 10^{-3}} = \mathbf{3.93}$$

For a practical laboratory experiment on parallel a.c. circuits and resonance, see Chapter 24, page 417.

Now try the following exercise

Exercise 95   Further problems on parallel resonance and Q-factor

1. A $0.15\,\mu F$ capacitor and a pure inductance of $0.01\,H$ are connected in parallel across a 10 V, variable frequency supply. Determine (a) the resonant frequency of the circuit, and (b) the current circulating in the capacitor and inductance.   [(a) 4.11 kHz (b) 38.74 mA]

2. A $30\,\mu F$ capacitor is connected in parallel with a coil of inductance 50 mH and unknown resistance R across a 120 V, 50 Hz supply. If the circuit has an overall power factor of 1 find (a) the value of R, (b) the current in the coil, and (c) the supply current.
    [(a) 37.68 Ω (b) 2.94 A (c) 2.714 A]

3. A coil of resistance $25\,\Omega$ and inductance 150 mH is connected in parallel with a $10\,\mu F$ capacitor across a 60 V, variable frequency supply. Calculate (a) the resonant frequency, (b) the dynamic resistance, (c) the current at resonance and (d) the Q-factor at resonance.
    [(a) 127.2 Hz (b) 600 Ω (c) 0.10 A (d) 4.80]

4. A coil having resistance R and inductance 80 mH is connected in parallel with a 5 nF capacitor across a 25 V, 3 kHz supply. Determine for the condition when the current is a minimum, (a) the resistance R of the coil, (b) the dynamic resistance, (c) the supply current, and (d) the Q-factor.
    [(a) 3.705 kΩ (b) 4.318 kΩ
    (c) 5.79 mA (d) 0.41]

5. A coil of resistance $1.5\,k\Omega$ and 0.25 H inductance is connected in parallel with a variable capacitance across a 10 V, 8 kHz supply. Calculate (a) the capacitance of the capacitor when the supply current is a minimum, (b) the dynamic resistance, and (c) the supply current.
    [(a) 1561 pF (b) 106.8 kΩ (c) 93.66 μA]

6. A parallel circuit as shown in Fig. 16.13 is tuned to resonance by varying capacitance C. Resistance, $R = 30\,\Omega$, inductance, $L = 400\,\mu H$, and the supply voltage, $V = 200\,V$, 5 MHz.

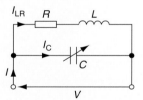

Figure 16.13

Calculate (a) the value of C to give resonance at 5 MHz, (b) the dynamic impedance, (c) the Q-factor, (d) the bandwidth, (e) the current in each branch, (f) the supply current, and (g) the power dissipated at resonance.
    [(a) 2.533 pF (b) 5.264 MΩ (c) 418.9
    (d) 11.94 kHz (e) $I_C = 15.915\angle 90°$ mA,
    $I_{LR} = 15.915\angle -89.863°$ mA (f) 38 μA
    (g) 7.60 mW]

16.7   Power factor improvement

From page 243, in any a.c. circuit, **power factor = $\cos\phi$**, where ϕ is the phase angle between supply current and supply voltage.

Industrial loads such as a.c. motors are essentially inductive (i.e. *R-L*) and may have a low power factor. For example, let a motor take a current of 50 A at a power factor of 0.6 lagging from a 240 V, 50 Hz supply, as shown in the circuit diagram of Fig. 16.14(a).

If power factor = 0.6 lagging, then:

$$\cos\phi = 0.6 \text{ lagging}$$

Hence,

$$\text{phase angle, } \phi = \cos^{-1}0.6 = 53.13° \text{ lagging}$$

Lagging means that *I* lags *V* (remember CIVIL), and the phasor diagram is as shown in Fig. 16.14(b).

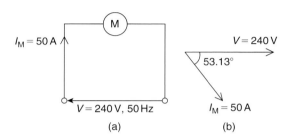

Figure 16.14

How can this power factor of 0.6 be 'improved' or 'corrected' to, say, unity?

Unity power factor means: $\cos\phi = 1$ from which, $\phi = 0$

So how can the circuit of Fig. 16.14(a) be modified so that the circuit phase angle is changed from 53.13° to 0°? The answer is to connect a capacitor in parallel with the motor as shown in Fig. 16.15(a).

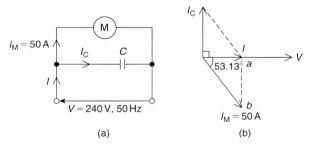

Figure 16.15

When a capacitor is connected in parallel with the inductive load, it takes a current shown as I_C. In the phasor diagram of Fig. 16.15(b), current I_C is shown leading the voltage *V* by 90° (again, remember CIVIL).

The supply current in Fig. 16.15(a) is shown as *I* and is now the phasor sum of I_M and I_C.

In the phasor diagram of Fig. 16.15(b), current *I* is shown as the phasor sum of I_M and I_C and is in phase with *V*, i.e. the circuit phase angle is 0°, which means that the power factor is cos 0° = 1.

Thus, by connecting a capacitor in parallel with the motor, the power factor has been improved from 0.6 lagging to unity.

From right angle triangles, cos 53.13°

$$= \frac{\text{adjacent}}{\text{hypotenuse}} = \frac{I}{50}$$

from which,   **supply current, $I = 50 \cos 53.13°$**

$$= 30\,\text{A}$$

Before the capacitor was connected, the supply current was 50 A. Now it is 30 A.

Herein lies **the advantage of power factor improvement – the supply current has been reduced.**

When power factor is improved, **the supply current is reduced, the supply system has lower losses** (i.e. lower I^2R losses) and therefore **cheaper running costs.**

Problem 11. In the circuit of Fig. 16.16, what value of capacitor is needed to improve the power factor from 0.6 lagging to unity?

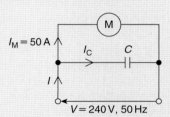

Figure 16.16

This is the same circuit as used above where the supply current was reduced from 50 A to 30 A by power factor improvement. In the phasor diagram of Fig. 16.17, current I_C needs to equal *ab* if *I* is to be in phase with *V*.

From right angle triangles, $\sin 53.13° = \dfrac{\text{opposite}}{\text{hypotenuse}}$

$$= \frac{ab}{50}$$

from which, $ab = 50 \sin 53.13° = 40\,\text{A}$

Hence, **a capacitor has to be of such a value as to take 40 A for the power factor to be improved from 0.6 to 1.**

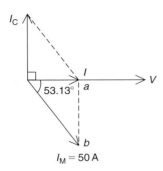

Figure 16.17

From a.c. theory, in the circuit of Fig. 16.16,

$$I_C = \frac{V}{X_c} = \frac{V}{\left(\dfrac{1}{2\pi f C}\right)} = 2\pi f C V$$

from which,

capacitance, $C = \dfrac{I_c}{2\pi f V} = \dfrac{40}{2\pi(50)(240)} = \mathbf{530.5\,\mu F}$

In **practical situations** a power factor of 1 is not normally required but a power factor in the region of **0.8** or better is usually aimed for. (Actually, a power factor of 1 means resonance!)

> **Problem 12.** An inductive load takes a current of 60 A at a power factor of 0.643 lagging when connected to a 240 V, 60 Hz supply. It is required to improve the power factor to 0.80 lagging by connecting a capacitor in parallel with the load. Calculate (a) the new supply current, (b) the capacitor current, and (c) the value of the power factor correction capacitor.

(a) A power factor of 0.643 means
$$\cos\phi_1 = 0.643$$
from which, $\phi_1 = \cos^{-1} 0.643 = 50°$

A power factor of 0.80 means
$$\cos\phi_2 = 0.80$$
from which, $\phi_2 = \cos^{-1} 0.80 = 36.87°$

The phasor diagram is shown in Fig. 16.18, where the new supply current I is shown by length Ob

From triangle Oac, $\cos 50° = \dfrac{Oa}{60}$ from which,
$$Oa = 60\,\cos 50° = 38.57\,\text{A}$$

From triangle Oab,
$$\cos 36.87° = \frac{Oa}{Ob} = \frac{38.57}{I}$$

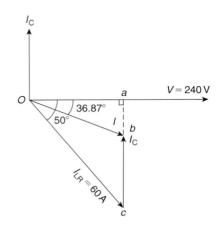

Figure 16.18

from which, **new supply current,**
$$I = \frac{38.57}{\cos 36.87} = \mathbf{48.21\,A}$$

(b) The new supply current I is the phasor sum of I_C and I_{LR}

Thus, if $I = I_C + I_{LR}$ then $I_C = I - I_{LR}$

i.e. **capacitor current,**
$$\begin{aligned}
I_C &= 48.21\angle -36.87° - 60\angle -50° \\
&= (38.57 - j28.93) - (38.57 - j45.96) \\
&= (0 + j17.03)\,\text{A} \quad \text{or} \quad \mathbf{17.03\angle 90°\,A}
\end{aligned}$$

(c) Current, $I_C = \dfrac{V}{X_c} = \dfrac{V}{\left(\dfrac{1}{2\pi f C}\right)} = 2\pi f C V$

from which, **capacitance,**
$$C = \frac{I_c}{2\pi f V} = \frac{17.03}{2\pi(60)(240)} = \mathbf{188.2\,\mu F}$$

> **Problem 13.** A 400 V alternator is supplying a load of 42 kW at a power factor of 0.7 lagging. Calculate (a) the kVA loading and (b) the current taken from the alternator. (c) If the power factor is now raised to unity find the new kVA loading.

(a) Power $= VI \cos\phi = (VI)$ (power factor)

Hence $VI = \dfrac{\text{power}}{\text{p.f.}} = \dfrac{42 \times 10^3}{0.7} = \mathbf{60\,kVA}$

(b) $VI = 60\,000$ VA

hence $I = \dfrac{60\,000}{V} = \dfrac{60\,000}{400} = \mathbf{150\,A}$

(c) The kVA loading remains at **60 kVA** irrespective of changes in power factor.

> **Problem 14.** A motor has an output of 4.8 kW, an efficiency of 80% and a power factor of 0.625 lagging when operated from a 240 V, 50 Hz supply. It is required to improve the power factor to 0.95 lagging by connecting a capacitor in parallel with the motor. Determine (a) the current taken by the motor, (b) the supply current after power factor correction, (c) the current taken by the capacitor, (d) the capacitance of the capacitor, and (e) the kvar rating of the capacitor.

(a) $\text{Efficiency} = \dfrac{\text{power output}}{\text{power input}}$

hence $\dfrac{80}{100} = \dfrac{4800}{\text{power input}}$

and power input $= \dfrac{4800}{0.8} = 6000 \text{ W}$

Hence, $6000 = V I_M \cos\phi = (240)(I_M)(0.625)$, since $\cos\phi = \text{p.f.} = 0.625$. Thus current taken by the motor,

$$I_M = \frac{6000}{(240)(0.625)} = \mathbf{40\,A}$$

The circuit diagram is shown in Fig. 16.19(a). The phase angle between I_M and V is given by: $\phi = \cos^{-1} 0.625 = 51.32°$, hence the phasor diagram is as shown in Fig. 16.19(b).

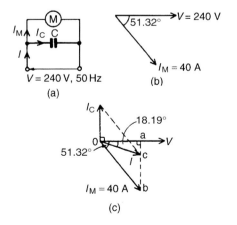

Figure 16.19

(b) When a capacitor C is connected in parallel with the motor a current I_C flows which leads V by 90°.

The phasor sum of I_M and I_C gives the supply current I, and has to be such as to change the circuit power factor to 0.95 lagging, i.e. a phase angle of $\cos^{-1} 0.95$ or 18.19° lagging, as shown in Fig. 16.19(c). The horizontal component of I_M (shown as oa)

$$= I_M \cos 51.32°$$
$$= 40 \cos 51.32° = 25 \text{ A}$$

The horizontal component of I (also given by oa)

$$= I \cos 18.19°$$
$$= 0.95 I$$

Equating the horizontal components gives: $25 = 0.95\,I$. Hence the supply current after p.f. correction,

$$I = \frac{25}{0.95} = \mathbf{26.32\,A}$$

(c) The vertical component of I_M (shown as ab)

$$= I_M \sin 51.32°$$
$$= 40 \sin 51.32° = 31.22 \text{ A}$$

The vertical component of I (shown as ac)

$$= I \sin 18.19°$$
$$= 26.32 \sin 18.19° = 8.22 \text{ A}$$

The magnitude of the capacitor current I_C (shown as bc) is given by

$$ab - ac \quad \text{i.e.} \quad I_C = 31.22 - 8.22 = \mathbf{23\,A}$$

(d) Current $I_C = \dfrac{V}{X_C} = \dfrac{V}{\left(\dfrac{1}{2\pi f C}\right)} = 2\pi f C V$

from which

$$C = \frac{I_C}{2\pi f V} = \frac{23}{2\pi(50)(240)} F = \mathbf{305\,\mu F}$$

(e) **kvar rating** of the capacitor

$$= \frac{V I_C}{1000} = \frac{(240)(23)}{1000} = \mathbf{5.52\,kvar}$$

In this problem the supply current has been reduced from 40 A to 26.32 A without altering the current or power taken by the motor. This means that the $I^2 R$ losses are reduced, and results in a saving of costs.

Problem 15. A 250 V, 50 Hz single-phase supply feeds the following loads (i) incandescent lamps taking a current of 10 A at unity power factor, (ii) fluorescent lamps taking 8 A at a power factor of 0.7 lagging, (iii) a 3 kVA motor operating at full load and at a power factor of 0.8 lagging and (iv) a static capacitor. Determine, for the lamps and motor, (a) the total current, (b) the overall power factor, and (c) the total power. (d) Find the value of the static capacitor to improve the overall power factor to 0.975 lagging.

A phasor diagram is constructed as shown in Fig. 16.20(a), where 8 A is lagging voltage V by $\cos^{-1} 0.7$, i.e. 45.57°, and the motor current is $(3000/250)$, i.e. 12 A lagging V by $\cos^{-1} 0.8$, i.e. 36.87°

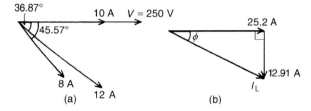

Figure 16.20

(a) The horizontal component of the currents

$$= 10\cos 0° + 12\cos 36.87° + 8\cos 45.57°$$

$$= 10 + 9.6 + 5.6 = 25.2 \text{ A}$$

The vertical component of the currents

$$= 10\sin 0° + 12\sin 36.87° + 8\sin 45.57°$$

$$= 0 + 7.2 + 5.713 = 12.91 \text{ A}$$

From Fig. 16.20(b), total current,

$$I_L = \sqrt{25.2^2 + 12.91^2} = \mathbf{28.31 \text{ A}} \text{ at a phase angle}$$
of $\phi = \tan^{-1}(12.91/25.2)$ i.e. 27.13° lagging.

(b) Power factor

$$= \cos\phi = \cos 27.13° = \mathbf{0.890 \text{ lagging}}$$

(c) Total power,

$$P = V I_L \cos\phi = (250)(28.31)(0.890)$$

$$= \mathbf{6.3 \text{ kW}}$$

(d) To improve the power factor, a capacitor is connected in parallel with the loads. The capacitor

takes a current I_C such that the supply current falls from 28.31 A to I, lagging V by $\cos^{-1} 0.975$, i.e. 12.84°. The phasor diagram is shown in Fig. 16.21.

$$oa = 28.31\cos 27.13° = I\cos 12.84°$$

hence $I = \dfrac{28.31\cos 27.13°}{\cos 12.84°} = 25.84 \text{ A}$

Current $I_C = bc = (ab - ac)$

$$= 28.31\sin 27.13° - 25.84\sin 12.84°$$

$$= 12.91 - 5.742 = 7.168 \text{ A}$$

$$I_C = \frac{V}{X_C} = \frac{V}{\left(\dfrac{1}{2\pi fc}\right)} = 2\pi fCV$$

Hence capacitance

$$C = \frac{I_C}{2\pi f V} = \frac{7.168}{2\pi (50)(250)} F = \mathbf{91.27 \,\mu F}$$

Thus to improve the power factor from 0.890 to 0.975 lagging a 91.27 μF capacitor is connected in parallel with the loads.

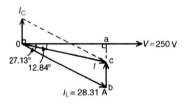

Figure 16.21

Now try the following exercises

Exercise 96   Further problems on power factor improvement

1. A 415 V alternator is supplying a load of 55 kW at a power factor of 0.65 lagging. Calculate (a) the kVA loading and (b) the current taken from the alternator. (c) If the power factor is now raised to unity find the new kVA loading.
   [(a) 84.6 kVA (b) 203.9 A (c) 84.6 kVA]

2. A single phase motor takes 30 A at a power factor of 0.65 lagging from a 240 V, 50 Hz

supply. Determine (a) the current taken by the capacitor connected in parallel to correct the power factor to unity, and (b) the value of the supply current after power factor correction.

[(a) 22.80 A (b) 19.50 A]

3. A 20 Ω non-reactive resistor is connected in series with a coil of inductance 80 mH and negligible resistance. The combined circuit is connected to a 200 V, 50 Hz supply. Calculate (a) the reactance of the coil, (b) the impedance of the circuit, (c) the current in the circuit, (d) the power factor of the circuit, (e) the power absorbed by the circuit, (f) the value of a power factor correction capacitor to produce a power factor of unity, and (g) the value of a power factor correction capacitor to produce a power factor of 0.9.

[(a) 25.13 Ω (b) 32.12$\angle$51.49° Ω
(c) 6.227$\angle$−51.49° A (d) 0.623
(e) 775.5 W (f) 77.56 μF (g) 47.67 μF]

4. A motor has an output of 6 kW, an efficiency of 75% and a power factor of 0.64 lagging when operated from a 250 V, 60 Hz supply. It is required to raise the power factor to 0.925 lagging by connecting a capacitor in parallel with the motor. Determine (a) the current taken by the motor, (b) the supply current after power factor correction, (c) the current taken by the capacitor, (d) the capacitance of the capacitor, and (e) the kvar rating of the capacitor.

[(a) 50 A (b) 34.59 A (c) 25.28 A
(d) 268.2 μF (e) 6.32 kvar]

5. A supply of 250 V, 80 Hz is connected across an inductive load and the power consumed is 2 kW, when the supply current is 10 A. Determine the resistance and inductance of the circuit. What value of capacitance connected in parallel with the load is needed to improve the overall power factor to unity?

[$R = 20\,\Omega$, $L = 29.84$ mH, $C = 47.75\,\mu$F]

6. A 200 V, 50 Hz single-phase supply feeds the following loads: (i) fluorescent lamps taking a current of 8 A at a power factor of 0.9 leading, (ii) incandescent lamps taking a current of 6 A at unity power factor, (iii) a motor taking a current of 12 A at a power factor of 0.65 lagging.

Determine the total current taken from the supply and the overall power factor. Find also the value of a static capacitor connected in parallel with the loads to improve the overall power factor to 0.98 lagging.

[21.74 A, 0.966 lagging, 21.74 μF]

Exercise 97 **Short answer questions on single-phase parallel a.c. circuits**

1. Draw a phasor diagram for a two-branch parallel circuit containing capacitance C in one branch and resistance R in the other, connected across a supply voltage V

2. Draw a phasor diagram for a two-branch parallel circuit containing inductance L and resistance R in one branch and capacitance C in the other, connected across a supply voltage V

3. Draw a phasor diagram for a two-branch parallel circuit containing inductance L in one branch and capacitance C in the other for the condition in which inductive reactance is greater than capacitive reactance

4. State two methods of determining the phasor sum of two currents

5. State two formulae which may be used to calculate power in a parallel circuit

6. State the condition for resonance for a two-branch circuit containing capacitance C in parallel with a coil of inductance L and resistance R

7. Develop a formula for the resonant frequency in an LR–C parallel circuit, in terms of resistance R, inductance L and capacitance C

8. What does Q-factor of a parallel circuit mean?

9. Develop a formula for the current at resonance in an LR–C parallel circuit in terms of resistance R, inductance L, capacitance C and supply voltage V

Section 2

10. What is dynamic resistance? State a formula for dynamic resistance

11. Explain a simple method of improving the power factor of an inductive circuit

12. Why is it advantageous to improve power factor?

Exercise 98 Multi-choice questions on single-phase parallel a.c. circuits
(Answers on page 421)

A two-branch parallel circuit containing a $10\,\Omega$ resistance in one branch and a $100\,\mu F$ capacitor in the other, has a 120 V, $2/3\pi$ kHz supply connected across it. Determine the quantities stated in questions 1 to 8, selecting the correct answer from the following list:

(a) 24 A   (b) $6\,\Omega$

(c) $7.5\,k\Omega$ (d) 12 A

(e) $\tan^{-1}\frac{3}{4}$ leading   (f) 0.8 leading

(g) $7.5\,\Omega$ (h) $\tan^{-1}\frac{4}{3}$ leading

(i) 16 A   (j) $\tan^{-1}\frac{5}{3}$ lagging

(k) 1.44 kW   (l) 0.6 leading

(m) $12.5\,\Omega$ (n) 2.4 kW

(o) $\tan^{-1}\frac{4}{3}$ lagging   (p) 0.6 lagging

(q) 0.8 lagging   (r) 1.92 kW

(s) 20 A

1. The current flowing in the resistance

2. The capacitive reactance of the capacitor

3. The current flowing in the capacitor

4. The supply current

5. The supply phase angle

6. The circuit impedance

7. The power consumed by the circuit

8. The power factor of the circuit

9. A two-branch parallel circuit consists of a 15 mH inductance in one branch and a $50\,\mu F$ capacitor in the other across a 120 V, $1/\pi$ kHz supply. The supply current is:

    (a) 8 A leading by $\dfrac{\pi}{2}$ rad

    (b) 16 A lagging by $90°$

(c) 8 A lagging by $90°$

(d) 16 A leading by $\dfrac{\pi}{2}$ rad

10. The following statements, taken correct to 2 significant figures, refer to the circuit shown in Fig. 16.22. Which are false?

    (a) The impedance of the R–L branch is $5\,\Omega$
    (b) $I_{LR} = 50$ A
    (c) $I_C = 20$ A
    (d) $L = 0.80$ H

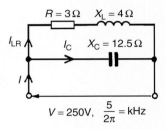

Figure 16.22

    (e) $C = 16\,\mu F$
    (f) The 'in-phase' component of the supply current is 30 A
    (g) The 'quadrature' component of the supply current is 40 A
    (h) $I = 36$ A
    (i) Circuit phase $= 33°41'$ leading
    (j) Circuit impedance $= 6.9\,\Omega$
    (k) Circuit power factor $= 0.83$ lagging
    (l) Power consumed $= 9.0$ kW

11. Which of the following statements is false?

    (a) The supply current is a minimum at resonance in a parallel circuit
    (b) The Q-factor at resonance in a parallel circuit is the voltage magnification
    (c) Improving power factor reduces the current flowing through a system
    (d) The circuit impedance is a maximum at resonance in a parallel circuit

12. An LR–C parallel circuit has the following component values: $R = 10\,\Omega$, $L = 10$ mH, $C = 10\,\mu F$ and $V = 100$ V. Which of the following statements is false?

    (a) The resonant frequency f_r is $1.5/\pi$ kHz
    (b) The current at resonance is 1 A
    (c) The dynamic resistance is $100\,\Omega$
    (d) The circuit Q-factor at resonance is 30

13. The magnitude of the impedance of the circuit shown in Fig. 16.23 is:
    (a) $7\,\Omega$ (b) $5\,\Omega$
    (c) $2.4\,\Omega$ (d) $1.71\,\Omega$

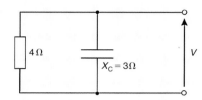

Figure 16.23

14. In the circuit shown in Fig. 16.24, the magnitude of the supply current I is:
    (a) 17A   (b) 7A
    (c) 15A   (d) 23A

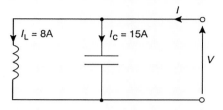

Figure 16.24

Chapter 17

Filter networks

At the end of this chapter you should be able to:

- appreciate the purpose of a filter network
- understand basic types of filter sections, i.e. low-pass, high-pass, band-pass and band-stop filters
- define cut-off frequency, two-port networks and characteristic impedance
- design low- and high-pass filter sections given nominal impedance and cut-off frequency
- determine the values of components comprising a band-pass filter given cut-off frequencies
- appreciate the difference between ideal and practical filter characteristics

17.1 Introduction

Attenuation is a reduction or loss in the magnitude of a voltage or current due to its transmission over a line. A **filter** is a network designed to pass signals having frequencies within certain bands (called **pass-bands)** with little attenuation, but greatly attenuates signals within other bands (called **attenuation bands** or **stop-bands**).

A filter is frequency sensitive and is thus composed of reactive elements. Since certain frequencies are to be passed with minimal loss, ideally the inductors and capacitors need to be pure components since the presence of resistance results in some attenuation at all frequencies.

Between the pass-band of a filter, where ideally the attenuation is zero, and the attenuation band, where ideally the attenuation is infinite, is the **cut-off frequency**, this being the frequency at which the attenuation changes from zero to some finite value.

A filter network containing no source of power is termed **passive**, and one containing one or more power sources is known as an **active** filter network.

Filters are used for a variety of purposes in nearly every type of electronic communications and control equipment. The bandwidths of filters used in communications systems vary from a fraction of a hertz to many megahertz, depending on the application.

There are four basic types of filter sections:

(a) low-pass

(b) high-pass

(c) band-pass

(d) band-stop

17.2 Two-port networks and characteristic impedance

Networks in which electrical energy is fed in at one pair of terminals and taken out at a second pair of terminals are called **two-port networks**. The network between the input port and the output port is a transmission network for which a known relationship exists between the input and output currents and voltages.

Figure 17.1(a) shows a **T-network**, which is termed **symmetrical** if $Z_A = Z_B$, and Fig. 17.1(b) shows a **π-network** which is symmetrical if $Z_E = Z_F$.

If $Z_A \neq Z_B$ in Fig. 17.1(a) and $Z_E \neq Z_F$ in Fig. 17.1(b), the sections are termed **asymmetrical**.

DOI: 10.1016/B978-0-08-089056-2.00017-6

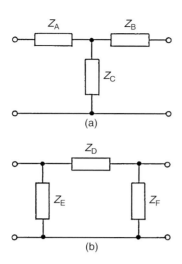

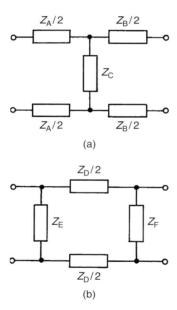

Figure 17.1

Figure 17.2

Both networks shown have one common terminal, which may be earthed, and are therefore said to be **unbalanced**. The **balanced** form of the T-network is shown in Fig. 17.2(a) and the balanced form of the π-network shown in Fig. 17.2(b).

The input impedance of a network is the ratio of voltage to current at the input terminals. With a two-port network the input impedance often varies according to the load impedance across the output terminals. For any passive two-port network it is found that a particular value of load impedance can always be found which will produce an input impedance having the same

value as the load impedance. This is called the **iterative impedance** for an asymmetrical network and its value depends on which pair of terminals is taken to be the input and which the output (there are thus two values of iterative impedance, one for each direction).

For a symmetrical network there is only one value for the iterative impedance and this is called the **characteristic impedance** Z_0 of the symmetrical two-port network.

17.3 Low-pass filters

Figure 17.3 shows simple unbalanced T- and π-section filters using series inductors and shunt capacitors. If either section is connected into a network and a continuously increasing frequency is applied, each would have a frequency-attenuation characteristic as shown in Fig. 17.4. This is an ideal characteristic and assumes pure reactive elements. All frequencies are seen to be passed from zero up to a certain value without attenuation, this value being shown as f_c, the cut-off frequency; all values of frequency above f_c are attenuated. It is for this reason that the networks shown in Fig. 17.3(a) and (b) are known as **low-pass filters**.

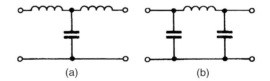

Figure 17.3

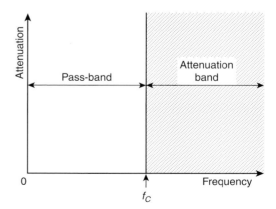

Figure 17.4

The electrical circuit diagram symbol for a low-pass filter is shown in Fig. 17.5.

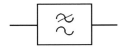

Figure 17.5

Summarising, **a low-pass filter is one designed to pass signals at frequencies below a specified cut-off frequency.**

In practise, the characteristic curve of a low-pass prototype filter section looks more like that shown in Fig. 17.6. The characteristic may be improved somewhat closer to the ideal by connecting two or more identical sections in cascade. This produces a much sharper cut-off characteristic, although the attenuation in the pass-band is increased a little.

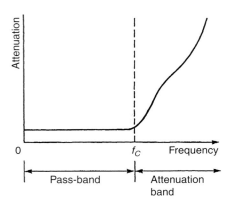

Figure 17.6

When rectifiers are used to produce the d.c. supplies of electronic systems, a large ripple introduces undesirable noise and may even mask the effect of the signal voltage. Low-pass filters are added to smooth the output voltage waveform, this being one of the most common applications of filters in electrical circuits.

Filters are employed to isolate various sections of a complete system and thus to prevent undesired interactions. For example, the insertion of low-pass decoupling filters between each of several amplifier stages and a common power supply reduces interaction due to the common power supply impedance.

Cut-off frequency and nominal impedance calculations

A low-pass symmetrical T-network and a low-pass symmetrical π-network are shown in Fig. 17.7. It may

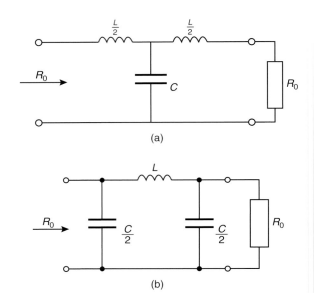

Figure 17.7

be shown that the cut-off frequency, f_c, for each section is the same, and is given by:

$$f_c = \frac{1}{\pi\sqrt{LC}} \qquad (1)$$

When the frequency is very low, the characteristic impedance is purely resistive. This value of characteristic impedance is known as the **design impedance** or the **nominal impedance** of the section and is often given the symbol R_0, where

$$R_0 = \sqrt{\frac{L}{C}} \qquad (2)$$

Problem 1. Determine the cut-off frequency and the nominal impedance for the low-pass T-connected section shown in Fig. 17.8.

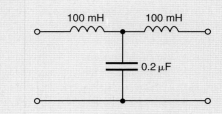

Figure 17.8

Comparing Fig. 17.8 with the low-pass section of Fig. 17.7(a), shows that:

$$\frac{L}{2} = 100\,\text{mH},$$

i.e. inductance, $L = 200\,\text{mH} = 0.2\,\text{H}$,

and capacitance $C = 0.2\,\mu\text{F} = 0.2 \times 10^{-6}\,\text{F}$.

From equation (1), **cut-off frequency**,

$$f_c = \frac{1}{\pi\sqrt{LC}}$$

$$= \frac{1}{\pi\sqrt{(0.2 \times 0.2 \times 10^{-6})}} = \frac{10^3}{\pi(0.2)}$$

i.e. $f_c = 1592\,\text{Hz}$ or $1.592\,\text{kHz}$

From equation (2), **nominal impedance**,

$$R_0 = \sqrt{\frac{L}{C}} = \sqrt{\frac{0.2}{0.2 \times 10^{-6}}}$$

$$= 1000\,\Omega \quad \text{or} \quad 1\,\text{k}\Omega$$

Problem 2.   Determine the cut-off frequency and the nominal impedance for the low-pass π-connected section shown in Fig. 17.9.

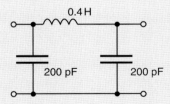

0.4 H

200 pF   200 pF

Figure 17.9

Comparing Fig. 17.9 with the low-pass section of Fig. 17.7(b), shows that:

$$\frac{C}{2} = 200\,\text{pF},$$

i.e. capacitance, $C = 400\,\text{pF} = 400 \times 10^{-12}\,\text{F}$,

and inductance $L = 0.4\,\text{H}$.

From equation (1), **cut-off frequency**,

$$f_c = \frac{1}{\pi\sqrt{LC}}$$

$$= \frac{1}{\pi\sqrt{(0.4 \times 400 \times 10^{-12})}} = \frac{10^6}{\pi\sqrt{160}}$$

i.e. $f_c = 25.16\,\text{kHz}$

From equation (2), **nominal impedance**,

$$R_0 = \sqrt{\frac{L}{C}} = \sqrt{\frac{0.4}{400 \times 10^{-12}}} = 31.62\,\text{k}\Omega$$

To determine values of L and C given R_0 and f_c

If the values of the nominal impedance R_0 and the cut-off frequency f_c are known for a low-pass T- or π-section, it is possible to determine the values of inductance and capacitance required to form the section. It may be shown that:

$$\text{capacitance } C = \frac{1}{\pi R_0 f_c} \tag{3}$$

and $$\text{inductance } L = \frac{R_0}{\pi f_c} \tag{4}$$

Problem 3.   A filter section is to have a characteristic impedance at zero frequency of $600\,\Omega$ and a cut-off frequency of 5 MHz. Design (a) a low-pass T-section filter, and (b) a low-pass π-section filter to meet these requirements.

The characteristic impedance at zero frequency is the nominal impedance R_0, i.e. $R_0 = 600\,\Omega$; cut-off frequency $f_c = 5\,\text{MHz} = 5 \times 10^6\,\text{Hz}$.

From equation (3), capacitance,

$$C = \frac{1}{\pi R_0 f_c} = \frac{1}{\pi(600)(5 \times 10^6)}\,\text{F}$$

$$= 1.06 \times 10^{-10}\,\text{F} = 106\,\text{pF}$$

From equation (4), inductance,

$$L = \frac{R_0}{\pi f_c} = \frac{600}{\pi(5 \times 10^6)}\,\text{H}$$

$$= 3.82 \times 10^{-5} = 38.2\,\mu\text{H}$$

Section 2

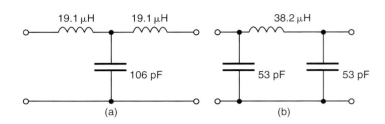

Figure 17.10

(a) A low-pass T-section filter is shown in Fig. 17.10(a), where the series arm inductances are each $\dfrac{L}{2}$ (see Fig. 17.7(a)), i.e. $\dfrac{38.2}{2} = 19.1\,\mu\text{H}$

(b) A low-pass π-section filter is shown in Fig. 17.10(b), where the shunt arm capacitances are each $\dfrac{C}{2}$ (see Fig. 17.7(b)), i.e. $\dfrac{106}{2} = 53\,\text{pF}$

Now try the following exercise

Exercise 99   Further problems on low-pass filter sections

1. Determine the cut-off frequency and the nominal impedance of each of the low-pass filter sections shown in Fig. 17.11.
   [(a) 1592 Hz; 5 kΩ (b) 9545 Hz; 600 Ω]

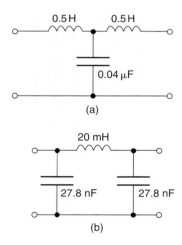

Figure 17.11

2. A filter section is to have a characteristic impedance at zero frequency of 500 Ω and a cut-off frequency of 1 kHz. Design (a) a low-pass T-section filter, and (b) a low-pass π-section filter to meet these requirements.
   [(a) Each series arm 79.60 mH shunt arm 0.6366 μF
   (b) Series arm 159.2 mH, each shunt arm 0.3183 μF]

3. Determine the value of capacitance required in the shunt arm of a low-pass T-section if the inductance in each of the series arms is 40 mH and the cut-off frequency of the filter is 2.5 kHz.   [0.203 μF]

4. The nominal impedance of a low-pass π-section filter is 600 Ω. If the capacitance in each of the shunt arms is 0.1 μF determine the inductance in the series arm.   [72 mH]

17.4   High-pass filters

Figure 17.12 shows simple unbalanced T- and π-section filters using series capacitors and shunt inductors. If either section is connected into a network and a continuously increasing frequency is applied, each would have a frequency-attenuation characteristic as shown in Fig. 17.13.

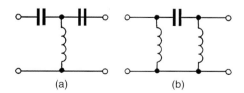

Figure 17.12

Once again this is an ideal characteristic assuming pure reactive elements. All frequencies below the

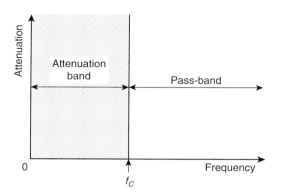

Figure 17.13

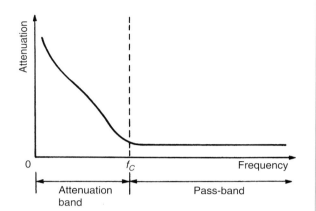

Figure 17.15

cut-off frequency f_c are seen to be attenuated and all frequencies above f_c are passed without loss.

It is for this reason that the networks shown in Figs 17.12(a) and (b) are known as **high-pass filters**. The electrical circuit diagram symbol for a high-pass filter is shown in Fig. 17.14.

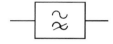

Figure 17.14

Summarising, **a high-pass filter is one designed to pass signals at frequencies above a specified cut-off frequency**.

The characteristic shown in Fig. 17.13 is ideal in that it is assumed that there is no attenuation at all in the pass-bands and infinite attenuation in the attenuation band. Both of these conditions are impossible to achieve in practice. Due to resistance, mainly in the inductive elements the attenuation in the pass-band will not be zero, and in a practical filter section the attenuation in the attenuation band will have a finite value. In addition to the resistive loss there is often an added loss due to mismatching.

Ideally when a filter is inserted into a network it is matched to the impedance of that network. However the characteristic impedance of a filter section will vary with frequency and the termination of the section may be an impedance that does not vary with frequency in the same way.

Figure 17.13 showed an ideal high-pass filter section characteristic of attenuation against frequency. In practise, the characteristic curve of a high-pass prototype filter section would look more like that shown in Fig. 17.15.

Cut-off frequency and nominal impedance calculations

A high-pass symmetrical T-network and a high-pass symmetrical π-network are shown in Fig. 17.16. It may be shown that the cut-off frequency, f_c, for each section is the same, and is given by:

$$f_c = \frac{1}{4\pi\sqrt{LC}} \tag{5}$$

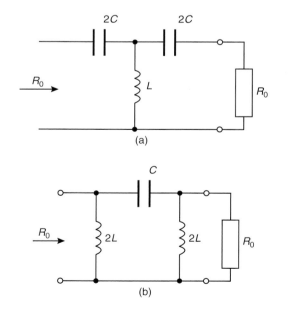

Figure 17.16

When the frequency is very high, the characteristic impedance is purely resistive. This value of characteristic impedance is then the **nominal imped-ance** of the section and is given by:

$$R_0 = \sqrt{\frac{L}{C}} \qquad (6)$$

Problem 4. Determine the cut-off frequency and the nominal impedance for the high-pass T-connected section shown in Fig. 17.17.

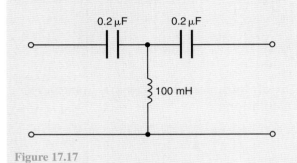

Figure 17.17

Comparing Fig. 17.17 with the high-pass section of Fig. 17.16(a), shows that:

$$2C = 0.2\,\mu F,$$

i.e. capacitance, $C = 0.1\,\mu F = 0.1 \times 10^{-6}$,

and inductance, $L = 100\,mH = 0.1\,H$.

From equation (5), **cut-off frequency**,

$$f_c = \frac{1}{4\pi\sqrt{LC}}$$

$$= \frac{1}{4\pi\sqrt{(0.1 \times 0.1 \times 10^{-6})}} = \frac{10^3}{4\pi(0.1)}$$

i.e. $f_c = 796\,Hz$

From equation (6), **nominal impedance**,

$$R_0 = \sqrt{\frac{L}{C}} = \sqrt{\frac{0.1}{0.1 \times 10^{-6}}}$$

$$= 1000\,\Omega \quad \text{or} \quad 1\,k\Omega$$

Problem 5. Determine the cut-off frequency and the nominal impedance for the high-pass π-connected section shown in Fig. 17.18.

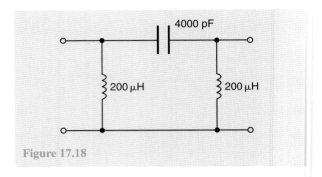

Figure 17.18

Comparing Fig. 17.18 with the high-pass section of Fig. 17.16(b), shows that:

$$2L = 200\,\mu H,$$

i.e. inductance, $L = 100\,\mu H = 10^{-4}\,H$,

and capacitance, $C = 4000\,pF = 4 \times 10^{-9}\,F$.

From equation (5), **cut-off frequency**,

$$f_c = \frac{1}{4\pi\sqrt{LC}}$$

$$= \frac{1}{4\pi\sqrt{(10^{-4} \times 4 \times 10^{-9})}} = 1.26 \times 10^5$$

i.e. $f_c = 126\,kHz$

From equation (6), **nominal impedance**,

$$R_0 = \sqrt{\frac{L}{C}} = \sqrt{\frac{10^{-4}}{4 \times 10^{-9}}}$$

$$= \sqrt{\frac{10^5}{4}} = 158\,\Omega$$

To determine values of *L* and *C* given R_0 and f_c

If the values of the nominal impedance R_0 and the cut-off frequency f_c are known for a high-pass T- or π-section, it is possible to determine the values of inductance and capacitance required to form the section. It may be shown that:

$$\text{capacitance } C = \frac{1}{4\pi R_0 f_c} \qquad (7)$$

and $\qquad$ inductance $L = \dfrac{R_0}{4\pi f_c}$ $\qquad$ (8)

Problem 6. A filter section is required to pass all frequencies above 25 kHz and to have a nominal impedance of 600 Ω. Design (a) a high-pass T-section filter, and (b) a high-pass π-section filter to meet these requirements.

Cut-off frequency $f_c = 25\,\text{kHz} = 25 \times 10^3\,\text{Hz}$, and nominal impedance, $R_0 = 600\,\Omega$.

From equation (7), capacitance,

$$C = \frac{1}{4\pi R_0 f_c} = \frac{1}{4\pi (600)(25 \times 10^3)}\,\text{F}$$

$$= \frac{10^{12}}{4\pi (600)(25 \times 10^3)}\,\text{pF}$$

$$= 5305\,\text{pF} \quad \text{or} \quad 5.305\,\text{nF}$$

From equation (8), inductance,

$$L = \frac{R_0}{4\pi f_c} = \frac{600}{4\pi (25 \times 10^3)}$$

$$= 0.00191\,\text{H} = 1.91\,\text{mH}$$

(a) A high-pass T-section filter is shown in Fig. 17.19(a), where the series arm capacitances

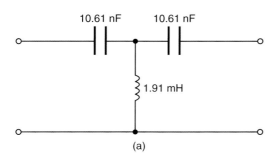

10.61 nF   10.61 nF

1.91 mH

(a)

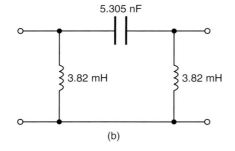

5.305 nF

3.82 mH   3.82 mH

(b)

Figure 17.19

are each $2C$ (see Fig. 17.16(a)), i.e. $2 \times 5.305 = 10.61\,\text{nF}$

(b) A high-pass π-section filter is shown in Fig. 17.19(b), where the shunt arm inductances are each $2L$ (see Fig. 17.6(b)), i.e. $2 \times 1.91 = 3.82\,\text{mH}$.

Now try the following exercise

Exercise 100 **Further problems on high-pass filter sections**

1. Determine the cut-off frequency and the nominal impedance of each of the high-pass filter sections shown in Fig. 17.20.
   [(a) 22.51 kHz; 14.14 kΩ
   (b) 281.3 Hz; 1414 Ω]

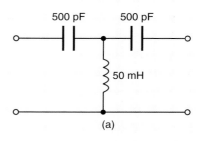

500 pF   500 pF

50 mH

(a)

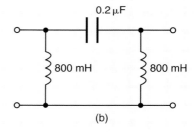

0.2 μF

800 mH   800 mH

(b)

Figure 17.20

2. A filter section is required to pass all frequencies above 4 kHz and to have a nominal impedance 750 Ω. Design (a) an appropriate high-pass T section filter, and (b) an appropriate high-pass π-section filter to meet these requirements.
   [(a) Each series arm = 53.06 nF, shunt arm = 14.92 mH
   (b) Series arm = 26.53 nF, each shunt arm = 29.84 mH]

3. The inductance in each of the shunt arms of a high-pass π-section filter is 50 mH. If the nominal impedance of the section is 600 Ω, determine the value of the capacitance in the series arm. [69.44 nF]

4. Determine the value of inductance required in the shunt arm of a high-pass T-section filter if in each series arm it contains a 0.5 μF capacitor. The cut-off frequency of the filter section is 1500 Hz. [11.26 mH]

17.5 Band-pass filters

A **band-pass filter is one designed to pass signals with frequencies between two specified cut-off frequencies**. The characteristic of an ideal band-pass filter is shown in Fig. 17.21.

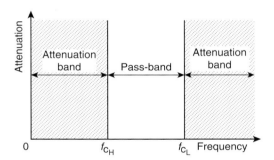

Figure 17.21

Such a filter may be formed by cascading a high-pass and a low-pass filter. f_{C_H} is the cut-off frequency of the high-pass filter and f_{C_L} is the cut-off frequency of the low-pass filter. As can be seen, for a band-pass filter $f_{C_L} > f_{C_H}$, the pass-band being given by the difference between these values.

The electrical circuit diagram symbol for a band-pass filter is shown in Fig. 17.22.

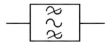

Figure 17.22

A typical practical characteristic for a band-pass filter is shown in Fig. 17.23.

Crystal and ceramic devices are used extensively as band-pass filters. They are common in the intermediate-frequency amplifiers of v.h.f. radios where a precisely

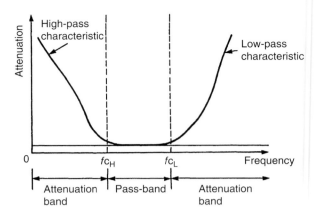

Figure 17.23

defined bandwidth must be maintained for good performance.

Problem 7. A band-pass filter is comprised of a low-pass T-section filter having a cut-off frequency of 15 kHz, connected in series with a high-pass T-section filter having a cut-off frequency of 10 kHz. The terminating impedance of the filter is 600 Ω. Determine the values of the components comprising the composite filter.

For the low-pass T-section filter:

$$f_{C_L} = 15\,000\,\text{Hz}$$

From equation (3), capacitance,

$$C = \frac{1}{\pi R_0 f_c} = \frac{1}{\pi (600)(15\,000)}$$

$$= 35.4 \times 10^{-9} = 35.4\,\text{nF}$$

From equation (4), inductance,

$$L = \frac{R_0}{\pi f_c} = \frac{600}{\pi (15\,000)}$$

$$= 0.01273\,\text{H} = 12.73\,\text{mH}$$

Thus, from Fig. 17.7(a), the series arm inductances are each $\frac{L}{2}$ i.e.

$$\frac{12.73}{2} = \mathbf{6.37\,mH}$$

and the shunt arm capacitance is **35.4 nF**.

For the high-pass T-section filter:

$$f_{C_H} = 10\,000\,\text{Hz}$$

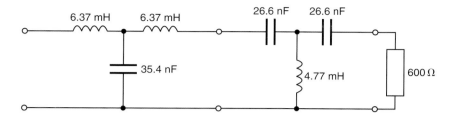

Figure 17.24

From equation (7), capacitance,

$$C = \frac{1}{4\pi R_0 f_c} = \frac{1}{4\pi(600)(10\,000)}$$

$$= 1.33 \times 10^{-8} = 13.3\,\text{nF}$$

From equation (8), inductance,

$$L = \frac{R_0}{4\pi f_c} = \frac{600}{4\pi(10\,000)}$$

$$= 4.77 \times 10^{-3} = 4.77\,\text{mH}.$$

Thus, from Fig. 17.16(a), the series arm capacitances are each $2C$,

i.e. $\qquad 2 \times 13.3 = \mathbf{26.6\,nF}$

and the shunt arm inductance is **4.77 mH**. The composite, band-pass filter is shown in Fig. 17.24.

The attenuation against frequency characteristic will be similar to Fig. 17.23 where $f_{C_H} = 10\,\text{kHz}$ and $f_{C_L} = 15\,\text{kHz}$.

Now try the following exercise

Exercise 101   Further problems on band-pass filters

1. A band-pass filter is comprised of a low-pass T-section filter having a cut-off frequency of 20 kHz, connected in series with a high-pass T-section filter having a cut-off frequency of 8 kHz. The terminating impedance of the filter is 600 Ω. Determine the values of the components comprising the composite filter.

[Low-pass T-section: each series arm 4.77 mH, shunt arm 26.53 nF
High-pass T-section: each series arm 33.16 nF, shunt arm 5.97 mH]

2. A band-pass filter is comprised of a low-pass π-section filter having a cut-off frequency of 50 kHz, connected in series with a high-pass π-section filter having a cut-off frequency of 40 kHz. The terminating impedance of the filter is 620 Ω. Determine the values of the components comprising the composite filter.

[Low-pass π-section: series arm 3.95 mH, each shunt arm 5.13 nF
High-pass π-section: series arm 3.21 nF, each shunt arm 2.47 mH]

17.6   Band-stop filters

A **band-stop filter is one designed to pass signals with all frequencies except those between two specified cut-off frequencies**. The characteristic of an ideal band-stop filter is shown in Fig. 17.25.

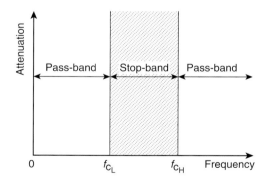

Figure 17.25

Such a filter may be formed by connecting a high-pass and a low-pass filter in parallel. As can be seen, for a band-stop filter $f_{C_H} > f_{C_L}$, the stop-band being given by the difference between these values.

The electrical circuit diagram symbol for a band-stop filter is shown in Fig. 17.26.

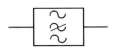

Figure 17.26

A typical practical characteristic for a band-stop filter is shown in Fig. 17.27.

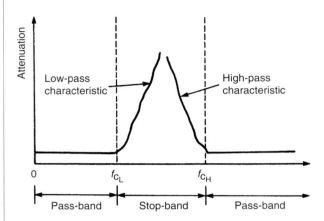

Figure 17.27

Sometimes, as in the case of interference from 50 Hz power lines in an audio system, the exact frequency of a spurious noise signal is known. Usually such interference is from an odd harmonic of 50 Hz, for example, 250 Hz. A sharply tuned band-stop filter, designed to attenuate the 250 Hz noise signal, is used to minimise the effect of the output. A high-pass filter with cut-off frequency greater than 250 Hz would also remove the interference, but some of the lower frequency components of the audio signal would be lost as well.

Filter design can be a complicated area. For more, see *Electrical Circuit Theory and Technology*.

Now try the following exercises

Exercise 102   Short answer questions
                on filters

1. Define a filter

2. Define the cut-off frequency for a filter

3. Define a two-port network

4. Define characteristic impedance for a two-port network

5. A network designed to pass signals at frequencies below a specified cut-off frequency is called a ...... filter

6. A network designed to pass signals with all frequencies except those between two specified cut-off frequencies is called a ...... filter

7. A network designed to pass signals with frequencies between two specified cut-off frequencies is called a ...... filter

8. A network designed to pass signals at frequencies above a specified cut-off frequency is called a ...... filter

9. State one application of a low-pass filter

10. Sketch (a) an ideal, and (b) a practical attenuation/frequency characteristic for a low-pass filter

11. Sketch (a) an ideal, and (b) a practical attenuation/frequency characteristic for a high-pass filter

12. Sketch (a) an ideal, and (b) a practical attenuation/frequency characteristic for a band-pass filter

14. State one application of a band-pass filter

13. Sketch (a) an ideal, and (b) a practical attenuation/frequency characteristic for a band-stop filter

15. State one application of a band-stop filter

Exercise 103   Multi-choice questions on
                filters
                (Answers on page 421)

1. A network designed to pass signals with all frequencies except those between two specified cut-off frequencies is called a:
   (a) low-pass filter   (b) high-pass filter
   (c) band-pass filter   (d) band-stop filter

2. A network designed to pass signals at frequencies above a specified cut-off frequency is called a:
   (a) low-pass filter   (b) high-pass filter
   (c) band-pass filter   (d) band-stop filter

3. A network designed to pass signals at frequencies below a specified cut-off frequency is called a:
   (a) low-pass filter   (b) high-pass filter
   (c) band-pass filter   (d) band-stop filter

4. A network designed to pass signals with frequencies between two specified cut-off frequencies is called a:
   (a) low-pass filter   (b) high-pass filter
   (c) band-pass filter   (d) band-stop filter

5. A low-pass T-connected symmetrical filter section has an inductance of 200 mH in each of its series arms and a capacitance of 0.5 μF in its shunt arm. The cut-off frequency of the filter is:
   (a) 1007 Hz   (b) 251.6 Hz
   (c) 711.8 Hz   (d) 177.9 Hz

6. A low-pass π-connected symmetrical filter section has an inductance of 200 mH in its series arm and capacitances of 400 pF in each of its shunt arms. The cut-off frequency of the filter is:
   (a) 25.16 kHz   (b) 6.29 kHz
   (c) 17.79 kHz   (d) 35.59 kHz

The following refers to questions 7 and 8.

A filter section is to have a nominal impedance of 620 Ω and a cut-off frequency of 2 MHz.

7. A low-pass T-connected symmetrical filter section is comprised of:
   (a) 98.68 μH in each series arm, 128.4 pF in shunt arm
   (b) 49.34 μH in each series arm, 256.7 pF in shunt arm
   (c) 98.68 μH in each series arm, 256.7 pF in shunt arm
   (d) 49.34 μH in each series arm, 128.4 pF in shunt arm

8. A low-pass π-connected symmetrical filter section is comprised of:
   (a) 98.68 μH in each series arm, 128.4 pF in shunt arm
   (b) 49.34 μH in each series arm, 256.7 pF in shunt arm

   (c) 98.68 μH in each series arm, 256.7 pF in shunt arm
   (d) 49.34 μH in each series arm, 128.4 pF in shunt arm

9. A high-pass T-connected symmetrical filter section has capacitances of 400 nF in each of its series arms and an inductance of 200 mH in its shunt arm. The cut-off frequency of the filter is:
   (a) 1592 Hz   (b) 1125 Hz
   (c) 281 Hz   (d) 398 Hz

10. A high-pass π-connected symmetrical filter section has a capacitance of 5000 pF in its series arm and inductances of 500 μH in each of its shunt arms. The cut-off frequency of the filter is:
    (a) 201.3 kHz   (b) 71.18 kHz
    (c) 50.33 kHz   (d) 284.7 kHz

The following refers to questions 11 and 12.

A filter section is required to pass all frequencies above 50 kHz and to have a nominal impedance of 650 Ω.

11. A high-pass T-connected symmetrical filter section is comprised of:
    (a) Each series arm 2.45 nF, shunt arm 1.03 mH
    (b) Each series arm 4.90 nF, shunt arm 2.08 mH
    (c) Each series arm 2.45 nF, shunt arm 2.08 mH
    (d) Each series arm 4.90 nF, shunt arm 1.03 mH

12. A high-pass π-connected symmetrical filter section is comprised of:
    (a) Series arm 4.90 nF, and each shunt arm 1.04 mH
    (b) Series arm 4.90 nF, and each shunt arm 2.07 mH
    (c) Series arm 2.45 nF, and each shunt arm 2.07 mH
    (d) Series arm 2.45 nF, and each shunt arm 1.04 mH

Section 2

Chapter 18

D.C. transients

At the end of this chapter you should be able to:

- understand the term 'transient'

- describe the transient response of capacitor and resistor voltages, and current in a series $C - R$ d.c. circuit

- define the term 'time constant'

- calculate time constant in a $C - R$ circuit

- draw transient growth and decay curves for a $C - R$ circuit

- use equations $v_C = V(1 - e^{-t/\tau})$, $v_R = Ve^{-t/\tau}$ and $i = Ie^{-t/\tau}$ for a $C - R$ circuit

- describe the transient response when discharging a capacitor

- describe the transient response of inductor and resistor voltages, and current in a series $L - R$ d.c. circuit

- calculate time constant in an $L - R$ circuit

- draw transient growth and decay curves for an $L - R$ circuit

- use equations $v_L = Ve^{-t/\tau}$, $v_R = V(1 - e^{-t/\tau})$ and $i = I(1 - e^{-t/\tau})$

- describe the transient response for current decay in an $L - R$ circuit

- understand the switching of inductive circuits

- describe the effects of time constant on a rectangular waveform via integrator and differentiator circuits

18.1 Introduction

When a d.c. voltage is applied to a capacitor C and resistor R connected in series, there is a short period of time immediately after the voltage is connected, during which the current flowing in the circuit and voltages across C and R are changing.

Similarly, when a d.c. voltage is connected to a circuit having inductance L connected in series with resistance R, there is a short period of time immediately after the voltage is connected, during which the current flowing in the circuit and the voltages across L and R are changing. These changing values are called **transients**.

18.2 Charging a capacitor

(a) The circuit diagram for a series connected $C - R$ circuit is shown in Fig. 18.1. When switch S is closed then by Kirchhoff's voltage law:

$$V = v_C + v_R \tag{1}$$

(b) The battery voltage V is constant. The capacitor voltage v_C is given by q/C, where q is the charge on the capacitor. The voltage drop across R is given by iR, where i is the current flowing in the circuit.

DOI: 10.1016/B978-0-08-089056-2.00018-8

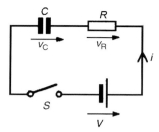

Figure 18.1

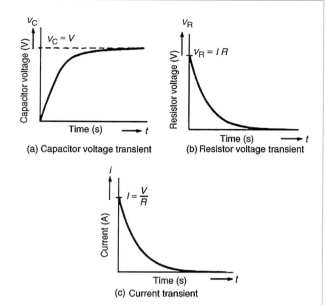

(a) Capacitor voltage transient
(b) Resistor voltage transient

(c) Current transient

Figure 18.2

Hence at all times:

$$V = \frac{q}{C} + iR \qquad (2)$$

At the instant of closing S, (initial circuit condition), assuming there is no initial charge on the capacitor, q_0 is zero, hence v_{Co} is zero. Thus from Equation (1), $V = 0 + v_{Ro}$, i.e. $v_{Ro} = V$. This shows that the resistance to current is solely due to R, and the initial current flowing, $i_0 = I = V/R$.

(c) A short time later at time t_1 seconds after closing S, the capacitor is partly charged to, say, q_1 coulombs because current has been flowing. The voltage v_{C1} is now (q_1/C) volts. If the current flowing is i_1 amperes, then the voltage drop across R has fallen to $i_1 R$ volts. Thus, equation (2) is now $V = (q_1/C) + i_1 R$.

(d) A short time later still, say at time t_2 seconds after closing the switch, the charge has increased to q_2 coulombs and v_C has increased to (q_2/C) volts. Since $V = v_C + v_R$ and V is a constant, then v_R decreases to $i_2 R$, Thus v_C is increasing and i and v_R are decreasing as time increases.

(e) Ultimately, a few seconds after closing S, (i.e. at the final or **steady-state** condition), the capacitor is fully charged to, say, Q coulombs, current no longer flows, i.e. $i = 0$, and hence $v_R = iR = 0$. It follows from equation (1) that $v_C = V$.

(f) Curves showing the changes in v_C, v_R and i with time are shown in Fig. 18.2.
The curve showing the variation of v_C with time is called an **exponential growth curve** and the graph is called the 'capacitor voltage/time' characteristic. The curves showing the variation of v_R and i with time are called **exponential decay curves**, and the graphs are called 'resistor voltage/time' and 'current/time' characteristics respectively. (The name 'exponential' shows that

the shape can be expressed mathematically by an exponential mathematical equation, as shown in Section 18.4.)

18.3   Time constant for a $C - R$ circuit

(a) If a constant d.c. voltage is applied to a series connected $C - R$ circuit, a transient curve of capacitor voltage v_C is as shown in Fig. 18.2(a).

(b) With reference to Fig. 18.3, let the constant voltage supply be replaced by a variable voltage supply at time t_1 seconds. Let the voltage be varied so that the **current** flowing in the circuit is **constant**.

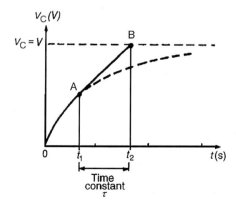

Figure 18.3

(c) Since the current flowing is a constant, the curve will follow a tangent, AB, drawn to the curve at point A.

(d) Let the capacitor voltage v_C reach its final value of V at time t_2 seconds.

(e) The time corresponding to $(t_2 - t_1)$ seconds is called the **time constant** of the circuit, denoted by the Greek letter 'tau', τ. The value of the time constant is CR seconds, i.e. for a series connected $C - R$ circuit,

$$\text{time constant } \tau = CR \text{ seconds}$$

Since the variable voltage mentioned in paragraph (b) above can be applied at any instant during the transient change, it may be applied at $t = 0$, i.e. at the instant of connecting the circuit to the supply. If this is done, then the time constant of the circuit may be defined as: *'the time taken for a transient to reach its final state if the initial rate of change is maintained'*.

18.4 Transient curves for a $C - R$ circuit

There are two main methods of drawing transient curves graphically, these being:

(a) the **tangent method** – this method is shown in Problem 1

(b) the **initial slope and three point method**, which is shown in Problem 2, and is based on the following properties of a transient exponential curve:

(i) for a growth curve, the value of a transient at a time equal to one time constant is 0.632 of its steady-state value (usually taken as 63 per cent of the steady-state value), at a time equal to two and a half time constants is 0.918 of its steady-state value (usually taken as 92 per cent of its steady-state value) and at a time equal to five time constants is equal to its steady-state value,

(ii) for a decay curve, the value of a transient at a time equal to one time constant is 0.368 of its initial value (usually taken as 37 per cent of its initial value), at a time equal to two and a half time constants is 0.082 of its initial value (usually taken as 8 per cent of its initial value) and at a time equal to five time constants is equal to zero.

The transient curves shown in Fig. 18.2 have mathematical equations, obtained by solving the differential equations representing the circuit. The equations of the curves are:

growth of capacitor voltage,

$$v_C = V(1 - e^{-t/CR}) = V(1 - e^{-t/\tau})$$

decay of resistor voltage,

$$v_R = Ve^{-t/CR} = Ve^{-t/\tau} \quad \text{and}$$

decay of resistor voltage,

$$i = Ie^{-t/CR} = Ie^{-t/\tau}$$

Problem 1. A $15\,\mu\text{F}$ uncharged capacitor is connected in series with a $47\,\text{k}\Omega$ resistor across a $120\,\text{V}$, d.c. supply. Use the tangential graphical method to draw the capacitor voltage/time characteristic of the circuit. From the characteristic, determine the capacitor voltage at a time equal to one time constant after being connected to the supply, and also two seconds after being connected to the supply. Also, find the time for the capacitor voltage to reach one half of its steady-state value.

To construct an exponential curve, the time constant of the circuit and steady-state value need to be determined.

$$\text{Time constant} = CR = 15\,\mu\text{F} \times 47\,\text{k}\Omega$$
$$= 15 \times 10^{-6} \times 47 \times 10^{3}$$
$$= 0.705\,\text{s}$$

Steady-state value of $v_C = V$, i.e. $v_C = 120\,\text{V}$.

With reference to Fig. 18.4, the scale of the horizontal axis is drawn so that it spans at least five time constants, i.e. 5×0.705 or about 3.5 seconds. The scale of the vertical axis spans the change in the capacitor voltage, that is, from 0 to $120\,\text{V}$. A broken line AB is drawn corresponding to the final value of v_C.

Point C is measured along AB so that AC is equal to 1τ, i.e. AC $= 0.705\,\text{s}$. Straight line OC is drawn. Assuming that about five intermediate points are needed to draw the curve accurately, a point D is selected on OC corresponding to a v_C value of about $20\,\text{V}$. DE is drawn vertically. *EF* is made to correspond to 1τ, i.e. EF $= 0.705\,\text{s}$. A straight line is drawn joining DF. This procedure of

(a) drawing a vertical line through point selected,

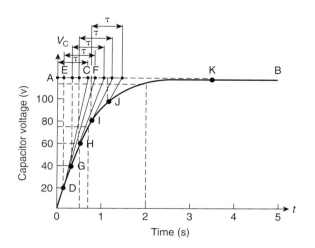

Figure 18.4

(b) at the steady-state value, drawing a horizontal line corresponding to 1τ, and

(c) joining the first and last points,

is repeated for v_C values of 40, 60, 80 and 100 V, giving points G, H, I and J.

The capacitor voltage effectively reaches its steady-state value of 120 V after a time equal to five time constants, shown as point K. Drawing a smooth curve through points 0, D, G, H, I, J and K gives the exponential growth curve of capacitor voltage.

From the graph, the value of capacitor voltage at a time equal to the time constant is about **75 V**. It is a characteristic of all exponential growth curves, that after a time equal to one time constant, the value of the transient is 0.632 of its steady-state value. In this problem, $0.632 \times 120 = 75.84$ V. Also from the graph, when t is two seconds, v_C is about **115** Volts. [This value may be checked using the equation $v_C = V(1 - e^{-t/\tau})$, where $V = 120$ V, $\tau = 0.705$ s and $t = 2$ s. This calculation gives $v_C = 112.97$ V.]

The time for v_C to rise to one half of its final value, i.e. 60 V, can be determined from the graph and is about **0.5 s**. [This value may be checked using $v_C = V(1 - e^{-t/\tau})$ where $V = 120$ V, $v_C = 60$ V and $\tau = 0.705$ s, giving $t = 0.489$ s.]

Problem 2. A $4\,\mu\mathrm{F}$ capacitor is charged to 24 V and then discharged through a $220\,\mathrm{k\Omega}$ resistor. Use the 'initial slope and three point' method to draw: (a) the capacitor voltage/time characteristic, (b) the resistor voltage/time characteristic, and (c) the current/time characteristic, for the transients which occur. From the characteristics determine the value

of capacitor voltage, resistor voltage and current 1.5 s after discharge has started.

To draw the transient curves, the time constant of the circuit and steady-state values are needed.

$$\text{Time constant, } \tau = CR$$

$$= 4 \times 10^{-6} \times 220 \times 10^{3}$$

$$= 0.88\,\text{s}$$

Initially, capacitor voltage $v_C = v_R = 24$ V,

$$i = \frac{V}{R} = \frac{24}{220 \times 10^{3}}$$

$$= 0.109\,\text{mA}$$

Finally, $v_C = v_R = i = 0$.

(a) The exponential decay of capacitor voltage is from 24 V to 0 V in a time equal to five time constants, i.e. $5 \times 0.88 = 4.4$ s. With reference to Fig. 18.5, to construct the decay curve:

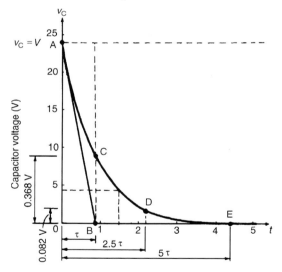

Figure 18.5

(i) the horizontal scale is made so that it spans at least five time constants, i.e. 4.4 s,

(ii) the vertical scale is made to span the change in capacitor voltage, i.e. 0 to 24 V,

(iii) point A corresponds to the initial capacitor voltage, i.e. 24 V,

(iv) OB is made equal to one time constant and line AB is drawn; this gives the initial slope of the transient,

(v) the value of the transient after a time equal to one time constant is 0.368 of the initial value, i.e. $0.368 \times 24 = 8.83$ V; a vertical line is drawn through B and distance BC is made equal to 8.83 V,

(vi) the value of the transient after a time equal to two and a half time constants is 0.082 of the initial value, i.e. $0.082 \times 24 = 1.97$ V, shown as point D in Fig. 18.5,

(vii) the transient effectively dies away to zero after a time equal to five time constants, i.e. 4.4 s, giving point E.

The smooth curve drawn through points A, C, D and E represents the decay transient. At 1.5 s after decay has started, $v_C \approx \mathbf{4.4\,V}$.
[This may be checked using $v_C = V e^{-t/\tau}$, where $V = 24$, $t = 1.5$ and $\tau = 0.88$, giving $v_C = 4.36$ V]

(b) The voltage drop across the resistor is equal to the capacitor voltage when a capacitor is discharging through a resistor, thus the resistor voltage/time characteristic is identical to that shown in Fig. 18.5 Since $v_R = v_C$, then at 1.5 seconds after decay has started, $v_R \approx \mathbf{4.4\,V}$ (see (vii) above).

(c) The current/time characteristic is constructed in the same way as the capacitor voltage/time characteristic, shown in part (a), and is as shown in Fig. 18.6. The values are:

point A: initial value of current $= 0.109$ mA

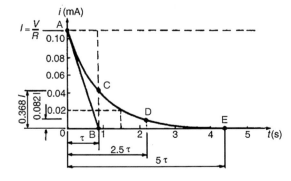

Figure 18.6

point C: at $1\,\tau, i = 0.368 \times 0.109 = 0.040$ mA
point D: at $2.5\,\tau, i = 0.082 \times 0.109 = 0.009$ mA
point E: at $5\,\tau, i = 0$

Hence the current transient is as shown. At a time of 1.5 s, the value of current, from the characteristic is **0.02 mA**

[This may be checked using $i = I e^{(-t/\tau)}$ where $I = 0.109$, $t = 1.5$ and $\tau = 0.88$, giving $i = 0.0198$ mA or 19.8 μA]

Problem 3. A 20 μF capacitor is connected in series with a 50 kΩ resistor and the circuit is connected to a 20 V, d.c. supply. Determine: (a) the initial value of the current flowing, (b) the time constant of the circuit, (c) the value of the current one second after connection, (d) the value of the capacitor voltage two seconds after connection, and (e) the time after connection when the resistor voltage is 15 V.

Parts (c), (d) and (e) may be determined graphically, as shown in Problems 1 and 2 or by calculation as shown below.
$V = 20$ V, $C = 20$ μF $= 20 \times 10^{-6}$ F,
$R = 50$ kΩ $= 50 \times 10^{3}$ V

(a) The initial value of the current flowing is
$$I = \frac{V}{R} = \frac{20}{50 \times 10^3} = \mathbf{0.4\,mA}$$

(b) From Section 18.3 the time constant,
$$\tau = CR = (20 \times 10^{-6})(50 \times 10^3) = \mathbf{1\,s}$$

(c) Current, $i = I e^{-t/\tau}$ and working in mA units,
$$i = 0.4 e^{-1/1} = 0.4 \times 0.368 = \mathbf{0.147\,mA}$$

(d) Capacitor voltage,
$$\mathbf{v_C} = V(1 - e^{-t/\tau}) = 20(1 - e^{-2/1})$$
$$= 20(1 - 0.135) = 20 \times 0.865$$
$$= \mathbf{18.3\,V}$$

(e) Resistor voltage, $v_R = V e^{-t/\tau}$
Thus $15 = 20 e^{-t/1}$, $15/20 = e^{-t}$ from which $e^t = 20/15 = 4/3$

Taking natural logarithms of each side of the equation gives
$$t = \ln \frac{4}{3} = \ln 1.3333 \text{ i.e. } \mathbf{time,\, t = 0.288\,s}$$

Problem 4. A circuit consists of a resistor connected in series with a 0.5 μF capacitor and has a time constant of 12 ms. Determine: (a) the value of the resistor, and (b) the capacitor voltage, 7 ms after connecting the circuit to a 10 V supply.

(a) The time constant $\tau = CR$, hence

$$R = \frac{\tau}{C}$$

$$= \frac{12 \times 10^{-3}}{0.5 \times 10^{-6}}$$

$$= 24 \times 10^3 = \textbf{24 k}\Omega$$

(b) The equation for the growth of capacitor voltage is: $v_C = V(1 - e^{-t/\tau})$
Since $\tau = 12\,\text{ms} = 12 \times 10^{-3}\,\text{s}$, $V = 10\,\text{V}$ and $t = 7\,\text{ms} = 7 \times 10^{-3}\,\text{s}$, then

$$v_C = 10(1 - e^{-7 \times 10^{-3}/12 \times 10^{-3}})$$

$$= 10(1 - e^{-0.583})$$

$$= 10(1 - 0.558) = \textbf{4.42 V}$$

Alternatively, the value of v_C when t is 7 ms may be determined using the growth characteristic as shown in Problem 1.

Problem 5.   A circuit consists of a $10\,\mu\text{F}$ capacitor connected in series with a $25\,\text{k}\Omega$ resistor with a switchable 100 V d.c. supply. When the supply is connected, calculate (a) the time constant, (b) the maximum current, (c) the voltage across the capacitor after 0.5 s, (d) the current flowing after one time constant, (e) the voltage across the resistor after 0.1 s, (f) the time for the capacitor voltage to reach 45 V, and (g) the initial rate of voltage rise.

(a) **Time constant,**
$$\tau = C \times R = 10 \times 10^{-6} \times 25 \times 10^3 = \textbf{0.25 s}$$

(b) Current is a maximum when the circuit is first connected and is only limited by the value of resistance in the circuit, i.e.

$$I_m = \frac{V}{R} = \frac{100}{25 \times 10^3} = \textbf{4 mA}$$

(c) Capacitor voltage, $v_C = V_m(1 - e^{-t/\tau})$
When time, $t = 0.5\,\text{s}$, then
$$v_C = 100(1 - e^{-0.5/0.25}) = 100(0.8647) = \textbf{86.47 V}$$

(d) Current, $i = I_m e^{-t/\tau}$
and when $t = \tau$,
current, $i = 4e^{-\tau/\tau} = 4e^{-1} = \textbf{1.472 mA}$

Alternatively, after one time constant the capacitor voltage will have risen to 63.2% of the supply voltage and the current will have fallen to 63.2% of

its final value, i.e. 36.8% of I_m. Hence, $i = 36.8\%$ of $4 = 0.368 \times 4 = \textbf{1.472 mA}$

(e) The voltage across the resistor, $v_R = V e^{-t/\tau}$
When $t = 0.1\,\text{s}$,
resistor voltage, $v_R = 100 e^{-0.1/0.25} = \textbf{67.03 V}$

(f) Capacitor voltage, $v_C = V_m(1 - e^{-t/\tau})$
When the capacitor voltage reaches 45 V, then:

$$45 = 100(1 - e^{-t/0.25})$$

from which, $\dfrac{45}{100} = 1 - e^{-t/0.25}$

and $e^{-t/0.25} = 1 - \dfrac{45}{100} = 0.55$

Hence, $-\dfrac{t}{0.25} = \ln 0.55$

and **time, t $= -0.25 \ln 0.55 = \textbf{0.149 s}$**

(g) **Initial rate of voltage rise** $= \dfrac{V}{\tau} = \dfrac{100}{0.25} = \textbf{400 V/s}$

(i.e. gradient of the tangent at $t = 0$)

18.5 Discharging a capacitor

When a capacitor is charged (i.e. with the switch in position A in Fig. 18.7), and the switch is then moved to position B, the electrons stored in the capacitor keep the current flowing for a short time. Initially, at the instant of moving from A to B, the current flow is such that the capacitor voltage v_C is balanced by an equal and opposite voltage $v_R = iR$. Since initially $v_C = v_R = V$, then $i = I = V/R$. During the transient decay, by applying Kirchhoff's voltage law to Fig. 18.7, $v_C = v_R$.

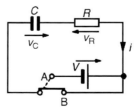

Finally the transients decay exponentially to zero, i.e. $v_C = v_R = 0$. The transient curves representing the voltages and current are as shown in Fig. 18.8.

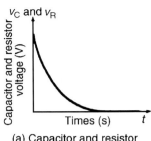

(a) Capacitor and resistor voltage transient

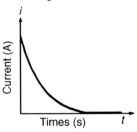

(b) Current transient

Figure 18.8

The equations representing the transient curves during the discharge period of a series connected $C - R$ circuit are:

decay of voltage,
$$v_C = v_R = Ve^{(-t/CR)} = Ve^{(-t/\tau)}$$

decay of current, $i = Ie^{(-t/CR)} = Ie^{(-t/\tau)}$

When a capacitor has been disconnected from the supply it may still be charged and it may retain this charge for some considerable time. Thus precautions must be taken to ensure that the capacitor is automatically discharged after the supply is switched off. This is done by connecting a high value resistor across the capacitor terminals.

Problem 6. A capacitor is charged to 100 V and then discharged through a 50 kΩ resistor. If the time constant of the circuit is 0.8 s. Determine: (a) the value of the capacitor, (b) the time for the capacitor voltage to fall to 20 V, (c) the current flowing when the capacitor has been discharging for 0.5 s, and (d) the voltage drop across the resistor when the capacitor has been discharging for one second.

Parts (b), (c) and (d) of this problem may be solved graphically as shown in Problems 1 and 2 or by calculation as shown below.

$V = 100\,\text{V}, \tau = 0.8\,\text{s}, R = 50\,\text{k}\Omega = 50 \times 10^3\,\Omega$

(a) Since time constant, $\tau = CR$, capacitance,

$$C = \frac{\tau}{R} = \frac{0.8}{50 \times 10^3} = \mathbf{16\,\mu F}$$

(b) Since $v_C = Ve^{-t/\tau}$ then $20 = 100e^{-t/0.8}$ from which $1/5 = e^{-t/0.8}$
Thus $e^{t/0.8} = 5$ and taking natural logarithms of each side, gives $t/0.8 = \ln 5$ and time, $t = 0.8 \ln 5 = \mathbf{1.29\,s}$.

(c) $i = Ie^{-t/\tau}$ where the initial current flowing,

$$I = \frac{V}{R} = \frac{100}{50 \times 10^3} = 2\,\text{mA}$$

Working in mA units,

$$i = Ie^{-t/\tau} = 2e^{(-0.5/0.8)}$$
$$= 2e^{-0.625} = 2 \times 0.535 = \mathbf{1.07\,mA}$$

(d) $v_R = v_C = Ve^{-t/\tau} = 100e^{-1/0.8}$
$$= 100e^{-1.25} = 100 \times 0.287 = \mathbf{28.7\,V}$$

Problem 7. A 0.1 μF capacitor is charged to 200 V before being connected across a 4 kΩ resistor. Determine (a) the initial discharge current, (b) the time constant of the circuit, and (c) the minimum time required for the voltage across the capacitor to fall to less than 2 V.

(a) Initial discharge current,

$$i = \frac{V}{R} = \frac{200}{4 \times 10^3} = \mathbf{0.05\,A} \quad \text{or} \quad \mathbf{50\,mA}$$

(b) Time constant $\tau = CR = 0.1 \times 10^{-6} \times 4 \times 10^3$
$$= \mathbf{0.0004\,s} \quad \text{or} \quad \mathbf{0.4\,ms}$$

(c) The minimum time for the capacitor voltage to fall to less than 2 V, i.e. less than 2/200 or 1 per cent of the initial value is given by 5τ. $5\tau = 5 \times 0.4 = \mathbf{2\,ms}$

In a d.c. circuit, a capacitor blocks the current except during the times that there are changes in the supply voltage.

For a practical laboratory experiment on the charging and discharging of a capacitor, see Chapter 24, page 419.

Now try the following exercise

Exercise 104   Further problems on
transients in series
connected C − R circuits

1. An uncharged capacitor of $0.2\,\mu F$ is connected to a 100 V, d.c. supply through a resistor of $100\,k\Omega$. Determine, either graphically or by calculation the capacitor voltage 10 ms after the voltage has been applied.

    [39.35 V]

2. A circuit consists of an uncharged capacitor connected in series with a $50\,k\Omega$ resistor and has a time constant of 15 ms. Determine either graphically or by calculation (a) the capacitance of the capacitor and (b) the voltage drop across the resistor 5 ms after connecting the circuit to a 20 V, d.c. supply.

    [(a) $0.3\,\mu F$ (b) 14.33 V]

3. A $10\,\mu F$ capacitor is charged to 120 V and then discharged through a $1.5\,M\Omega$ resistor. Determine either graphically or by calculation the capacitor voltage 2 s after discharging has commenced. Also find how long it takes for the voltage to fall to 25 V.

    [105.0 V, 23.53 s]

4. A capacitor is connected in series with a voltmeter of resistance $750\,k\Omega$ and a battery. When the voltmeter reading is steady the battery is replaced with a shorting link. If it takes 17 s for the voltmeter reading to fall to two-thirds of its original value, determine the capacitance of the capacitor.   [$55.9\,\mu F$]

5. When a $3\,\mu F$ charged capacitor is connected to a resistor, the voltage falls by 70 per cent in 3.9 s. Determine the value of the resistor.

    [$1.08\,M\Omega$]

6. A $50\,\mu F$ uncharged capacitor is connected in series with a $1\,k\Omega$ resistor and the circuit is switched to a 100 V, d.c. supply. Determine:
    (a) the initial current flowing in the circuit,
    (b) the time constant,
    (c) the value of current when t is 50 ms and
    (d) the voltage across the resistor 60 ms after closing the switch.

    [(a) 0.1 A (b) 50 ms
    (c) 36.8 mA (d) 30.1 V]

7. An uncharged $5\,\mu F$ capacitor is connected in series with a $30\,k\Omega$ resistor across a 110 V, d.c. supply. Determine the time constant of the circuit, the initial charging current, the current flowing 120 ms after connecting to the supply.
    [150 ms, 3.67 mA, 1.65 mA]

8. An uncharged $80\,\mu F$ capacitor is connected in series with a $1\,k\Omega$ resistor and is switched across a 110 V supply. Determine the time constant of the circuit and the initial value of current flowing. Determine also the value of current flowing after (a) 40 ms and (b) 80 ms.
    [80 ms, 0.11 A (a) 66.7 mA (b) 40.5 mA]

9. A resistor of $0.5\,M\Omega$ is connected in series with a $20\,\mu F$ capacitor and the capacitor is charged to 200 V. The battery is replaced instantaneously by a conducting link. Draw a graph showing the variation of capacitor voltage with time over a period of at least 6 time constants. Determine from the graph the approximate time for the capacitor voltage to fall to 75 V.   [9.8 s]

10. A $60\,\mu F$ capacitor is connected in series with a $10\,k\Omega$ resistor and connected to a 120 V d.c. supply. Calculate (a) the time constant, (b) the initial rate of voltage rise, (c) the initial charging current, and (d) the time for the capacitor voltage to reach 50 V.
    [(a) 0.60 s (b) 200 V/s
    (c) 12 mA (d) 0.323 s]

11. If a 200 V d.c. supply is connected to a $2.5\,M\Omega$ resistor and a $2\,\mu F$ capacitor in series. Calculate
    (a) the current flowing 4 s after connecting,
    (b) the voltage across the resistor after 4 s, and
    (c) the energy stored in the capacitor after 4 s.
    [(a) $35.95\,\mu A$ (b) 89.87 V
    (c) 12.13 mJ]

12. (a) In the circuit shown in Fig. 18.9, with the switch in position 1, the capacitor is uncharged. If the switch is moved to position 2 at time $t = 0$ s, calculate the (i) initial current through the $0.5\,M\Omega$ resistor, (ii) the voltage across the capacitor when $t = 1.5$ s, and (iii) the time taken for the voltage across the capacitor to reach 12 V.

(b) If at the time $t = 1.5\,$s, the switch is moved to position 3, calculate (i) the initial current through the $1\,$MΩ resistor, (ii) the energy stored in the capacitor $3.5\,$s later (i.e. when $t = 5\,$s).

(c) Sketch a graph of the voltage across the capacitor against time from $t = 0$ to $t = 5\,$s, showing the main points.

[(a)(i) $80\,\mu$A (ii) $18.05\,$V (iii) $0.892\,$s
(b)(i) $40\,\mu$A (ii) $48.30\,\mu$J]

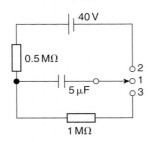

Figure 18.9

18.6 Camera flash

The internal workings of a camera flash are an example of the application of $C - R$ circuits. When a camera is first switched on, a battery slowly charges a capacitor to its full potential via a $C - R$ circuit. When the capacitor is fully charged, an indicator (red light) typically lets the photographer know that the flash is ready for use. Pressing the shutter button quickly discharges the capacitor through the flash (i.e. a resistor). The current from the capacitor is responsible for the bright light that is emitted. The flash rapidly draws current in order to emit the bright light. The capacitor must then be discharged before the flash can be used again.

18.7 Current growth in an $L - R$ circuit

(a) The circuit diagram for a series connected $L - R$ circuit is shown in Fig. 18.10. When switch S is closed, then by Kirchhoff's voltage law:

$$V = v_L + v_R \qquad (3)$$

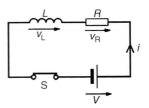

Figure 18.10

(b) The battery voltage V is constant. The voltage across the inductance is the induced voltage, i.e.

$$v_L = L \times \frac{\text{change of current}}{\text{change of time}} = L\frac{\mathrm{d}i}{\mathrm{d}t}$$

The voltage drop across R, v_R is given by iR. Hence, at all times:

$$V = L\frac{\mathrm{d}i}{\mathrm{d}t} + iR \qquad (4)$$

(c) At the instant of closing the switch, the rate of change of current is such that it induces an e.m.f. in the inductance which is equal and opposite to V, hence $V = v_L + 0$, i.e. $v_L = V$. From equation (3), because $v_L = V$, then $v_R = 0$ and $i = 0$.

(d) A short time later at time t_1 seconds after closing S, current i_1 is flowing, since there is a rate of change of current initially, resulting in a voltage drop of $i_1 R$ across the resistor. Since V (which is constant) $= v_L + v_R$ the induced e.m.f. is reduced, and equation (4) becomes:

$$V = L\frac{\mathrm{d}i_1}{\mathrm{d}t_1} + i_1 R$$

(e) A short time later still, say at time t_2 seconds after closing the switch, the current flowing is i_2, and the voltage drop across the resistor increases to $i_2 R$. Since v_R increases, v_L decreases.

(f) Ultimately, a few seconds after closing S, the current flow is entirely limited by R, the rate of change of current is zero and hence v_L is zero. Thus $V = iR$. Under these conditions, steady-state current flows, usually signified by I. Thus, $I = V/R$, $v_R = IR$ and $v_L = 0$ at steady-state conditions.

(g) Curves showing the changes in v_L, v_R and i with time are shown in Fig. 18.11 and indicate that v_L is a maximum value initially (i.e. equal to V), decaying exponentially to zero, whereas v_R and i grow exponentially from zero to their steady-state values of V and $I = V/R$ respectively.

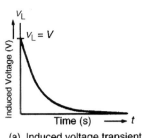
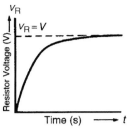

(a) Induced voltage transient   (b) Resistor voltage transient

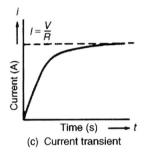

(c) Current transient

Figure 18.11

18.8   Time constant for an $L - R$ circuit

With reference to Section 18.3, the time constant of a series connected $L - R$ circuit is defined in the same way as the time constant for a series connected $C - R$ circuit. Its value is given by:

$$\text{time constant}, \tau = \frac{L}{R} \text{ seconds}$$

18.9   Transient curves for an $L - R$ circuit

Transient curves representing the induced voltage/time, resistor voltage/time and current/time characteristics may be drawn graphically, as outlined in Section 18.4. A method of construction is shown in Problem 8.

Each of the transient curves shown in Fig. 18.11 have mathematical equations, and these are:

decay of induced voltage,

$$v_{\text{L}} = Ve^{(-Rt/L)} = Ve^{(-t/\tau)}$$

growth of resistor voltage,

$$v_{\text{R}} = V(1 - e^{-Rt/L}) = V(1 - e^{-t/\tau})$$

growth of current flow,

$$i = I(1 - e^{-Rt/L}) = I(1 - e^{-t/\tau})$$

The application of these equations is shown in Problem 10.

> **Problem 8.**   A relay has an inductance of 100 mH and a resistance of 20 Ω. It is connected to a 60 V, d.c. supply. Use the 'initial slope and three point' method to draw the current/time characteristic and hence determine the value of current flowing at a time equal to two time constants and the time for the current to grow to 1.5 A.

Before the current/time characteristic can be drawn, the time constant and steady-state value of the current have to be calculated.

Time constant,

$$\tau = \frac{L}{R} = \frac{10 \times 10^{-3}}{20} = 5 \text{ ms}$$

Final value of current,

$$I = \frac{V}{R} = \frac{60}{20} = 3 \text{ A}$$

The method used to construct the characteristic is the same as that used in Problem 2

(a)   The scales should span at least five time constants (horizontally), i.e. 25 ms, and 3 A (vertically)

(b)   With reference to Fig. 18.12, the initial slope is obtained by making AB equal to 1 time constant, (i.e. 5 ms), and joining OB.

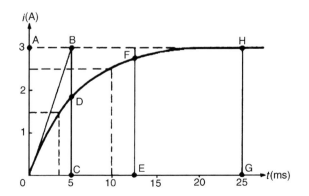

Figure 18.12

(c)   At a time of 1 time constant,
      CD is $0.632 \times I = 0.632 \times 3 = 1.896$ A.
      At a time of 2.5 time constants,
      EF is $0.918 \times I = 0.918 \times 3 = 2.754$ A.
      At a time of 5 time constants, GH is $I = 3$ A.

Section 2

(d) A smooth curve is drawn through points 0, D, F and H and this curve is the current/time characteristic.

From the characteristic, when $t = 2\tau$, $i \approx \textbf{2.6 A}$. [This may be checked by calculation using $i = I(1 - e^{-t/\tau})$, where $I = 3$ and $t = 2\tau$, giving $i = 2.59$ A.] Also, when the current is 1.5 A, the corresponding time is about **3.6 ms**. [Again, this may be checked by calculation, using $i = I(1 - e^{-t/\tau})$ where $i = 1.5$, $I = 3$ and $\tau = 5$ ms, giving $t = 3.466$ ms.]

> **Problem 9.** A coil of inductance 0.04 H and resistance 10 Ω is connected to a 120 V, d.c. supply. Determine (a) the final value of current, (b) the time constant of the circuit, (c) the value of current after a time equal to the time constant from the instant the supply voltage is connected, (d) the expected time for the current to rise to within 1 per cent of its final value.

(a) Final steady current, $I = \dfrac{V}{R} = \dfrac{120}{10} = \textbf{12 A}$

(b) Time constant of the circuit,

$$\tau = \frac{L}{R} = \frac{0.004}{10} = \textbf{0.004 s or 4 ms}$$

(c) In the time τ s the current rises to 63.2 per cent of its final value of 12 A, i.e. in 4 ms the current rises to $0.632 \times 12 = \textbf{7.58 A}$.

(d) The expected time for the current to rise to within 1 per cent of its final value is given by 5τ s, i.e. $5 \times 4 = \textbf{20 ms}$.

> **Problem 10.** The winding of an electromagnet has an inductance of 3 H and a resistance of 15 Ω. When it is connected to a 120 V, d.c. supply, calculate: (a) the steady-state value of current flowing in the winding, (b) the time constant of the circuit, (c) the value of the induced e.m.f. after 0.1 s, (d) the time for the current to rise to 85 per cent of its final value, and (e) the value of the current after 0.3 s.

(a) The steady-state value of current,

$$I = \frac{V}{R} = \frac{120}{15} = \textbf{8 A}$$

(b) The time constant of the circuit,

$$\tau = \frac{L}{R} = \frac{3}{15} = \textbf{0.2 s}$$

Parts (c), (d) and (e) of this problem may be determined by drawing the transients graphically, as shown in Problem 8 or by calculation as shown below.

(c) The induced e.m.f., v_L is given by $v_L = Ve^{-t/\tau}$. The d.c. voltage V is 120 V, t is 0.1 s and τ is 0.2 s, hence

$$v_L = 120e^{-0.1/0.2} = 120e^{-0.5}$$
$$= 120 \times 0.6065 = \textbf{72.78 V}$$

(d) When the current is 85 per cent of its final value, $i = 0.85 I$. Also, $i = I(1 - e^{-t/\tau})$, thus

$$0.85 I = I(1 - e^{-t/\tau})$$
$$0.85 = 1 - e^{-t/\tau}$$

$\tau = 0.2$, hence

$$0.85 = 1 - e^{-t/0.2}$$
$$e^{-t/0.2} = 1 - 0.85 = 0.15$$
$$e^{t/0.2} = \frac{1}{0.15} = 6.\dot{6}$$

Taking natural logarithms of each side of this equation gives:

$$\ln e^{t/0.2} = \ln 6.\dot{6}$$

and by the laws of logarithms

$$\frac{t}{0.2} \ln e = \ln 6.\dot{6}$$

$\ln e = 1$, hence **time** $t = 0.2 \ln 6.\dot{6} = \textbf{0.379 s}$

(e) The current at any instant is given by $i = I(1 - e^{-t/\tau})$. When $I = 8$, $t = 0.3$ and $\tau = 0.2$, then

$$\textbf{i} = 8(1 - e^{-0.3/0.2}) = 8(1 - e^{-1.5})$$
$$= 8(1 - 0.2231) = 8 \times 0.7769 = \textbf{6.215 A}$$

18.10 Current decay in an $L - R$ circuit

When a series connected $L - R$ circuit is connected to a d.c. supply as shown with S in position A of Fig. 18.13, a current $I = V/R$ flows after a short time, creating a magnetic field ($\Phi \propto I$) associated with the inductor. When S is moved to position B, the current value decreases, causing a decrease in the strength of the magnetic field. Flux linkages occur, generating a voltage v_L, equal to $L(di/dt)$. By Lenz's law, this voltage keeps current i flowing in the circuit, its value being limited by R. Since $V = v_L + v_R$, $0 = v_L + v_R$ and $v_L = -v_R$, i.e. v_L and

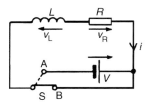

Figure 18.13

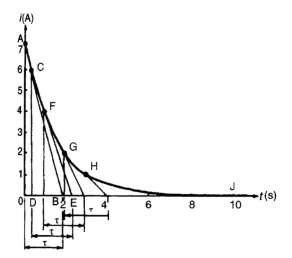

Figure 18.14

v_R are equal in magnitude but opposite in direction. The current decays exponentially to zero and since v_R is proportional to the current flowing, v_R decays exponentially to zero. Since $v_L = v_R$, v_L also decays exponentially to zero. The curves representing these transients are similar to those shown in Fig. 18.9.

The equations representing the decay transient curves are:

decay of voltages,

$$v_L = v_R = Ve^{(-Rt/L)} = Ve^{(-t/\tau)}$$

decay of current, $i = Ie^{(-Rt/L)} = Ie^{(-t/\tau)}$

> **Problem 11.** The field winding of a 110 V, d.c. motor has a resistance of 15 Ω and a time constant of 2 s. Determine the inductance and use the tangential method to draw the current/time characteristic when the supply is removed and replaced by a shorting link. From the characteristic determine (a) the current flowing in the winding 3 s after being shorted-out and (b) the time for the current to decay to 5 A.

Since the time constant, $\tau = (L/R)$, $L = R\tau$ i.e. inductance $L = 15 \times 2 = \mathbf{30\,H}$

The current/time characteristic is constructed in a similar way to that used in Problem 1

(i) The scales should span at least five time constants horizontally, i.e. 10 s, and $I = V/R = 110/15 = 7.\dot{3}$ A vertically

(ii) With reference to Fig. 18.14, the initial slope is obtained by making OB equal to 1 time constant, (i.e. 2 s), and joining AB

(iii) At, say, $i = 6$ A, let C be the point on AB corresponding to a current of 6 A. Make DE equal to 1 time constant, (i.e. 2 s), and join CE

(iv) Repeat the procedure given in (iii) for current values of, say, 4 A, 2 A and 1 A, giving points F, G and H

(v) Point J is at five time constants, when the value of current is zero.

(vi) Join points A, C, F, G, H and J with a smooth curve. This curve is the current/time characteristic.

(a) From the current/time characteristic, when $t = 3$ s, $i = \mathbf{1.3\,A}$ [This may be checked by calculation using $i = Ie^{-t/\tau}$, where $I = 7.\dot{3}$, $t = 3$ and $\tau = 2$, giving $i = 1.64$ A]. The discrepancy between the two results is due to relatively few values, such as C, F, G and H, being taken.

(b) From the characteristic, when $i = 5$ A, $t = \mathbf{0.70\,s}$ [This may be checked by calculation using $i = Ie^{-t/\tau}$, where $i = 5$, $I = 7.\dot{3}$, $\tau = 2$, giving $t = 0.766$ s]. Again, the discrepancy between the graphical and calculated values is due to relatively few values such as C, F, G and H being taken.

> **Problem 12.** A coil having an inductance of 6 H and a resistance of $R\,\Omega$ is connected in series with a resistor of 10 Ω to a 120 V, d.c. supply. The time constant of the circuit is 300 ms. When steady-state conditions have been reached, the supply is replaced instantaneously by a short-circuit. Determine: (a) the resistance of the coil, (b) the current flowing in the circuit one second after the shorting link has been placed in the circuit, and (c) the time taken for the current to fall to 10 per cent of its initial value.

(a) The time constant,

$$\tau = \frac{\text{circuit inductance}}{\text{total circuit resistance}} = \frac{L}{R + 10}$$

Section 2

Thus $R = \dfrac{L}{\tau} - 10 = \dfrac{6}{0.3} - 10 = \mathbf{10\,\Omega}$

Parts (b) and (c) may be determined graphically as shown in Problems 8 and 11 or by calculation as shown below.

(b) The steady-state current,

$$I = \frac{V}{R} = \frac{120}{10 + 10} = 6\,\text{A}$$

The transient current after 1 second,

$$i = I e^{-t/\tau} = 6 e^{-1/0.3}$$

Thus $i = 6 e^{-3.\dot{3}} = 6 \times 0.03567$
$$= \mathbf{0.214\,A}$$

(c) 10 per cent of the initial value of the current is $(10/100) \times 6$, i.e. 0.6 A. Using the equation

$$i = I e^{-t/\tau} \text{ gives}$$

$$0.6 = 6 e^{-t/0.3}$$

i.e. $\quad \dfrac{0.6}{6} = e^{-t/0.3}$

or $\quad e^{t/0.3} = \dfrac{6}{0.6} = 10$

Taking natural logarithms of each side of this equation gives:

$$\frac{t}{0.3} = \ln 10$$

from which, time, $t = \mathbf{0.3\ln 10 = 0.691\,s}$

Problem 13. An inductor has a negligible resistance and an inductance of 200 mH and is connected in series with a 1 kΩ resistor to a 24 V, d.c. supply. Determine the time constant of the circuit and the steady-state value of the current flowing in the circuit. Find (a) the current flowing in the circuit at a time equal to one time constant, (b) the voltage drop across the inductor at a time equal to two time constants, and (c) the voltage drop across the resistor after a time equal to three time constants.

The time constant,

$$\tau = \frac{L}{R} = \frac{0.2}{1000} = \mathbf{0.2\,ms}$$

The steady-state current

$$I = \frac{V}{R} = \frac{24}{1000} = \mathbf{24\,mA}$$

(a) The transient current,

$$i = I(1 - e^{-t/\tau}) \quad \text{and} \quad t = 1\tau.$$

Working in mA units gives,

$$i = 24(1 - e^{-(1\tau/\tau)}) = 24(1 - e^{-1})$$
$$= 24(1 - 0.368) = \mathbf{15.17\,mA}$$

(b) The voltage drop across the inductor, $v_L = V e^{-t/\tau}$

When $t = 2\tau$, $v_L = 24 e^{-2\tau/\tau} = 24 e^{-2}$
$$= \mathbf{3.248\,V}$$

(c) The voltage drop across the resistor,
$v_R = V(1 - e^{-t/\tau})$

When $t = 3\tau$, $v_R = 24(1 - e^{-3\tau/\tau})$
$$= 24(1 - e^{-3})$$
$$= \mathbf{22.81\,V}$$

Now try the following exercise

Exercise 105   **Further problems on transients in series $L - R$ circuits**

1. A coil has an inductance of 1.2 H and a resistance of 40 Ω and is connected to a 200 V, d.c. supply. Either by drawing the current/time characteristic or by calculation determine the value of the current flowing 60 ms after connecting the coil to the supply.   [4.32 A]

2. A 25 V d.c. supply is connected to a coil of inductance 1 H and resistance 5 Ω. Either by using a graphical method to draw the exponential growth curve of current or by calculation determine the value of the current flowing 100 ms after being connected to the supply.   [1.97 A]

3. An inductor has a resistance of 20 Ω and an inductance of 4 H. It is connected to a 50 V d.c. supply. Calculate (a) the value of current flowing after 0.1 s and (b) the time for the current to grow to 1.5 A.   [(a) 0.984 A (b) 0.183 s]

4. The field winding of a 200 V d.c. machine has a resistance of 20 Ω and an inductance of 500 mH. Calculate:

(a) the time constant of the field winding,
(b) the value of current flow one time constant after being connected to the supply, and
(c) the current flowing 50 ms after the supply has been switched on

[(a) 25 ms (b) 6.32 A (c) 8.65 A]

5. A circuit comprises an inductor of 9 H of negligible resistance connected in series with a 60 Ω resistor and a 240 V d.c. source. Calculate (a) the time constant, (b) the current after 1 time constant, (c) the time to develop maximum current, (d) the time for the current to reach 2.5 A, and (e) the initial rate of change of current.

[(a) 0.15 s (b) 2.528 A (c) 0.75 s
(d) 0.147 s (e) 26.67 A/s]

6. In the inductive circuit shown in Fig. 18.15, the switch is moved from position A to position B until maximum current is flowing. Calculate (a) the time taken for the voltage across the resistance to reach 8 volts, (b) the time taken for maximum current to flow in the circuit, (c) the energy stored in the inductor when maximum current is flowing, and (d) the time for current to drop to 750 mA after switching to position C.

[(a) 64.38 ms (b) 0.20 s
(c) 0.20 J (d) 7.67 ms]

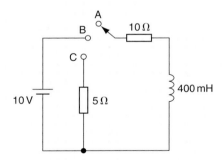

Figure 18.15

18.11 Switching inductive circuits

Energy stored in the magnetic field of an inductor exists because a current provides the magnetic field. When the d.c. supply is switched off the current falls rapidly, the magnetic field collapses causing a large induced e.m.f. which will either cause an arc across the switch contacts or will break down the insulation between adjacent turns of the coil. The high induced e.m.f. acts in a direction which tends to keep the current flowing, i.e. in the same direction as the applied voltage. The energy from the magnetic field will thus be aided by the supply voltage in maintaining an arc, which could cause severe damage to the switch. To reduce the induced e.m.f. when the supply switch is opened, a discharge resistor R_D is connected in parallel with the inductor as shown in Fig. 18.16. The magnetic field energy is dissipated as heat in R_D and R and arcing at the switch contacts is avoided.

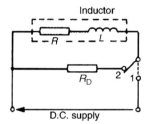

Figure 18.16

18.12 The effects of time constant on a rectangular waveform

Integrator circuit

By varying the value of either C or R in a series-connected $C-R$ circuit, the time constant ($\tau = CR$), of a circuit can be varied. If a rectangular waveform varying from $+E$ to $-E$ is applied to a $C-R$ circuit as shown in Fig. 18.17, output waveforms of the capacitor voltage have various shapes, depending on the value of R. When R is small, $\tau = CR$ is small and an output waveform such as that shown in Fig. 18.18(a) is obtained. As the value of R is increased, the waveform changes to that shown in Fig. 18.18(b). When R is large,

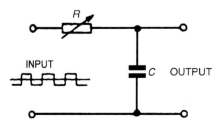

Figure 18.17

the waveform is as shown in Fig. 18.18(c), the circuit then being described as an **integrator circuit**.

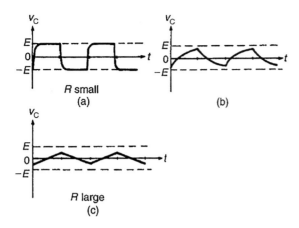

Figure 18.18

Differentiator circuit

If a rectangular waveform varying from $+E$ to $-E$ is applied to a series connected $C - R$ circuit and the waveform of the voltage drop across the resistor is observed, as shown in Fig. 18.19, the output waveform alters as R is varied due to the time constant, $(\tau = CR)$, altering.

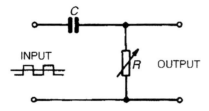

Figure 18.19

When R is small, the waveform is as shown in Fig. 18.20(a), the voltage being generated across R by the capacitor discharging fairly quickly. Since the change in capacitor voltage is from $+E$ to $-E$, the change in discharge current is $2E/R$, resulting in

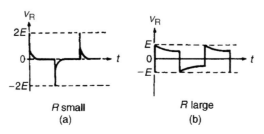

Figure 18.20

a change in voltage across the resistor of $2E$. This circuit is called a **differentiator circuit**. When R is large, the waveform is as shown in Fig. 18.20(b).

Now try the following exercises

A capacitor of capacitance C farads is connected in series with a resistor of R ohms and is switched across a constant voltage d.c. supply of V volts. After a time of t seconds, the current flowing is i amperes. Use this data to answer questions 1 to 10.

1. The voltage drop across the resistor at time t seconds is $v_R = \ldots\ldots$

2. The capacitor voltage at time t seconds is $v_C = \ldots\ldots$

3. The voltage equation for the circuit is $V = \ldots\ldots$

4. The time constant for the circuit is $\tau = \ldots\ldots$

5. The final value of the current flowing is $\ldots\ldots$

6. The initial value of the current flowing is $I = \ldots\ldots$

7. The final value of capacitor voltage is $\ldots\ldots$

8. The initial value of capacitor voltage is $\ldots\ldots$

9. The final value of the voltage drop across the resistor is $\ldots\ldots$

10. The initial value of the voltage drop across the resistor is $\ldots\ldots$

A capacitor charged to V volts is disconnected from the supply and discharged through a resistor of R ohms. Use this data to answer questions 11 to 15.

11. The initial value of current flowing is $I = \ldots\ldots$

12. The approximate time for the current to fall to zero in terms of C and R is $\ldots\ldots$ seconds

13. If the value of resistance R is doubled, the time for the current to fall to zero is $\ldots\ldots$ when compared with the time in question 12 above

14. The approximate fall in the value of the capacitor voltage in a time equal to one time constant is ...... per cent

15. The time constant of the circuit is given by ...... seconds

An inductor of inductance L henrys and negligible resistance is connected in series with a resistor of resistance R ohms and is switched across a constant voltage d.c. supply of V volts. After a time interval of t seconds, the transient current flowing is i amperes. Use this data to answer questions 16 to 25.

16. The induced e.m.f., v_L, opposing the current flow when $t = 0$ is ......

17. The voltage drop across the resistor when $t = 0$ is $v_R = $ ......

18. The current flowing when $t = 0$ is ......

19. V, v_R and v_L are related by the equation $V = $ ......

20. The time constant of the circuit in terms of L and R is ......

21. The steady-state value of the current is reached in practise in a time equal to ...... seconds

22. The steady-state voltage across the inductor is ...... volts

23. The final value of the current flowing is ...... amperes

24. The steady-state resistor voltage is ...... volts

25. The e.m.f. induced in the inductor during the transient in terms of current, time and inductance is ...... volts

A series-connected $L - R$ circuit carrying a current of I amperes is suddenly short-circuited to allow the current to decay exponentially. Use this data to answer questions 26 to 30.

26. The current will fall to ...... per cent of its final value in a time equal to the time constant

27. The voltage equation of the circuit is ......

28. The time constant of the circuit in terms of L and R is ......

29. The current reaches zero in a time equal to ...... seconds

30. If the value of R is halved, the time for the current to fall to zero is ...... when compared with the time in question 29

31. With the aid of a circuit diagram, explain briefly the effects on the waveform of the capacitor voltage of altering the value of resistance in a series connected $C - R$ circuit, when a rectangular wave is applied to the circuit

32. What do you understand by the term 'integrator circuit' ?

33. With reference to a rectangular wave applied to a series connected $C - R$ circuit, explain briefly the shape of the waveform when R is small and hence what you understand by the term 'differentiator circuit'

Exercise 107   Multi-choice questions on d.c. transients
(Answers on page 421)

An uncharged $2\,\mu F$ capacitor is connected in series with a $5\,M\Omega$ resistor to a $100\,V$, constant voltage, d.c. supply. In questions 1 to 7, use this data to select the correct answer from those given below:

(a) $10\,ms$ (b) $100\,V$ (c) $10\,s$
(d) $10\,V$ (e) $20\,\mu A$ (f) $1\,s$
(g) $0\,V$ (h) $50\,V$ (i) $1\,ms$
(j) $50\,\mu A$ (k) $20\,mA$ (l) $0\,A$

1. Determine the time constant of the circuit

2. Determine the final voltage across the capacitor

3. Determine the initial voltage across the resistor

4. Determine the final voltage across the resistor

5. Determine the initial voltage across the capacitor

6. Determine the initial current flowing in the circuit

7. Determine the final current flowing in the circuit

In questions 8 and 9, a series connected $C - R$ circuit is suddenly connected to a d.c. source of V volts. Which of the statements is false ?

8. (a) The initial current flowing is given by V/R
   (b) The time constant of the circuit is given by CR
   (c) The current grows exponentially
   (d) The final value of the current is zero

9. (a) The capacitor voltage is equal to the voltage drop across the resistor
   (b) The voltage drop across the resistor decays exponentially
   (c) The initial capacitor voltage is zero
   (d) The initial voltage drop across the resistor is IR, where I is the steady-state current

10. A capacitor which is charged to V volts is discharged through a resistor of R ohms. Which of the following statements is false?
    (a) The initial current flowing is V/R amperes
    (b) The voltage drop across the resistor is equal to the capacitor voltage
    (c) The time constant of the circuit is CR seconds
    (d) The current grows exponentially to a final value of V/R amperes

An inductor of inductance 0.1 H and negligible resistance is connected in series with a 50 Ω resistor to a 20 V d.c. supply. In questions 11 to 15, use this data to determine the value required, selecting your answer from those given below:
(a) 5 ms   (b) 12.6 V   (c) 0.4 A
(d) 500 ms (e) 7.4 V   (f) 2.5 A
(g) 2 ms   (h) 0 V   (i) 0 A
(j) 20 V

11. The value of the time constant of the circuit

12. The approximate value of the voltage across the resistor after a time equal to the time constant

13. The final value of the current flowing in the circuit

14. The initial value of the voltage across the inductor

15. The final value of the steady-state voltage across the inductor

16. The time constant for a circuit containing a capacitance of 100 nF in series with a 5 Ω resistance is:
    (a) 0.5 μs (b) 20 ns (c) 5 μs (d) 50 μs

17. The time constant for a circuit containing an inductance of 100 mH in series with a resistance of 4 Ω is:
    (a) 25 ms (b) 400 s (c) 0.4 s (d) 40 s

18. The graph shown in Fig. 18.21 represents the growth of current in an $L - R$ series circuit connected to a d.c. voltage V volts. The equation for the graph is:
    (a) $i = I(1 - e^{-Rt/L})$ (b) $i = Ie^{-Li/t}$
    (c) $i = Ie^{-Rt/L}$ (d) $i = I(1 - e^{RL/t})$

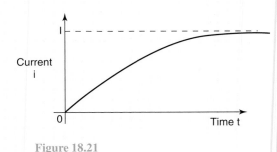

Figure 18.21

Chapter 19

Operational amplifiers

At the end of this chapter you should be able to:

- recognize the main properties of an operational amplifier
- understand op amp parameters input bias current and offset current and voltage
- define and calculate common-mode rejection ratio
- appreciate slew rate
- explain the principle of operation, draw the circuit diagram symbol and calculate gain for the following operational amplifiers:

  inverter

  non-inverter

  voltage follower (or buffer)

  summing

  voltage comparator

  integrator

  differentiator

- understand digital to analogue conversion
- understand analogue to digital conversion

19.1 Introduction to operational amplifiers

Operational Amplifiers (usually called **'op amps'**) were originally made from discrete components, being designed to solve mathematical equations electronically, by performing operations such as addition and division in analogue computers. Now produced in integrated-circuit (IC) form, op amps have many uses, with one of the most important being as a high-gain d.c. and a.c. voltage amplifier.

The **main properties** of an op amp include:

(i) a very high open-loop voltage gain A_o of around 10^5 for d.c. and low frequency a.c., which decreases with frequency increase

(ii) a very high input impedance, typically $10^6\,\Omega$ to $10^{12}\,\Omega$, such that current drawn from the device, or the circuit supplying it, is very small and the input voltage is passed on to the op amp with little loss

(iii) a very low output impedance, around $100\,\Omega$, such that its output voltage is transferred efficiently to any load greater than a few kilohms. The **circuit diagram symbol** for an op amp is shown in Fig. 19.1. It has one output, V_o, and two inputs; the **inverting input**, V_1 is marked $-$, and the non-**inverting input**, V_2, is marked $+$

The operation of an op amp is most convenient from a dual balanced d.c. power supply $\pm V_s$ (i.e. $+V_s$, 0, $-V_s$); the centre point of the supply, i.e. $0\,V$, is

DOI: 10.1016/B978-0-08-089056-2.00019-X

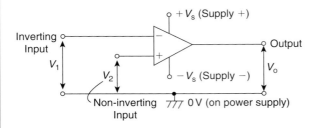

Figure 19.1

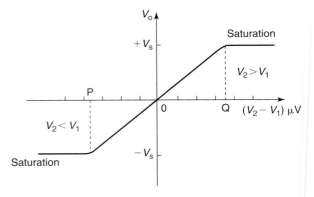

Figure 19.2

common to the input and output circuits and is taken as their voltage reference level. The power supply connections are not usually shown in a circuit diagram.

An op amp is basically a **differential** voltage amplifier, i.e. it amplifies the difference between input voltages V_1 and V_2. Three situations are possible:

(i) if $V_2 > V_1$, V_0 is positive

(ii) if $V_2 < V_1$, V_0 is negative

(iii) if $V_2 = V_1$, V_0 is zero

In general, $V_0 = A_0(V_2 - V_1)$

or $A_0 = \dfrac{V_0}{V_2 - V_1}$ (1)

where A_0 is the open-loop voltage gain.

> **Problem 1.** A differential amplifier has an open-loop voltage gain of 120. The input signals are 2.45 V and 2.35 V. Calculate the output voltage of the amplifier.

From equation (1), **output voltage**,

$$V_0 = A_0(V_2 - V_1) = 120(2.45 - 2.35)$$

$$= (120)(0.1) = \mathbf{12\,V}$$

Transfer characteristic

A typical **voltage characteristic** showing how the output V_0 varies with the input $(V_2 - V_1)$ is shown in Fig. 19.2.

It is seen from Fig. 19.2 that only within the very small input range P0Q is the output directly proportional to the input; it is in this range that the op amp behaves linearly and there is minimum distortion of the amplifier output. Inputs outside the linear range cause saturation and the output is then close to the maximum value, i.e. $+V_s$ or $-V_s$. The limited linear behaviour is due to the very high

open-loop gain A_0, and the higher it is the greater is the limitation.

Negative feedback

Operational amplifiers nearly always use **negative feedback**, obtained by feeding back some, or all, of the output to the inverting (−) input (as shown in Fig. 19.5 in the next section). The feedback produces an output voltage that opposes the one from which it is taken. This reduces the new output of the amplifier and the resulting closed-loop gain A is then less than the open-loop gain A_0. However, as a result, a wider range of voltages can be applied to the input for amplification. As long as $A_0 \gg A$, negative feedback gives:

(i) a constant and predictable voltage gain A,

(ii) reduced distortion of the output, and

(iii) better frequency response.

The advantages of using negative feedback outweigh the accompanying loss of gain which is easily increased by using two or more op amp stages.

Bandwidth

The open-loop voltage gain of an op amp is not constant at all frequencies; because of capacitive effects it falls at high frequencies. Figure 19.3 shows the gain/bandwidth characteristic of a 741 op amp. At frequencies below 10 Hz the gain is constant, but at higher frequencies the gain falls at a constant rate of 6 dB/octave (equivalent to a rate of 20 dB per decade) to 0 dB. The gain-bandwidth product for any amplifier is the linear voltage gain multiplied by the bandwidth at that gain. The value of frequency at which the

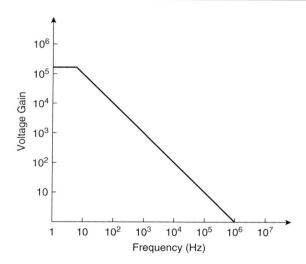

Figure 19.3

open-loop gain has fallen to unity is called the transition frequency f_T.

$$f_T = \text{closed-loop voltage gain} \times \text{bandwidth} \qquad (2)$$

In Fig. 19.3, $f_T = 10^6$ Hz or 1 MHz; a gain of 20 dB (i.e. $20 \log_{10} 10$) gives a 100 kHz bandwidth, whilst a gain of 80 dB (i.e. $20 \log_{10} 10^4$) restricts the bandwidth to 100 Hz.

19.2 Some op amp parameters

Input bias current

The input bias current, I_B, is the average of the currents into the two input terminals with the output at zero volts, which is typically around 80 nA (i.e. 80×10^{-9} A) for a 741 op amp. The input bias current causes a volt drop across the equivalent source impedance seen by the op amp input.

Input offset current

The input offset current, I_{os}, of an op amp is the difference between the two input currents with the output at zero volts. In a 741 op amp, I_{os} is typically 20 nA.

Input offset voltage

In the ideal op amp, with both inputs at zero there should be zero output. Due to imbalances within the amplifier this is not always the case and a small output voltage results. The effect can be nullified by applying a small offset voltage, V_{os}, to the amplifier. In a 741 op amp, V_{os} is typically 1 mV.

Common-mode rejection ratio

The output voltage of an op amp is proportional to the difference between the voltages applied to its two input terminals. Ideally, when the two voltages are equal, the output voltages should be zero. A signal applied to both input terminals is called a common-mode signal and it is usually an unwanted noise voltage. The ability of an op amp to suppress common-mode signals is expressed in terms of its common-mode rejection ratio (CMRR), which is defined by:

$$\text{CMRR} = 20 \log_{10} \left(\frac{\text{differential}}{\text{common-mode}} \right) \text{dB} \qquad (3)$$

In a 741 op amp, the CMRR is typically 90 dB. The common-mode gain, A_{com}, is defined as:

$$A_{com} = \frac{V_o}{V_{com}} \qquad (4)$$

where V_{com} is the common input signal.

Problem 2. Determine the common-mode gain of an op amp that has a differential voltage gain of 150×10^3 and a CMRR of 90 dB.

From equation (3),

$$\text{CMRR} = 20 \log_{10} \left(\frac{\text{differential}}{\text{common-mode}} \right) \text{dB}$$

Hence $\quad 90 = 20 \log_{10} \left(\dfrac{150 \times 10^3}{\text{common-mode}} \right)$

from which

$$4.5 = \log_{10} \left(\frac{150 \times 10^3}{\text{common-mode}} \right)$$

and $\quad 10^{4.5} = \dfrac{150 \times 10^3}{\text{common-mode}}$

Hence, **common-mode gain** $= \dfrac{150 \times 10^3}{10^{4.5}} = \mathbf{4.74}$

> **Problem 3.** A differential amplifier has an open-loop voltage gain of 120 and a common input signal of 3.0 V to both terminals. An output signal of 24 mV results. Calculate the common-mode gain and the CMRR.

From equation (4), the common-mode gain,

$$\mathbf{A}_{com} = \frac{V_o}{V_{com}} = \frac{24 \times 10^{-3}}{3.0} = 8 \times 10^{-3} = \mathbf{0.008}$$

From equation (3), the

$$\mathbf{CMRR} = 20 \log_{10} \left(\frac{\text{differential voltage gain}}{\text{common-mode gain}} \right) \text{dB}$$

$$= 20 \log_{10} \left(\frac{120}{0.008} \right)$$

$$= 20 \log_{10} 15\,000 = \mathbf{83.52\,dB}$$

Slew rate

The slew rate of an op amp is the maximum rate of change of output voltage following a step input voltage. Figure 19.4 shows the effects of slewing; it causes the output voltage to change at a slower rate than the input, such that the output waveform is a distortion of the input waveform. 0.5 V/μs is a typical value for the slew rate.

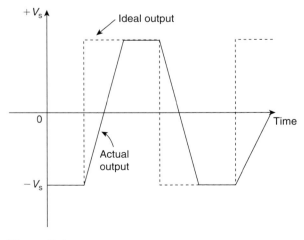

Figure 19.4

19.3 Op amp inverting amplifier

The basic circuit for an inverting amplifier is shown in Fig. 19.5 where the input voltage V_i (a.c. or d.c.) to be amplified is applied via resistor R_i to the inverting ($-$) terminal; the output voltage V_o is therefore in anti-phase with the input. The non-inverting ($+$) terminal is held at 0 V. Negative feedback is provided by the feedback resistor, R_f, feeding back a certain fraction of the output voltage to the inverting terminal.

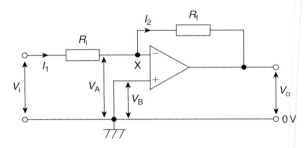

Figure 19.5

Amplifier gain

In an **ideal op amp** two assumptions are made, these being that:

(i) each input draws zero current from the signal source, i.e. their input impedances are infinite, and

(ii) the inputs are both at the same potential if the op amp is not saturated, i.e. $V_A = V_B$ in Fig. 19.5

In Fig. 19.5, $V_B = 0$, hence $V_A = 0$ and point X is called a **virtual earth**. Thus,

$$I_1 = \frac{V_i - 0}{R_i}$$

and

$$I_2 = \frac{0 - V_o}{R_f}$$

However, $I_1 = I_2$ from assumption (i) above. Hence

$$\frac{V_i}{R_i} = \frac{-V_o}{R_f}$$

the negative sign showing that V_o is negative when V_i is positive, and vice versa.

The **closed-loop gain** A is given by:

$$A = \frac{V_o}{V_i} = \frac{-R_f}{R_i} \tag{5}$$

This shows that the gain of the amplifier depends only on the two resistors, which can be made with precise values, and not on the characteristics of the op amp, which may vary from sample to sample.

For example, if $R_i = 10\,k\Omega$ and $R_f = 100\,k\Omega$, then the closed-loop gain,

$$A = \frac{-R_f}{R_i} = \frac{-100 \times 10^3}{10 \times 10^3} = -10$$

Thus an input of 100 mV will cause an output change of 1 V.

Input impedance

Since point X is a virtual earth (i.e. at 0 V), R_i may be considered to be connected between the inverting ($-$) input terminal and 0 V. The input impedance of the circuit is therefore R_i in parallel with the much greater input impedance of the op amp, i.e. effectively R_i. The circuit input impedance can thus be controlled by simply changing the value of R_i.

Problem 4. In the inverting amplifier of Fig. 19.5, $R_i = 1\,k\Omega$ and $R_f = 2\,k\Omega$. Determine the output voltage when the input voltage is: (a) +0.4 V (b) −1.2 V.

From equation (5),

$$V_o = \left(\frac{-R_f}{R_i}\right) V_i$$

(a) When $V_i = +0.4\,V$,

$$V_o = \left(\frac{-2000}{1000}\right)(+0.4) = -0.8\,V$$

(b) When $V_i = -1.2\,V$,

$$V_o = \left(\frac{-2000}{1000}\right)(-1.2) = +2.4\,V$$

Problem 5. The op amp shown in Fig. 19.6 has an input bias current of 100 nA at 20 °C. Calculate (a) the voltage gain, and (b) the output offset

---

voltage due to the input bias current. (c) How can the effect of input bias current be minimised?

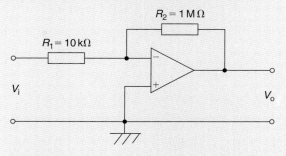

Figure 19.6

Comparing Fig. 19.6 with Fig. 19.5, gives $R_i = 10\,k\Omega$ and $R_f = 1\,M\Omega$

(a) From equation (5), **voltage gain**,

$$A = \frac{-R_f}{R_i} = \frac{-1 \times 10^6}{10 \times 10^3} = -100$$

(b) The input bias current, I_B, causes a volt drop across the equivalent source impedance seen by the op amp input, in this case, R_i and R_f in parallel. Hence, the offset voltage, V_{os}, at the input due to the 100 nA input bias current, I_B, is given by:

$$V_{os} = I_B \left(\frac{R_i R_f}{R_i + R_f}\right)$$

$$= (100 \times 10^{-9})\left(\frac{10 \times 10^3 \times 1 \times 10^6}{(10 \times 10^3) + (1 \times 10^6)}\right)$$

$$= (10^{-7})(9.9 \times 10^3) = 9.9 \times 10^{-4}$$

$$= 0.99\,mV$$

(c) The effect of input bias current can be minimised by ensuring that both inputs 'see' the same driving resistance. This means that **a resistance of value of 9.9 kΩ** (from part (b)) **should be placed between the non-inverting (+) terminal and earth** in Fig. 19.6

Problem 6. Design an inverting amplifier to have a voltage gain of 40 dB, a closed-loop bandwidth of 5 kHz and an input resistance of 10 kΩ.

Section 2

The voltage gain of an op amp, in decibels, is given by:

$$\text{gain in decibels} = 20 \log_{10} (\text{voltage gain})$$

from Chapter 10.

Hence $\qquad 40 = 20 \log_{10} A$

from which, $\qquad 2 = \log_{10} A$

and $\qquad A = 10^2 = 100$

With reference to Fig. 19.5, and from equation (5),

$$A = \left| \frac{R_f}{R_i} \right|$$

i.e. $\qquad 100 = \dfrac{R_f}{10 \times 10^3}$

Hence $\qquad R_f = 100 \times 10 \times 10^3 = 1\,M\Omega$

From equation (2), Section 19.1,

$$\textbf{frequency} = \text{gain} \times \text{bandwidth}$$

$$= 100 \times 5 \times 10^3$$

$$= \mathbf{0.5\,MHz} \text{ or } \mathbf{500\,kHz}$$

Now try the following exercise

Exercise 108 Further problems on operational amplifiers

1. A differential amplifier has an open-loop voltage gain of 150 when the input signals are 3.55 V and 3.40 V. Determine the output voltage of the amplifier. [22.5 V]

2. Calculate the differential voltage gain of an op amp that has a common-mode gain of 6.0 and a CMRR of 80 dB. $[6 \times 10^4]$

3. A differential amplifier has an open-loop voltage gain of 150 and a common input signal of 4.0 V to both terminals. An output signal of 15 mV results. Determine the common-mode gain and the CMRR. $[3.75 \times 10^{-3}, 92.04\,dB]$

4. In the inverting amplifier of Fig. 19.5 (on page 298), $R_i = 1.5\,k\Omega$ and $R_f = 2.5\,k\Omega$.

Determine the output voltage when the input voltage is: (a) +0.6 V (b) −0.9 V
[(a) −1.0 V (b) +1.5 V]

5. The op amp shown in Fig. 19.7 has an input bias current of 90 nA at 20°C. Calculate (a) the voltage gain, and (b) the output offset voltage due to the input bias current.
[(a) −80 (b) 1.33 mV]

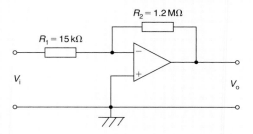

Figure 19.7

6. Determine (a) the value of the feedback resistor, and (b) the frequency for an inverting amplifier to have a voltage gain of 45 dB, a closed-loop bandwidth of 10 kHz and an input resistance of 20 kΩ.
[(a) 3.56 MΩ (b) 1.78 MHz]

19.4 Op amp non-inverting amplifier

The basic circuit for a non-inverting amplifier is shown in Fig. 19.8 where the input voltage V_i (a.c. or d.c.) is applied to the non-inverting (+) terminal of the op amp. This produces an output V_o that is in phase with the input. Negative feedback is obtained by feeding back to the inverting (−) terminal, the fraction of V_o developed across R_i in the voltage divider formed by R_f and R_i across V_o.

Amplifier gain

In Fig. 19.8, let the feedback factor,

$$\beta = \frac{R_i}{R_i + R_f}$$

It may be shown that for an amplifier with open-loop gain A_o, the closed-loop voltage gain A is given by:

$$A = \frac{A_o}{1 + \beta A_o}$$

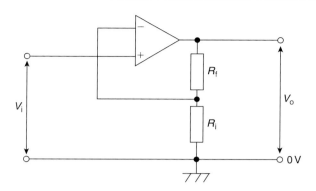

Figure 19.8

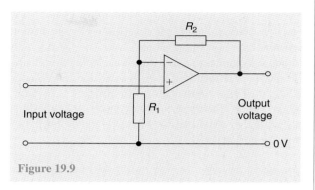

Figure 19.9

For a typical op amp, $A_o = 10^5$, thus βA_o is large compared with 1, and the above expression approximates to:

$$A = \frac{A_o}{\beta A_o} = \frac{1}{\beta} \qquad (6)$$

Hence $\qquad A = \dfrac{V_o}{V_i} = \dfrac{R_i + R_f}{R_i} = 1 + \dfrac{R_f}{R_i} \qquad (7)$

For example, if $R_i = 10\,\text{k}\Omega$ and $R_f = 100\,\text{k}\Omega$, then

$$A = 1 + \frac{100 \times 10^3}{10 \times 10^3} = 1 + 10 = \mathbf{11}$$

Again, the gain depends only on the values of R_i and R_f and is independent of the open-loop gain A_o.

Input impedance

Since there is no virtual earth at the non-inverting (+) terminal, the input impedance is much higher (– typically 50 MΩ) than that of the inverting amplifier. Also, it is unaffected if the gain is altered by changing R_f and/or R_i. This non-inverting amplifier circuit gives good matching when the input is supplied by a high impedance source.

Problem 7. For the op amp shown in Fig. 19.9, $R_1 = 4.7\,\text{k}\Omega$ and $R_2 = 10\,\text{k}\Omega$. If the input voltage is $-0.4\,\text{V}$, determine (a) the voltage gain (b) the output voltage.

The op amp shown in Fig. 19.9 is a non-inverting amplifier, similar to Fig. 19.8

(a) From equation (7), **voltage gain**,

$$A = 1 + \frac{R_f}{R_i} = 1 + \frac{R_2}{R_1} = 1 + \frac{10 \times 10^3}{4.7 \times 10^3}$$
$$= 1 + 2.13 = \mathbf{3.13}$$

(b) Also from equation (7), **output voltage**,

$$V_o = \left(1 + \frac{R_2}{R_1}\right) V_i = (3.13)(-0.4) = \mathbf{-1.25\,V}$$

19.5 Op amp voltage-follower

The **voltage-follower** is a special case of the non-inverting amplifier in which 100% negative feedback is obtained by connecting the output directly to the inverting (−) terminal, as shown in Fig. 19.10. Thus R_f in Fig. 19.8 is zero and R_i is infinite.

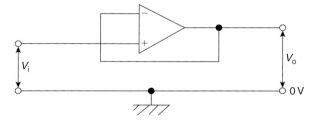

Figure 19.10

From equation (6), $A = 1/\beta$ (when A_o is very large). Since all of the output is fed back, $\beta = 1$ and $A \approx 1$. Thus the voltage gain is nearly 1 and $V_o = V_i$ to within a few millivolts.

The circuit of Fig. 19.10 is called a voltage-follower since, as with its transistor emitter-follower equivalent,

V_o follows V_i. It has an extremely high input impedance and a low output impedance. Its main use is as a **buffer amplifier,** giving current amplification, to match a high impedance source to a low impedance load. For example, it is used as the input stage of an analogue voltmeter where the highest possible input impedance is required so as not to disturb the circuit under test; the output voltage is measured by a relatively low impedance moving-coil meter.

19.6 Op amp summing amplifier

Because of the existence of the virtual earth point, an op amp can be used to add a number of voltages (d.c. or a.c.) when connected as a multi-input inverting amplifier. This, in turn, is a consequence of the high value of the open-loop voltage gain A_o. Such circuits may be used as 'mixers' in audio systems to combine the outputs of microphones, electric guitars, pick-ups, etc. They are also used to perform the mathematical process of addition in analogue computing.

The circuit of an op amp summing amplifier having three input voltages V_1, V_2 and V_3 applied via input resistors R_1, R_2 and R_3 is shown in Fig. 19.11. If it is assumed that the inverting ($-$) terminal of the op amp draws no input current, all of it passing through R_f, then:

$$I = I_1 + I_2 + I_3$$

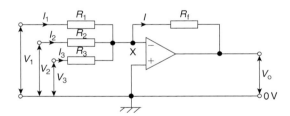

Figure 19.11

Since X is a virtual earth (i.e. at $0\,V$), it follows that:

$$\frac{-V_o}{R_f} = \frac{V_1}{R_1} + \frac{V_2}{R_2} + \frac{V_3}{R_3}$$

Hence

$$V_o = -\left(\frac{R_f}{R_1}V_1 + \frac{R_f}{R_2}V_2 + \frac{R_f}{R_3}V_3\right)$$

$$= -R_f\left(\frac{V_1}{R_1} + \frac{V_2}{R_2} + \frac{V_3}{R_3}\right) \qquad (8)$$

The three input voltages are thus added and amplified if R_f is greater than each of the input resistors; 'weighted'

summation is said to have occurred. Alternatively, the input voltages are added and attenuated if R_f is less than each input resistor.

For example, if

$$\frac{R_f}{R_1} = 4 \qquad \frac{R_f}{R_2} = 3$$

and

$$\frac{R_f}{R_3} = 1$$

and $V_1 = V_2 = V_3 = +1\,V$, then

$$V_o = -\left(\frac{R_f}{R_1}V_1 + \frac{R_f}{R_2}V_2 + \frac{R_f}{R_3}V_3\right)$$

$$= -(4+3+1) = -\mathbf{8\,V}$$

If $R_1 = R_2 = R_3 = R_i$, the input voltages are amplified or attenuated equally, and

$$V_o = -\frac{R_f}{R_i}(V_1 + V_2 + V_3)$$

If, also, $R_i = R_f$ then $V_o = -(V_1 + V_2 + V_3)$.

The virtual earth is also called the **summing point** of the amplifier. It isolates the inputs from one another so that each behaves as if none of the others existed and none feeds any of the other inputs even though all the resistors are connected at the inverting ($-$) input.

Problem 8. For the summing op amp shown in Fig. 19.12, determine the output voltage, V_o.

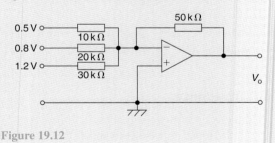

Figure 19.12

From equation (8),

$$V_o = -R_f\left(\frac{V_1}{R_1} + \frac{V_2}{R_2} + \frac{V_3}{R_3}\right)$$

$$= -(50 \times 10^3)\left(\frac{0.5}{10 \times 10^3} + \frac{0.8}{20 \times 10^3} + \frac{1.2}{30 \times 10^3}\right)$$

$$= -(50 \times 10^3)\,(5 \times 10^{-5} + 4 \times 10^{-5} + 4 \times 10^{-5})$$

$$= -(50 \times 10^3)\,(13 \times 10^{-5})$$

$$= -\mathbf{6.5\,V}$$

19.7 Op amp voltage comparator

If both inputs of the op amp shown in Fig. 19.13 are used simultaneously, then from equation (1), page 296, the output voltage is given by:

$$V_o = A_o(V_2 - V_1)$$

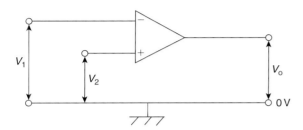

Figure 19.13

When $V_2 > V_1$ then V_o is positive, its maximum value being the positive supply voltage $+V_s$, which it has when $(V_2 - V_1) \geq V_s/A_o$. The op amp is then saturated. For example, if $V_s = +9$ V and $A_o = 10^5$, then saturation occurs when

$$(V_2 - V_1) \geq \frac{9}{10^5}$$

i.e. when V_2 exceeds V_1 by $90\,\mu$V and $V_o \approx 9$ V.

When $V_1 > V_2$, then V_o is negative and saturation occurs if V_1 exceeds V_2 by V_s/A_o i.e. around $90\,\mu$V in the above example; in this case, $V_o \approx -V_s = -9$ V.

A small change in $(V_2 - V_1)$ therefore causes V_o to switch between near $+V_s$ and near to $-V_s$ and enables the op amp to indicate when V_2 is greater or less than V_1, i.e. to act as a **differential amplifier** and compare two voltages. It does this in an electronic digital voltmeter.

> **Problem 9.** Devise a light-operated alarm circuit using an op amp, a LDR, a LED and a ± 15 V supply.

A typical light-operated alarm circuit is shown in Fig. 19.14.

Resistor R and the light dependent resistor (LDR) form a voltage divider across the $+15/0/-15$ V supply. The op amp compares the voltage V_1 at the voltage divider junction, i.e. at the inverting $(-)$ input, with that at the non-inverting $(+)$ input, i.e. with V_2, which is 0 V. In the dark the resistance of the LDR is much greater than that of R, so more of the 30 V across the voltage divider is dropped across the LDR, causing V_1 to fall below 0 V. Now $V_2 > V_1$ and the output voltage V_o switches from near -15 V to near $+15$ V and the light emitting diode (LED) lights.

19.8 Op amp integrator

The circuit for the op amp integrator shown in Fig. 19.15 is the same as for the op amp inverting amplifier shown in Fig. 19.5, but feedback occurs via a capacitor C, rather than via a resistor.

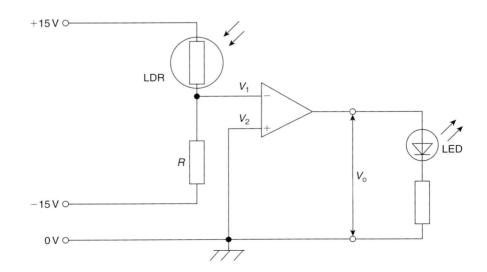

Figure 19.14

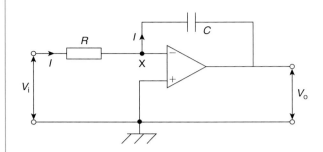

Figure 19.15

The output voltage is given by:

$$V_o = -\frac{1}{CR} \int V_i \, dt \qquad (9)$$

Since the inverting $(-)$ input is used in Fig. 19.15, V_o is negative if V_i is positive, and vice versa, hence the negative sign in equation (9).

Since X is a virtual earth in Fig. 19.15, i.e. at 0 V, the voltage across R is V_i and that across C is V_o. Assuming again that none of the input current I enters the op amp inverting $(-)$ input, then all of current I flows through C and charges it up. If V_i is constant, I will be a constant value given by $I = V_i/R$. Capacitor C therefore charges at a constant rate and the potential of the output side of C $(= V_o$, since its input side is zero) charges so that the feedback path absorbs I. If Q is the charge on C at time t and the p.d. across it (i.e. the output voltage) changes from 0 to V_o in that time then:

$$Q = -V_o C = It$$

(from Chapter 6)

i.e.
$$-V_o C = \frac{V_i}{R} t$$

i.e.
$$V = -\frac{1}{CR} V_i t$$

This result is the same as would be obtained from

$$V_o = -\frac{1}{CR} \int V_i \, dt$$

if V_i is a constant value.
For example, if the input voltage $V_i = -2$ V and, say, $CR = 1$ s, then

$$V_o = -(-2) t = 2t$$

A graph of V_o/t will be ramp function as shown in Fig. 19.16 ($V_o = 2t$ is of the straight line form $y = mx + c$; in this case $y = V_o$ and $x = t$, gradient, $m = 2$ and vertical axis intercept $c = 0$). V_o rises

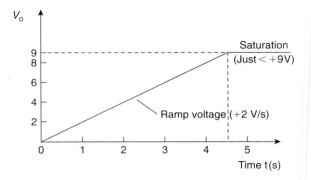

Figure 19.16

steadily by $+2V/s$ in Fig. 19.16, and if the power supply is, say, ± 9 V, then V_o reaches $+9$ V after 4.5 s when the op amp saturates.

> **Problem 10.** A steady voltage of -0.75 V is applied to an op amp integrator having component values of $R = 200\,\text{k}\Omega$ and $C = 2.5\,\mu\text{F}$. Assuming that the initial capacitor charge is zero, determine the value of the output voltage 100 ms after application of the input.

From equation (9), output voltage,

$$V_o = -\frac{1}{CR} \int V_i \, dt$$

$$= -\frac{1}{(2.5 \times 10^{-6})(200 \times 10^3)} \int (-0.75) \, dt$$

$$= -\frac{1}{0.5} \int (-0.75) \, dt = -2[-0.75t]$$

$$= +1.5t$$

When time $t = 100$ ms,
output voltage, $V_o = (1.5)(100 \times 10^{-3}) = \mathbf{0.15\,V}$.

19.9 Op amp differential amplifier

The circuit for an op amp differential amplifier is shown in Fig. 19.17 where voltages V_1 and V_2 are applied to its two input terminals and the difference between these voltages is amplified.

(i) Let V_1 volts be applied to terminal 1 and 0 V be applied to terminal 2. The difference in the potentials at the inverting $(-)$ and non-inverting $(+)$ op amp inputs is practically zero and hence the inverting terminal must be at zero potential. Then

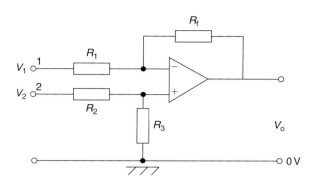

Figure 19.17

$I_1 = V_1/R_1$. Since the op amp input resistance is high, this current flows through the feedback resistor R_f. The volt drop across R_f, which is the output voltage

$$V_o = \frac{V_1}{R_1} R_f$$

hence, the closed loop voltage gain A is given by:

$$A = \frac{V_o}{V_1} = -\frac{R_f}{R_1} \quad (10)$$

(ii) By similar reasoning, if V_2 is applied to terminal 2 and 0 V to terminal 1, then the voltage appearing at the non-inverting terminal will be

$$\left(\frac{R_3}{R_2 + R_3}\right) V_2 \text{ volts.}$$

This voltage will also appear at the inverting (−) terminal and thus the voltage across R_1 is equal to

$$-\left(\frac{R_3}{R_2 + R_3}\right) V_2 \text{ volts.}$$

Now the output voltage,

$$V_o = \left(\frac{R_3}{R_2 + R_3}\right) V_2$$
$$+ \left[-\left(\frac{R_3}{R_2 + R_3}\right) V_2\right]\left(\frac{-R_f}{R_1}\right)$$

and the voltage gain,

$$A = \frac{V_o}{V_2}$$
$$= \left(\frac{R_3}{R_2 + R_3}\right) + \left[-\left(\frac{R_3}{R_2 + R_3}\right)\right]\left(-\frac{R_f}{R_1}\right)$$

i.e. $\quad A = \frac{V_o}{V_2} = \left(\frac{R_3}{R_2 + R_3}\right)\left(1 + \frac{R_f}{R_1}\right) \quad (11)$

(iii) Finally, if the voltages applied to terminals 1 and 2 are V_1 and V_2 respectively, then the difference between the two voltages will be amplified.

If $V_1 > V_2$, then:

$$V_o = (V_1 - V_2)\left(-\frac{R_f}{R_1}\right) \quad (12)$$

If $V_2 > V_1$, then:

$$V_o = (V_2 - V_1)\left(\frac{R_3}{R_2 + R_3}\right)\left(1 + \frac{R_f}{R_1}\right) \quad (13)$$

Problem 11. In the differential amplifier shown in Fig. 19.17, $R_1 = 10\,k\Omega$, $R_2 = 10\,k\Omega$, $R_3 = 100\,k\Omega$ and $R_f = 100\,k\Omega$. Determine the output voltage V_o if:
(a) $V_1 = 5\,mV$ and $V_2 = 0$
(b) $V_1 = 0$ and $V_2 = 5\,mV$
(c) $V_1 = 50\,mV$ and $V_2 = 25\,mV$
(d) $V_1 = 25\,mV$ and $V_2 = 50\,mV$.

(a) From equation (10),

$$V_o = -\frac{R_f}{R_1} V_1 = -\left(\frac{100 \times 10^3}{10 \times 10^3}\right)(5)\,mV$$
$$= -50\,mV$$

(b) From equation (11),

$$V_o = \left(\frac{R_3}{R_2 + R_3}\right)\left(1 + \frac{R_f}{R_1}\right) V_2$$
$$= \left(\frac{100}{110}\right)\left(1 + \frac{100}{10}\right)(5)\,mV = +50\,mV$$

(c) $V_1 > V_2$ hence from equation (12),

$$V_o = (V_1 - V_2)\left(-\frac{R_f}{R_1}\right)$$
$$= (50 - 25)\left(-\frac{100}{10}\right)mV = -250\,mV$$

(d) $V_2 > V_1$ hence from equation (13),

$$V_o = (V_2 - V_1)\left(\frac{R_3}{R_2 + R_3}\right)\left(1 + \frac{R_f}{R_1}\right)$$
$$= (50 - 25)\left(\frac{100}{100 + 10}\right)\left(1 + \frac{100}{10}\right)mV$$
$$= (25)\left(\frac{100}{110}\right)(11) = +250\,mV$$

Section 2

Now try the following exercise

Exercise 109 Further problems on operational amplifiers

1. If the input voltage for the op amp shown in Fig. 19.18, is -0.5 V, determine (a) the voltage gain (b) the output voltage

    [(a) 3.21 (b) -1.60 V]

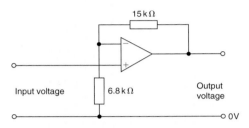

Figure 19.18

2. In the circuit of Fig. 19.19, determine the value of the output voltage, V_o, when (a) $V_1 = +1$ V and $V_2 = +3$ V (b) $V_1 = +1$ V and $V_2 = -3$ V   [(a) -10 V (b) $+5$ V]

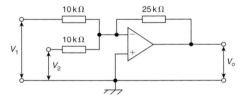

Figure 19.19

3. For the summing op amp shown in Fig. 19.20, determine the output voltage, V_o

    [-3.9 V]

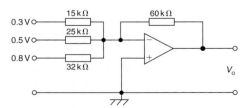

Figure 19.20

4. A steady voltage of -1.25 V is applied to an op amp integrator having component values of $R = 125$ kΩ and $C = 4.0\,\mu$F. Calculate the value of the output voltage 120 ms after applying the input, assuming that the initial capacitor charge is zero.   [0.3 V]

5. In the differential amplifier shown in Fig. 19.21, determine the output voltage, V_o, if: (a) $V_1 = 4$ mV and $V_2 = 0$ (b) $V_1 = 0$ and $V_2 = 6$ mV (c) $V_1 = 40$ mV and $V_2 = 30$ mV (d) $V_1 = 25$ mV and $V_2 = 40$ mV.

    [(a) -60 mV (b) $+90$ mV (c) -150 mV (d) $+225$ mV]

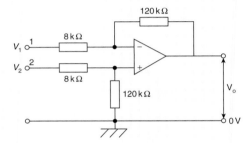

Figure 19.21

19.10 Digital to analogue (D/A) conversion

There are a number of situations when digital signals have to be converted to analogue ones. For example, a digital computer often needs to produce a graphical display on the screen; this involves using a D/A converter to change the two-level digital output voltage from the computer, into a continuously varying analogue voltage for the input to the cathode ray tube, so that it can deflect the electron beam to produce screen graphics.

A binary weighted resistor D/A converter is shown in Fig. 19.22 for a four-bit input. The values of the resistors, R, $2R$, $4R$, $8R$ increase according to the binary scale – hence the name of the converter. The circuit uses an op amp as a **summing amplifier** (see Section 19.6) with a feedback resistor R_f. Digitally controlled electronic switches are shown as S_1 to S_4. Each switch connects the resistor in series with it to a fixed reference voltage V_{REF} when the input bit controlling it is a 1 and to ground (0 V) when it is a 0. The input voltages V_1 to V_4 applied to the op amp by the four-bit

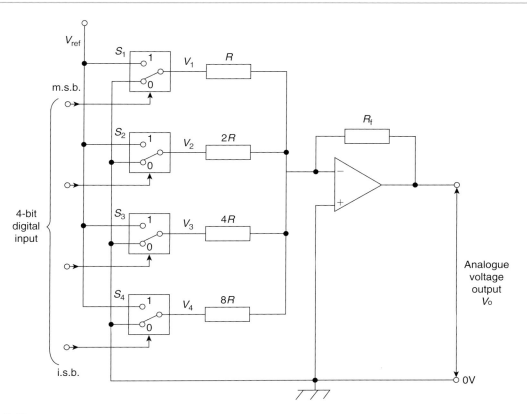

Figure 19.22

input via the resistors therefore have one of two values, i.e. either V_{REF} or 0 V.

From equation (8), page 302, the analogue output voltage V_o is given by:

$$V_o = -\left(\frac{R_f}{R}V_1 + \frac{R_f}{2R}V_2 + \frac{R_f}{4R}V_3 + \frac{R_f}{8R}V_4\right)$$

Let $R_f = R = 1\,k\Omega$, then:

$$V_o = -\left(V_1 + \frac{1}{2}V_2 + \frac{1}{4}V_3 + \frac{1}{8}V_4\right)$$

With a four-bit input of 0001 (i.e. decimal 1), S_4 connects $8R$ to V_{REF}, i.e. $V_4 = V_{REF}$, and S_1, S_2 and S_3 connect R, $2R$ and $4R$ to 0 V, making $V_1 = V_2 = V_3 = 0$. Let $V_{REF} = -8\,V$, then output voltage,

$$V_o = -\left(0 + 0 + 0 + \frac{1}{8}(-8)\right) = +1\,V$$

With a four-bit input of 0101 (i.e. decimal 5), S_2 and S_4 connects $2R$ and $8R$ to V_{REF}, i.e. $V_2 = V_4 = V_{REF}$, and S_1 and S_3 connect R and $4R$ to 0 V, making $V_1 = V_3 = 0$.

Again, if $V_{REF} = -8\,V$, then output voltage,

$$V_o = -\left(0 + \frac{1}{2}(-8) + 0 + \frac{1}{8}(-8)\right) = +5\,V$$

If the input is 0111 (i.e. decimal 7), the output voltage will be 7 V, and so on. From these examples, it is seen that the analogue output voltage, V_o, is directly proportional to the digital input. V_o has a 'stepped' waveform, the waveform shape depending on the binary input. A typical waveform is shown in Fig. 19.23.

19.11   Analogue to digital (A/D) conversion

In a digital voltmeter, its input is in analogue form and the reading is displayed digitally. This is an example where an analogue to digital converter is needed.

A block diagram for a four-bit counter type A/D conversion circuit is shown in Fig. 19.24. An op amp is again used, in this case as a **voltage comparator** (see Section 19.7). The analogue input voltage V_2, shown in

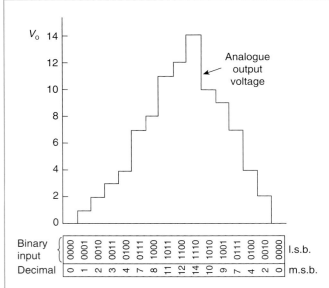

Figure 19.23

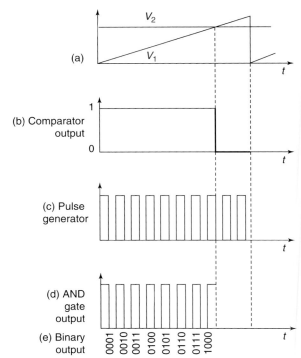

Fig. 19.25(a) as a steady d.c. voltage, is applied to the non-inverting (+) input, whilst a sawtooth voltage V_1 supplies the inverting (−) input.

The output from the comparator is applied to one input of an AND gate and is a 1 (i.e. 'high') until V_1 equals or exceeds V_2, when it then goes to 0 (i.e. 'low') as shown in Fig. 19.25(b). The other input of the AND gate is fed by a steady train of pulses from a pulse generator, as shown in Fig. 19.25(c). When both inputs to the AND gate are 'high', the gate 'opens' and gives a 'high' output, i.e. a pulse, as shown in Fig. 19.25(d). The time taken by V_1 to reach V_2 is proportional to the analogue voltage if the ramp is linear. The output pulses from the AND gate are recorded by a binary counter

Figure 19.25

and, as shown in Fig. 19.25(e), are the digital equivalent of the analogue input voltage V_2. In practise, the ramp generator is a D/A converter which takes its digital input from the binary counter, shown by the broken lines in Fig. 19.24. As the counter advances through its normal binary sequence, a staircase waveform with equal steps (i.e. a ramp) is built up at the output of the D/A converter (as shown by the first few steps in Fig. 19.23.

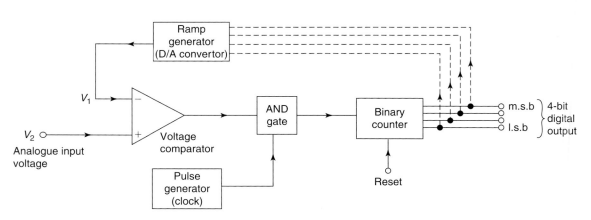

Figure 19.24

Now try the following exercises

Exercise 110   **Short answer questions on operational amplifiers**

1. List three main properties of an op amp

2. Sketch a typical voltage characteristic showing how the output voltage varies with the input voltage for an op amp

3. What effect does negative feedback have when applied to an op amp

4. Sketch a typical gain/bandwidth characteristic for an op amp

5. With reference to an op amp explain the parameters input bias current, input offset current and input offset voltage

6. Define common-mode rejection ratio

7. Explain the principle of operation of an op amp inverting amplifier

8. In an inverting amplifier, the closed-loop gain A is given by: $A = \ldots\ldots$

9. Explain the principle of operation of an op amp non-inverting amplifier

10. In a non-inverting amplifier, the closed-loop gain A is given by: $A = \ldots\ldots$

11. Explain the principle of operation of an op amp voltage-follower (or buffer)

12. Explain the principle of operation of an op amp summing amplifier

13. In a summing amplifier having three inputs, the output voltage V_0 is given by: $V_0 = \ldots\ldots$

14. Explain the principle of operation of an op amp voltage comparator

15. Explain the principle of operation of an op amp integrator

16. In an op amp integrator, the output voltage V_0 is given by: $V_0 = \ldots\ldots$

17. Explain the principle of operation of an op amp differential amplifier

18. Explain the principle of operation of a binary weighted resistor digital to analogue converter using a four-bit input

19. Explain the principle of operation of a four-bit counter type analogue to digital converter

Exercise 111   **Multi-choice questions on operational amplifiers**
(Answers on page 421)

1. A differential amplifier has an open-loop voltage gain of 100. The input signals are 2.5 V and 2.4 V. The output voltage of the amplifier is:
   (a) -10 V   (b) 1 mV
   (c) 10 V   (d) 1 kV

2. Which of the following statements relating to operational amplifiers is true?
   (a) It has a high open-loop voltage gain at low frequency, a low input impedance and low output impedance
   (b) It has a high open-loop voltage gain at low frequency, a high input impedance and low output impedance
   (c) It has a low open-loop voltage gain at low frequency, a high input impedance and low output impedance
   (d) It has a high open-loop voltage gain at low frequency, a low input impedance and high output impedance

3. A differential amplifier has a voltage gain of 120×10^3 and a common-mode rejection ratio of 100 dB. The common-mode gain of the operational amplifier is:
   (a) 1.2×10^3 (b) 1.2
   (c) 1.2×10^{10} (d) 1.2×10^{-5}

4. The output voltage, V_0, in the amplifier shown in Fig. 19.26 is:
   (a) -0.2 V   (b) $+1.8$ V
   (c) $+0.2$ V   (d) -1.8 V

5. The 3 kΩ resistor in Fig. 19.26 is replaced by one of value 0.1 MΩ. If the op amp has an input bias current of 80 nA, the output offset voltage is:
   (a) $79.2\,\mu$V   (b) $8\,\mu$V
   (c) 8 mV   (d) 80.2 nV

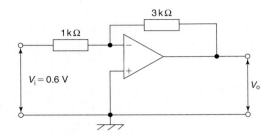

Figure 19.26

6. In the op amp shown in Fig. 19.27, the voltage gain is:
   (a) −3   (b) +4
   (c) +3   (d) −4

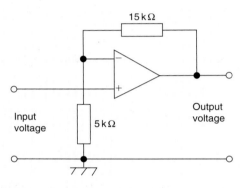

Figure 19.27

7. For the op amp shown in Fig. 19.28, the output voltage, V_o, is:
   (a) −1.2 V   (b) +5 V
   (c) +2 V   (d) −5 V

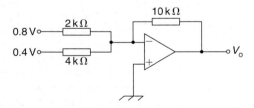

Figure 19.28

8. A steady voltage of −1.0 V is applied to an op amp integrator having component values of $R = 100\,k\Omega$ and $C = 10\,\mu F$. The value of the output voltage 10 ms after applying the input voltage is:
   (a) +10 mV   (b) −1 mV
   (c) −10 mV   (d) +1 mV

9. In the differential amplifier shown in Fig. 19.29, the output voltage, V_o, is:
   (a) +1.28 mV   (b) 1.92 mV
   (c) −1.28 mV   (d) +5 μV

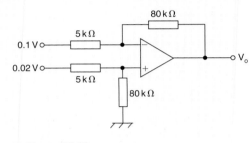

Figure 19.29

10. Which of the following statements is false?
    (a) A digital computer requires a D/A converter
    (b) When negative feedback is used in an op amp, a constant and predictable voltage gain results
    (c) A digital voltmeter requires a D/A converter
    (d) The value of frequency at which the open-loop gain has fallen to unity is called the transition frequency

This revision test covers the material contained in Chapters 15 to 19. *The marks for each question are shown in brackets at the end of each question.*

1. The power taken by a series inductive circuit when connected to a 100 V, 100 Hz supply is 250 W and the current is 5 A. Calculate (a) the resistance, (b) the impedance, (c) the reactance, (d) the power factor, and (e) the phase angle between voltage and current. (9)

2. A coil of resistance 20 Ω and inductance 200 mH is connected in parallel with a 4 μF capacitor across a 50 V, variable frequency supply. Calculate (a) the resonant frequency, (b) the dynamic resistance, (c) the current at resonance, and (d) the Q-factor at resonance. (10)

3. A series circuit comprises a coil of resistance 30 Ω and inductance 50 mH, and a 2500 pF capacitor. Determine the Q-factor of the circuit at resonance. (4)

4. The winding of an electromagnet has an inductance of 110 mH and a resistance of 5.5 Ω. When it is connected to a 110 V, d.c. supply, calculate (a) the steady-state value of current flowing in the winding, (b) the time constant of the circuit, (c) the value of the induced e.m.f. after 0.01 s, (d) the time for the current to rise to 75 per cent of it's final value, and (e) the value of the current after 0.02 s. (11)

5. A single-phase motor takes 30 A at a power factor of 0.65 lagging from a 300 V, 50 Hz supply. Calculate (a) the current taken by a capacitor connected in parallel with the motor to correct the power factor to unity, and (b) the value of the supply current after power factor correction. (7)

6. For the summing operational amplifier shown in Fig. RT5.1, determine the value of the output voltage, V_O (3)

7. In the differential amplifier shown in Fig. RT5.2, determine the output voltage, V_O when:
    (a) $V_1 = 4$ mV and $V_2 = 0$
    (b) $V_1 = 0$ and $V_2 = 5$ mV
    (c) $V_1 = 20$ mV and $V_2 = 10$ mV (6)

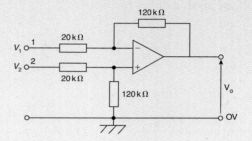

Figure RT5.2

8. A filter section is to have a characteristic impedance at zero frequency of 600 Ω and a cut-off frequency of 2.5 MHz. Design (a) a low-pass T-section filter, and (b) a low-pass π-section filter to meet these requirements. (6)

9. Determine the cut-off frequency and the nominal impedance for a high-pass π-connected section having a 5 nF capacitor in its series arm and inductances of 1 mH in each of its shunt arms. (4)

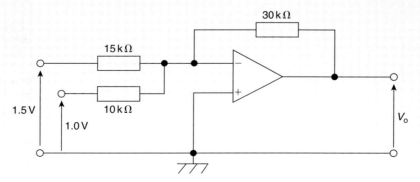

Figure RT5.1

Formulae for further electrical and electronic principles

A.C. Theory:

$$T = \frac{1}{f} \quad \text{or} \quad f = \frac{1}{T}$$

$$I = \sqrt{\frac{i_1^2 + i_2^2 + i_2^2 + \cdots + i_n^2}{n}}$$

For a sine wave: $I_{AV} = \frac{2}{\pi} I_m$ or $0.637\, I_m$

$$I = \frac{1}{\sqrt{2}} I_m \quad \text{or} \quad 0.707\, I_m$$

Form factor $= \dfrac{\text{r.m.s.}}{\text{average}}$ Peak factor $= \dfrac{\text{maximum}}{\text{r.m.s.}}$

General sinusoidal voltage: $v = V_m \sin(\omega t \pm \phi)$

Single-phase circuits:

$$X_L = 2\pi f L \qquad X_C = \frac{1}{2\pi f C}$$

$$Z = \frac{V}{I} = \sqrt{(R^2 + X^2)}$$

Series resonance: $f_r = \dfrac{1}{2\pi\sqrt{LC}}$

$$Q = \frac{V_L}{V} \quad \text{or} \quad \frac{V_C}{V} = \frac{2\pi f_r L}{R} = \frac{1}{2\pi f_r CR} = \frac{1}{R}\sqrt{\frac{L}{C}}$$

$$Q = \frac{f_r}{f_2 - f_1} \quad \text{or} \quad (f_2 - f_1) = \frac{f_r}{Q}$$

Parallel resonance (LR-C circuit):

$$f_r = \frac{1}{2\pi}\sqrt{\frac{1}{LC} - \frac{R^2}{L^2}}$$

$$I_r = \frac{VRC}{L} \qquad R_D = \frac{L}{CR}$$

$$Q = \frac{2\pi f_r L}{R} = \frac{I_C}{I_r}$$

$$P = VI\cos\phi \quad \text{or} \quad I^2 R \qquad S = VI \qquad Q = VI\sin\phi$$

$$\text{power factor} = \cos\phi = \frac{R}{Z}$$

Filter networks:

Low-pass T or π:

$$f_C = \frac{1}{\pi\sqrt{LC}} \qquad R_0 = \sqrt{\frac{L}{C}}$$

$$C = \frac{1}{\pi R_0 f_C} \qquad L = \frac{R_0}{\pi f_C}$$

See Fig. F1

High-pass T or π:

$$f_C = \frac{1}{4\pi\sqrt{LC}} \qquad R_0 = \sqrt{\frac{L}{C}}$$

$$C = \frac{1}{4\pi R_0 f_C} \qquad L = \frac{R_0}{4\pi f_C}$$

See Fig. F2

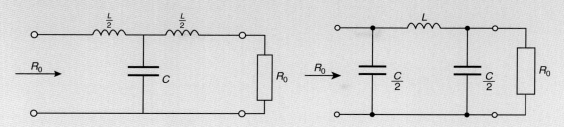

Figure F1

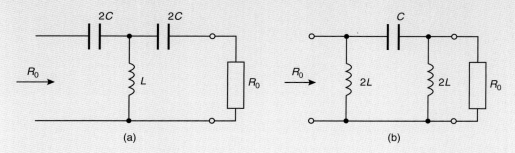

(a)   (b)

Figure F2

D.C. Transients:

C–R circuit $\tau = CR$

Charging: $v_C = V(1 - e^{-t/CR})$

$v_r = Ve^{-t/CR}$

$i = Ie^{-t/CR}$

Discharging: $v_C = v_R = Ve^{-t/CR}$

$i = Ie^{-t/CR}$

L–R circuit $\tau = \dfrac{L}{R}$

Current growth: $v_L = Ve^{-Rt/L}$

$v_R = V(1 - e^{-Rt/L})$

$i = I(1 - e^{-Rt/L})$

Current decay: $v_L = v_R = Ve^{-Rt/L}$

$i = Ie^{-Rt/L}$

Operational amplifiers:

$$CMRR = 20\log_{10}\left(\frac{\text{differential voltage gain}}{\text{common-mode gain}}\right)dB$$

Inverter: $A = \dfrac{V_o}{V_i} = \dfrac{-R_f}{R_i}$

Non-inverter: $A = \dfrac{V_o}{V_i} = 1 + \dfrac{R_f}{R_i}$

Summing: $V_o = -R_f\left(\dfrac{V_1}{R_1} + \dfrac{V_2}{R_2} + \dfrac{V_3}{R_3}\right)$

Integrator: $V_o = -\dfrac{1}{CR}\displaystyle\int V_i\,dt$

Differential:

If $V_1 > V_2$: $V_o = (V_1 - V_2)\left(-\dfrac{R_f}{R_1}\right)$

If $V_2 > V_1$: $V_o = (V_2 - V_1)\left(\dfrac{R_3}{R_2 + R_3}\right)\left(1 + \dfrac{R_f}{R_1}\right)$

Section 2

Electrical Power Technology

Chapter 20

Three-phase systems

At the end of this chapter you should be able to:

- describe a single-phase supply
- describe a three-phase supply
- understand a star connection, and recognise that $I_L = I_p$ and $V_L = \sqrt{3}V_p$
- draw a complete phasor diagram for a balanced, star connected load
- understand a delta connection, and recognise that $V_L = V_p$ and $I_L = \sqrt{3}I_p$
- draw a phasor diagram for a balanced, delta connected load
- calculate power in three-phase systems using $P = \sqrt{3}\,V_L I_L \cos\phi$
- appreciate how power is measured in a three-phase system, by the one, two and three-wattmeter methods
- compare star and delta connections
- appreciate the advantages of three-phase systems

20.1 Introduction

Generation, transmission and distribution of electricity via the National Grid system is accomplished by three-phase alternating currents.

The voltage induced by a single coil when rotated in a uniform magnetic field is shown in Fig. 20.1 and is known as a **single-phase voltage**. Most consumers are fed by means of a single-phase a.c. supply. Two wires are used, one called the live conductor (usually coloured red) and the other is called the neutral conductor (usually coloured black). The neutral is usually connected via protective gear to earth, the earth wire being coloured green. The standard voltage for a single-phase a.c. supply is 240 V. The majority of single-phase supplies are obtained by connection to a three-phase supply (see Fig. 20.5, page 319).

20.2 Three-phase supply

A three-phase supply is generated when three coils are placed 120° apart and the whole rotated in a uniform magnetic field as shown in Fig. 20.2(a). The result is three independent supplies of equal voltages which are each displaced by 120° from each other as shown in Fig. 20.2(b).

(i) The convention adopted to identify each of the phase voltages is: R-red, Y-yellow, and B-blue, as shown in Fig. 20.2

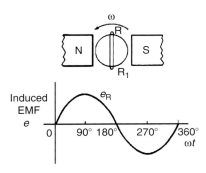

Figure 20.1

DOI: 10.1016/B978-0-08-089056-2.00020-6

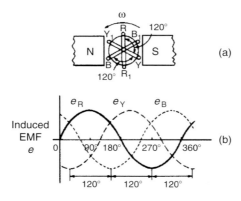

Figure 20.2

(ii) The **phase-sequence** is given by the sequence in which the conductors pass the point initially taken by the red conductor. The national standard phase sequence is R, Y, B.

A three-phase a.c. supply is carried by three conductors, called **'lines'** which are coloured red, yellow and blue. The currents in these conductors are known as line currents (I_L) and the p.d.'s between them are known as line voltages (V_L). A fourth conductor, called the **neutral** (coloured black, and connected through protective devices to earth) is often used with a three-phase supply. If the three-phase windings shown in Fig. 20.2 are kept independent then six wires are needed to connect a supply source (such as a generator) to a load (such as motor). To reduce the number of wires it is usual to interconnect the three phases. There are two ways in which this can be done, these being:

(a) a **star connection**, and (b) a **delta**, or **mesh, connection**. Sources of three-phase supplies, i.e. alternators, are usually connected in star, whereas three-phase transformer windings, motors and other loads may be connected either in star or delta.

20.3 Star connection

(i) A **star-connected load** is shown in Fig. 20.3 where the three line conductors are each connected to a load and the outlets from the loads are joined together at N to form what is termed the **neutral point** or the **star point**.

(ii) The voltages, V_R, V_Y and V_B are called **phase voltages** or line to neutral voltages. Phase voltages are generally denoted by V_p.

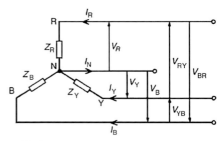

Figure 20.3

(iii) The voltages, V_{RY}, V_{YB} and V_{BR} are called **line voltages**.

(iv) From Fig. 20.3 it can be seen that the phase currents (generally denoted by I_p) are equal to their respective line currents I_R, I_Y and I_B, i.e. for a star connection:

$$I_L = I_p$$

(v) For a balanced system:

$$I_R = I_Y = I_B, \quad V_R = V_Y = V_B$$
$$V_{RY} = V_{YB} = V_{BR}, \quad Z_R = Z_Y = Z_B$$

and the current in the neutral conductor, $I_N = 0$. When a star-connected system is balanced, then the neutral conductor is unnecessary and is often omitted.

(vi) The line voltage, V_{RY}, shown in Fig. 20.4(a) is given by $V_{RY} = V_R - V_Y$ (V_Y is negative since it is in the opposite direction to V_{RY}). In the phasor diagram of Fig. 20.4(b), phasor V_Y is reversed (shown by the broken line) and then added phasorially to V_R (i.e. $V_{RY} = V_R + (-V_Y)$). By trigonometry, or by measurement, $V_{RY} = \sqrt{3}\, V_R$, i.e. for a balanced star connection:

$$V_L = \sqrt{3}\, V_p$$

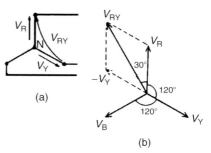

Figure 20.4

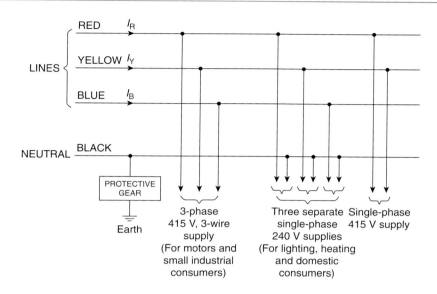

Figure 20.5

(See Problem 3 following for a complete phasor diagram of a star-connected system.)

(vii) The star connection of the three phases of a supply, together with a neutral conductor, allows the use of two voltages – the phase voltage and the line voltage. A 4-wire system is also used when the load is not balanced. The standard electricity supply to consumers in Great Britain is 415/240 V, 50 Hz, 3-phase, 4-wire alternating current, and a diagram of connections is shown in Fig. 20.5.

For most of the 20th century, the **supply voltage in the UK in domestic premises has been 240 V a.c.** (r.m.s.) at 50 Hz. In 1988, a European-wide agreement was reached to change the various national voltages, which ranged at the time from 220 V to 240 V, to a common European standard of **230 V**.

As a result, the standard nominal supply voltage in domestic single-phase 50 Hz installations in the UK has been 230 V since 1995. However, as an interim measure, electricity suppliers can work with an asymmetric voltage tolerance of 230 V +10%/−6% (i.e. 216.2 V to 253 V). The old standard was 240 V ±6% (i.e. 225.6 V to 254.4 V), which is mostly contained within the new range, and so in practice suppliers have had no reason to actually change voltages.

Similarly, the **three-phase voltage** in the UK had been for many years **415 V** ±6% (i.e. 390 V to 440 V). European harmonisation required this to be changed to **400 V** +10%/−6% (i.e. 376 V to 440 V). Again, since the present supply voltage of 415 V lies within this range, supply companies are unlikely to reduce their voltages in the near future.

Many of the calculations following are based on the 240 V/415 V supply voltages which have applied for many years and are likely to continue to do so.

> **Problem 1.** Three loads, each of resistance 30 Ω, are connected in star to a 415 V, 3-phase supply. Determine (a) the system phase voltage, (b) the phase current and (c) the line current.

A '415 V, 3-phase supply' means that 415 V is the line voltage, V_L

(a) For a star connection, $V_L = \sqrt{3} V_p$. Hence phase voltage, $V_p = V_L/\sqrt{3} = 415/\sqrt{3} = \mathbf{239.6\,V}$ or **240 V**, correct to 3 significant figures.

(b) Phase current, $I_p = V_p/R_p = 240/30 = \mathbf{8\,A}$

(c) For a star connection, $I_p = I_L$ hence the line current, $\mathbf{I_L = 8\,A}$

> **Problem 2.** A star-connected load consists of three identical coils each of resistance 30 Ω and inductance 127.3 mH. If the line current is 5.08 A, calculate the line voltage if the supply frequency is 50 Hz.

Inductive reactance

$$X_L = 2\pi f L = 2\pi(50)(127.3 \times 10^{-3}) = 40\,\Omega$$

Impedance of each phase

$$Z_p = \sqrt{R^2 + X_L^2} = \sqrt{30^2 + 40^2} = 50\,\Omega$$

For a star connection

$$I_L = I_p = \frac{V_p}{Z_p}$$

Hence phase voltage,

$$V_p = I_p Z_p = (5.08)(50) = 254\,V$$

Line voltage

$$V_L = \sqrt{3}\,V_p = \sqrt{3}(254) = \mathbf{440\,V}$$

> **Problem 3.** A balanced, three-wire, star-connected, 3-phase load has a phase voltage of 240 V, a line current of 5 A and a lagging power factor of 0.966. Draw the complete phasor diagram.

The phasor diagram is shown in Fig. 20.6.

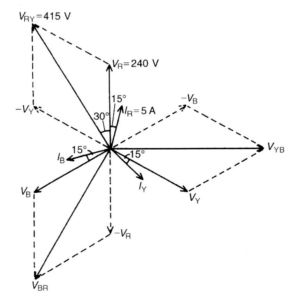

Figure 20.6

Procedure to construct the phasor diagram:

(i) Draw $V_R = V_Y = V_B = 240\,V$ and spaced $120°$ apart. (Note that V_R is shown vertically upwards – this however is immaterial for it may be drawn in any direction.)

(ii) Power factor $= \cos\phi = 0.966$ lagging. Hence the load phase angle is given by $\cos^{-1}0.966$, i.e. $15°$

lagging. Hence $I_R = I_Y = I_B = 5\,A$, lagging V_R, V_Y and V_B respectively by $15°$.

(iii) $V_{RY} = V_R - V_Y$ (phasorially). Hence V_Y is reversed and added phasorially to V_R. By measurement, $V_{RY} = 415\,V$ (i.e. $\sqrt{3} \times 240$) and leads V_R by $30°$. Similarly, $V_{YB} = V_Y - V_B$ and $V_{BR} = V_B - V_R$

> **Problem 4.** A 415 V, 3-phase, 4 wire, star-connected system supplies three resistive loads as shown in Fig. 20.7. Determine (a) the current in each line and (b) the current in the neutral conductor.

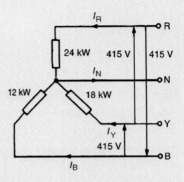

Figure 20.7

(a) For a star-connected system $V_L = \sqrt{3}\,V_p$, hence

$$V_p = \frac{V_L}{\sqrt{3}} = \frac{415}{\sqrt{3}} = 240\,V$$

Since current $I = $ power $P/$voltage V for a resistive load then

$$I_R = \frac{P_R}{V_R} = \frac{24\,000}{240} = \mathbf{100\,A}$$

$$I_Y = \frac{P_Y}{V_Y} = \frac{18\,000}{240} = \mathbf{75\,A}$$

and $$I_B = \frac{P_B}{V_B} = \frac{12\,000}{240} = \mathbf{50\,A}$$

(b) The three line currents are shown in the phasor diagram of Fig. 20.8. Since each load is resistive the currents are in phase with the phase voltages and are hence mutually displaced by $120°$. The current in the neutral conductor is given by $I_N = I_R + I_Y + I_B$ phasorially.

Figure 20.9 shows the three line currents added phasorially. oa represents I_R in magnitude and direction. From the nose of oa, ab is drawn representing I_Y in

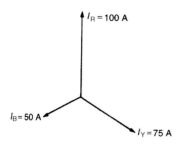

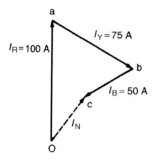

Figure 20.8

Figure 20.9

magnitude and direction. From the nose of ab, bc is drawn representing I_B in magnitude and direction. oc represents the resultant, I_N By measurement, $I_N = 43\,A$.

Alternatively, by calculation, considering I_R at $90°$, I_B at $210°$ and I_Y at $330°$:

Total horizontal component

$= 100\cos 90° + 75\cos 330° + 50\cos 210° = 21.65$

Total vertical component

$= 100\sin 90° + 75\sin 330° + 50\sin 210° = 37.50$

Hence magnitude of $I_N = \sqrt{21.65^2 + 37.50^2} = \mathbf{43.3\,A}$

Now try the following exercise

Exercise 112   Further problems on star connections

1. Three loads, each of resistance $50\,\Omega$ are connected in star to a 400 V, 3-phase supply. Determine (a) the phase voltage, (b) the phase current, and (c) the line current.
   [(a) 231 V (b) 4.62 A (c) 4.62 A]

2. A star-connected load consists of three identical coils, each of inductance 159.2 mH and resistance $50\,\Omega$. If the supply frequency is 50 Hz and the line current is 3 A determine (a) the phase voltage and (b) the line voltage.
   [(a) 212 V (b) 367 V]

3. Three identical capacitors are connected in star to a 400 V, 50 Hz 3-phase supply. If the line current is 12 A determine the capacitance of each of the capacitors.   [165.4 µF]

4. Three coils each having resistance $6\,\Omega$ and inductance L H are connected in star to a 415 V, 50 Hz, 3-phase supply. If the line current is 30 A, find the value of L.   [16.78 mH]

5. A 400 V, 3-phase, 4 wire, star-connected system supplies three resistive loads of 15 kW, 20 kW and 25 kW in the red, yellow and blue phases respectively. Determine the current flowing in each of the four conductors.
   $[I_R = 64.95\,A, I_Y = 86.60\,A,$
   $I_B = 108.25\,A, I_N = 37.50\,A]$

20.4   Delta connection

(i) A **delta (or mesh) connected load** is shown in Fig. 20.10 where the end of one load is connected to the start of the next load.

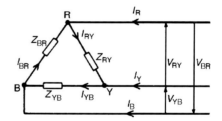

Figure 20.10

(ii) From Fig. 20.10, it can be seen that the line voltages V_{RY}, V_{YB} and V_{BR} are the respective phase voltages, i.e. for a delta connection:

$$V_L = V_p$$

(iii) Using Kirchhoff's current law in Fig. 20.10, $I_R = I_{RY} - I_{BR} = I_{RY} + (-I_{BR})$. From the phasor diagram shown in Fig. 20.11, by trigonometry or by measurement, $I_R = \sqrt{3}\,I_{RY}$, i.e. for a delta connection:

$$I_L = \sqrt{3}I_p$$

Problem 5.   Three identical coils each of resistance $30\,\Omega$ and inductance 127.3 mH are connected in delta to a 440 V, 50 Hz, 3-phase supply. Determine (a) the phase current, and (b) the line current.

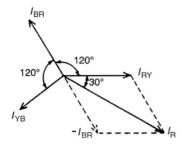

Figure 20.11

Phase impedance, $Z_p = 50\,\Omega$ (from Problem 2) and for a delta connection, $V_p = V_L$

(a)   Phase current,

$$I_p = \frac{V_p}{Z_p} = \frac{V_L}{Z_p} = \frac{440}{50} = \textbf{8.8 A}$$

(b)   For a delta connection,

$$I_L = \sqrt{3}\,I_p = \sqrt{3}(8.8) = \textbf{15.24 A}$$

Thus when the load is connected in delta, three times the line current is taken from the supply than is taken if connected in star.

Problem 6.   Three identical capacitors are connected in delta to a 415 V, 50 Hz, 3-phase supply. If the line current is 15 A, determine the capacitance of each of the capacitors.

For a delta connection $I_L = \sqrt{3}\,I_p$. Hence phase current,

$$I_p = \frac{I_L}{\sqrt{3}} = \frac{15}{\sqrt{3}} = 8.66\,\text{A}$$

Capacitive reactance per phase,

$$X_C = \frac{V_p}{I_p} = \frac{V_L}{I_p}$$

(since for a delta connection $V_L = V_p$). Hence

$$X_C = \frac{415}{8.66} = 47.92\,\Omega$$

$X_C = 1/2\pi f C$, from which capacitance,

$$C = \frac{1}{2\pi f X_C} = \frac{2}{2\pi(50)(47.92)}\,\text{F} = \textbf{66.43}\,\mu\text{F}$$

$3\,\Omega$ and inductive reactance $4\,\Omega$ are connected (i) in star and (ii) in delta to a 415 V, 3-phase supply. Calculate for each connection (a) the line and phase voltages and (b) the phase and line currents.

(i)   **For a star connection:** $I_L = I_p$ and $V_L = \sqrt{3}\,V_p$.

   (a)   A 415 V, 3-phase supply means that the line voltage, $V_L = \textbf{415 V}$

   Phase voltage,

$$V_p = \frac{V_L}{\sqrt{3}} = \frac{415}{\sqrt{3}} = \textbf{240 V}$$

   (b)   Impedance per phase,

$$Z_p = \sqrt{R^2 + X_L^2} = \sqrt{3^2 + 4^2} = 5\,\Omega$$

   Phase current,

$$I_p = V_p/Z_p = 240/5 = \textbf{48 A}$$

   Line current,

$$I_L = I_p = \textbf{48 A}$$

(ii)   **For a delta connection:** $V_L = V_p$ and $I_L = \sqrt{3}\,I_p$.

   (a)   Line voltage, $V_L = 415\,\text{V}$

   Phase voltage, $V_p = V_L = \textbf{415 V}$

   (b)   Phase current,

$$I_p = \frac{V_p}{Z_p} = \frac{415}{5} = \textbf{83 A}$$

   Line current,

$$I_L = \sqrt{3}\,I_p = \sqrt{3}(83) = \textbf{144 A}$$

Now try the following exercise

Exercise 113   Further problems on delta connections

1.   Three loads, each of resistance $50\,\Omega$ are connected in delta to a 400 V, 3-phase supply. Determine (a) the phase voltage, (b) the phase current, and (c) the line current.

[(a) 400 V (b) 8 A (c) 13.86 A]

2. Three inductive loads each of resistance $75\,\Omega$ and inductance $318.4\,$mH are connected in delta to a $415\,$V, $50\,$Hz, 3-phase supply. Determine (a) the phase voltage, (b) the phase current, and (c) the line current.
[(a) 415 V (b) 3.32 A (c) 5.75 A]

3. Three identical capacitors are connected in delta to a $400\,$V, $50\,$Hz 3-phase supply. If the line current is $12\,$A determine the capacitance of each of the capacitors. [$55.13\,\mu$F]

4. Three coils each having resistance $6\,\Omega$ and inductance $L\,H$ are connected in delta, to a $415\,$V, $50\,$Hz, 3-phase supply. If the line current is $30\,$A, find the value of L.
[73.84 mH]

5. A 3-phase, star-connected alternator delivers a line current of $65\,$A to a balanced delta-connected load at a line voltage of $380\,$V. Calculate (a) the phase voltage of the alternator, (b) the alternator phase current, and (c) the load phase current.
[(a) 219.4 V (b) 65 A (c) 37.53 A]

6. Three $24\,\mu$F capacitors are connected in star across a $400\,$V, $50\,$Hz, 3-phase supply. What value of capacitance must be connected in delta in order to take the same line current? [$8\,\mu$F]

20.5 Power in three-phase systems

The power dissipated in a three-phase load is given by the sum of the power dissipated in each phase. If a load is balanced then the total power P is given by: $P = 3 \times$ power consumed by one phase.

The power consumed in one phase $= I_p^2 R_p$ or $V_p I_p \cos\phi$ (where ϕ is the phase angle between V_p and I_p).
For a star connection,

$$V_p = \frac{V_L}{\sqrt{3}} \quad \text{and} \quad I_p = I_L$$

hence

$$P = 3\frac{V_L}{\sqrt{3}}I_L \cos\phi = \sqrt{3}\,V_L I_L \cos\phi$$

For a delta connection,

$$V_p = V_L \quad \text{and} \quad I_p = \frac{I_L}{\sqrt{3}}$$

hence

$$P = 3V_L\frac{I_L}{\sqrt{3}}\cos\phi = \sqrt{3}\,V_L I_L \cos\phi$$

Hence for either a star or a delta balanced connection the total power P is given by:

$$P = \sqrt{3}V_L I_L \cos\phi \text{ watts}$$
$$\text{or } P = 3I_p^2 R_p \text{ watts}$$

Total volt-amperes

$$S = \sqrt{3}V_L I_L \text{ volt-amperes}$$

Problem 8. Three $12\,\Omega$ resistors are connected in star to a $415\,$V, 3-phase supply. Determine the total power dissipated by the resistors.

Power dissipated, $P = \sqrt{3}\,V_L I_L \cos\phi$ or $P = 3I_p^2 R_p$
Line voltage, $V_L = 415\,$V and phase voltage

$$V_p = \frac{415}{\sqrt{3}} = 240\,\text{V}$$

(since the resistors are star-connected). Phase current,

$$I_p = \frac{V_p}{Z_p} = \frac{V_p}{R_p} = \frac{240}{12} = 20\,\text{A}$$

For a star connection

$$I_L = I_p = 20\,\text{A}$$

For a purely resistive load, the power

$$\text{factor} = \cos\phi = 1$$

Hence power

$$\mathbf{P} = \sqrt{3}\,V_L I_L \cos\phi = \sqrt{3}(415)(20)(1)$$
$$= \mathbf{14.4\,kW}$$

or power

$$\mathbf{P} = 3I_p^2 R_p = 3(20)^2(12) = \mathbf{14.4\,kW}$$

> **Problem 9.** The input power to a 3-phase a.c. motor is measured as 5 kW. If the voltage and current to the motor are 400 V and 8.6 A respectively, determine the power factor of the system.

Power $P = 5000$ W,

$$\text{line voltage } V_L = 400 \text{ V},$$
$$\text{line current, } I_L = 8.6 \text{ A and}$$
$$\text{power, } P = \sqrt{3}\, V_L I_L \cos\phi$$

Hence

$$\textbf{power factor} = \cos\phi = \frac{P}{\sqrt{3}\, V_L I_L}$$

$$= \frac{5000}{\sqrt{3}(400)(8.6)} = \textbf{0.839}$$

> **Problem 10.** Three identical coils, each of resistance $10\,\Omega$ and inductance 42 mH are connected (a) in star and (b) in delta to a 415 V, 50 Hz, 3-phase supply. Determine the total power dissipated in each case.

(a) **Star connection**

Inductive reactance,

$$X_L = 2\pi f L = 2\pi(50)(42 \times 10^{-3}) = 13.19\,\Omega.$$

Phase impedance,

$$Z_p = \sqrt{R^2 + X_L^2} = \sqrt{10^2 + 13.19^2} = 16.55\,\Omega.$$

Line voltage,

$$V_L = 415 \text{ V}$$

and phase voltage,

$$V_P = V_L/\sqrt{3} = 415/\sqrt{3} = 240 \text{ V}.$$

Phase current,

$$I_p = V_p/Z_p = 240/16.55 = 14.50 \text{ A}.$$

Line current,

$$I_L = I_p = 14.50 \text{ A}.$$

Power factor $= \cos\phi = R_p/Z_p = 10/16.55$
$$= 0.6042 \text{ lagging}.$$

Power dissipated,

$$P = \sqrt{3}\, V_L I_L \cos\phi = \sqrt{3}(415)(14.50)(0.6042)$$
$$= \textbf{6.3 kW}$$

(Alternatively,

$$P = 3I_p^2 R_p = 3(14.50)^2(10) = \textbf{6.3 kW})$$

(b) **Delta connection**

$$V_L = V_p = 415 \text{ V},$$
$$Z_p = 16.55\,\Omega, \cos\phi = 0.6042$$

lagging (from above).

Phase current,

$$I_p = V_p/Z_p = 415/16.55 = 25.08 \text{ A}$$

Line current,

$$I_L = \sqrt{3} I_p = \sqrt{3}(25.08) = 43.44 \text{ A}$$

Power dissipated,

$$P = \sqrt{3}\, V_L I_L \cos\phi$$
$$= \sqrt{3}(415)(43.44)(0.6042) = \textbf{18.87 kW}$$

(Alternatively,

$$P = 3I_p^2 R_p = 3(25.08)^2(10) = \textbf{18.87 kW})$$

Hence loads connected in delta dissipate three times the power than when connected in star, and also take a line current three times greater.

> **Problem 11.** A 415 V, 3-phase a.c. motor has a power output of 12.75 kW and operates at a power factor of 0.77 lagging and with an efficiency of 85 per cent. If the motor is delta-connected, determine (a) the power input, (b) the line current, and (c) the phase current.

(a) Efficiency = power output/power input. Hence $85/100 = 12750/\text{power input}$ from which,

$$\textbf{power input} = \frac{12750 \times 100}{85}$$
$$= \textbf{15000 W or 15 kW}$$

(b) Power, $P = \sqrt{3}\, V_L I_L \cos\phi$, hence **line current**,

$$I_L = \frac{P}{\sqrt{3}(415)(0.77)}$$

$$= \frac{15\,000}{\sqrt{3}(415)(0.77)} = \textbf{27.10 A}$$

(c) For a delta connection, $I_L = \sqrt{3}\, I_p$, hence **phase current**,

$$I_p = \frac{I_L}{\sqrt{3}} = \frac{27.10}{\sqrt{3}} = \textbf{15.65 A}$$

Now try the following exercise

Exercise 114   Further problems on power in three-phase systems

1. Determine the total power dissipated by three $20\,\Omega$ resistors when connected (a) in star and (b) in delta to a $440\,\text{V}$, 3-phase supply.
    [(a) 9.68 kW (b) 29.04 kW]

2. Determine the power dissipated in the circuit of Problem 2, Exercise 112, page 321.
    [1.35 kW]

3. A balanced delta-connected load has a line voltage of $400\,\text{V}$, a line current of $8\,\text{A}$ and a lagging power factor of 0.94. Draw a complete phasor diagram of the load. What is the total power dissipated by the load?   [5.21 kW]

4. Three inductive loads, each of resistance $4\,\Omega$ and reactance $9\,\Omega$ are connected in delta. When connected to a 3-phase supply the loads consume $1.2\,\text{kW}$. Calculate (a) the power factor of the load, (b) the phase current, (c) the line current, and (d) the supply voltage.
    [(a) 0.406 (b) 10 A (c) 17.32 A (d) 98.53 V]

5. The input voltage, current and power to a motor is measured as $415\,\text{V}$, $16.4\,\text{A}$ and $6\,\text{kW}$ respectively. Determine the power factor of the system.   [0.509]

6. A $440\,\text{V}$, 3-phase a.c. motor has a power output of $11.25\,\text{kW}$ and operates at a power factor of 0.8 lagging and with an efficiency of 84 per cent. If the motor is delta connected determine (a) the power input, (b) the line current, and (c) the phase current.
    [(a) 13.39 kW (b) 21.97 A (c) 12.68 A]

20.6 Measurement of power in three-phase systems

Power in three-phase loads may be measured by the following methods:

(i) **One-wattmeter method for a balanced load**

Wattmeter connections for both star and delta are shown in Fig. 20.12.

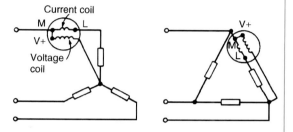

Figure 20.12

Total power $= 3 \times$ wattmeter reading

(ii) **Two-wattmeter method for balanced or unbalanced loads**

A connection diagram for this method is shown in Fig. 20.13 for a star-connected load. Similar connections are made for a delta-connected load.

Total power $=$ sum of wattmeter readings

$$= P_1 + P_2$$

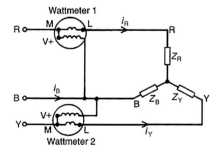

Figure 20.13

The power factor may be determined from:

$$\tan\phi = \sqrt{3}\left(\frac{P_1 - P_2}{P_1 + P_2}\right)$$

(see Problems 12 and 15 to 18).

Section 3

It is possible, depending on the load power factor, for one wattmeter to have to be 'reversed' to obtain a reading. In this case it is taken as a negative reading (see Problem 17).

(iii) **Three-wattmeter method for a three-phase, 4-wire system for balanced and unbalanced loads** (see Fig. 20.14).

$$\text{Total power} = P_1 + P_2 + P_3$$

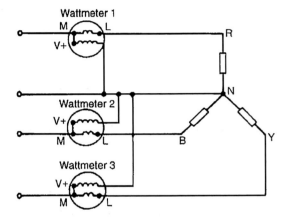

Figure 20.14

Problem 12. (a) Show that the total power in a 3-phase, 3-wire system using the two-wattmeter method of measurement is given by the sum of the wattmeter readings. Draw a connection diagram. (b) Draw a phasor diagram for the two-wattmeter method for a balanced load. (c) Use the phasor diagram of part (b) to derive a formula from which the power factor of a 3-phase system may be determined using only the wattmeter readings.

(a) A connection diagram for the two-wattmeter method of a power measurement is shown in Fig. 20.15 for a star-connected load.

Total instantaneous power, $p = e_R i_R + e_Y i_Y + e_B i_B$ and in any 3-phase system $i_R + i_Y + i_B = 0$; hence $i_B = -i_R - i_Y$ Thus,

$$p = e_R i_R + e_Y i_Y + e_B(-i_R - i_Y)$$

$$= (e_R - e_B)i_R + (e_Y - e_B)i_Y$$

However, $(e_R - e_B)$ is the p.d. across wattmeter 1 in Fig. 20.15 and $(e_Y - e_B)$ is the p.d. across

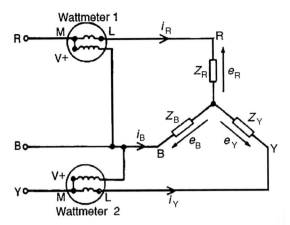

Figure 20.15

wattmeter 2. Hence total instantaneous power,

$$p = (\text{wattmeter 1 reading})$$
$$+ (\text{wattmeter 2 reading})$$
$$= p_1 + p_2$$

The moving systems of the wattmeters are unable to follow the variations which take place at normal frequencies and they indicate the mean power taken over a cycle. Hence the total power, $P = P_1 + P_2$ for balanced or unbalanced loads.

(b) The phasor diagram for the two-wattmeter method for a balanced load having a lagging current is shown in Fig. 20.16, where $V_{RB} = V_R - V_B$ and $V_{YB} = V_Y - V_B$ (phasorially).

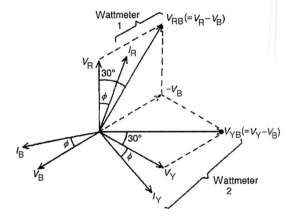

Figure 20.16

(c) Wattmeter 1 reads $V_{RB} I_R \cos(30° - \phi) = P_1$

Wattmeter 2 reads $V_{YB} I_Y \cos(30° + \phi) = P_2$

$$\frac{P_1}{P_2} = \frac{V_{RB} I_R \cos(30° - \phi)}{V_{YB} I_Y \cos(30° + \phi)} = \frac{\cos(30° - \phi)}{\cos(30° + \phi)}$$

since $I_R = I_Y$ and $V_{RB} = V_{YB}$ for a balanced load. Hence

$$\frac{P_1}{P_2} = \frac{\cos 30° \cos \phi + \sin 30° \sin \phi}{\cos 30° \cos \phi - \sin 30° \sin \phi}$$

(from compound angle formulae, see '*Engineering Mathematics*').

Dividing throughout by $\cos 30° \cos \phi$ gives:

$$\frac{P_1}{P_2} = \frac{1 + \tan 30° \tan \phi}{1 - \tan 30° \tan \phi}$$

$$= \frac{1 + \frac{1}{\sqrt{3}} \tan \phi}{1 - \frac{1}{\sqrt{3}} \tan \phi}$$

$$\left(\text{since } \frac{\sin \phi}{\cos \phi} = \tan \phi \right)$$

Cross-multiplying gives:

$$P_1 - \frac{P_1}{\sqrt{3}} \tan \phi = P_2 + \frac{P_2}{\sqrt{3}} \tan \phi$$

Hence

$$P_1 - P_2 = (P_1 + P_2) \frac{\tan \phi}{\sqrt{3}}$$

from which

$$\boldsymbol{\tan \phi = \sqrt{3} \left(\frac{P_1 - P_2}{P_1 + P_2} \right)}$$

ϕ, $\cos \phi$ and thus power factor can be determined from this formula.

Problem 13. A 400 V, 3-phase star connected alternator supplies a delta-connected load, each phase of which has a resistance of 30 Ω and inductive reactance 40 Ω. Calculate (a) the current supplied by the alternator and (b) the output power and the kVA of the alternator, neglecting losses in the line between the alternator and load.

A circuit diagram of the alternator and load is shown in Fig. 20.17.

(a) Considering the load:

Phase current, $I_p = V_p / Z_p$

$V_p = V_L$ for a delta connection,

hence $V_p = 400$ V.

Phase impedance,

$$Z_p = \sqrt{R_p^2 + X_L^2} = \sqrt{30^2 + 40^2} = 50\,\Omega.$$

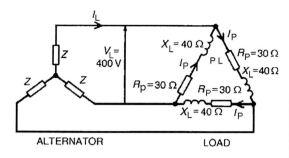

Figure 20.17

Hence $I_p = V_p / Z_p = 400/50 = 8$ A.

For a delta-connection, line current,

$$I_L = \sqrt{3}\, I_p = \sqrt{3}(8) = 13.86\,A.$$

Hence **13.86 A is the current supplied by the alternator**.

(b) Alternator output power is equal to the power dissipated by the load i.e.

$$P = \sqrt{3}\, V_L I_L \cos \phi$$

where $\cos \phi = R_p / Z_p = 30/50 = 0.6$

Hence $P = \sqrt{3}(400)(13.86)(0.6)$

$$= \mathbf{5.76\,kW}.$$

Alternator output kVA,

$$S = \sqrt{3}\, V_L I_L = \sqrt{3}(400)(13.86)$$

$$= \mathbf{9.60\,kVA}.$$

Problem 14. Each phase of a delta-connected load comprises a resistance of 30 Ω and an 80 μF capacitor in series. The load is connected to a 400 V, 50 Hz, 3-phase supply. Calculate (a) the phase current, (b) the line current, (c) the total power dissipated, and (d) the kVA rating of the load. Draw the complete phasor diagram for the load.

(a) Capacitive reactance,

$$X_C = \frac{1}{2\pi f C} = \frac{1}{2\pi (50)(80 \times 10^{-6})} = 39.79\,\Omega$$

Phase impedance,

$$Z_p = \sqrt{R_p^2 + X_c^2} = \sqrt{30^2 + 39.79^2} = 49.83\,\Omega.$$

Power factor $= \cos \phi = R_p / Z_p$

$$= 30/49.83 = 0.602$$

Hence $\phi = \cos^{-1} 0.602 = 52.99°$ leading.

Phase current,

$$I_p = V_p/Z_p \quad \text{and} \quad V_p = V_L$$

for a delta connection. Hence

$$I_p = 400/49.83 = \mathbf{8.027\,A}$$

(b) Line current, $I_L = \sqrt{3}\,I_p$ for a delta-connection. Hence $I_L = \sqrt{3}(8.027) = \mathbf{13.90\,A}$

(c) Total power dissipated,

$$P = \sqrt{3}\,V_L I_L \cos\phi$$

$$= \sqrt{3}(400)(13.90)(0.602) = \mathbf{5.797\,kW}$$

(d) Total kVA,

$$S = \sqrt{3}\,V_L I_L = \sqrt{3}(400)(13.90) = \mathbf{9.630\,kVA}$$

The phasor diagram for the load is shown in Fig. 20.18.

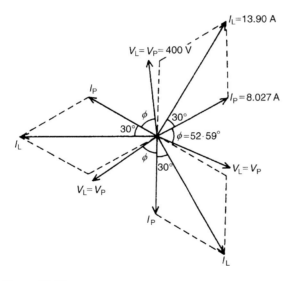

$I_L = 13.90$ A
$V_L = V_p = 400$ V
I_p
$30°$
$30°$
I_L
$I_p = 8.027$ A
$\phi = 52·59°$
$30°$
$V_L = V_p$
ϕ
$V_L = V_p$
I_p
I_L

Figure 20.18

Problem 15. Two wattmeters are connected to measure the input power to a balanced 3-phase load by the two-wattmeter method. If the instrument readings are 8 kW and 4 kW, determine (a) the total power input and (b) the load power factor.

(a) Total input power,

$$P = P_1 + P_2 = 8 + 4 = \mathbf{12\,kW}$$

(b) $\tan\phi = \sqrt{3}\left(\dfrac{P_1 - P_2}{P_1 + P_2}\right) = \sqrt{3}\left(\dfrac{8-4}{8+4}\right)$

$$= \sqrt{3}\left(\frac{4}{12}\right) = \sqrt{3}\left(\frac{1}{3}\right) = \frac{1}{\sqrt{3}}$$

Hence $\phi = \tan^{-1}\dfrac{1}{\sqrt{3}} = 30°$

Power factor $= \cos\phi = \cos 30° = \mathbf{0.866}$

Problem 16. Two wattmeters connected to a 3-phase motor indicate the total power input to be 12 kW. The power factor is 0.6. Determine the readings of each wattmeter.

If the two wattmeters indicate P_1 and P_2 respectively then

$$P_1 + P_2 = 12\,\text{kW} \tag{1}$$

$$\tan\phi = \sqrt{3}\left(\frac{P_1 - P_2}{P_1 + P_2}\right)$$

and power factor $= 0.6 = \cos\phi$.
Angle $\phi = \cos^{-1} 0.6 = 53.13°$ and $\tan 53.13° = 1.3333$.
Hence

$$1.3333 = \sqrt{3}\left(\frac{P_1 - P_2}{12}\right)$$

from which,

$$P_1 - P_2 = \frac{12(1.3333)}{\sqrt{3}}$$

i.e. $\qquad P_1 - P_2 = 9.237\,\text{kW} \tag{2}$

Adding equations (1) and (2) gives:

$$2P_1 = 21.237$$

i.e. $\qquad P_1 = \dfrac{21.237}{2}$

$$= 10.62\,\text{kW}$$

Hence **wattmeter 1 reads 10.62 kW**
From equation (1), **wattmeter 2 reads**
$(12 - 10.62) = 1.38\,\text{kW}$

Problem 17. Two wattmeters indicate 10 kW and 3 kW respectively when connected to measure the input power to a 3-phase balanced load, the reverse switch being operated on the meter indicating the 3 kW reading. Determine (a) the input power and (b) the load power factor.

Since the reversing switch on the wattmeter had to be operated the 3 kW reading is taken as -3 kW

(a) Total input power,

$$P = P_1 + P_2 = 10 + (-3) = \textbf{7 kW}$$

(b) $\tan\phi = \sqrt{3}\left(\dfrac{P_1 - P_2}{P_1 + P_2}\right) = \sqrt{3}\left(\dfrac{10 - (-3)}{10 + (-3)}\right)$

$$= \sqrt{3}\left(\dfrac{13}{7}\right) = 3.2167$$

Angle $\phi = \tan^{-1}3.2167 = 72.73°$

Power factor $= \cos\phi = \cos 72.73° = \textbf{0.297}$

Problem 18. Three similar coils, each having a resistance of $8\,\Omega$ and an inductive reactance of $8\,\Omega$ are connected (a) in star and (b) in delta, across a 415 V, 3-phase supply. Calculate for each connection the readings on each of two wattmeters connected to measure the power by the two-wattmeter method.

(a) **Star connection:** $V_L = \sqrt{3}\,V_p$ and $I_L = I_p$

Phase voltage, $V_p = \dfrac{V_L}{\sqrt{3}} = \dfrac{415}{\sqrt{3}}$

and phase impedance,

$$Z_p = \sqrt{R_p^2 + X_L^2} = \sqrt{8^2 + 8^2} = 11.31\,\Omega$$

Hence phase current,

$$I_p = \dfrac{V_p}{Z_p} = \dfrac{\frac{415}{\sqrt{3}}}{11.31} = 21.18\,\text{A}$$

Total power,

$$P = 3I_p^2 R_p = 3(21.18)^2(8) = 10766\,\text{W}$$

If wattmeter readings are P_1 and P_2 then:

$$P_1 + P_2 = 10766 \tag{1}$$

Since $R_p = 8\,\Omega$ and $X_L = 8\,\Omega$, then phase angle $\phi = 45°$ (from impedance triangle).

$$\tan\phi = \sqrt{3}\left(\dfrac{P_1 - P_2}{P_1 + P_2}\right)$$

hence $\tan 45° = \dfrac{\sqrt{3}(P_1 - P_2)}{10766}$

from which

$$P_1 - P_2 = \dfrac{(10766)(1)}{\sqrt{3}} = 6216\,\text{W} \tag{2}$$

Adding equations (1) and (2) gives:

$2P_1 = 10766 + 6216 = 16982\,\text{W}$

Hence $P_1 = 8491\,\text{W}$

From equation (1), $P_2 = 10766 - 8491 = 2275\,\text{W}$.

When the coils are star-connected the wattmeter readings are thus 8.491 kW and 2.275 kW

(b) **Delta connection:** $V_L = V_p$ and $I_L = \sqrt{3}\,I_p$

Phase current, $I_p = \dfrac{V_p}{Z_p} = \dfrac{415}{11.31} = 36.69\,\text{A}$.

Total power,

$$P = 3I_p^2 R_p = 3(36.69)^2(8) = 32310\,\text{W}$$

Hence $P_1 + P_2 = 32310\,\text{W}$ \qquad(3)

$\tan\phi = \sqrt{3}\left(\dfrac{P_1 - P_2}{P_1 + P_2}\right)$ thus $1 = \dfrac{\sqrt{3}(P_1 - P_2)}{32310}$

from which,

$$P_1 - P_2 = \dfrac{32310}{\sqrt{3}} = 18650\,\text{W} \tag{4}$$

Adding equations (3) and (4) gives:

$2P_1 = 50960$ from which $P_1 = 25480\,\text{W}$.

From equation (3), $P_2 = 32310 - 25480$
$$= 6830\,\text{W}$$

When the coils are delta-connected the wattmeter readings are thus 25.48 kW and 6.83 kW

Now try the following exercise

Exercise 115 Further problems on the measurement of power in 3-phase circuits

1. Two wattmeters are connected to measure the input power to a balanced three-phase load. If the wattmeter readings are 9.3 kW and 5.4 kW determine (a) the total output power, and (b) the load power factor.
    [(a) 14.7 kW (b) 0.909]

2. 8 kW is found by the two-wattmeter method to be the power input to a 3-phase motor. Determine the reading of each wattmeter if the power factor of the system is 0.85.

[5.431 kW, 2.569 kW]

3. When the two-wattmeter method is used to measure the input power of a balanced load, the readings on the wattmeters are 7.5 kW and 2.5 kW, the connections to one of the coils on the meter reading 2.5 kW having to be reversed. Determine (a) the total input power, and (b) the load power factor.

[(a) 5 kW (b) 0.277]

4. Three similar coils, each having a resistance of 4.0 Ω and an inductive reactance of 3.46 Ω are connected (a) in star and (b) in delta across a 400 V, 3-phase supply. Calculate for each connection the readings on each of two wattmeters connected to measure the power by the two-wattmeter method.

[(a) 17.15 kW, 5.73 kW
(b) 51.46 kW, 17.18 kW]

5. A 3-phase, star-connected alternator supplies a delta-connected load, each phase of which has a resistance of 15 Ω and inductive reactance 20 Ω. If the line voltage is 400 V, calculate (a) the current supplied by the alternator and (b) the output power and kVA rating of the alternator, neglecting any losses in the line between the alternator and the load.

[(a) 27.71 A (b) 11.52 kW, 19.20 kVA]

6. Each phase of a delta-connected load comprises a resistance of 40 Ω and a 40 μF capacitor in series. Determine, when connected to a 415 V, 50 Hz, 3-phase supply (a) the phase current, (b) the line current, (c) the total power dissipated, and (d) the kVA rating of the load.

[(a) 4.66 A (b) 8.07 A
(c) 2.605 kW (d) 5.80 kVA]

20.7 Comparison of star and delta connections

(i) Loads connected in delta dissipate three times more power than when connected in star to the same supply.

(ii) For the same power, the phase currents must be the same for both delta and star connections (since power $= 3I_p^2 R_p$), hence the line current in the delta-connected system is greater than the line current in the corresponding star-connected system. To achieve the same phase current in a star-connected system as in a delta-connected system, the line voltage in the star system is $\sqrt{3}$ times the line voltage in the delta system. Thus for a given power transfer, a delta system is associated with larger line currents (and thus larger conductor cross-sectional area) and a star system is associated with a larger line voltage (and thus greater insulation).

20.8 Advantages of three-phase systems

Advantages of three-phase systems over single-phase supplies include:

(i) For a given amount of power transmitted through a system, the three-phase system requires conductors with a smaller cross-sectional area. This means a saving of copper (or aluminium) and thus the original installation costs are less.

(ii) Two voltages are available (see Section 20.3 (vii))

(iii) Three-phase motors are very robust, relatively cheap, generally smaller, have self-starting properties, provide a steadier output and require little maintenance compared with single-phase motors.

Now try the following exercises

Exercise 116 Short answer questions on three-phase systems

1. Explain briefly how a three-phase supply is generated

2. State the national standard phase sequence for a three-phase supply

3. State the two ways in which phases of a three-phase supply can be interconnected to reduce the number of conductors used compared with three single-phase systems

4. State the relationships between line and phase currents and line and phase voltages for a star-connected system

5. When may the neutral conductor of a star-connected system be omitted?

6. State the relationships between line and phase currents and line and phase voltages for a delta-connected system

7. What is the standard electricity supply to domestic consumers in Great Britain?

8. State two formulae for determining the power dissipated in the load of a three-phase balanced system

9. By what methods may power be measured in a three-phase system?

10. State a formula from which power factor may be determined for a balanced system when using the two-wattmeter method of power measurement

11. Loads connected in star dissipate ...... the power dissipated when connected in delta and fed from the same supply

12. Name three advantages of three-phase systems over single-phase systems

Exercise 117   **Multi-choice questions on three-phase systems**
(Answers on page 421)

Three loads, each of $10\,\Omega$ resistance, are connected in star to a 400 V, 3-phase supply. Determine the quantities stated in questions 1 to 5, selecting answers from the following list:

(a) $\dfrac{40}{\sqrt{3}}$ A   (b) $\sqrt{3}(16)\,$kW   (c) $\dfrac{400}{\sqrt{3}}$ V

(d) $\sqrt{3}(40)$ A   (e) $\sqrt{3}(400)$ V   (f) 16 kW

(g) 400 V   (h) 48 kW   (i) 40 A

1. Line voltage
2. Phase voltage
3. Phase current
4. Line current
5. Total power dissipated in the load
6. Which of the following statements is false?
  (a) For the same power, loads connected in delta have a higher line voltage and a smaller line current than loads connected in star
  (b) When using the two-wattmeter method of power measurement the power factor is unity when the wattmeter readings are the same
  (c) A.c. may be distributed using a single-phase system with two wires, a three-phase system with three wires or a three-phase system with four wires
  (d) The national standard phase sequence for a three-phase supply is R, Y, B

Three loads, each of resistance $16\,\Omega$ and inductive reactance $12\,\Omega$ are connected in delta to a 400 V, 3-phase supply. Determine the quantities stated in questions 7 to 12, selecting the correct answer from the following list:

(a) $4\,\Omega$ (b) $\sqrt{3}(400)$ V   (c) $\sqrt{3}(6.4)\,$kW

(d) 20 A   (e) 6.4 kW   (f) $\sqrt{3}(20)$ A

(g) $20\,\Omega$ (h) $\dfrac{20}{\sqrt{3}}$ V   (i) $\dfrac{400}{\sqrt{3}}$ V

(j) 19.2 kW   (k) 100 A   (l) 400 V

(m) $28\,\Omega$

7. Phase impedance
8. Line voltage
9. Phase voltage
10. Phase current
11. Line current
12. Total power dissipated in the load
13. The phase voltage of a delta-connected three-phase system with balanced loads is 240 V. The line voltage is:
  (a) 720 V   (b) 440 V
  (c) 340 V   (d) 240 V
14. A 4-wire three-phase star-connected system has a line current of 10 A. The phase current is:
  (a) 40 A   (b) 10 A
  (c) 20 A   (d) 30 A
15. The line voltage of a 4-wire three-phase star-connected system is 11 kV. The phase voltage is:
  (a) 19.05 kV   (b) 11 kV
  (c) 6.35 kV   (d) 7.78 kV

Section 3

16. In the two-wattmeter method of measurement power in a balanced three-phase system readings of P_1 and P_2 watts are obtained. The power factor may be determined from:

    (a) $\sqrt{3}\left(\dfrac{P_1 + P_2}{P_1 - P_2}\right)$ (b) $\sqrt{3}\left(\dfrac{P_1 - P_2}{P_1 + P_2}\right)$

    (c) $\dfrac{(P_1 - P_2)}{\sqrt{3}(P_1 + P_2)}$ (d) $\dfrac{(P_1 + P_2)}{\sqrt{3}(P_1 - P_2)}$

17. The phase voltage of a 4-wire three-phase star-connected system is 110 V. The line voltage is:

    (a) 440 V (b) 330 V
    (c) 191 V (d) 110 V

Chapter 21

Transformers

At the end of this chapter you should be able to:

- understand the principle of operation of a transformer
- understand the term 'rating' of a transformer
- use $V_1/V_2 = N_1/N_2 = I_2/I_1$ in calculations on transformers
- construct a transformer no-load phasor diagram and calculate magnetising and core loss components of the no-load current
- state the e.m.f. equation for a transformer $E = 4.44\,f\,\Phi_m N$ and use it in calculations
- construct a transformer on-load phasor diagram for an inductive circuit assuming the volt drop in the windings is negligible
- describe transformer construction
- derive the equivalent resistance, reactance and impedance referred to the primary of a transformer
- understand voltage regulation
- describe losses in transformers and calculate efficiency
- appreciate the concept of resistance matching and how it may be achieved
- perform calculations using $R_1 = (N_1/N_2)^2 R_L$
- describe an auto transformer, its advantages/disadvantages and uses
- describe an isolating transformer, stating uses
- describe a three-phase transformer
- describe current and voltage transformers

21.1 Introduction

A transformer is a device which uses the phenomenon of mutual induction (see Chapter 9) to change the values of alternating voltages and currents. In fact, one of the main advantages of a.c. transmission and distribution is the ease with which an alternating voltage can be increased or decreased by transformers.

Losses in transformers are generally low and thus efficiency is high. Being static they have a long life and are very stable.

Transformers range in size from the miniature units used in electronic applications to the large power transformers used in power stations; the principle of operation is the same for each.

A transformer is represented in Fig. 21.1(a) as consisting of two electrical circuits linked by a common

DOI: 10.1016/B978-0-08-089056-2.00021-8

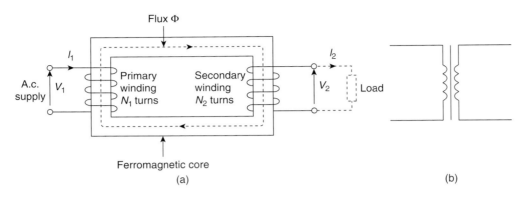

Figure 21.1

ferromagnetic core. One coil is termed the **primary winding** which is connected to the supply of electricity, and the other the **secondary winding**, which may be connected to a load. A circuit diagram symbol for a transformer is shown in Fig. 21.1(b).

21.2 Transformer principle of operation

When the secondary is an open-circuit and an alternating voltage V_1 is applied to the primary winding, a small current – called the no-load current I_0 – flows, which sets up a magnetic flux in the core. This alternating flux links with both primary and secondary coils and induces in them e.m.f.'s of E_1 and E_2 respectively by mutual induction.

The induced e.m.f. E in a coil of N turns is given by $E = -N(d\Phi/dt)$ volts, where $\frac{d\Phi}{dt}$ is the rate of change of flux. In an ideal transformer, the rate of change of flux is the same for both primary and secondary and thus $E_1/N_1 = E_2/N_2$ i.e. **the induced e.m.f. per turn is constant**.

Assuming no losses, $E_1 = V_1$ and $E_2 = V_2$

Hence $\qquad \dfrac{V_1}{N_1} = \dfrac{V_2}{N_2}$ or $\dfrac{V_1}{V_2} = \dfrac{N_1}{N_2}$ (1)

(V_1/V_2) is called the voltage ratio and (N_1/N_2) the turns ratio, or the '**transformation ratio**' of the transformer. If N_2 is less than N_1 then V_2 is less than V_1 and the device is termed a **step-down transformer**. If N_2 is greater then N_1 then V_2 is greater than V_1 and the device is termed a **step-up transformer**.

When a load is connected across the secondary winding, a current I_2 flows. In an ideal transformer losses are neglected and a transformer is considered to be 100 per cent efficient. Hence input power = output power,

or $V_1 I_1 = V_2 I_2$ i.e. in an ideal transformer, the **primary and secondary ampere-turns are equal**

Thus $\qquad \dfrac{V_1}{V_2} = \dfrac{I_2}{I_1}$ (2)

Combining equations (1) and (2) gives:

$$\frac{V_1}{V_2} = \frac{N_1}{N_2} = \frac{I_2}{I_1}$$ (3)

The **rating** of a transformer is stated in terms of the volt-amperes that it can transform without overheating. With reference to Fig. 21.1(a), the transformer rating is either $V_1 I_1$ or $V_2 I_2$, where I_2 is the full-load secondary current.

> **Problem 1.** A transformer has 500 primary turns and 3000 secondary turns. If the primary voltage is 240 V, determine the secondary voltage, assuming an ideal transformer.

For an ideal transformer, voltage ratio = turns ratio i.e.

$$\frac{V_1}{V_2} = \frac{N_1}{N_2} \quad \text{hence} \quad \frac{240}{V_2} = \frac{500}{3000}$$

Thus secondary voltage

$$V_2 = \frac{(240)(3000)}{500} = \textbf{1440\,V or 1.44\,kV}$$

> **Problem 2.** An ideal transformer with a turns ratio of 2:7 is fed from a 240 V supply. Determine its output voltage.

A turns ratio of 2:7 means that the transformer has 2 turns on the primary for every 7 turns on the secondary (i.e. a step-up transformer); thus $(N_1/N_2) = (2/7)$.

For an ideal transformer, $(N_1/N_2) = (V_1/V_2)$ hence $(2/7) = (240/V_2)$. Thus the secondary voltage

$$V_2 = \frac{(240)(7)}{2} = \textbf{840 V}$$

Problem 3. An ideal transformer has a turns ratio of 8:1 and the primary current is 3 A when it is supplied at 240 V. Calculate the secondary voltage and current.

A turns ratio of 8:1 means $(N_1/N_2) = (1/8)$ i.e. a step-down transformer.

$$\left(\frac{N_1}{N_2}\right) = \left(\frac{V_1}{V_2}\right) \text{ or secondary voltage}$$

$$V_2 = V_1 \left(\frac{N_1}{N_2}\right) = 240 \left(\frac{1}{8}\right) = \textbf{30 volts}$$

Also, $\left(\dfrac{N_1}{N_2}\right) = \left(\dfrac{I_2}{I_1}\right)$ hence secondary current

$$I_2 = I_1 \left(\frac{N_1}{N_2}\right) = 3 \left(\frac{8}{1}\right) = \textbf{24 A}$$

Problem 4. An ideal transformer, connected to a 240 V mains, supplies a 12 V, 150 W lamp. Calculate the transformer turns ratio and the current taken from the supply.

$V_1 = 240$ V, $V_2 = 12$ V,
$I_2 = (P/V_2) = (150/12) = 12.5$ A.

$$\textbf{Turns ratio} = \frac{N_1}{N_2} = \frac{V_1}{V_2} = \frac{240}{12} = \textbf{20}$$

$\left(\dfrac{V_1}{V_2}\right) = \left(\dfrac{I_2}{I_1}\right)$, from which,

$$I_1 = I_2 \left(\frac{V_2}{V_1}\right) = 12.5 \left(\frac{12}{240}\right)$$

Hence current taken from the supply,

$$I_1 = \frac{12.5}{20} = \textbf{0.625 A}$$

Problem 5. A 12 Ω resistor is connected across the secondary winding of an ideal transformer whose secondary voltage is 120 V. Determine the primary voltage if the supply current is 4 A.

Secondary current $I_2 = (V_2/R_2) = (120/12) = 10$ A. $(V_1/V_2) = (I_2/I_1)$, from which the primary voltage

$$V_1 = V_2 \left(\frac{I_2}{I_1}\right) = 120 \left(\frac{10}{4}\right) = \textbf{300 volts}$$

Problem 6. A 5 kVA single-phase transformer has a turns ratio of 10:1 and is fed from a 2.5 kV supply. Neglecting losses, determine (a) the full-load secondary current, (b) the minimum load resistance which can be connected across the secondary winding to give full load kVA, (c) the primary current at full load kVA.

(a) $N_1/N_2 = 10/1$ and $V_1 = 2.5$ kV $= 2500$ V.

Since $\left(\dfrac{N_1}{N_2}\right) = \left(\dfrac{V_1}{V_2}\right)$, secondary voltage

$$V_2 = V_1 \left(\frac{N_2}{N_1}\right) = 2500 \left(\frac{1}{10}\right) = 250 \text{ V}$$

The transformer rating in volt-amperes $= V_2 I_2$ (at full load) i.e. $5000 = 250 I_2$

Hence full-load secondary current,
$I_2 = (5000/250) = \textbf{20 A}$.

(b) Minimum value of load resistance,

$$R_L = \left(\frac{V_2}{V_1}\right) = \left(\frac{250}{20}\right) = \textbf{12.5 }\Omega.$$

(c) $\left(\dfrac{N_1}{N_2}\right) = \left(\dfrac{I_2}{I_1}\right)$ from which primary current

$$I_1 = I_2 \left(\frac{N_1}{N_2}\right) = 20 \left(\frac{1}{10}\right) = \textbf{2 A}$$

Now try the following exercise

Exercise 118 **Further problems on the transformer principle of operation**

1. A transformer has 600 primary turns connected to a 1.5 kV supply. Determine the number of secondary turns for a 240 V output voltage, assuming no losses. [96]

2. An ideal transformer with a turns ratio of 2:9 is fed from a 220 V supply. Determine its output voltage. [990 V]

3. A transformer has 800 primary turns and 2000 secondary turns. If the primary voltage is 160 V, determine the secondary voltage assuming an ideal transformer. [400 V]

Section 3

4. An ideal transformer with a turns ratio of 3:8 has an output voltage of 640 V. Determine its input voltage. [240 V]

5. An ideal transformer has a turns ratio of 12:1 and is supplied at 192 V. Calculate the secondary voltage. [16 V]

6. A transformer primary winding connected across a 415 V supply has 750 turns. Determine how many turns must be wound on the secondary side if an output of 1.66 kV is required. [3000 turns]

7. An ideal transformer has a turns ratio of 15:1 and is supplied at 180 V when the primary current is 4 A. Calculate the secondary voltage and current. [12 V, 60 A]

8. A step-down transformer having a turns ratio of 20:1 has a primary voltage of 4 kV and a load of 10 kW. Neglecting losses, calculate the value of the secondary current. [50 A]

9. A transformer has a primary to secondary turns ratio of 1:15. Calculate the primary voltage necessary to supply a 240 V load. If the load current is 3 A determine the primary current. Neglect any losses. [16 V, 45 A]

10. A 10 kVA, single-phase transformer has a turns ratio of 12:1 and is supplied from a 2.4 kV supply. Neglecting losses, determine (a) the full-load secondary current, (b) the minimum value of load resistance which can be connected across the secondary winding without the kVA rating being exceeded, and (c) the primary current. [(a) 50 A (b) 4 Ω (c) 4.17 A]

11. A 20 Ω resistance is connected across the secondary winding of a single-phase power transformer whose secondary voltage is 150 V. Calculate the primary voltage and the turns ratio if the supply current is 5 A, neglecting losses. [225 V, 3:2]

21.3 Transformer no-load phasor diagram

The core flux is common to both primary and secondary windings in a transformer and is thus taken as the reference phasor in a phasor diagram. On no-load the primary winding takes a small no-load current I_0 and since, with losses neglected, the primary winding is a pure inductor, this current lags the applied voltage V_1 by 90°. In the phasor diagram assuming no losses, shown in Fig. 21.2(a), current I_0 produces the flux and is drawn in phase with the flux. The primary induced e.m.f. E_1 is in phase opposition to V_1 (by Lenz's law) and is shown 180° out of phase with V_1 and equal in magnitude. The secondary induced e.m.f. is shown for a 2:1 turns ratio transformer.

A no-load phasor diagram for a practical transformer is shown in Fig. 21.2(b). If current flows then losses will occur. When losses are considered then the no-load current I_0 is the phasor sum of two components – (i) I_M, the magnetising component, in phase with the flux, and (ii) I_C, the core loss component (supplying the hysteresis and eddy current losses). From Fig. 21.2(b):

No-load current, $I_0 = \sqrt{I_M^2 + I_C^2}$ where

$I_M = I_0 \sin\phi_0$ and $I_C = I_0 \cos\phi_0$.

Power factor on no-load $= \cos\phi_0 = (I_C/I_0)$.
The total core losses (i.e. iron losses) $= V_1 I_0 \cos\phi_0$

Problem 7. A 2400 V/400 V single-phase transformer takes a no-load current of 0.5 A and the core loss is 400 W. Determine the values of the magnetising and core loss components of the no-load current. Draw to scale the no-load phasor diagram for the transformer.

$V_1 = 2400$ V, $V_2 = 400$ V and $I_0 = 0.5$ A Core loss (i.e. iron loss) $= 400 = V_1 I_0 \cos\phi_0$.

i.e. $400 = (2400)(0.5)\cos\phi_0$

Hence $\cos\phi_0 = \dfrac{400}{(2400)(0.5)} = 0.3333$

$\phi_0 = \cos^{-1} 0.3333 = 70.53°$

The no-load phasor diagram is shown in Fig. 21.3
Magnetising component,
$I_M = I_0 \sin\phi_0 = 0.5 \sin 70.53° = \mathbf{0.471\,A}$.
Core loss component, $I_C = I_0 \cos\phi_0 = 0.5 \cos 70.53°$
$= \mathbf{0.167\,A}$

Problem 8. A transformer takes a current of 0.8 A when its primary is connected to a 240 volt, 50 Hz supply, the secondary being on open circuit. If the power absorbed is 72 watts, determine (a) the iron loss current, (b) the power factor on no-load, and (c) the magnetising current.

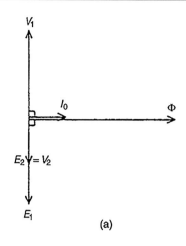

Figure 21.2

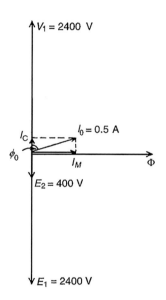

Figure 21.3

$I_0 = 0.8\,\text{A}$ and $V = 240\,\text{V}$

(a) Power absorbed = total core loss $= 72 = V_1 I_0 \cos\phi_0$. Hence $72 = 240 I_0 \cos\phi_0$ and iron loss current, $I_c = I_0 \cos\phi_0 = 72/240 = \textbf{0.30 A}$

(b) Power factor at no load,

$$\cos\phi_0 = \frac{I_C}{I_0} = \frac{0.3}{0.8} = \textbf{0.375}$$

(c) From the right-angled triangle in Fig. 21.2(b) and using Pythagoras' theorem, $I_0^2 = I_C^2 + I_M^2$ from which, magnetising current,

$$I_M = \sqrt{I_0^2 - I_C^2} = \sqrt{0.8^2 - 0.3^2} = \textbf{0.74 A}$$

Now try the following exercise

Exercise 119   Further problems on the no-load phasor diagram

1. A 500 V/100 V, single-phase transformer takes a full-load primary current of 4 A. Neglecting losses, determine (a) the full-load secondary current, and (b) the rating of the transformer.

   [(a) 20 A (b) 2 kVA]

2. A 3300 V/440 V, single-phase transformer takes a no-load current of 0.8 A and the iron loss is 500 W. Draw the no-load phasor diagram and determine the values of the magnetising and core loss components of the no-load current.   [0.786 A, 0.152 A]

3. A transformer takes a current of 1 A when its primary is connected to a 300 V, 50 Hz supply, the secondary being on open-circuit. If the power absorbed is 120 watts, calculate (a) the iron loss current, (b) the power factor on no-load, and (c) the magnetising current.

   [(a) 0.40 A (b) 0.40 (c) 0.917 A]

21.4   E.m.f. equation of a transformer

The magnetic flux Φ set up in the core of a transformer when an alternating voltage is applied to its primary winding is also alternating and is sinusoidal.

Let Φ_m be the maximum value of the flux and f be the frequency of the supply. The time for 1 cycle of the alternating flux is the periodic time T, where $T = (1/f)$ seconds.

The flux rises sinusoidally from zero to its maximum value in $(1/4)$ cycle, and the time for $(1/4)$ cycle is $(1/4f)$ seconds. Hence the average rate of change of flux $= (\Phi_m/(1/4f)) = 4f\Phi_m$ Wb/s, and since 1 Wb/s $= 1$ volt, the average e.m.f. induced in each turn $= 4f\Phi_m$ volts. As the flux Φ varies sinusoidally, then a sinusoidal e.m.f. will be induced in each turn of both primary and secondary windings.

For a sine wave,

$$\text{form factor} = \frac{\text{r.m.s. value}}{\text{average value}}$$

$$= 1.11 \text{ (see Chapter 14)}$$

Hence r.m.s. value $=$ form factor $\times$ average value $= 1.11 \times$ average value. Thus r.m.s. e.m.f. induced in each turn

$$= 1.11 \times 4f\Phi_m \text{ volts}$$

$$= 4.44f\Phi_m \text{ volts}$$

Therefore, r.m.s. value of e.m.f. induced in primary,

$$E_1 = 4.44f\Phi_m N_1 \text{ volts} \tag{4}$$

and r.m.s. value of e.m.f. induced in secondary,

$$E_2 = 4.44f\Phi_m N_2 \text{ volts} \tag{5}$$

Dividing equation (4) by equation (5) gives:

$$\left(\frac{E_1}{E_2}\right) = \left(\frac{N_1}{N_2}\right)$$

as previously obtained in Section 21.2

Problem 9. A 100 kVA, 4000 V/200 V, 50 Hz single-phase transformer has 100 secondary turns. Determine (a) the primary and secondary current, (b) the number of primary turns, and (c) the maximum value of the flux.

$V_1 = 4000$ V, $V_2 = 200$ V, $f = 50$ Hz, $N_2 = 100$ turns

(a) Transformer rating $= V_1 I_1 = V_2 I_2 = 100\,000$ VA
Hence primary current,

$$I_1 = \frac{100\,000}{V_1} = \frac{100\,000}{4000} = 25 \text{ A}$$

and secondary current,

$$I_2 = \frac{100\,000}{V_2} = \frac{100\,000}{200} = 500 \text{ A}$$

(b) From equation (3), $\dfrac{V_1}{V_2} = \dfrac{N_1}{N_2}$ from which, primary turns,

$$N_1 = \left(\frac{V_1}{V_2}\right)(N_2) = \left(\frac{4000}{200}\right)(100) = 2000 \text{ turns}$$

(c) From equation (5), $E_2 = 4.44f\Phi_m N_2$ from which, maximum flux,

$$\Phi_m = \frac{E}{4.44fN_2}$$

$$= \frac{200}{(4.44)(50)(100)} \text{ (assuming } E_2 = V_2\text{)}$$

$$= 9.01 \times 10^{-3} \text{ Wb or } 9.01 \text{ mWb}$$

[Alternatively, equation (4) could have been used, where

$$E_1 = 4.44f\Phi_m N_1 \text{ from which,}$$

$$\Phi_m = \frac{4000}{(4.44)(50)(2000)} \text{ (assuming } E_1 = V_1\text{)}$$

$$= 9.01 \text{ mWb as above]}$$

Problem 10. A single-phase, 50 Hz transformer has 25 primary turns and 300 secondary turns. The cross-sectional area of the core is 300 cm^2. When the primary winding is connected to a 250 V supply, determine (a) the maximum value of the flux density in the core, and (b) the voltage induced in the secondary winding.

(a) From equation (4),
e.m.f. $E_1 = 4.44f\Phi_m N_1$ volts
i.e. $250 = 4.44(50)\Phi_m(25)$ from which, maximum flux density,

$$\Phi_m = \frac{250}{(4.44)(50)(25)} \text{Wb} = 0.04505 \text{ Wb}$$

However, $\Phi_m = B_m \times A$, where $B_m = $ maximum flux density in the core and $A = $ cross-sectional area of the core (see Chapter 7). Hence
$B_m \times 300 \times 10^{-4} = 0.04505$ from which,

$$\textbf{maximum flux density, } B_m = \frac{0.04505}{300 \times 10^{-4}}$$

$$= 1.50 \text{ T}$$

(b) $\dfrac{V_1}{V_2} = \dfrac{N_1}{N_2}$ from which, $V_2 = V_1 \left(\dfrac{N_2}{N_1}\right)$ i.e. voltage induced in the secondary winding,

$$V_2 = (250)\left(\dfrac{300}{25}\right) = \mathbf{3000\,V}\text{ or }\mathbf{3kV}$$

Problem 11. A single-phase 500 V/100 V, 50 Hz transformer has a maximum core flux density of 1.5 T and an effective core cross-sectional area of $50\,\text{cm}^2$. Determine the number of primary and secondary turns.

The e.m.f. equation for a transformer is $E = 4.44\,f\,\Phi_m N$ and maximum flux, $\Phi_m = B \times A = (1.5)(50 \times 10^{-4}) = 75 \times 10^{-4}\,\text{Wb}$

Since $E_1 = 4.44\,f\,\Phi_m N_1$ then primary turns,

$$N_1 = \dfrac{E_1}{4.44\,f\,\Phi_m} = \dfrac{500}{(4.44)(50)(75 \times 10^{-4})}$$
$$= \mathbf{300\ turns}$$

Since $E_2 = 4.4\,f\,\Phi_m N_2$ then secondary turns,

$$N_2 = \dfrac{E_2}{4.44\,f\,\Phi_m} = \dfrac{100}{(4.44)(50)(75 \times 10^{-4})}$$
$$= \mathbf{60\ turns}$$

Problem 12. A 4500 V/225 V, 50 Hz single-phase transformer is to have an approximate e.m.f. per turn of 15 V and operate with a maximum flux of 1.4 T. Calculate (a) the number of primary and secondary turns and (b) the cross-sectional area of the core.

(a) E.m.f. per turn $= \dfrac{E_1}{N_1} = \dfrac{E_2}{N_2} = 15$

Hence primary turns, $N_1 = \dfrac{E_1}{15} = \dfrac{4500}{15} = \mathbf{300}$

and secondary turns, $N_2 = \dfrac{E_2}{15} = \dfrac{255}{15} = \mathbf{15}$

(b) E.m.f. $E_1 = 4.44\,f\,\Phi_m N_1$ from which,

$$\Phi_m = \dfrac{E_1}{4.44\,f\,N_1} = \dfrac{4500}{(4.44)(50)(300)} = 0.0676\,\text{Wb}$$

Now flux, $\Phi_m = B_m \times A$, where A is the cross-sectional area of the core,

hence area, $\quad \mathbf{A} = \left(\dfrac{\Phi_m}{B_m}\right) = \left(\dfrac{0.0676}{1.4}\right)$
$$= \mathbf{0.0483\,m^2}\text{ or }\mathbf{483\,cm^2}$$

Now try the following exercise

Exercise 120   Further problems on the transformer e.m.f. equation

1. A 60 kVA, 1600 V/100 V, 50 Hz, single-phase transformer has 50 secondary windings. Calculate (a) the primary and secondary current, (b) the number of primary turns, and (c) the maximum value of the flux.
   [(a) 37.5 A, 600 A (b) 800 (c) 9.0 mWb]

2. A single-phase, 50 Hz transformer has 40 primary turns and 520 secondary turns. The cross-sectional area of the core is $270\,\text{cm}^2$. When the primary winding is connected to a 300 volt supply, determine (a) the maximum value of flux density in the core, and (b) the voltage induced in the secondary winding.
   [(a) 1.25 T (b) 3.90 kV]

3. A single-phase 800 V/100 V, 50 Hz transformer has a maximum core flux density of 1.294 T and an effective cross-sectional area of $60\,\text{cm}^2$. Calculate the number of turns on the primary and secondary windings.
   [464, 58]

4. A 3.3 kV/110 V, 50 Hz, single-phase transformer is to have an approximate e.m.f. per turn of 22 V and operate with a maximum flux of 1.25 T. Calculate (a) the number of primary and secondary turns, and (b) the cross-sectional area of the core.
   [(a) 150, 5 (b) $792.8\,\text{cm}^2$]

21.5 Transformer on-load phasor diagram

If the voltage drop in the windings of a transformer are assumed negligible, then the terminal voltage V_2 is the same as the induced e.m.f. E_2 in the secondary. Similarly, $V_1 = E_1$. Assuming an equal number of turns on primary and secondary windings, then $E_1 = E_2$, and let the load have a lagging phase angle ϕ_2.

In the phasor diagram of Fig. 21.4, current I_2 lags V_2 by angle ϕ_2. When a load is connected across the secondary winding a current I_2 flows in the secondary winding. The resulting secondary e.m.f. acts so as to tend to reduce the core flux. However this does not happen since reduction of the core flux reduces E_1,

Section 3

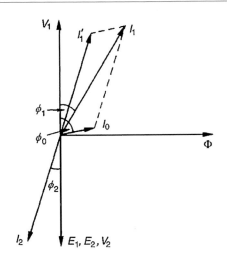

Figure 21.4

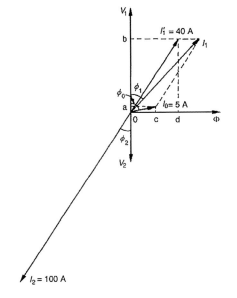

Figure 21.5

hence a reflected increase in primary current I_1' occurs which provides a restoring m.m.f. Hence at all loads, primary and secondary m.m.f.'s are equal, but in opposition, and the core flux remains constant. I_1' is sometimes called the 'balancing' current and is equal, but in the opposite direction, to current I_2 as shown in Fig. 21.4. I_0, shown at a phase angle ϕ_0 to V_1, is the no-load current of the transformer (see Section 21.3).

The phasor sum of I_1' and I_0 gives the supply current I_1 and the phase angle between V_1 and I_1 is shown as ϕ_1.

> **Problem 13.** A single-phase transformer has 2000 turns on the primary and 800 turns on the secondary. Its no-load current is 5 A at a power factor of 0.20 lagging. Assuming the volt drop in the windings is negligible, determine the primary current and power factor when the secondary current is 100 A at a power factor of 0.85 lagging.

Let I_1' be the component of the primary current which provides the restoring m.m.f. Then

$$I_1' N_1 = I_2 N_2$$

i.e.

$$I_1'(2000) = (100)(800)$$

from which,

$$I_1' = \frac{(100)(800)}{2000}$$

$$= 40\,\text{A}$$

If the power factor of the secondary is 0.85, then $\cos\phi_2 = 0.85$, from which, $\phi_2 = \cos^{-1} 0.85 = 31.8°$.

If the power factor on no-load is 0.20, then $\cos\phi_0 = 0.2$ and $\phi_0 = \cos^{-1} 0.2 = 78.5°$.

In the phasor diagram shown in Fig. 21.5, $I_2 = 100\,\text{A}$ is shown at an angle of $\phi = 31.8°$ to V_2 and $I_1' = 40\,\text{A}$ is shown in anti-phase to I_2.

The no-load current $I_0 = 5\,\text{A}$ is shown at an angle of $\phi_0 = 78.5°$ to V_1. Current I_1 is the phasor sum of I_1' and I_0, and by drawing to scale, $I_1 = 44\,\text{A}$ and angle $\phi_1 = 37°$.

By calculation,

$$I_1 \cos\phi_1 = 0a + 0b$$

$$= I_0 \cos\phi_0 + I_1' \cos\phi_2$$

$$= (5)(0.2) + (40)(0.85)$$

$$= 35.0\,\text{A}$$

and

$$I_1 \sin\phi_1 = 0c + 0d$$

$$= I_0 \sin\phi_0 + I_1' \sin\phi_2$$

$$= (5)\sin 78.5° + (40)\sin 31.8°$$

$$= 25.98\,\text{A}$$

Hence the magnitude of $I_1 = \sqrt{35.0^2 + 25.98^2} = $ **43.59 A** and $\tan\phi_1 = (25.98/35.0)$ from which, $\phi_1 = \tan^{-1}(25.98/35.0) = \mathbf{36.59°}$. Hence the power factor of the primary $= \cos\phi_1 = \cos 36.59° = \mathbf{0.80}$

Now try the following exercise

Exercise 121   A further problem on the
transformer on-load

1. A single-phase transformer has 2400 turns on
    the primary and 600 turns on the secondary.
    Its no-load current is 4 A at a power factor of
    0.25 lagging. Assuming the volt drop in the
    windings is negligible, calculate the primary
    current and power factor when the secondary
    current is 80 A at a power factor of 0.8 lagging.
    [23.26 A, 0.73]

21.6 Transformer construction

(i)   There are broadly two types of single-phase
      double-wound transformer constructions – the
      core type and the **shell type**, as shown in Fig. 21.6.
      The low and high voltage windings are wound as
      shown to reduce leakage flux.

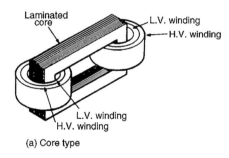

(a) Core type

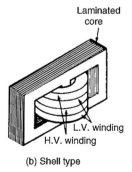

(b) Shell type

Figure 21.6

(ii) For **power transformers**, rated possibly at sev-
      eral MVA and operating at a frequency of 50 Hz
      in Great Britain, the core material used is usually
      laminated silicon steel or stalloy, the lamina-
      tions reducing eddy currents and the silicon steel
      keeping hysteresis loss to a minimum.

      Large power transformers are used in the main dis-
      tribution system and in industrial supply circuits.
      Small power transformers have many applica-
      tions, examples including welding and rectifier
      supplies, domestic bell circuits, imported washing
      machines, and so on.

(iii) For **audio frequency (a.f.) transformers**, rated
      from a few mVA to no more than 20 VA, and oper-
      ating at frequencies up to about 15 kHz, the small
      core is also made of laminated silicon steel. A typ-
      ical application of a.f. transformers is in an audio
      amplifier system.

(iv) **Radio frequency (r.f.) transformers**, operating
      in the MHz frequency region have either an air
      core, a ferrite core or a dust core. Ferrite is a
      ceramic material having magnetic properties sim-
      ilar to silicon steel, but having a high resistivity.
      Dust cores consist of fine particles of carbonyl iron
      or permalloy (i.e. nickel and iron), each particle
      of which is insulated from its neighbour. Appli-
      cations of r.f. transformers are found in radio and
      television receivers.

(v)   Transformer **windings** are usually of enamel-
      insulated copper or aluminium.

(vi) **Cooling** is achieved by air in small transformers
      and oil in large transformers.

21.7 Equivalent circuit of a transformer

Figure 21.7 shows an equivalent circuit of a transformer.
R_1 and R_2 represent the resistances of the primary and
secondary windings and X_1 and X_2 represent the reactances of the primary and secondary windings, due to
leakage flux.

The core losses due to hysteresis and eddy currents are
allowed for by resistance R which takes a current I_C, the
core loss component of the primary current. Reactance
X takes the magnetising component I_m. In a simplified
equivalent circuit shown in Fig. 21.8, R and X are omitted since the no-load current I_0 is normally only about
3–5 per cent of the full-load primary current.

It is often convenient to assume that all of the
resistance and reactance as being on one side of the
transformer. Resistance R_2 in Fig. 21.8 can be replaced

Section 3

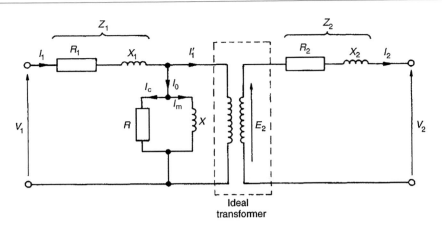

Figure 21.7

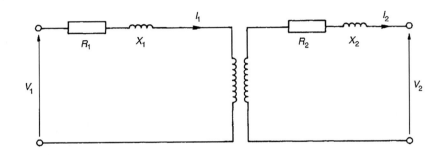

Figure 21.8

by inserting an additional resistance R'_2 in the primary circuit such that the power absorbed in R'_2 when carrying the primary current is equal to that in R_2 due to the secondary current, i.e.

$$I_1^2 R'_2 = I_2^2 R_2$$

from which, $\quad R'_2 = R_2 \left(\dfrac{I_2}{I_1}\right)^2 = R_2 \left(\dfrac{V_1}{V_2}\right)^2$

Then the total equivalent resistance in the primary circuit R_e is equal to the primary and secondary resistances of the actual transformer.

Hence $R_e = R_1 + R'_2$

i.e. $\qquad R_e = R_1 + R_2 \left(\dfrac{V_1}{V_2}\right)^2 \qquad (6)$

By similar reasoning, the equivalent reactance in the primary circuit is given by $X_e = X_1 + X'_2$

i.e. $\qquad X_e = X_1 + X_2 \left(\dfrac{V_1}{V_2}\right)^2 \qquad (7)$

The equivalent impedance Z_e of the primary and secondary windings referred to the primary is given by

$$Z_e = \sqrt{R_e^2 + X_e^2} \qquad (8)$$

If ϕ_e is the phase angle between I_1 and the volt drop $I_1 Z_e$ then

$$\cos \phi_e = \frac{R_e}{Z_e} \qquad (9)$$

The simplified equivalent circuit of a transformer is shown in Fig. 21.9.

Problem 14. A transformer has 600 primary turns and 150 secondary turns. The primary and secondary resistances are 0.25 Ω and 0.01 Ω respectively and the corresponding leakage reactances are 1.0 Ω and 0.04 Ω respectively. Determine (a) the equivalent resistance referred to the primary winding, (b) the equivalent reactance referred to the primary winding, (c) the equivalent impedance referred to the primary winding, and (d) the phase angle of the impedance.

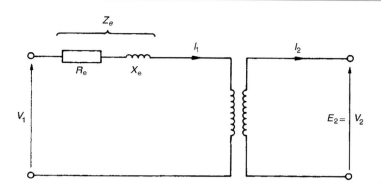

Figure 21.9

(a) From equation (6), equivalent resistance

$$R_e = R_1 + R_2 \left(\frac{V_1}{V_2}\right)^2$$

i.e. $R_e = 0.25 + 0.01 \left(\frac{600}{150}\right)^2$

$$= \mathbf{0.41\,\Omega} \text{ since } \frac{N_1}{N_2} = \frac{V_1}{V_2}$$

(b) From equation (7), equivalent reactance,

$$X_e = X_1 + X_2 \left(\frac{V_1}{V_2}\right)^2$$

i.e. $X_e = 1.0 + 0.04 \left(\frac{600}{150}\right)^2 = \mathbf{1.64\,\Omega}$

(c) From equation (8), equivalent impedance,

$$Z_e = \sqrt{R_e^2 + X_e^2} = \sqrt{0.41^2 + 1.64^2} = \mathbf{1.69\,\Omega}$$

(d) From equation (9),

$$\cos\phi_e = \frac{R_e}{Z_e} = \frac{0.41}{1.69}$$

Hence $\phi_e = \cos^{-1}\dfrac{0.41}{1.69} = \mathbf{75.96°}$

Now try the following exercise

Exercise 122   A further problem on the equivalent circuit of a transformer

1. A transformer has 1200 primary turns and 200 secondary turns. The primary and secondary resistances are $0.2\,\Omega$ and $0.02\,\Omega$ respectively and the corresponding leakage reactances are $1.2\,\Omega$ and $0.05\,\Omega$ respectively. Calculate

(a) the equivalent resistance, reactance and impedance referred to the primary winding, and (b) the phase angle of the impedance.
[(a) $0.92\,\Omega$, $3.0\,\Omega$, $3.14\,\Omega$ (b) $72.95°$]

21.8   Regulation of a transformer

When the secondary of a transformer is loaded, the secondary terminal voltage, V_2, falls. As the power factor decreases, this voltage drop increases. This is called the **regulation of the transformer** and it is usually expressed as a percentage of the secondary no-load voltage, E_2. For full-load conditions:

$$\text{Regulation} = \left(\frac{E_2 - V_2}{E_2}\right) \times 100\% \qquad (10)$$

The fall in voltage, $(E_2 - V_2)$, is caused by the resistance and reactance of the windings. Typical values of voltage regulation are about 3% in small transformers and about 1% in large transformers.

Problem 15.   A 5 kVA, 200 V/400 V, single-phase transformer has a secondary terminal voltage of 387.6 volts when loaded. Determine the regulation of the transformer.

From equation (10):

$$\text{regulation} = \left(\frac{\begin{array}{c}\text{No-load secondary voltage} -\\ \text{terminal voltage on load}\end{array}}{\text{no-load secondary voltage}}\right) \times 100\%$$

$$= \left(\frac{400 - 387.6}{400}\right) \times 100\%$$

$$= \left(\frac{12.4}{400}\right) \times 100\%$$

$$= \mathbf{3.1\%}$$

Section 3

Problem 16. The open-circuit voltage of a transformer is 240 V. A tap-changing device is set to operate when the percentage regulation drops below 2.5%. Determine the load voltage at which the mechanism operates.

$$\text{Regulation} = \left(\frac{\begin{array}{c}\text{No-load secondary voltage} - \\ \text{terminal voltage on load}\end{array}}{\text{no-load secondary voltage}} \right) \times 100\%$$

Hence $\qquad 2.5 = \left(\dfrac{240 - V_2}{240} \right) \times 100\%$

$\therefore \qquad \dfrac{(2.5)(240)}{100} = 240 - V_2$

i.e. $\qquad 6 = 240 - V_2$

from which, **load voltage, $V_2 = 240 - 6 = \mathbf{234\,volts}$**

Now try the following exercise

Exercise 123   Further problems on regulation

1. A 6 kVA, 100 V/500 V, single-phase transformer has a secondary terminal voltage of 487.5 volts when loaded. Determine the regulation of the transformer.   [2.5%]

2. A transformer has an open-circuit voltage of 110 volts. A tap-changing device operates when the regulation falls below 3%. Calculate the load voltage at which the tap-changer operates.   [106.7 volts]

21.9 Transformer losses and efficiency

There are broadly two sources of **losses in transformers** on load, these being copper losses and iron losses.

(a) **Copper losses** are variable and result in a heating of the conductors, due to the fact that they possess resistance. If R_1 and R_2 are the primary

and secondary winding resistances then the total copper loss is $I_1^2 R_1 + I_2^2 R_2$

(b) **Iron losses** are constant for a given value of frequency and flux density and are of two types – hysteresis loss and eddy current loss.

   (i) **Hysteresis loss** is the heating of the core as a result of the internal molecular structure reversals which occur as the magnetic flux alternates. The loss is proportional to the area of the hysteresis loop and thus low loss nickel iron alloys are used for the core since their hysteresis loops have small areas. (See Chapter 7)

   (ii) **Eddy current loss** is the heating of the core due to e.m.f.'s being induced not only in the transformer windings but also in the core. These induced e.m.f.'s set up circulating currents, called eddy currents. Owing to the low resistance of the core, eddy currents can be quite considerable and can cause a large power loss and excessive heating of the core. Eddy current losses can be reduced by increasing the resistivity of the core material or, more usually, by laminating the core (i.e. splitting it into layers or leaves) when very thin layers of insulating material can be inserted between each pair of laminations. This increases the resistance of the eddy current path, and reduces the value of the eddy current.

Transformer efficiency,

$$\eta = \frac{\text{output power}}{\text{input power}} = \frac{\text{input power} - \text{losses}}{\text{input power}}$$

i.e. $\qquad \eta = 1 - \dfrac{\text{losses}}{\text{input power}} \qquad\qquad (11)$

and is usually expressed as a percentage. It is not uncommon for power transformers to have efficiencies of between 95% and 98%

Output power $= V_2 I_2 \cos\phi_2$
Total losses $=$ copper loss $+$ iron losses,
and input power $=$ output power $+$ losses

Problem 17. A 200 kVA rated transformer has a full-load copper loss of 1.5 kW and an iron loss of 1 kW. Determine the transformer efficiency at full load and 0.85 power factor.

Efficiency, $\eta = \dfrac{\text{output power}}{\text{input power}}$

$= \dfrac{\text{input power} - \text{losses}}{\text{input power}}$

$= 1 - \dfrac{\text{losses}}{\text{input power}}$

Full-load output power $= VI\cos\phi = (200)(0.85)$
$= 170\,\text{kW}.$
Total losses $= 1.5 + 1.0 = 2.5\,\text{kW}$
Input power $=$ output power $+$ losses
$= 170 + 2.5 = 172.5\,\text{kW}.$

Hence efficiency $= \left(1 - \dfrac{2.5}{172.5}\right) = 1 - 0.01449$
$= 0.9855$ or $\mathbf{98.55\%}$

Problem 18. Determine the efficiency of the transformer in Problem 17 at half full load and 0.85 power factor.

Half full-load power output $= (1/2)(200)(0.85) = 85\,\text{kW}.$
Copper loss (or I^2R loss) is proportional to current squared. Hence the copper loss at half full load is:
$\left(\frac{1}{2}\right)^2 (1500) = 375\,\text{W}$
Iron loss $= 1000\,\text{W}$ (constant)
Total losses $= 375 + 1000 = 1375\,\text{W}$ or $1.375\,\text{kW}.$
Input power at half full load
$=$ output power at half full load $+$ losses
$= 85 + 1.375 = 86.375\,\text{kW}.$
Hence

efficiency $= 1 - \dfrac{\text{losses}}{\text{input power}}$

$= \left(1 - \dfrac{1.375}{86.375}\right)$

$= 1 - 0.01592$

$= 0.9841$ or $\mathbf{98.41\%}$

Problem 19. A 400 kVA transformer has a primary winding resistance of $0.5\,\Omega$ and a secondary winding resistance of $0.001\,\Omega$. The iron loss is $2.5\,\text{kW}$ and the primary and secondary voltages are $5\,\text{kV}$ and $320\,\text{V}$ respectively. If the power factor of the load is 0.85, determine the efficiency of the transformer (a) on full load, and (b) on half load.

(a) Rating $= 400\,\text{kVA} = V_1 I_1 = V_2 I_2$. Hence primary current,

$$I_1 = \dfrac{400 \times 10^3}{V_1} = \dfrac{400 \times 10^3}{5000} = 80\,\text{A}$$

and secondary current,

$$I_2 = \dfrac{400 \times 10^3}{V_2} = \dfrac{400 \times 10^3}{320} = 1250\,\text{A}$$

Total copper loss $= I_1^2 R_1 + I_2^2 R_2$,
(where $R_1 = 0.5\,\Omega$ and $R_2 = 0.001\,\Omega$)

$= (80)^2 (0.5) + (1250)^2 (0.001)$

$= 3200 + 1562.5 = 4762.5$ watts

On full load, total loss $=$ copper loss $+$ iron loss

$= 4762.5 + 2500 = 7262.5\,\text{W} = 7.2625\,\text{kW}$

Total output power on full load

$= V_2 I_2 \cos\phi_2 = (400 \times 10^3)(0.85) = 340\,\text{kW}$

Input power $=$ output power $+$ losses
$= 340\,\text{kW} + 7.2625\,\text{kW}$
$= 347.2625\,\text{kW}$

Efficiency, $\eta = \left(1 - \dfrac{\text{losses}}{\text{input power}}\right) \times 100\%$

$= \left(1 - \dfrac{7.2625}{347.2625}\right) \times 100\%$

$= \mathbf{97.91\%}$

(b) Since the copper loss varies as the square of the current, then total copper loss on half load $= 4762.5 \times \left(\frac{1}{2}\right)^2 = 1190.625\,\text{W}$. Hence total loss on half load $= 1190.625 + 2500 = 3690.625\,\text{W}$ or $3.691\,\text{kW}.$
Output power on half full load $= \left(\frac{1}{2}\right)(340)$
$= 170\,\text{kW}.$
Input power on half full load
$=$ output power $+$ losses

$= 170\,\text{kW} + 3.691\,\text{kW}$

$= 173.691\,\text{kW}$

Hence efficiency at half full load,

$$\eta = \left(1 - \frac{\text{losses}}{\text{input power}}\right) \times 100\%$$

$$= \left(1 - \frac{3.691}{173.691}\right) \times 100\% = \mathbf{97.87\%}$$

Maximum efficiency

It may be shown that the efficiency of a transformer is a maximum when the variable copper loss (i.e. $I_1^2 R_1 + I_2^2 R_2$) is equal to the constant iron losses.

Problem 20. A 500 kVA transformer has a full-load copper loss of 4 kW and an iron loss of 2.5 kW. Determine (a) the output kVA at which the efficiency of the transformer is a maximum, and (b) the maximum efficiency, assuming the power factor of the load is 0.75.

(a) Let x be the fraction of full load kVA at which the efficiency is a maximum. The corresponding total copper loss $= (4\,\text{kW})(x^2)$. At maximum efficiency, copper loss = iron loss. Hence $4x^2 = 2.5$ from which $x^2 = 2.5/4$ and $x = \sqrt{2.5/4} = 0.791$. Hence **the output kVA at maximum efficiency** $= 0.791 \times 500 = \mathbf{395.5\,kVA}$.

(b) Total loss at maximum efficiency
$$= 2 \times 2.5 = 5\,\text{kW}$$
Output power $= 395.5\,\text{kVA} \times \text{p.f.}$
$$= 395.5 \times 0.75 = 296.625\,\text{kW}$$
Input power $=$ output power $+$ losses
$$= 296.625 + 5 = 301.625\,\text{kW}$$

Maximum efficiency,

$$\eta = \left(1 - \frac{\text{losses}}{\text{input power}}\right) \times 100\%$$

$$= \left(1 - \frac{5}{301.625}\right) \times 100\% = \mathbf{98.34\%}$$

Now try the following exercise

Exercise 124 Further problems on losses and efficiency

1. A single-phase transformer has a voltage ratio of 6:1 and the h.v. winding is supplied at 540 V.

The secondary winding provides a full load current of 30 A at a power factor of 0.8 lagging. Neglecting losses, find (a) the rating of the transformer, (b) the power supplied to the load, (c) the primary current.
[(a) 2.7 kVA (b) 2.16 kW (c) 5 A]

2. A single-phase transformer is rated at 40 kVA. The transformer has full-load copper losses of 800 W and iron losses of 500 W. Determine the transformer efficiency at full load and 0.8 power factor. [96.10%]

3. Determine the efficiency of the transformer in problem 2 at half full load and 0.8 power factor. [95.81%]

4. A 100 kVA, 2000 V/400 V, 50 Hz, single-phase transformer has an iron loss of 600 W and a full-load copper loss of 1600 W. Calculate its efficiency for a load of 60 kW at 0.8 power factor. [97.56%]

5. Determine the efficiency of a 15 kVA transformer for the following conditions:
   (i) full-load, unity power factor
   (ii) 0.8 full-load, unity power factor
   (iii) half full-load, 0.8 power factor
   Assume that iron losses are 200 W and the full-load copper loss is 300 W.
   [(a) 96.77% (ii) 96.84% (iii) 95.62%]

6. A 300 kVA transformer has a primary winding resistance of 0.4 Ω and a secondary winding resistance of 0.0015 Ω. The iron loss is 2 kW and the primary and secondary voltages are 4 kV and 200 V respectively. If the power factor of the load is 0.78, determine the efficiency of the transformer (a) on full load, and (b) on half load. [(a) 96.84% (b) 97.17%]

7. A 250 kVA transformer has a full-load copper loss of 3 kW and an iron loss of 2 kW. Calculate (a) the output kVA at which the efficiency of the transformer is a maximum, and (b) the maximum efficiency, assuming the power factor of the load is 0.80.
[(a) 204.1 kVA (b) 97.61%]

21.10 Resistance matching

Varying a load resistance to be equal, or almost equal, to the source internal resistance is called **matching**. Examples where resistance matching is important include coupling an aerial to a transmitter or receiver, or in coupling a loudspeaker to an amplifier, where coupling transformers may be used to give maximum power transfer.

With d.c. generators or secondary cells, the internal resistance is usually very small. In such cases, if an attempt is made to make the load resistance as small as the source internal resistance, overloading of the source results.

A method of achieving maximum power transfer between a source and a load (see Section 13.9, page 204), is to adjust the value of the load resistance to 'match' the source internal resistance. A transformer may be used as a **resistance matching device** by connecting it between the load and the source.

The reason why a transformer can be used for this is shown below. With reference to Fig. 21.10:

$$R_L = \frac{V_2}{I_2} \quad \text{and} \quad R_1 = \frac{V_1}{I_1}$$

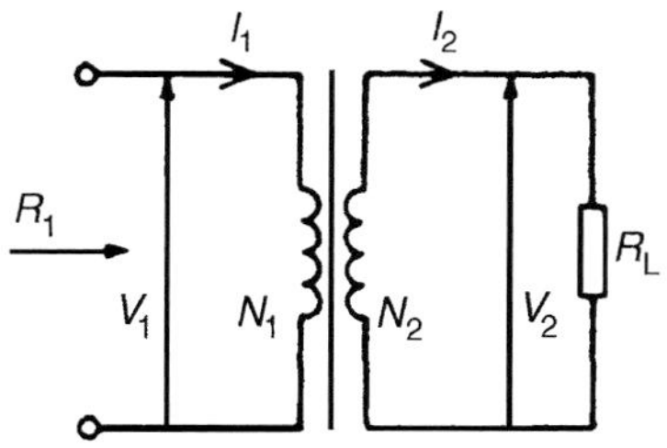

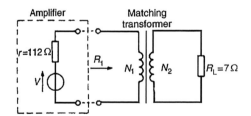

Figure 21.10

For an ideal transformer,

$$V_1 = \left(\frac{N_1}{N_2}\right) V_2$$

and

$$I_1 = \left(\frac{N_2}{N_1}\right) I_2$$

Thus the equivalent input resistance R_1 of the transformer is given by:

$$R_1 = \frac{V_1}{I_1} = \frac{\left(\dfrac{N_1}{N_2}\right) V_2}{\left(\dfrac{N_2}{N_1}\right) I_2}$$

$$= \left(\frac{N_1}{N_2}\right)^2 \left(\frac{V_2}{I_2}\right) = \left(\frac{N_1}{N_2}\right)^2 R_L$$

i.e.

$$R_1 = \left(\frac{N_1}{N_2}\right)^2 R_L$$

Hence by varying the value of the turns ratio, the equivalent input resistance of a transformer can be 'matched' to the internal resistance of a load to achieve maximum power transfer.

Problem 21. A transformer having a turns ratio of 4:1 supplies a load of resistance $100\,\Omega$. Determine the equivalent input resistance of the transformer.

From above, the equivalent input resistance,

$$R_1 = \left(\frac{N_1}{N_2}\right)^2 R_L$$

$$= \left(\frac{4}{1}\right)^2 (100) = \mathbf{1600\,\Omega}$$

Problem 22. The output stage of an amplifier has an output resistance of $112\,\Omega$. Calculate the optimum turns ratio of a transformer which would match a load resistance of $7\,\Omega$ to the output resistance of the amplifier.

The circuit is shown in Fig. 21.11.

Figure 21.11

The equivalent input resistance, R_1 of the transformer needs to be $112\,\Omega$ for maximum power transfer.

$$R_1 = \left(\frac{N_1}{N_2}\right)^2 R_L$$

Hence

$$\left(\frac{N_1}{N_2}\right)^2 = \frac{R_1}{R_L} = \frac{112}{7} = 16$$

i.e.

$$\frac{N_1}{N_2} = \sqrt{16} = 4$$

Hence the optimum turns ratio is 4:1

Problem 23. Determine the optimum value of load resistance for maximum power transfer if the load is connected to an amplifier of output resistance $150\,\Omega$ through a transformer with a turns ratio of 5:1

The equivalent input resistance R_1 of the transformer needs to be $150\,\Omega$ for maximum power transfer.

$$R_1 = \left(\frac{N_1}{N_2}\right)^2 R_L$$

from which, $$\boldsymbol{R_L = R_1 \left(\frac{N_2}{N_1}\right)^2}$$

$$= 150\left(\tfrac{1}{5}\right)^2 = \boldsymbol{6\,\Omega}$$

Problem 24. A single-phase, $220\,V/1760\,V$ ideal transformer is supplied from a $220\,V$ source through a cable of resistance $2\,\Omega$. If the load across the secondary winding is $1.28\,k\Omega$ determine (a) the primary current flowing and (b) the power dissipated in the load resistor.

The circuit diagram is shown in Fig. 21.12

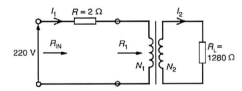

Figure 21.12

(a) Turns ratio

$$\left(\frac{N_1}{N_2}\right) = \left(\frac{V_1}{V_2}\right) = \left(\frac{220}{1760}\right) = \left(\frac{1}{8}\right)$$

Equivalent input resistance of the transformer.

$$R_1 = \left(\frac{N_1}{N_2}\right)^2 R_L = \left(\frac{1}{8}\right)^2 (1.28 \times 10^3) = 20\,\Omega$$

Total input resistance,

$$R_{IN} = R + R_1 = 2 + 20 = 22\,\Omega$$

Primary current,

$$\boldsymbol{I_1} = \frac{V_1}{R_{IN}} = \frac{220}{22} = \boldsymbol{10\,A}$$

(b) For an ideal transformer

$$\frac{V_1}{V_2} = \frac{I_2}{I_1}$$

from which,

$$I_2 = I_1\left(\frac{V_1}{V_2}\right) = 10\left(\frac{220}{1760}\right) = 1.25\,A$$

Power dissipated in load resistor R_L,

$$\boldsymbol{P} = I_2^2 R_L = (1.25)^2(1.28 \times 10^3)$$

$$= \boldsymbol{2000\ watts}\ \text{or}\ \boldsymbol{2\,kW}$$

Problem 25. An a.c. source of $24\,V$ and internal resistance $15\,k\Omega$ is matched to a load by a 25:1 ideal transformer. Determine (a) the value of the load resistance and (b) the power dissipated in the load.

The circuit diagram is shown in Fig. 21.13

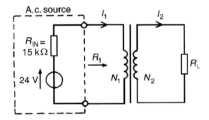

Figure 21.13

(a) For maximum power transfer R_1 needs to be equal to $15\,k\Omega$.

$$R_1 = \left(\frac{N_1}{N_2}\right)^2 R_L$$

from which, load resistance,

$$\boldsymbol{R_L} = R_1\left(\frac{N_2}{N_1}\right)^2 = (15\,000)\left(\frac{1}{25}\right)^2 = \boldsymbol{24\,\Omega}$$

(b) The total input resistance when the source is connected to the matching transformer is $R_{IN} + R_1$ i.e. $15\,k\Omega + 15\,k\Omega = 30\,k\Omega$.

Primary current,

$$I_1 = \frac{V}{30\,000} = \frac{24}{30\,000} = 0.8\,mA$$

$N_1/N_2 = I_2/I_1$ from which, $I_2 = I_1(N_1/N_2) = (0.8 \times 10^{-3})(25/1) = 20 \times 10^{-3}\,A$.

Power dissipated in the load R_L,

$$P = I_2^2 R_L = (20 \times 10^{-3})^2 (24)$$
$$= 9600 \times 10^{-6} \, \text{W} = \textbf{9.6 mW}$$

Now try the following exercise

Exercise 125 Further problems on resistance matching

1. A transformer having a turns ratio of 8:1 supplies a load of resistance 50 Ω. Determine the equivalent input resistance of the transformer.
    [3.2 kΩ]

2. What ratio of transformer turns is required to make a load of resistance 30 Ω appear to have a resistance of 270 Ω? [3:1]

3. Determine the optimum value of load resistance for maximum power transfer if the load is connected to an amplifier of output resistance 147 Ω through a transformer with a turns ratio of 7:2. [12 Ω]

4. A single-phase, 240 V/2880 V ideal transformer is supplied from a 240 V source through a cable of resistance 3 Ω. If the load across the secondary winding is 720 Ω determine (a) the primary current flowing and (b) the power dissipated in the load resistance.
    [(a) 30 A (b) 4.5 kW]

5. A load of resistance 768 Ω is to be matched to an amplifier which has an effective output resistance of 12 Ω. Determine the turns ratio of the coupling transformer. [1:8]

6. An a.c. source of 20 V and internal resistance 20 kΩ is matched to a load by a 16:1 single-phase transformer. Determine (a) the value of the load resistance and (b) the power dissipated in the load.
    [(a) 78.13 Ω (b) 5 mW]

21.11 Auto transformers

An auto transformer is a transformer which has part of its winding common to the primary and secondary circuits. Fig. 21.14(a) shows the circuit for a double-wound transformer and Fig. 21.14(b) that for an auto

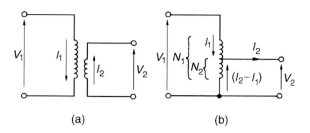

(a)   (b)

Figure 21.14

transformer. The latter shows that the secondary is actually part of the primary, the current in the secondary being $(I_2 - I_1)$. Since the current is less in this section, the cross-sectional area of the winding can be reduced, which reduces the amount of material necessary. Figure 21.15 shows the circuit diagram symbol for an auto transformer.

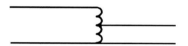

Figure 21.15

> **Problem 26.** A single-phase auto transformer has a voltage ratio 320 V:250 V and supplies a load of 20 kVA at 250 V. Assuming an ideal transformer, determine the current in each section of the winding.

Rating $= 20 \, \text{kVA} = V_1 I_1 = V_2 I_2$
Hence primary current,

$$I_1 = \frac{20 \times 10^3}{V_1} = \frac{20 \times 10^3}{320} = \textbf{62.5 A}$$

and secondary current,

$$I_2 = \frac{20 \times 10^3}{V_2} = \frac{20 \times 10^3}{250} = \textbf{80 A}$$

Hence current in common part of the winding
$= 80 - 62.5 = \textbf{17.5 A}$
The current flowing in each section of the transformer is shown in Fig. 21.16.

Saving of copper in an auto transformer

For the same output and voltage ratio, the auto transformer requires less copper than an ordinary double-wound transformer. This is explained below.

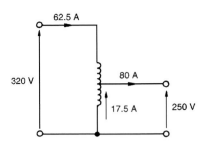

Figure 21.16

The volume, and hence weight, of copper required in a winding is proportional to the number of turns and to the cross-sectional area of the wire. In turn this is proportional to the current to be carried, i.e. volume of copper is proportional to NI.

Volume of copper in an auto transformer

$$\propto (N_1 - N_2)I_1 + N_2(I_2 - I_1)$$

see Fig. 21.14(b)

$$\propto N_1 I_1 - N_2 I_1 + N_2 I_2 - N_2 I_1$$

$$\propto N_1 I_1 + N_2 I_2 - 2N_2 I_1$$

$$\propto 2N_1 I_1 - 2N_2 I_1 \quad (\text{since } N_2 I_2 = N_1 I_1)$$

Volume of copper in a double-wound transformer

$$\propto N_1 I_1 + N_2 I_2 \propto 2N_1 I_1$$

(again, since $N_2 I_2 = N_1 I_1$). Hence

$$\frac{\begin{array}{c}\text{volume of copper in}\\ \text{an auto transformer}\\ \hline \text{volume of copper in a}\\ \text{double-wound transformer}\end{array}}{} = \frac{2N_1 I_1 - 2N_2 I_1}{2N_1 I_1}$$

$$= \frac{2N_1 I_1}{2N_1 I_1} - \frac{2N_2 I_1}{2N_1 I_1}$$

$$= 1 - \frac{N_2}{N_1}$$

If $(N_2/N_1) = x$ then

(volume of copper in an auto transformer)
$= (1 - x)$ (volume of copper in a double-
wound transformer) (12)

If, say, $x = (4/5)$ then (volume of copper in auto transformer)

$$= \left(1 - \tfrac{4}{5}\right) \begin{array}{l}\text{(volume of copper in a}\\ \text{double-wound transformer)}\end{array}$$

$$= \tfrac{1}{5} \text{ (volume in double-wound transformer)}$$

i.e. a saving of 80%.

Similarly, if $x = (1/4)$, the saving is 25 per cent, and so on. The closer N_2 is to N_1, the greater the saving in copper.

Problem 27. Determine the saving in the volume of copper used in an auto transformer compared with a double-wound transformer for (a) a 200 V:150 V transformer, and (b) a 500 V:100 V transformer.

(a) For a 200 V:150 V transformer,

$$x = \frac{V_2}{V_1} = \frac{150}{200} = 0.75$$

Hence from equation (12), (volume of copper in auto transformer)

$= (1 - 0.75)$ (volume of copper in double-wound transformer)

$= (0.25)$ (volume of copper in double-wound transformer)

$= 25\%$ (of copper in a double-wound transformer)

Hence the saving is 75%

(b) For a 500 V:100 V transformer,

$$x = \frac{V_2}{V_1} = \frac{100}{500} = 0.2$$

Hence, (volume of copper in auto transformer)

$= (1 - 0.2)$ (volume of copper in double-wound transformer)

$= (0.8)$ (volume in double-wound transformer)

$= 80\%$ of copper in a double-wound transformer

Hence the saving is 20%.

Now try the following exercise

Exercise 126 Further problems on the auto transformer

1. A single-phase auto transformer has a voltage ratio of 480 V:300 V and supplies a load of 30 kVA at 300 V. Assuming an ideal

transformer, calculate the current in each section of the winding.

$$[I_1 = 62.5 \, \text{A}, \ I_2 = 100 \, \text{A}, (I_2 - I_1) = 37.5 \, \text{A}]$$

2. Calculate the saving in the volume of copper used in an auto transformer compared with a double-wound transformer for (a) a 300 V: 240 V transformer, and (b) a 400 V:100 V transformer. [(a) 80% (b) 25%]

Advantages of auto transformers

The advantages of auto transformers over double-wound transformers include:

1. a saving in cost since less copper is needed (see above)

2. less volume, hence less weight

3. a higher efficiency, resulting from lower I^2R losses

4. a continuously variable output voltage is achievable if a sliding contact is used

5. a smaller percentage voltage regulation.

Disadvantages of auto transformers

The primary and secondary windings are not electrically separate, hence if an open-circuit occurs in the secondary winding the full primary voltage appears across the secondary.

Uses of auto transformers

Auto transformers are used for reducing the voltage when starting induction motors (see Chapter 23) and for interconnecting systems that are operating at approximately the same voltage.

21.12   Isolating transformers

Transformers not only enable current or voltage to be transformed to some different magnitude but provide a means of isolating electrically one part of a circuit from another when there is no electrical connection between primary and secondary windings. An **isolating transformer** is a 1:1 ratio transformer with several important applications, including bathroom shaver-sockets, portable electric tools, model railways, and so on.

21.13   Three-phase transformers

Three-phase double-wound transformers are mainly used in power transmission and are usually of the core type. They basically consist of three pairs of single-phase windings mounted on one core, as shown in Fig. 21.17, which gives a considerable saving in the amount of iron used. The primary and secondary windings in Fig. 21.17 are wound on top of each other in the form of concentric cylinders, similar to that shown in Fig. 21.6(a). The windings may be with the primary delta-connected and the secondary star-connected, or star-delta, star-star or delta-delta, depending on its use.

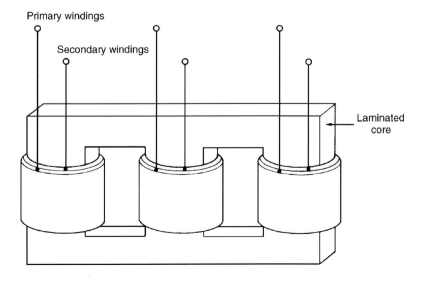

Primary windings
Secondary windings
Laminated core

Figure 21.17

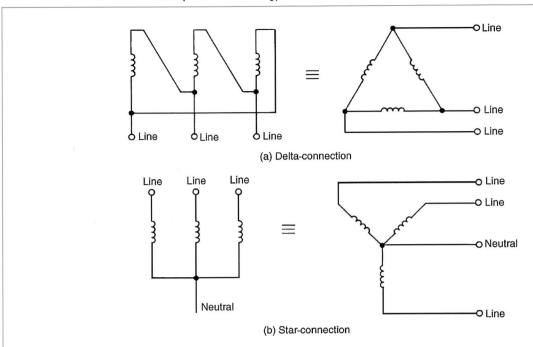

Figure 21.18

A delta-connection is shown in Fig. 21.18(a) and a star-connection in Fig. 21.18(b).

Problem 28. A three-phase transformer has 500 primary turns and 50 secondary turns. If the supply voltage is 2.4 kV find the secondary line voltage on no-load when the windings are connected (a) star-delta, (b) delta-star.

(a) For a star-connection, $V_L = \sqrt{3}\,V_p$ (see Chapter 20). Primary phase voltage,

$$V_p = \frac{V_{L1}}{\sqrt{3}} = \frac{2400}{\sqrt{3}} = 1385.64 \text{ volts.}$$

For a delta-connection, $V_L = V_p$
$N_1/N_2 = V_1/V_2$ from which, secondary phase voltage,

$$\mathbf{V_{p2}} = V_{p1}\left(\frac{N_2}{N_1}\right) = (1385.64)\left(\frac{50}{500}\right)$$

$$= \mathbf{138.6\,volts}$$

(b) For a delta-connection, $V_L = V_p$ hence, primary phase voltage $V_{p1} = 2.4\,kV = 2400$ volts. Secondary phase voltage,

$$V_{p2} = V_{p1}\left(\frac{N_2}{N_1}\right) = (2400)\left(\frac{50}{500}\right) = 240 \text{ volts}$$

For a star-connection, $V_L = \sqrt{3}\,V_p$ hence, the secondary line voltage, $V_{L2} = \sqrt{3}(240) = \mathbf{416\,volts}$.

Now try the following exercise

Exercise 127   A further problem on the three-phase transformer

1. A three-phase transformer has 600 primary turns and 150 secondary turns. If the supply voltage is 1.5 kV determine the secondary line voltage on no-load when the windings are connected (a) delta-star (b) star-delta.
    [(a) 649.5 V (b) 216.5 V]

21.14   Current transformers

For measuring currents in excess of about 100 A a current transformer is normally used. With a d.c. moving-coil ammeter the current required to give full-scale deflection is very small – typically a few milliamperes. When larger currents are to be measured a shunt resistor is added to the circuit (see Chapter 10). However, even with shunt resistors added it is not possible to measure very large currents. When a.c. is being measured a shunt

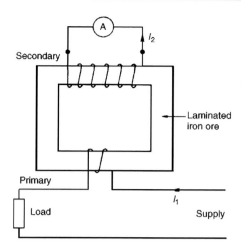

Figure 21.19

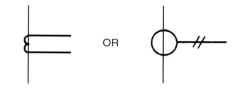

Figure 21.20

cannot be used since the proportion of the current which flows in the meter will depend on its impedance, which varies with frequency.

In a double-wound transformer:

$$\frac{I_1}{I_2} = \frac{N_2}{N_1}$$

from which,

$$\text{secondary current } I_2 = I_1 \left(\frac{N_2}{N_1}\right)$$

In current transformers the primary usually consists of one or two turns whilst the secondary can have several hundred turns. A typical arrangement is shown in Fig. 21.19.

If, for example, the primary has 2 turns and the secondary 200 turns, then if the primary current is 500 A,

$$\text{secondary current, } I_2 = I_1 \left(\frac{N_2}{N_1}\right) = (500) \left(\frac{2}{200}\right)$$
$$= 5 \text{ A}$$

Current transformers isolate the ammeter from the main circuit and allow the use of a standard range of ammeters giving full-scale deflections of 1 A, 2 A or 5 A.

For very large currents the transformer core can be mounted around the conductor or bus-bar. Thus the primary then has just one turn.

It is very important to short-circuit the secondary winding before removing the ammeter. This is because if current is flowing in the primary, dangerously high voltages could be induced in the secondary should it be open-circuited.

Current transformer circuit diagram symbols are shown in Fig. 21.20.

Problem 29. A current transformer has a single turn on the primary winding and a secondary winding of 60 turns. The secondary winding is connected to an ammeter with a resistance of 0.15 Ω. The resistance of the secondary winding is 0.25 Ω. If the current in the primary winding is 300 A, determine (a) the reading on the ammeter, (b) the potential difference across the ammeter and (c) the total load (in VA) on the secondary.

(a) Reading on the ammeter,

$$I_2 = I_1 \left(\frac{N_1}{N_2}\right) = 300 \left(\frac{1}{60}\right) = \textbf{5 A}.$$

(b) P.d. across the ammeter $= I_2 R_A$, (where R_A is the ammeter resistance) $= (5)(0.15) = \textbf{0.75 volts}$.

(c) Total resistance of secondary circuit

$$= 0.15 + 0.25 = 0.40 \, \Omega.$$

Induced e.m.f. in secondary $= (5)(0.40) = 2.0$ V.

Total load on secondary $= (2.0)(5) = \textbf{10 VA}.$

Now try the following exercise

Exercise 128   A further problem on the current transformer

1. A current transformer has two turns on the primary winding and a secondary winding of 260 turns. The secondary winding is connected to an ammeter with a resistance of 0.2 Ω. The resistance of the secondary winding is 0.3 Ω. If the current in the primary winding is 650 A, determine (a) the reading on the ammeter, (b) the potential difference across the ammeter, and (c) the total load in VA on the secondary.

[(a) 5 A (b) 1 V (c) 7.5 VA]

Section 3

21.15 Voltage transformers

For measuring voltages in excess of about 500 V it is often safer to use a voltage transformer. These are normal double-wound transformers with a large number of turns on the primary, which is connected to a high voltage supply, and a small number of turns on the secondary. A typical arrangement is shown in Fig. 21.21.

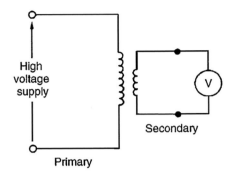

Figure 21.21

Since

$$\frac{V_1}{V_2} = \frac{N_1}{N_2}$$

the **secondary voltage**,

$$V_2 = \frac{V_1 N_2}{V_1}$$

Thus if the arrangement in Fig. 21.21 has 4000 primary turns and 20 secondary turns then for a voltage of 22 kV on the primary, the voltage on the secondary,

$$V_2 = V_1 \left(\frac{N_2}{N_1}\right) = (22\,000)\left(\frac{20}{4000}\right) = \textbf{110 volts}$$

Now try the following exercises

Exercise 129   Short answer questions on transformers

1. What is a transformer?

2. Explain briefly how a voltage is induced in the secondary winding of a transformer

3. Draw the circuit diagram symbol for a transformer

4. State the relationship between turns and voltage ratios for a transformer

5. How is a transformer rated?

6. Briefly describe the principle of operation of a transformer

7. Draw a phasor diagram for an ideal transformer on no-load

8. State the e.m.f. equation for a transformer

9. Draw an on-load phasor diagram for an ideal transformer with an inductive load

10. Name two types of transformer construction

11. What core material is normally used for power transformers

12. Name three core materials used in r.f. transformers

13. State a typical application for (a) a.f. transformers (b) r.f. transformers

14. How is cooling achieved in transformers?

15. State the expressions for equivalent resistance and reactance of a transformer, referred to the primary

16. Define regulation of a transformer

17. Name two sources of loss in a transformer

18. What is hysteresis loss? How is it minimised in a transformer?

19. What are eddy currents? How may they be reduced in transformers?

20. How is efficiency of a transformer calculated?

21. What is the condition for maximum efficiency of a transformer?

22. What does 'resistance matching' mean?

23. State a practical application where matching would be used

24. Derive a formula for the equivalent resistance of a transformer having a turns ratio of $N_1:N_2$ and load resistance R_L

25. What is an auto transformer?

26. State three advantages and one disadvantage of an auto transformer compared with a double-wound transformer

Section 3

27. In what applications are auto transformers used?

28. What is an isolating transformer? Give two applications

29. Describe briefly the construction of a three-phase transformer

30. For what reason are current transformers used?

31. Describe how a current transformer operates

32. For what reason are voltage transformers used?

33. Describe how a voltage transformer operates

Exercise 130   Multi-choice questions on transformers

(Answers on page 421)

1. The e.m.f. equation of a transformer of secondary turns N_2, magnetic flux density B_m, magnetic area of core a, and operating at frequency f is given by:

    (a) $E_2 = 4.44 N_2 B_m a f$ volts

    (b) $E_2 = 4.44 \dfrac{N_2 B_m f}{a}$ volts

    (c) $E_2 = \dfrac{N_2 B_m f}{a}$ volts

    (d) $E_2 = 1.11 N_2 B_m \, a f$ volts

2. In the auto-transformer shown in Fig. 21.22, the current in section PQ is:
    (a) 3.3 A (b) 1.7 A (c) 5 A (d) 1.6 A

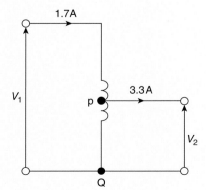

Figure 21.22

3. A step-up transformer has a turns ratio of 10. If the output current is 5 A, the input current is:
    (a) 50 A   (b) 5 A
    (c) 2.5 A   (d) 0.5 A

4. A 440 V/110 V transformer has 1000 turns on the primary winding. The number of turns on the secondary is:
    (a) 550   (b) 250
    (c) 4000   (d) 25

5. An advantage of an auto-transformer is that:
    (a) it gives a high step-up ratio
    (b) iron losses are reduced
    (c) copper loss is reduced
    (d) it reduces capacitance between turns

6. A 1 kV/250 V transformer has 500 turns on the secondary winding. The number of turns on the primary is:
    (a) 2000   (b) 125
    (c) 1000   (d) 250

7. The core of a transformer is laminated to:
    (a) limit hysteresis loss
    (b) reduce the inductance of the windings
    (c) reduce the effects of eddy current loss
    (d) prevent eddy currents from occurring

8. The power input to a mains transformer is 200 W. If the primary current is 2.5 A, the secondary voltage is 2 V and assuming no losses in the transformer, the turns ratio is:
    (a) 40:1 step down   (b) 40:1 step up
    (c) 80:1 step down   (d) 80:1 step up

9. A transformer has 800 primary turns and 100 secondary turns. To obtain 40 V from the secondary winding the voltage applied to the primary winding must be:
    (a) 5 V   (b) 320 V
    (c) 2.5 V   (d) 20 V

A 100 kVA, 250 V/10 kV, single-phase transformer has a full-load copper loss of 800 W and an iron loss of 500 W. The primary winding contains 120 turns. For the statements in questions 10 to 16, select the correct answer from the following list:

(a) 81.3 kW   (b) 800 W   (c) 97.32%
(d) 80 kW   (e) 3   (f) 4800
(g) 1.3 kW   (h) 98.40%   (i) 100 kW
(j) 98.28%   (k) 200 W   (l) 101.3 kW
(m) 96.38%   (n) 400 W

10. The total full-load losses

11. The full-load output power at 0.8 power factor

12. The full-load input power at 0.8 power factor

13. The full-load efficiency at 0.8 power factor

14. The half full-load copper loss

15. The transformer efficiency at half full load, 0.8 power factor

16. The number of secondary winding turns

17. Which of the following statements is false?
    (a) In an ideal transformer, the volts per turn are constant for a given value of primary voltage
    (b) In a single-phase transformer, the hysteresis loss is proportional to frequency
    (c) A transformer whose secondary current is greater than the primary current is a step-up transformer
    (d) In transformers, eddy current loss is reduced by laminating the core

18. An ideal transformer has a turns ratio of 1:5 and is supplied at 200 V when the primary current is 3 A. Which of the following statements is false?
    (a) The turns ratio indicates a step-up transformer
    (b) The secondary voltage is 40 V
    (c) The secondary current is 15 A
    (d) The transformer rating is 0.6 kVA
    (e) The secondary voltage is 1 kV
    (f) The secondary current is 0.6 A

19. Iron losses in a transformer are due to:
    (a) eddy currents only
    (b) flux leakage
    (c) both eddy current and hysteresis losses
    (d) the resistance of the primary and secondary windings

20. A load is to be matched to an amplifier having an effective internal resistance of 10 Ω via a coupling transformer having a turns ratio of 1:10. The value of the load resistance for maximum power transfer is:
    (a) 100 Ω   (b) 1 kΩ
    (c) 100 mΩ   (d) 1 mΩ

This revision test covers the material contained in Chapters 20 to 21. *The marks for each question are shown in brackets at the end of each question.*

1. Three identical coils each of resistance $40\,\Omega$ and inductive reactance $30\,\Omega$ are connected (i) in star, and (ii) in delta to a $400\,V$, three-phase supply. Calculate for each connection (a) the line and phase voltages, (b) the phase and line currents, and (c) the total power dissipated. (12)

2. Two wattmeters are connected to measure the input power to a balanced three-phase load by the two-wattmeter method. If the instrument readings are $10\,kW$ and $6\,kW$, determine (a) the total power input, and (b) the load power factor. (5)

3. An ideal transformer connected to a $250\,V$ mains, supplies a $25\,V$, $200\,W$ lamp. Calculate the transformer turns ratio and the current taken from the supply. (5)

4. A $200\,kVA$, $8000\,V/320\,V$, $50\,Hz$ single-phase transformer has 120 secondary turns. Determine (a) the primary and secondary currents, (b) the number of primary turns, and (c) the maximum value of flux. (9)

5. Determine the percentage regulation of an $8\,kVA$, $100\,V/200\,V$, single-phase transformer when its secondary terminal voltage is $194\,V$ when loaded. (3)

6. A $500\,kVA$ rated transformer has a full-load copper loss of $4\,kW$ and an iron loss of $3\,kW$. Determine the transformer efficiency (a) at full load and 0.80 power factor, and (b) at half full load and 0.80 power factor. (10)

7. Determine the optimum value of load resistance for maximum power transfer if the load is connected to an amplifier of output resistance $288\,\Omega$ through a transformer with a turns ratio $6:1$ (3)

8. A single-phase auto transformer has a voltage ratio of $250\,V:200\,V$ and supplies a load of $15\,kVA$ at $200\,V$. Assuming an ideal transformer, determine the current in each section of the winding. (3)

Chapter 22

D.C. machines

At the end of this chapter you should be able to:

- distinguish between the function of a motor and a generator
- describe the action of a commutator
- describe the construction of a d.c. machine
- distinguish between wave and lap windings
- understand shunt, series and compound windings of d.c. machines
- understand armature reaction
- calculate generated e.m.f. in an armature winding using $E = 2p\Phi nZ/c$
- describe types of d.c. generator and their characteristics
- calculate generated e.m.f. for a generator using $E = V + I_a R_a$
- state typical applications of d.c. generators
- list d.c. machine losses and calculate efficiency
- calculate back e.m.f. for a d.c. motor using $E = V - I_a R_a$
- calculate the torque of a d.c. motor using $T = EI_a/2\pi n$ and $T = p\Phi ZI_a/\pi c$
- describe types of d.c. motor and their characteristics
- state typical applications of d.c. motors
- describe a d.c. motor starter
- describe methods of speed control of d.c. motors
- list types of enclosure for d.c. motors

22.1   Introduction

When the input to an electrical machine is electrical energy, (seen as applying a voltage to the electrical terminals of the machine), and the output is mechanical energy, (seen as a rotating shaft), the machine is called an electric **motor**. Thus an electric motor converts electrical energy into mechanical energy.

The principle of operation of a motor is explained in Section 8.4, page 97. When the input to an electrical machine is mechanical energy, (seen as, say, a diesel motor, coupled to the machine by a shaft), and the output is electrical energy, (seen as a voltage appearing at the electrical terminals of the machine), the machine is called a **generator**. Thus, a generator converts mechanical energy to electrical energy.

The principle of operation of a generator is explained in Section 9.2, page 103.

22.2   The action of a commutator

In an electric motor, conductors rotate in a uniform magnetic field. A single-loop conductor mounted between

DOI: 10.1016/B978-0-08-089056-2.00022-X

permanent magnets is shown in Fig. 22.1. A voltage is applied at points A and B in Fig. 22.1(a).

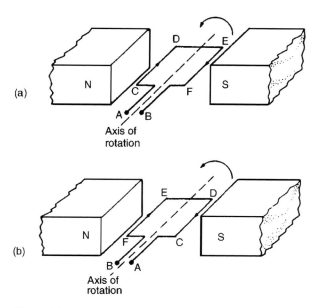

Figure 22.1

A force, F, acts on the loop due to the interaction of the magnetic field of the permanent magnets and the magnetic field created by the current flowing in the loop. This force is proportional to the flux density, B, the current flowing, I, and the effective length of the conductor, l, i.e. $F = BIl$. The force is made up of two parts, one acting vertically downwards due to the current flowing from C to D and the other acting vertically upwards due to the current flowing from E to F (from Fleming's left-hand rule). If the loop is free to rotate, then when it has rotated through 180°, the conductors are as shown in Fig. 22.1(b). For rotation to continue in the same direction, it is necessary for the current flow to be as shown in Fig. 22.1(b), i.e. from D to C and from F to E. This apparent reversal in the direction of current flow is achieved by a process called **commutation**.

With reference to Fig. 22.2(a), when a direct voltage is applied at A and B, then as the single-loop conductor rotates, current flow will always be away from the commutator for the part of the conductor adjacent to the N-pole and towards the commutator for the part of the conductor adjacent to the S-pole. Thus the forces act to give continuous rotation in an anticlockwise direction. The arrangement shown in Fig. 22.2(a) is called a 'two-segment' commutator and the voltage is applied to the rotating segments by stationary **brushes**, (usually carbon blocks), which slide on the commutator material, (usually copper), when rotation takes place.

In practice, there are many conductors on the rotating part of a d.c. machine and these are attached to many commutator segments. A schematic diagram of a multi-segment commutator is shown in Fig. 22.2(b).

Poor commutation results in sparking at the trailing edge of the brushes. This can be improved by using **interpoles** (situated between each pair of main poles), high resistance brushes, or using brushes spanning several commutator segments.

22.3 D.C. machine construction

The basic parts of any d.c. machine are shown in Fig. 22.3, and comprise:

(a) a stationary part called the **stator** having,
   (i) a steel ring called the **yoke**, to which are attached
   (ii) the magnetic **poles**, around which are the
   (iii) **field windings**, i.e. many turns of a conductor wound round the pole core; current passing through this conductor creates an electromagnet, (rather than the permanent magnets shown in Figs 22.1 and 22.2),

(b) a rotating part called the **armature** mounted in bearings housed in the stator and having,
   (iv) a laminated cylinder of iron or steel called the **core**, on which teeth are cut to house the

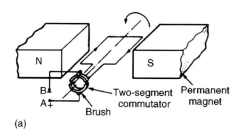

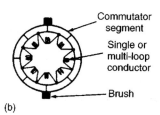

Figure 22.2

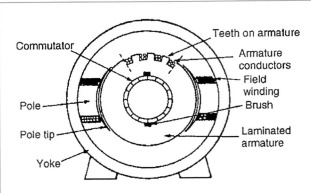

Figure 22.3

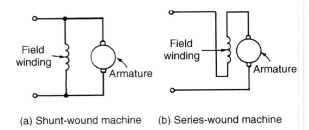

(a) Shunt-wound machine   (b) Series-wound machine

Figure 22.4

(v) **armature winding**, i.e. a single or multi-loop conductor system, and

(vi) the **commutator**, (see Section 22.2)

Armature windings can be divided into two groups, depending on how the wires are joined to the commutator. These are called **wave windings** and **lap windings**.

(a) In **wave windings** there are two paths in parallel irrespective of the number of poles, each path supplying half the total current output. Wave wound generators produce high voltage, low current outputs.

(b) In **lap windings** there are as many paths in parallel as the machine has poles. The total current output divides equally between them. Lap wound generators produce high current, low voltage output.

22.4 Shunt, series and compound windings

When the field winding of a d.c. machine is connected in parallel with the armature, as shown in Fig. 22.4(a), the machine is said to be **shunt** wound. If the field winding is connected in series with the armature, as shown in Fig. 22.4(b), then the machine is said to be **series** wound. A **compound** wound machine has a combination of series and shunt windings.

Depending on whether the electrical machine is series wound, shunt wound or compound wound, it behaves differently when a load is applied. The behaviour of a d.c. machine under various conditions is shown by means of graphs, called characteristic curves or just **characteristics**. The characteristics shown in the following sections are theoretical, since they neglect the effects of armature reaction.

Armature reaction is the effect that the magnetic field produced by the armature current has on the magnetic field produced by the field system. In a generator, armature reaction results in a reduced output voltage, and in a motor, armature reaction results in increased speed.

A way of overcoming the effect of armature reaction is to fit compensating windings, located in slots in the pole face.

22.5 E.m.f. generated in an armature winding

Let Z = number of armature conductors,
       Φ = useful flux per pole, in webers,
       p = number of **pairs** of poles
and n = armature speed in rev/s

The e.m.f. generated by the armature is equal to the e.m.f. generated by one of the parallel paths. Each conductor passes $2p$ poles per revolution and thus cuts $2p\Phi$ webers of magnetic flux per revolution. Hence flux cut by one conductor per second = $2p\Phi n$ Wb and so the average e.m.f. E generated per conductor is given by:

$$E2p\Phi n \text{ volts}$$

(since 1 volt = 1 Weber per second)

Let c = number of parallel paths through the winding between positive and negative brushes

$$c = 2 \quad \text{for a wave winding}$$

$$c = 2p \quad \text{for a lap winding}$$

The number of conductors in series in each path = Z/c
The total e.m.f. between

brushes = (average e.m.f./conductor) (number of conductors in series per path)

$$= 2p\Phi nZ/c$$

i.e.   generated e.m.f. $E = \dfrac{2p\Phi nZ}{c}$ volts   (1)

Since Z, p and c are constant for a given machine, then $E \propto \Phi n$. However $2\pi n$ is the angular velocity ω in radians per second, hence the generated e.m.f. is proportional to Φ and ω,

i.e.   generated e.m.f. $E \propto \Phi \omega$ (2)

Problem 1. An 8-pole, wave-connected armature has 600 conductors and is driven at 625 rev/min. If the flux per pole is 20 mWb, determine the generated e.m.f.

$Z = 600$, $c = 2$ (for a wave winding), $p = 4$ pairs, $n = 625/60$ rev/s and $\Phi = 20 \times 10^{-3}$ Wb.
Generated e.m.f.

$$E = \frac{2p\Phi nZ}{c}$$

$$= \frac{2(4)(20 \times 10^{-3})\left(\dfrac{625}{60}\right)(600)}{2}$$

$$= \mathbf{500\,volts}$$

Problem 2. A 4-pole generator has a lap-wound armature with 50 slots with 16 conductors per slot. The useful flux per pole is 30 mWb. Determine the speed at which the machine must be driven to generate an e.m.f. of 240 V.

$E = 240$ V, $c = 2p$ (for a lap winding), $Z = 50 \times 16 = 800$ and $\Phi = 30 \times 10^{-3}$ Wb.
Generated e.m.f.

$$E = \frac{2p\Phi nZ}{c} = \frac{2p\Phi nZ}{2p} = \Phi nZ$$

Rearranging gives, speed,

$$n = \frac{E}{\Phi Z} = \frac{240}{(30 \times 10^{-3})(800)}$$

$$= \mathbf{10\,rev/s}\ \text{or}\ \mathbf{600\,rev/min}$$

Problem 3. An 8-pole, lap-wound armature has 1200 conductors and a flux per pole of 0.03 Wb. Determine the e.m.f. generated when running at 500 rev/min.

Generated e.m.f.,

$$E = \frac{2p\Phi nZ}{c}$$

$$= \frac{2p\Phi nZ}{2p} \text{ for a lap-wound machine,}$$

i.e. $E = \Phi nZ$

$$= (0.03)\left(\frac{500}{60}\right)(1200)$$

$$= \mathbf{300\,volts}$$

Problem 4. Determine the generated e.m.f. in Problem 3 if the armature is wave-wound.

Generated e.m.f.

$$E = \frac{2p\Phi nZ}{c}$$

$$= \frac{2p\Phi nZ}{2} \quad \text{(since } c = 2 \text{ for wave-wound)}$$

$$= p\Phi nZ = (4)(\Phi nZ)$$

$$= (4)(300) \text{ from Problem 3}$$

$$= \mathbf{1200\,volts}$$

Problem 5. A d.c. shunt-wound generator running at constant speed generates a voltage of 150 V at a certain value of field current. Determine the change in the generated voltage when the field current is reduced by 20 per cent, assuming the flux is proportional to the field current.

The generated e.m.f. E of a generator is proportional to $\Phi \omega$, i.e. is proportional to Φn, where Φ is the flux and n is the speed of rotation. It follows that $E = k\Phi n$, where k is a constant.

At speed n_1 and flux Φ_1, $E_1 = k\Phi_1 n_1$
At speed n_2 and flux Φ_2, $E_2 = k\Phi_2 n_2$

Thus, by division:

$$\frac{E_1}{E_2} = \frac{k\Phi_1 n_1}{k\Phi_2 n_2} = \frac{\Phi_1 n_1}{\Phi_2 n_2}$$

The initial conditions are $E_1 = 150$ V, $\Phi = \Phi_1$ and $n = n_1$. When the flux is reduced by 20 per cent, the new value of flux is $80/100$ or 0.8 of the initial value, i.e. $\Phi_2 = 0.8\Phi_1$. Since the generator is running at constant speed, $n_2 = n_1$

Thus $$\frac{E_1}{E_2} = \frac{\Phi_1 n_1}{\Phi_2 n_2} = \frac{\Phi_1 n_1}{0.8\Phi_1 n_2} = \frac{1}{0.8}$$

that is, $E_2 = 150 \times 0.8 = 120$ V

Thus, a reduction of 20 per cent in the value of the flux **reduces the generated voltage to 120 V** at constant speed.

Problem 6. A d.c. generator running at 30 rev/s generates an e.m.f. of 200 V. Determine the percentage increase in the flux per pole required to generate 250 V at 20 rev/s.

From equation (2), generated e.m.f., $E \propto \Phi\omega$ and since $\omega = 2\pi n$, $E \propto \Phi n$

Let $E_1 = 200$ V, $n_1 = 30$ rev/s

and flux per pole at this speed be Φ_1

Let $E_2 = 250$ V, $n_2 = 20$ rev/s

and flux per pole at this speed be Φ_2

Since $\quad E \propto \Phi n$ then $\dfrac{E_1}{E_2} = \dfrac{\Phi_1 n_1}{\Phi_2 n_2}$

Hence $\quad \dfrac{200}{250} = \dfrac{\Phi_1(30)}{\Phi_2(20)}$

from which, $\quad \Phi_2 = \dfrac{\Phi_1(30)(250)}{(20)(200)}$

$$= 1.875\Phi_1$$

Hence **the increase in flux per pole needs to be 87.5 per cent.**

Now try the following exercise

Exercise 131   Further problems on generator e.m.f.

1. A 4-pole, wave-connected armature of a d.c. machine has 750 conductors and is driven at 720 rev/min. If the useful flux per pole is 15 mWb, determine the generated e.m.f.
[270 volts]

2. A 6-pole generator has a lap-wound armature with 40 slots with 20 conductors per slot. The flux per pole is 25 mWb. Calculate the speed at which the machine must be driven to generate an e.m.f. of 300 V.   [15 rev/s or 900 rev/min]

3. A 4-pole armature of a d.c. machine has 1000 conductors and a flux per pole of 20 mWb. Determine the e.m.f. generated when running at 600 rev/min when the armature is (a) wave-wound (b) lap-wound.
[(a) 400 volts (b) 200 volts]

4. A d.c. generator running at 25 rev/s generates an e.m.f. of 150 V. Determine the percentage increase in the flux per pole required to generate 180 V at 20 rev/s.   [50%]

22.6   D.C. generators

D.C. generators are classified according to the method of their field excitation. These groupings are:

(i) **Separately-excited generators**, where the field winding is connected to a source of supply other than the armature of its own machine.

(ii) **Self-excited generators**, where the field winding receives its supply from the armature of its own machine, and which are sub-divided into (a) shunt, (b) series, and (c) compound wound generators.

22.7   Types of d.c. generator and their characteristics

(a) Separately-excited generator

A typical separately-excited generator circuit is shown in Fig. 22.5.

When a load is connected across the armature terminals, a load current I_a will flow. The terminal voltage V will fall from its open-circuit e.m.f. E due to a volt drop caused by current flowing through the armature resistance, shown as R_a.

i.e.   terminal voltage, $V = E - I_a R_a$

or   generated e.m.f., $E = V + I_a R_a$ $\qquad$ (3)

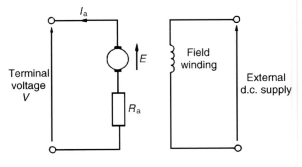

Figure 22.5

Problem 7. Determine the terminal voltage of a generator which develops an e.m.f. of 200 V and has an armature current of 30 A on load. Assume the armature resistance is 0.30 Ω.

With reference to Fig. 22.5, terminal voltage,

$$V = E - I_a R_a$$
$$= 200 - (30)(0.30)$$
$$= 200 - 9 = \textbf{191 volts}$$

Problem 8. A generator is connected to a 60 Ω load and a current of 8 A flows. If the armature resistance is 1 Ω determine (a) the terminal voltage, and (b) the generated e.m.f.

(a) Terminal voltage, $V = I_a R_L = (8)(60) = \textbf{480 volts}$

(b) Generated e.m.f.,

$$E = V + I_a R_a \quad \text{from equation (3)}$$
$$= 480 + (8)(1) = 480 + 8 = \textbf{488 volts}$$

Problem 9. A separately-excited generator develops a no-load e.m.f. of 150 V at an armature speed of 20 rev/s and a flux per pole of 0.10 Wb. Determine the generated e.m.f. when (a) the speed increases to 25 rev/s and the pole flux remains unchanged, (b) the speed remains at 20 rev/s and the pole flux is decreased to 0.08 Wb, and (c) the speed increases to 24 rev/s and the pole flux is decreased to 0.07 Wb.

(a) From Section 22.5, generated e.m.f. $E \propto \Phi n$

$$\text{from which,} \quad \frac{E_1}{E_2} = \frac{\Phi_1 N_1}{\Phi_2 N_2}$$

$$\text{Hence} \quad \frac{150}{E_2} = \frac{(0.10)(20)}{(0.1)(25)}$$

$$\text{from which,} \quad E_2 = \frac{(150)(0.10)(25)}{(0.10)(20)}$$

$$= \textbf{187.5 volts}$$

(b)
$$\frac{150}{E_3} = \frac{(0.10)(20)}{(0.08)(20)}$$

$$\text{from which, e.m.f.,} \quad E_3 = \frac{(150)(0.08)(20)}{(0.10)(20)}$$

$$= \textbf{120 volts}$$

(c)
$$\frac{150}{E_4} = \frac{(0.10)(20)}{(0.07)(24)}$$

$$\text{from which, e.m.f.,} \quad E_4 = \frac{(150)(0.07)(24)}{(0.10)(20)}$$

$$= \textbf{126 volts}$$

Characteristics

The two principal generator characteristics are the generated voltage/field current characteristics, called the **open-circuit characteristic** and the terminal voltage/load current characteristic, called the **load characteristic**. A typical separately-excited generator **open-circuit characteristic** is shown in Fig. 22.6(a) and a typical **load characteristic** is shown in Fig. 22.6(b).

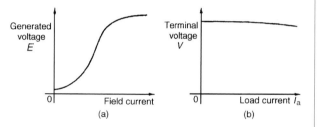

Figure 22.6

A separately-excited generator is used only in special cases, such as when a wide variation in terminal p.d. is required, or when exact control of the field current is necessary. Its disadvantage lies in requiring a separate source of direct current.

(b) Shunt-wound generator

In a shunt-wound generator the field winding is connected in parallel with the armature as shown in Fig. 22.7. The field winding has a relatively high resistance and therefore the current carried is only a fraction of the armature current.

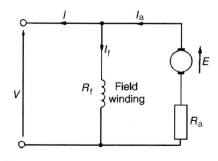

Figure 22.7

For the circuit shown in Fig. 22.7

$$\text{terminal voltage, } V = E - I_a R_a$$

or   generated e.m.f., $E = V + I_a R_a$

$I_a = I_f + I$ from Kirchhoff's current law, where I_a = armature current, I_f = field current ($= V/R_f$) and I = load current.

> **Problem 10.** A shunt generator supplies a 20 kW load at 200 V through cables of resistance, $R =$ 100 mΩ. If the field winding resistance, $R_f = 50\,\Omega$ and the armature resistance, $R_a = 40$ mΩ, determine (a) the terminal voltage, and (b) the e.m.f. generated in the armature.

(a)   The circuit is as shown in Fig. 22.8

$$\text{Load current, } I = \frac{20\,000 \text{ watts}}{200 \text{ volts}} = 100\,\text{A}$$

Volt drop in the cables to the load
$= IR = (100)(100 \times 10^{-3}) = 10\,\text{V}.$
Hence **terminal voltage, $V = 200 + 10 = 210$ volts.**

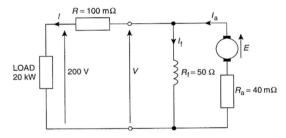

Figure 22.8

(b)   Armature current $I_a = I_f + I$

$$\text{Field current, } I_f = \frac{V}{R_f} = \frac{210}{50} = 4.2\,\text{A}$$

Hence $I_a = I_f + I = 4.2 + 100 = 104.2\,\text{A}$

Generated e.m.f. $E = V + I_a R_a$

$$= 210 + (104.2)(40 \times 10^{-3})$$
$$= 210 + 4.168$$
$$= \mathbf{214.17\,volts}$$

Characteristics

The generated e.m.f., E, is proportional to $\Phi\omega$, (see Section 22.5), hence at constant speed, since $\omega = 2\pi n$,

$E \propto \Phi$. Also the flux Φ is proportional to field current I_f until magnetic saturation of the iron circuit of the generator occurs. Hence the open circuit characteristic is as shown in Fig. 22.9(a).

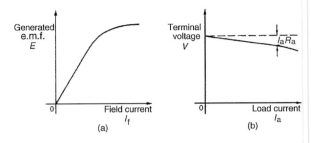

Figure 22.9

As the load current on a generator having constant field current and running at constant speed increases, the value of armature current increases, hence the armature volt drop, $I_a R_a$ increases. The generated voltage E is larger than the terminal voltage V and the voltage equation for the armature circuit is $V = E - I_a R_a$. Since E is constant, V decreases with increasing load. The load characteristic is as shown in Fig. 22.9(b). In practice, the fall in voltage is about 10 per cent between no-load and full-load for many d.c. shunt-wound generators.

The shunt-wound generator is the type most used in practice, but the load current must be limited to a value that is well below the maximum value. This then avoids excessive variation of the terminal voltage. Typical applications are with battery charging and motor car generators.

(c) Series-wound generator

In the series-wound generator the field winding is connected in series with the armature as shown in Fig. 22.10.

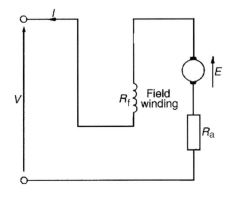

Figure 22.10

Characteristics

The load characteristic is the terminal voltage/current characteristic. The generated e.m.f. E is proportional to $\Phi\omega$ and at constant speed $\omega(=2\pi n)$ is a constant. Thus E is proportional to Φ. For values of current below magnetic saturation of the yoke, poles, air gaps and armature core, the flux Φ is proportional to the current, hence $E \propto I$. For values of current above those required for magnetic saturation, the generated e.m.f. is approximately constant. The values of field resistance and armature resistance in a series wound machine are small, hence the terminal voltage V is very nearly equal to E. A typical load characteristic for a series generator is shown in Fig. 22.11.

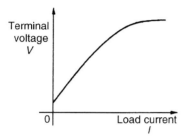

Figure 22.11

In a series-wound generator, the field winding is in series with the armature and it is not possible to have a value of field current when the terminals are open circuited, thus it is not possible to obtain an open-circuit characteristic.

Series-wound generators are rarely used in practise, but can be used as a 'booster' on d.c. transmission lines.

(d) Compound-wound generator

In the compound-wound generator two methods of connection are used, both having a mixture of shunt and series windings, designed to combine the advantages of each. Figure 22.12(a) shows what is termed a **long-shunt** compound generator, and Fig. 22.12(b) shows a

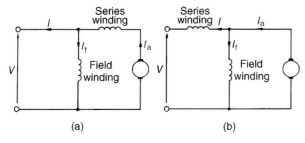

(a)   (b)

Figure 22.12

short-shunt compound generator. The latter is the most generally used form of d.c. generator.

> **Problem 11.** A short-shunt compound generator supplies 80 A at 200 V. If the field resistance, $R_f = 40\,\Omega$, the series resistance, $R_{Se} = 0.02\,\Omega$ and the armature resistance, $R_a = 0.04\,\Omega$, determine the e.m.f. generated.

The circuit is shown in Fig. 22.13.
Volt drop in series winding $= IR_{Se} = (80)(0.02)$

$$= 1.6\,V$$

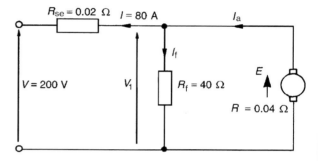

Figure 22.13

P.d. across the field winding $=$ p.d. across armature $= V_1 = 200 + 1.6 = 201.6\,V$

$$\text{Field current } I_f = \frac{V_1}{R_f} = \frac{201.6}{40} = 5.04\,A$$

Armature current, $I_a = I + I_f = 80 + 5.04 = 85.04\,A$

$$\textbf{Generated e.m.f., } E = V_1 + I_a R_a$$

$$= 201.6 + (85.04)(0.04)$$

$$= 201.6 + 3.4016$$

$$= \textbf{205 volts}$$

Characteristics

In cumulative-compound machines the magnetic flux produced by the series and shunt fields are additive. Included in this group are **over-compounded**, **level-compounded** and **under-compounded machines** – the degree of compounding obtained depending on the number of turns of wire on the series winding.

A large number of series winding turns results in an over-compounded characteristic, as shown in Fig. 22.14, in which the full-load terminal voltage exceeds the no-load voltage. A level-compound machine gives a full-load terminal voltage which is equal to the no-load voltage, as shown in Fig. 22.14.

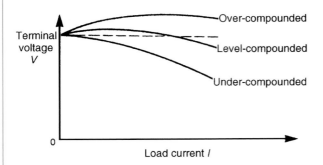

Figure 22.14

An under-compounded machine gives a full-load terminal voltage which is less than the no-load voltage, as shown in Fig. 22.14. However even this latter characteristic is a little better than that for a shunt generator alone. Compound-wound generators are used in electric arc welding, with lighting sets and with marine equipment.

Now try the following exercise

Exercise 132 **Further problems on the d.c. generator**

1. Determine the terminal voltage of a generator which develops an e.m.f. of 240 V and has an armature current of 50 A on load. Assume the armature resistance is 40 mΩ. [238 volts]

2. A generator is connected to a 50 Ω load and a current of 10 A flows. If the armature resistance is 0.5 Ω, determine (a) the terminal voltage, and (b) the generated e.m.f. [(a) 500 volts (b) 505 volts]

3. A separately excited generator develops a no-load e.m.f. of 180 V at an armature speed of 15 rev/s and a flux per pole of 0.20 Wb. Calculate the generated e.m.f. when:
   (a) the speed increases to 20 rev/s and the flux per pole remains unchanged
   (b) the speed remains at 15 rev/s and the pole flux is decreased to 0.125 Wb
   (c) the speed increases to 25 rev/s and the pole flux is decreased to 0.18 Wb.
   [(a) 240 volts (b) 112.5 volts (c) 270 volts]

4. A shunt generator supplies a 50 kW load at 400 V through cables of resistance 0.2 Ω. If the field winding resistance is 50 Ω and the armature resistance is 0.05 Ω, determine (a) the terminal voltage, (b) the e.m.f. generated in the armature. [(a) 425 volts (b) 431.68 volts]

5. A short-shunt compound generator supplies 50 A at 300 V. If the field resistance is 30 Ω, the series resistance 0.03 Ω and the armature resistance 0.05 Ω, determine the e.m.f. generated. [304.5 volts]

6. A d.c. generator has a generated e.m.f. of 210 V when running at 700 rev/min and the flux per pole is 120 mWb. Determine the generated e.m.f.
   (a) at 1050 rev/min, assuming the flux remains constant,
   (b) if the flux is reduced by one-sixth at constant speed, and
   (c) at a speed of 1155 rev/min and a flux of 132 mWb.
   [(a) 315 V (b) 175 V (c) 381.2 V]

7. A 250 V d.c. shunt-wound generator has an armature resistance of 0.1 Ω. Determine the generated e.m.f. when the generator is supplying 50 kW, neglecting the field current of the generator. [270 V]

22.8 D.C. machine losses

As stated in Section 22.1, a generator is a machine for converting mechanical energy into electrical energy and a motor is a machine for converting electrical energy into mechanical energy. When such conversions take place, certain losses occur which are dissipated in the form of heat.

The principal **losses of machines** are:

(i) **Copper loss**, due to I^2R heat losses in the armature and field windings.

(ii) **Iron (or core) loss**, due to hysteresis and eddy-current losses in the armature. This loss can be reduced by constructing the armature of silicon steel laminations having a high resistivity and low hysteresis loss. At constant speed, the iron loss is assumed constant.

(iii) **Friction and windage losses**, due to bearing and brush contact friction and losses due to air resistance against moving parts (called windage).

At constant speed, these losses are assumed to be constant.

(iv) **Brush contact loss** between the brushes and commutator. This loss is approximately proportional to the load current.

The total losses of a machine can be quite significant and operating efficiencies of between 80 per cent and 90 per cent are common.

22.9 Efficiency of a d.c. generator

The efficiency of an electrical machine is the ratio of the output power to the input power and is usually expressed as a percentage. The Greek letter, 'η' (eta) is used to signify efficiency and since the units are, power/power, then efficiency has no units. Thus

$$\text{efficiency, } \eta = \left(\frac{\text{output power}}{\text{input power}}\right) \times 100\%$$

If the total resistance of the armature circuit (including brush contact resistance) is R_a, then **the total loss in the armature circuit is $I_a^2 R_a$**

If the terminal voltage is V and the current in the shunt circuit is I_f, then **the loss in the shunt circuit is $I_f V$**

If the sum of the iron, friction and windage losses is C then **the total losses is given by: $I_a^2 R_a + I_f V + C$** ($I_a^2 R_a + I_f V$ is, in fact, the 'copper loss').

If the output current is I, then **the output power is VI**. Total input power $= VI + I_a^2 R_a + I_f V + C$. Hence

$$\textbf{efficiency, } \eta = \frac{\textbf{output}}{\textbf{input}}, \text{i.e.}$$

$$\eta = \left(\frac{VI}{VI + I_a^2 R_a + I_f V + C}\right) \times 100\% \qquad (4)$$

The **efficiency of a generator is a maximum** when the load is such that:

$$I_a^2 R_a = VI_f + C$$

i.e. when the variable loss = the constant loss

Problem 12. A 10 kW shunt generator having an armature circuit resistance of 0.75 Ω and a field

resistance of 125 Ω, generates a terminal voltage of 250 V at full load. Determine the efficiency of the generator at full load, assuming the iron, friction and windage losses amount to 600 W.

The circuit is shown in Fig. 22.15

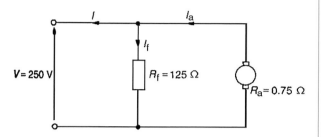

Figure 22.15

Output power $= 10\,000\,\text{W} = VI$ from which, load current $I = 10\,000/V = 10\,000/250 = 40\,\text{A}$.
Field current, $I_f = V/R_f = 250/125 = 2\,\text{A}$.
Armature current, $I_a = I_f + I = 2 + 40 = 42\,\text{A}$

$$\text{Efficiency, } \eta = \left(\frac{VI}{\begin{array}{c}VI + I_a^2 R \\ + I_f V + C\end{array}}\right) \times 100\%$$

$$= \left(\frac{10\,000}{\begin{array}{c}10\,000 + (42)^2(0.75) \\ + (2)(250) + 600\end{array}}\right) \times 100\%$$

$$= \left(\frac{10\,000}{12\,423}\right) \times 100\%$$

$$= \mathbf{80.50\%}$$

Now try the following exercise

Exercise 133   A further problem on the efficiency of a d.c. generator

1. A 15 kW shunt generator having an armature circuit resistance of 0.4 Ω and a field resistance of 100 Ω, generates a terminal voltage of 240 V at full load. Determine the efficiency of the generator at full load, assuming the iron, friction and windage losses amount to 1 kW.

[82.14%]

22.10 D.C. motors

The construction of a d.c. motor is the same as a d.c. generator. The only difference is that in a generator the generated e.m.f. is greater than the terminal voltage, whereas in a motor the generated e.m.f. is less than the terminal voltage.

D.C. motors are often used in power stations to drive emergency stand-by pump systems which come into operation to protect essential equipment and plant should the normal a.c. supplies or pumps fail.

Back e.m.f.

When a d.c. motor rotates, an e.m.f. is induced in the armature conductors. By Lenz's law this induced e.m.f. E opposes the supply voltage V and is called a **back e.m.f.**, and the supply voltage, V is given by:

$$V = E + I_aR_a \quad \text{or} \quad E = V - I_aR_a \quad (5)$$

> **Problem 13.** A d.c. motor operates from a 240 V supply. The armature resistance is 0.2 Ω. Determine the back e.m.f. when the armature current is 50 A.

For a motor, $V = E + I_aR_a$ hence back e.m.f.,

$$E = V - I_aR_a$$
$$= 240 - (50)(0.2)$$
$$= 240 - 10 = \textbf{230 volts}$$

> **Problem 14.** The armature of a d.c. machine has a resistance of 0.25 Ω and is connected to a 300 V supply. Calculate the e.m.f. generated when it is running: (a) as a generator giving 100 A, and (b) as a motor taking 80 A.

(a) As a generator, generated e.m.f.,

$$E = V + I_aR_a, \text{ from equation (3),}$$
$$= 300 + (100)(0.25)$$
$$= 300 + 25$$
$$= \textbf{325 volts}$$

(b) As a motor, generated e.m.f. (or back e.m.f.),

$$E = V - I_aR_a, \text{ from equation (5),}$$
$$= 300 - (80)(0.25)$$
$$= \textbf{280 volts}$$

Now try the following exercise

Exercise 134 Further problems on back e.m.f.

1. A d.c. motor operates from a 350 V supply. If the armature resistance is 0.4 Ω determine the back e.m.f. when the armature current is 60 A.
   [326 volts]

2. The armature of a d.c. machine has a resistance of 0.5 Ω and is connected to a 200 V supply. Calculate the e.m.f. generated when it is running (a) as a motor taking 50 A, and (b) as a generator giving 70 A.
   [(a) 175 volts (b) 235 volts]

3. Determine the generated e.m.f. of a d.c. machine if the armature resistance is 0.1 Ω and it (a) is running as a motor connected to a 230 V supply, the armature current being 60 A, and (b) is running as a generator with a terminal voltage of 230 V, the armature current being 80 A.
   [(a) 224 V (b) 238 V]

22.11 Torque of a d.c. motor

From equation (5), for a d.c. motor, the supply voltage V is given by

$$V = E + I_aR_a$$

Multiplying each term by current I_a gives:

$$VI_a = EI_a + I_a^2R_a$$

The term VI_a is the **total electrical power supplied to the armature**, the term $I_a^2R_a$ is the **loss due to armature resistance**, and the term EI_a is the **mechanical power developed by the armature**. If T is the torque, in newton metres, then the mechanical power developed is given by $T\omega$ watts (see 'Science for Engineering')

Hence $\quad T\omega = 2\pi nT = EI_a$

from which,

$$\text{torque } T = \frac{EI_a}{2\pi n} \text{ newton metres} \quad (6)$$

From Section 22.5, equation (1), the e.m.f. E generated is given by

$$E = \frac{2p\Phi nZ}{c}$$

Hence
$$2\pi nT = EI_a = \left(\frac{2p\Phi nZ}{c}\right)I_a$$

Hence torque
$$T = \frac{\left(\dfrac{2p\Phi nZ}{c}\right)}{2\pi n}I_a$$

i.e.
$$T = \frac{p\Phi ZI_a}{\pi c} \text{ newton metres} \qquad (7)$$

For a given machine, Z, c and p are fixed values

Hence
$$\text{torque, } T \propto \Phi I_a \qquad (8)$$

Problem 15. An 8-pole d.c. motor has a wave-wound armature with 900 conductors. The useful flux per pole is 25 mWb. Determine the torque exerted when a current of 30 A flows in each armature conductor.

$p = 4$, $c = 2$ for a wave winding,
$\Phi = 25 \times 10^{-3}$ Wb, $Z = 900$ and $I_a = 30$ A.
From equation (7),

$$\text{torque, } T = \frac{p\Phi ZI_a}{\pi c}$$
$$= \frac{(4)(25 \times 10^{-3})(900)(30)}{\pi(2)}$$
$$= \mathbf{429.7\,Nm}$$

Problem 16. Determine the torque developed by a 350 V d.c. motor having an armature resistance of $0.5\,\Omega$ and running at 15 rev/s. The armature current is 60 A.

$V = 350$ V, $R_a = 0.5\,\Omega$, $n = 15$ rev/s and $I_a = 60$ A.
Back e.m.f. $E = V - I_a R_a = 350 - (60)(0.5) = 320$ V.
From equation (6),

$$\text{torque, } T = \frac{EI_a}{2\pi n} = \frac{(320)(60)}{2\pi(15)} = \mathbf{203.7\,Nm}$$

Problem 17. A six-pole lap-wound motor is connected to a 250 V d.c. supply. The armature has 500 conductors and a resistance of $1\,\Omega$. The flux per pole is 20 mWb. Calculate (a) the speed and (b) the torque developed when the armature current is 40 A.

$V = 250$ V, $Z = 500$, $R_a = 1\,\Omega$, $\Phi = 20 \times 10^{-3}$ Wb, $I_a = 40$ A and $c = 2p$ for a lap winding

(a) Back e.m.f. $E = V - I_a R_a = 250 - (40)(1)$
$= 210$ V

$$\text{E.m.f. } E = \frac{2p\Phi nZ}{c}$$

i.e. $210 = \dfrac{2p(20 \times 10^{-3})n(500)}{2p} = 10n$

Hence **speed** $n = \dfrac{210}{10} = \mathbf{21\,rev/s}$ or (21×60)

$= \mathbf{1260\,rev/min}$

(b) **Torque** $T = \dfrac{EI_a}{2\pi n} = \dfrac{(210)(40)}{2\pi(21)} = \mathbf{63.66\,Nm}$

Problem 18. The shaft torque of a diesel motor driving a 100 V d.c. shunt-wound generator is 25 Nm. The armature current of the generator is 16 A at this value of torque. If the shunt field regulator is adjusted so that the flux is reduced by 15 per cent, the torque increases to 35 Nm. Determine the armature current at this new value of torque.

From equation (8), the shaft torque T of a generator is proportional to ΦI_a, where Φ is the flux and I_a is the armature current, or, $T = k\Phi I_a$, where k is a constant.
The torque at flux Φ_1 and armature current I_{a1} is $T_1 = k\Phi_1 I_{a1}$ Similarly, $T_2 = k\Phi_2 I_{a2}$

By division $\dfrac{T_1}{T_2} = \dfrac{k\Phi_1 I_{a1}}{k\Phi_2 I_{a2}} = \dfrac{\Phi_1 I_{a1}}{\Phi_2 I_{a2}}$

Hence $\dfrac{25}{35} = \dfrac{\Phi_1 \times 16}{0.85\Phi_1 \times I_{a2}}$

i.e. $I_{a2} = \dfrac{16 \times 35}{0.85 \times 25} = 26.35$ A

That is, **the armature current at the new value of torque is 26.35A**

Problem 19. A 100 V d.c. generator supplies a current of 15 A when running at 1500 rev/min. If the torque on the shaft driving the generator is 12 Nm, determine (a) the efficiency of the generator and (b) the power loss in the generator.

(a) From Section 22.9, the efficiency of a generator = output power/input power × 100 per cent. The output power is the electrical output, i.e. VI watts. The input power to a generator is the mechanical power in the shaft driving the generator, i.e. $T\omega$ or $T(2\pi n)$ watts, where T is the torque in Nm and n is speed of rotation in rev/s. Hence, for a generator,

$$\text{efficiency, } \eta = \frac{VI}{T(2\pi n)} \times 100\%$$

$$= \frac{(100)(15)(100)}{(12)(2\pi)\left(\dfrac{1500}{60}\right)}$$

i.e. **efficiency = 79.6%**

(b) The input power = output power + losses

Hence, $T(2\pi n) = VI + \text{losses}$

i.e. losses $= T(2\pi n) - VI$

$$= \left[(12)(2\pi)\left(\frac{1500}{60}\right)\right]$$

$$- [(100)(15)]$$

i.e. **power loss** = 1885 − 1500 = **385 W**

Now try the following exercise

Exercise 135   Further problems on losses, efficiency, and torque

1. The shaft torque required to drive a d.c. generator is 18.7 Nm when it is running at 1250 rev/min. If its efficiency is 87 per cent under these conditions and the armature current is 17.3 A, determine the voltage at the terminals of the generator.   [123.1 V]

2. A 220 V, d.c. generator supplies a load of 37.5 A and runs at 1550 rev/min. Determine the shaft torque of the diesel motor driving the generator, if the generator efficiency is 78 per cent.   [65.2 Nm]

3. A 4-pole d.c. motor has a wave-wound armature with 800 conductors. The useful flux per pole is 20 mWb. Calculate the torque exerted when a current of 40 A flows in each armature conductor.   [203.7 Nm]

4. Calculate the torque developed by a 240 V d.c. motor whose armature current is 50 A, armature resistance is 0.6 Ω and is running at 10 rev/s.   [167.1 Nm]

5. An 8-pole lap-wound d.c. motor has a 200 V supply. The armature has 800 conductors and a resistance of 0.8 Ω. If the useful flux per pole is 40 mWb and the armature current is 30 A, calculate (a) the speed and (b) the torque developed.   [(a) 5.5 rev/s or 330 rev/min (b) 152.8 Nm]

6. A 150 V d.c. generator supplies a current of 25 A when running at 1200 rev/min. If the torque on the shaft driving the generator is 35.8 Nm, determine (a) the efficiency of the generator, and (b) the power loss in the generator.   [(a) 83.4 per cent (b) 748.8 W]

22.12   Types of d.c. motor and their characteristics

(a) Shunt-wound motor

In the shunt-wound motor the field winding is in parallel with the armature across the supply as shown in Fig. 22.16.

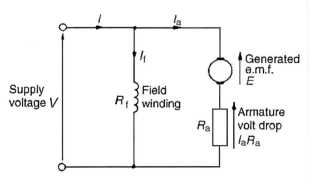

Figure 22.16

For the circuit shown in Fig. 22.16,

$$\text{Supply voltage, } V = E + I_a R_a$$

$$\text{or generated e.m.f., } E = V - I_a R_a$$

$$\text{Supply current, } I = I_a + I_f$$

from Kirchhoff's current law

Problem 20. A 240 V shunt motor takes a total current of 30 A. If the field winding resistance $R_f = 150\,\Omega$ and the armature resistance $R_a = 0.4\,\Omega$ determine (a) the current in the armature, and (b) the back e.m.f.

(a) Field current $I_f = \dfrac{V}{R_f} = \dfrac{240}{150} = 1.6\,\text{A}$

Supply current $I = I_a + I_f$
Hence armature current, $I_a = I - I_f = 30 - 1.6$
$$= \mathbf{28.4\,A}$$

(b) Back e.m.f.

$$E = V - I_a R_a = 240 - (28.4)(0.4) = \mathbf{228.64\,volts}$$

Characteristics

The two principal characteristics are the torque/armature current and speed/armature current relationships. From these, the torque/speed relationship can be derived.

(i) The theoretical torque/armature current characteristic can be derived from the expression $T \propto \Phi I_a$, (see Section 22.11). For a shunt-wound motor, the field winding is connected in parallel with the armature circuit and thus the applied voltage gives a constant field current, i.e. a shunt-wound motor is a constant flux machine. Since Φ is constant, it follows that $T \propto I_a$, and the characteristic is as shown in Fig. 22.17.

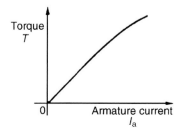

Figure 22.17

(ii) The armature circuit of a d.c. motor has resistance due to the armature winding and brushes, R_a ohms, and when armature current I_a is flowing through it, there is a voltage drop of $I_a R_a$ volts. In Fig. 22.16 the armature resistance is shown as a separate resistor in the armature circuit to help understanding. Also, even though the machine is a motor, because conductors are rotating in a magnetic field, a voltage, $E \propto \Phi \omega$, is generated by the armature conductors. From equation (5), $V = E + I_a R_a$ or $E = V - I_a R_a$ However, from Section 22.5, $E \propto \Phi n$, hence $n \propto E/\Phi$ i.e.

$$\text{speed of rotation, } n \propto \frac{E}{\Phi} \propto \frac{V - I_a R_a}{\Phi} \quad (9)$$

For a shunt motor, V, Φ and R_a are constants, hence as armature current I_a increases, $I_a R_a$ increases and $V - I_a R_a$ decreases, and the speed is proportional to a quantity which is decreasing and is as shown in Fig. 22.18. As the load on the shaft of the motor increases, I_a increases and the speed drops slightly. In practice, the speed falls by about 10 per cent between no-load and full-load on many d.c. shunt-wound motors. Due to this relatively small drop in speed, the d.c. shunt-wound motor is taken as basically being a constant-speed machine and may be used for driving lathes, lines of shafts, fans, conveyor belts, pumps, compressors, drilling machines and so on.

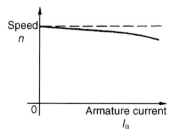

Figure 22.18

(iii) Since torque is proportional to armature current, (see (i) above), the theoretical speed/torque characteristic is as shown in Fig. 22.19.

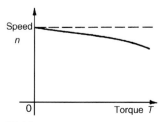

Figure 22.19

Section 3

Problem 21. A 200 V, d.c. shunt-wound motor has an armature resistance of 0.4 Ω and at a certain load has an armature current of 30 A and runs at 1350 rev/min. If the load on the shaft of the motor is increased so that the armature current increases to 45 A, determine the speed of the motor, assuming the flux remains constant.

The relationship $E \propto \Phi n$ applies to both generators and motors. For a motor, $E = V - I_a R_a$, (see equation (5))

Hence $E_1 = 200 - 30 \times 0.4 = 188 \, V$

and $E_2 = 200 - 45 \times 0.4 = 182 \, V$

The relationship

$$\frac{E_1}{E_2} = \frac{\Phi_1 n_1}{\Phi_2 n_2}$$

applies to both generators and motors. Since the flux is constant, $\Phi_1 = \Phi_2$. Hence

$$\frac{188}{182} = \frac{\Phi_1 \times \left(\dfrac{1350}{60}\right)}{\Phi_1 \times n_2}$$

i.e. $n_2 = \dfrac{22.5 \times 182}{188} = 21.78 \, \text{rev/s}$

Thus **the speed of the motor when the armature current is 45 A** is 21.78×60 rev/min i.e. **1307 rev/min**.

Problem 22. A 220 V, d.c. shunt-wound motor runs at 800 rev/min and the armature current is 30 A. The armature circuit resistance is 0.4 Ω. Determine (a) the maximum value of armature current if the flux is suddenly reduced by 10 per cent and (b) the steady-state value of the armature current at the new value of flux, assuming the shaft torque of the motor remains constant.

(a) For a d.c. shunt-wound motor, $E = V - I_a R_a$. Hence initial generated e.m.f., $E_1 = 220 = 30 \times 0.4 = 208 \, V$. The generated e.m.f. is also such that $E \propto \Phi n$, so at the instant the flux is reduced, the speed has not had time to change, and $E = 208 \times 90/100 - 187.2 \, V$. Hence, the voltage drop due to the armature resistance is $220 - 187.2$ i.e. 32.8 V. The **instantaneous value of the current** $= 32.8/0.4 = $ **82 A**. This increase

in current is about three times the initial value and causes an increase in torque, $(T \propto \Phi I_a)$. The motor accelerates because of the larger torque value until steady-state conditions are reached.

(b) $T \propto \Phi I_a$ and, since the torque is constant, $\Phi_1 I_{a1} = \Phi_2 I_{a2}$. The flux Φ is reduced by 10 per cent, hence $\Phi_2 = 0.9 \Phi_1$. Thus, $\Phi_1 \times 30 = 0.9 \Phi_1 \times I_{a2}$ i.e. the steady-state value of armature current, $I_{a2} = 30/0.9 = $ **33.33 A**.

(b) Series-wound motor

In the series-wound motor the field winding is in series with the armature across the supply as shown in Fig. 22.20.

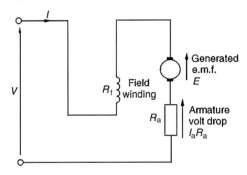

Figure 22.20

For the series motor shown in Fig. 22.20,

Supply voltage $V = E + I(R_a + R_f)$

or generated e.m.f. $E = V - I(R_a + R_f)$

Characteristics

In a series motor, the armature current flows in the field winding and is equal to the supply current, I.

(i) **The torque/current characteristic**
It is shown in Section 22.11 that torque $T \propto \Phi I_a$. Since the armature and field currents are the same current, I, in a series machine, then $T \propto \Phi I$ over a limited range, before magnetic saturation of the magnetic circuit of the motor is reached, (i.e. the linear portion of the B–H curve for the yoke, poles, air gap, brushes and armature in series). Thus $\Phi \propto I$ and $T \propto I^2$. After magnetic saturation, Φ almost becomes a constant and $T \propto I$. Thus the theoretical torque/current characteristic is as shown in Fig. 22.21.

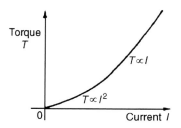

Figure 22.21

(ii) **The speed/current characteristic**

It is shown in equation (9) that

$$n \propto \frac{V - I_a R_a}{\Phi}$$

In a series motor, $I_a = I$ and below the magnetic saturation level, $\Phi \propto I$. Thus $n \propto (V - IR)/I$ where R is the combined resistance of the series field and armature circuit. Since IR is small compared with V, then an approximate relationship for the speed is $n \propto V/I \propto 1/I$ since V is constant. Hence the theoretical speed/current characteristic is as shown in Fig. 22.22. The high speed at small values of current indicate that this type of motor must not be run on very light loads and invariably, such motors are permanently coupled to their loads.

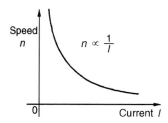

Figure 22.22

(iii) The theoretical **speed/torque characteristic** may be derived from (i) and (ii) above by obtaining the torque and speed for various values of current and plotting the co-ordinates on the speed/torque characteristics. A typical speed/torque characteristic is shown in Fig. 22.23.

A d.c. series motor takes a large current on starting and the characteristic shown in Fig. 22.21 shows that the series-wound motor has a large torque when the current is large. Hence these motors are used for traction (such as trains, milk delivery vehicles, etc.), driving fans and for cranes and hoists, where a large initial torque is required.

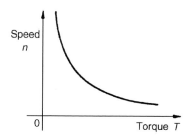

Figure 22.23

> **Problem 23.** A series motor has an armature resistance of $0.2\,\Omega$ and a series field resistance of $0.3\,\Omega$. It is connected to a 240 V supply and at a particular load runs at 24 rev/s when drawing 15 A from the supply. (a) Determine the generated e.m.f. at this load. (b) Calculate the speed of the motor when the load is changed such that the current is increased to 30 A. Assume that this causes a doubling of the flux.

(a) With reference to Fig. 22.20, generated e.m.f., E_1 at initial load, is given by

$$E_1 = V - I_a(R_a + R_f)$$
$$= 240 - (15)(0.2 + 0.3)$$
$$= 240 - 7.5 = \mathbf{232.5\,volts}$$

(b) When the current is increased to 30 A, the generated e.m.f. is given by:

$$E_2 = V - I_2(R_a + R_f)$$
$$= 240 - (30)(0.2 + 0.3)$$
$$= 240 - 15 = 225\,volts$$

Now e.m.f. $E \propto \Phi n$ thus

$$\frac{E_1}{E_2} = \frac{\Phi_1 n_1}{\Phi_2 n_2}$$

i.e. $\dfrac{232.5}{22.5} = \dfrac{\Phi_1(24)}{(2\Phi_1)n_2}$ since $\Phi_2 = 2\Phi_1$

Hence

$$\textbf{speed of motor, } n_2 = \frac{(24)(225)}{(232.5)(2)} = \mathbf{11.6\,rev/s}$$

As the current has been increased from 15 A to 30 A, the speed has decreased from 24 rev/s

Section 3

to 11.6 rev/s. Its speed/current characteristic is similar to Fig. 22.22.

(c) Compound-wound motor

There are two types of compound-wound motor:

(i) **Cumulative compound**, in which the series winding is so connected that the field due to it assists that due to the shunt winding.

(ii) **Differential compound**, in which the series winding is so connected that the field due to it opposes that due to the shunt winding.

Figure 22.24(a) shows a **long-shunt** compound motor and Fig. 22.24(b) a **short-shunt** compound motor.

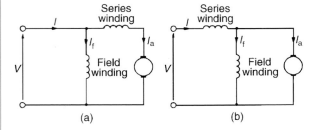

Figure 22.24

Characteristics

A compound-wound motor has both a series and a shunt field winding, (i.e. one winding in series and one in parallel with the armature), and is usually wound to have a characteristic similar in shape to a series-wound motor (see Figs 22.21–22.23). A limited amount of shunt winding is present to restrict the no-load speed to a safe value. However, by varying the number of turns on the series and shunt windings and the directions of the magnetic fields produced by these windings (assisting or opposing), families of characteristics may be obtained to suit almost all applications. Generally, compound-wound motors are used for heavy duties, particularly in applications where sudden heavy load may occur such as for driving plunger pumps, presses, geared lifts, conveyors, hoists and so on.

Typical compound motor torque and speed characteristics are shown in Fig. 22.25.

22.13 The efficiency of a d.c. motor

It was stated in Section 22.9, that the efficiency of a d.c. machine is given by:

$$\text{efficiency, } \eta = \frac{\text{output power}}{\text{input power}} \times 100\%$$

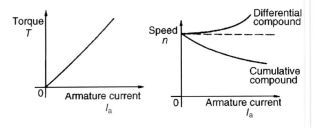

Figure 22.25

Also, the total losses $= I_a^2 R_a + I_f V + C$ (for a shunt motor) where C is the sum of the iron, friction and windage losses.

For a motor,

$$\text{the input power} = VI$$

$$\text{and the output power} = VI - \text{losses}$$

$$= VI - I_a^2 R_a - I_f V - C$$

Hence **efficiency**,

$$\eta = \left(\frac{VI - I_a^2 R_a - I_f V - C}{VI} \right) \times 100\% \qquad (10)$$

The **efficiency of a motor is a maximum** when the load is such that:

$$I_a^2 R_a = I_f V + C$$

Problem 24. A 320 V shunt motor takes a total current of 80 A and runs at 1000 rev/min. If the iron, friction and windage losses amount to 1.5 kW, the shunt field resistance is 40 Ω and the armature resistance is 0.2 Ω, determine the overall efficiency of the motor.

The circuit is shown in Fig. 22.26.
Field current, $I_f = V/R_f = 320/40 = 8$ A.
Armature current $I_a = I - I_f = 80 - 8 = 72$ A.
$C = $ iron, friction and windage losses $= 1500$ W.

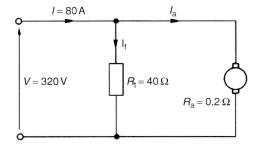

Figure 22.26

Efficiency,

$$\eta = \left(\frac{VI - I_a^2 R_a - I_f V - C}{VI}\right) \times 100\%$$

$$= \left(\frac{\begin{array}{c}(320)(80) - (72)^2 (0.2)\\ - (8)(320) - 1500\end{array}}{(320)(80)}\right) \times 100\%$$

$$= \left(\frac{25\,600 - 1036.8 - 2560 - 1500}{25\,600}\right) \times 100\%$$

$$= \left(\frac{20\,503.2}{25\,600}\right) \times 100\%$$

$$= \mathbf{80.1\%}$$

Problem 25.   A 250 V series motor draws a current of 40 A. The armature resistance is 0.15 Ω and the field resistance is 0.05 Ω. Determine the maximum efficiency of the motor.

The circuit is as shown in Fig. 22.27.
From equation (10), efficiency,

$$\eta = \left(\frac{VI - I_a^2 R_a - I_f V - C}{VI}\right) \times 100\%$$

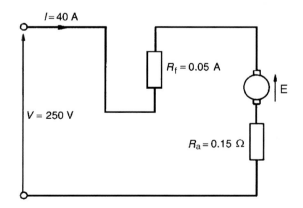

Figure 22.27

However for a series motor, $I_f = 0$ and the $I_a^2 R_a$ loss needs to be $I^2 (R_a + R_f)$. Hence efficiency,

$$\eta = \left(\frac{VI - I^2 (R_a + R_f) - C}{VI}\right) \times 100\%$$

For maximum efficiency $I^2 (R_a + R_f) = C$. Hence efficiency,

$$\eta = \left(\frac{VI - 2I^2 (R_a + R_f)}{VI}\right) \times 100\%$$

$$= \left(\frac{(250)(40) - 2(40)^2 (0.15 + 0.05)}{(250)(40)}\right) \times 100\%$$

$$= \left(\frac{10\,000 - 640}{10\,000}\right) \times 100\%$$

$$= \left(\frac{9360}{10\,000}\right) \times 100\% = \mathbf{93.6\%}$$

Problem 26.   A 200 V d.c. motor develops a shaft torque of 15 Nm at 1200 rev/min. If the efficiency is 80 per cent, determine the current supplied to the motor.

The efficiency of a motor $= \dfrac{\text{output power}}{\text{input power}} \times 100\%$.

The output power of a motor is the power available to do work at its shaft and is given by $T\omega$ or $T(2\pi n)$ watts, where T is the torque in Nm and n is the speed of rotation in rev/s. The input power is the electrical power in watts supplied to the motor, i.e. VI watts.
Thus for a motor,

efficiency, $\eta = \dfrac{T(2\pi n)}{VI} \times 100\%$

i.e. $80 = \left[\dfrac{(15)(2\pi n)\left(\dfrac{1200}{60}\right)}{(200)(I)}\right] \times 100$

Thus the current supplied,

$$I = \frac{(15)(2\pi)(20)(100)}{(200)(80)}$$

$$= \mathbf{11.8\,A}$$

Problem 27.   A d.c. series motor drives a load at 30 rev/s and takes a current of 10 A when the supply voltage is 400 V. If the total resistance of the motor is 2 Ω and the iron, friction and windage losses amount to 300 W, determine the efficiency of the motor.

Efficiency,

$$\eta = \left(\frac{VI - I^2R - C}{VI} \right) \times 100\%$$

$$= \left(\frac{(400)(10) - (10)^2(2) - 300}{(400)(10)} \right) \times 100\%$$

$$= \left(\frac{4000 - 200 - 300}{4000} \right) \times 100\%$$

$$= \left(\frac{3500}{4000} \right) \times 100\% = \mathbf{87.5\%}$$

Now try the following exercise

Exercise 136   Further problems on d.c. motors

1. A 240 V shunt motor takes a total current of 80 A. If the field winding resistance is 120 Ω and the armature resistance is 0.4 Ω, determine (a) the current in the armature, and (b) the back e.m.f.   [(a) 78 A (b) 208.8 V]

2. A d.c. motor has a speed of 900 rev/min when connected to a 460 V supply. Find the approximate value of the speed of the motor when connected to a 200 V supply, assuming the flux decreases by 30 per cent and neglecting the armature volt drop.   [559 rev/min]

3. A series motor having a series field resistance of 0.25 Ω and an armature resistance of 0.15 Ω, is connected to a 220 V supply and at a particular load runs at 20 rev/s when drawing 20 A from the supply. Calculate the e.m.f. generated at this load. Determine also the speed of the motor when the load is changed such that the current increases to 25 A. Assume the flux increases by 25 per cent.

    [212 V, 15.85 rev/s]

4. A 500 V shunt motor takes a total current of 100 A and runs at 1200 rev/min. If the shunt field resistance is 50 Ω, the armature resistance is 0.25 Ω and the iron, friction and windage losses amount to 2 kW, determine the overall efficiency of the motor.   [81.95 per cent]

5. A 250 V, series-wound motor is running at 500 rev/min and its shaft torque is 130 Nm.

If its efficiency at this load is 88 per cent, find the current taken from the supply.

    [30.94 A]

6. In a test on a d.c. motor, the following data was obtained. Supply voltage: 500 V, current taken from the supply: 42.4 A, speed: 850 rev/min, shaft torque: 187 Nm. Determine the efficiency of the motor correct to the nearest 0.5 per cent.   [78.5 per cent]

7. A 300 V series motor draws a current of 50 A. The field resistance is 40 mΩ and the armature resistance is 0.2 Ω. Determine the maximum efficiency of the motor.   [92 per cent]

8. A series motor drives a load at 1500 rev/min and takes a current of 20 A when the supply voltage is 250 V. If the total resistance of the motor is 1.5 Ω and the iron, friction and windage losses amount to 400 W, determine the efficiency of the motor.   [80 per cent]

9. A series-wound motor is connected to a d.c. supply and develops full-load torque when the current is 30 A and speed is 1000 rev/min. If the flux per pole is proportional to the current flowing, find the current and speed at half full-load torque, when connected to the same supply.   [21.2 A, 1415 rev/min]

22.14   D.C. motor starter

If a d.c. motor whose armature is stationary is switched directly to its supply voltage, it is likely that the fuses protecting the motor will burn out. This is because the armature resistance is small, frequently being less than one ohm. Thus, additional resistance must be added to the armature circuit at the instant of closing the switch to start the motor.

As the speed of the motor increases, the armature conductors are cutting flux and a generated voltage, acting in opposition to the applied voltage, is produced, which limits the flow of armature current. Thus the value of the additional armature resistance can then be reduced.

When at normal running speed, the generated e.m.f. is such that no additional resistance is required in the armature circuit. To achieve this varying resistance in the armature circuit on starting, a d.c. motor starter is used, as shown in Fig. 22.28.

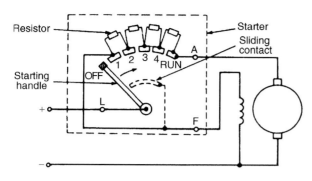

Figure 22.28

The starting handle is moved **slowly** in a clockwise direction to start the motor. For a shunt-wound motor, the field winding is connected to stud 1 or to L via a sliding contact on the starting handle, to give maximum field current, hence maximum flux, hence maximum torque on starting, since $T \propto \Phi I_a$. A similar arrangement without the field connection is used for series motors.

22.15 Speed control of d.c. motors

Shunt-wound motors

The speed of a shunt-wound d.c. motor, n, is proportional to

$$\frac{V - I_a R_a}{\Phi}$$

(see equation (9)). The speed is varied either by varying the value of flux, Φ, or by varying the value of R_a. The former is achieved by using a variable resistor in series with the field winding, as shown in Fig. 22.29(a) and such a resistor is called the **shunt field regulator**.

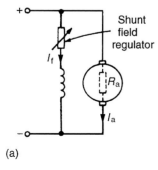
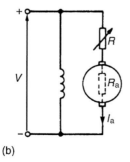

(a)   (b)

Figure 22.29

As the value of resistance of the shunt field regulator is increased, the value of the field current, I_f, is decreased.

This results in a decrease in the value of flux, Φ, and hence an increase in the speed, since $n \propto 1/\Phi$. Thus only speeds **above** that given without a shunt field regulator can be obtained by this method. Speeds **below** those given by

$$\frac{V - I_a R_a}{\Phi}$$

are obtained by increasing the resistance in the armature circuit, as shown in Fig. 22.29(b), where

$$n \propto \frac{V - I_a(R_a + R)}{\Phi}$$

Since resistor R is in series with the armature, it carries the full armature current and results in a large power loss in large motors where a considerable speed reduction is required for long periods.

These methods of speed control are demonstrated in the following worked problem.

Problem 28. A 500 V shunt motor runs at its normal speed of 10 rev/s when the armature current is 120 A. The armature resistance is 0.2 Ω.
(a) Determine the speed when the current is 60 A and a resistance of 0.5 Ω is connected in series with the armature, the shunt field remaining constant.
(b) Determine the speed when the current is 60 A and the shunt field is reduced to 80 per cent of its normal value by increasing resistance in the field circuit.

(a) With reference to Fig. 22.29(b), back e.m.f. at 120 A, $E_1 = V - I_a R_a = 500 - (120)(0.2)$

$$= 500 - 24 = 476 \text{ volts.}$$

When $I_a = 60$ A,

$$E_2 = 500 - (60)(0.2 + 0.5)$$

$$= 500 - (60)(0.7)$$

$$= 500 - 42 = 458 \text{ volts}$$

Now $\dfrac{E_1}{E_2} = \dfrac{\Phi_1 n_1}{\Phi_2 n_2}$

i.e. $\dfrac{476}{458} = \dfrac{\Phi_1(10)}{\Phi_1 n_2}$ since $\Phi_2 = \Phi_1$

from which,

speed $n_2 = \dfrac{(10)(458)}{476} = \mathbf{9.62 \, rev/s}$

(b) Back e.m.f. when $I_a = 60$ A,

$$E_3 = 500 - (60)(0.2)$$

$$= 500 - 12 = 488 \text{ volts}$$

Now $\dfrac{E_1}{E_3} = \dfrac{\Phi_1 n_1}{\Phi_3 n_3}$

i.e. $\dfrac{476}{488} = \dfrac{\Phi_1(10)}{0.8\Phi_1 n_3}$ since $\Phi_3 = 0.8\,\Phi_1$

from which,

$$\textbf{speed } n_3 = \dfrac{(10)(488)}{(0.8)(476)} = \textbf{12.82 rev/s}$$

Series-wound motors

The speed control of series-wound motors is achieved using either (a) field resistance, or (b) armature resistance techniques.

(a) The speed of a d.c. series-wound motor is given by:

$$n = k\left(\dfrac{V - IR}{\Phi}\right)$$

where k is a constant, V is the terminal voltage, R is the combined resistance of the armature and series field and Φ is the flux. Thus, a reduction in flux results in an increase in speed. This is achieved by putting a variable resistance in parallel with the field winding and reducing the field current, and hence flux, for a given value of supply current. A circuit diagram of this arrangement is shown in Fig. 22.30(a). A variable resistor connected in parallel with the series-wound field to control speed is called a **diverter**. Speeds above those given with no diverter are obtained by this method. Problem 29 below demonstrates this method.

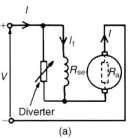
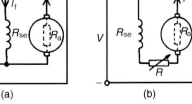

(a)   (b)

Figure 22.30

(b) Speeds below normal are obtained by connecting a variable resistor in series with the field winding and armature circuit, as shown in Fig. 22.30(b). This effectively increases the value of R in the equation

$$n = k\left(\dfrac{V - IR}{\Phi}\right)$$

and thus reduces the speed. Since the additional resistor carries the full supply current, a large power loss is associated with large motors in which a considerable speed reduction is required for long periods. This method is demonstrated in problem 30.

Problem 29. On full-load a 300 V series motor takes 90 A and runs at 15 rev/s. The armature resistance is 0.1 Ω and the series winding resistance is 50 mΩ. Determine the speed when developing full load torque but with a 0.2 Ω diverter in parallel with the field winding. (Assume that the flux is proportional to the field current.)

At 300 V, e.m.f.

$$E_1 = V - IR = V - I(R_a + R_{se})$$

$$= 300 - (90)(0.1 + 0.05)$$

$$= 300 - (90)(0.15)$$

$$= 300 - 13.5 = 286.5 \text{ volts}$$

With the 0.2 Ω diverter in parallel with R_{se} (see Fig. 22.30(a)), the equivalent resistance,

$$R = \dfrac{(0.2)(0.05)}{0.2 + 0.05} = \dfrac{(0.2)(0.05)}{0.25} = 0.04\,\Omega$$

By current division, current

$$I_1 \text{ (in Fig. 22.30(a))} = \left(\dfrac{0.2}{0.2 + 0.05}\right) I = 0.8\,I$$

Torque, $T \propto I_a \Phi$ and for full load torque,
$I_{a1}\Phi_1 = I_{a2}\Phi_2$.
Since flux is proportional to field current $\Phi_1 \propto I_{a1}$ and $\Phi_2 \propto 0.8\,I_{a2}$ then $(90)(90) = (I_{a2})(0.8\,I_{a2})$

from which, $\qquad I_{a2}^2 = \dfrac{90^2}{0.8}$

and $\qquad I_{a2} = \dfrac{90}{\sqrt{0.8}} = 100.62 \text{ A}$

Hence e.m.f. $E_2 = V - I_{a2}(R_a + R)$

$$= 300 - (100.62)(0.1 + 0.04)$$

$$= 300 - (100.62)(0.14)$$

$$= 300 - 14.087 = 285.9 \text{ volts}$$

Now e.m.f., $E \propto \Phi n$, from which,

$$\frac{E_1}{E_2} = \frac{\Phi_1 n_1}{\Phi_2 n_2} = \frac{I_{a1} n_1}{0.8 I_{a2} n_2}$$

Hence $\quad \dfrac{286.5}{285.9} = \dfrac{(90)(15)}{(0.8)(100.62)n_2}$

and $\quad$ **new speed, n_2** $= \dfrac{(285.9)(90)(15)}{(286.5)(0.8)(100.62)}$

$$= \mathbf{16.74 \, rev/s}$$

Thus the speed of the motor has increased from 15 rev/s (i.e. 900 rev/min) to 16.74 rev/s (i.e. 1004 rev/min) by inserting a 0.2 Ω diverter resistance in parallel with the series winding.

Problem 30. A series motor runs at 800 rev/min when the voltage is 400 V and the current is 25 A. The armature resistance is 0.4 Ω and the series field resistance is 0.2 Ω. Determine the resistance to be connected in series to reduce the speed to 600 rev/min with the same current.

With reference to Fig. 22.30(b), at 800 rev/min,

e.m.f., $\quad E_1 = V - I(R_a + R_{se})$

$$= 400 - (25)(0.4 + 0.2)$$

$$= 400 - (25)(0.6)$$

$$= 400 - 15 = 385 \text{ volts}$$

At 600 rev/min, since the current is unchanged, the flux is unchanged.
Thus $E \propto \Phi n$ or $E \propto n$ and

$$\frac{E_1}{E_2} = \frac{n_1}{n_2}$$

Hence $\quad \dfrac{385}{E_2} = \dfrac{800}{600}$

from which, $\quad E_2 = \dfrac{(385)(600)}{800} = 288.75 \text{ volts}$

and $\quad E_2 = V - I(R_a + R_{se} + R)$

Hence $\quad 288.75 = 400 - 25(0.4 + 0.2 + R)$

Rearranging gives:

$$0.6 + R = \frac{400 - 288.75}{25} = 4.45$$

from which, extra series resistance, $R = 4.45 - 0.6$ i.e.
R = 3.85 Ω.
Thus the addition of a series resistance of 3.85 Ω has reduced the speed from 800 rev/min to 600 rev/min.

Now try the following exercise

Exercise 137 **Further problems on the speed control of d.c. motors**

1. A 350 V shunt motor runs at its normal speed of 12 rev/s when the armature current is 90 A. The resistance of the armature is 0.3 Ω.
   (a) Find the speed when the current is 45 A and a resistance of 0.4 Ω is connected in series with the armature, the shunt field remaining constant.
   (b) Find the speed when the current is 45 A and the shunt field is reduced to 75 per cent of its normal value by increasing resistance in the field circuit.

   [(a) 11.83 rev/s (b) 16.67 rev/s]

2. A series motor runs at 900 rev/min when the voltage is 420 V and the current is 40 A. The armature resistance is 0.3 Ω and the series field resistance is 0.2 Ω. Calculate the resistance to be connected in series to reduce the speed to 720 rev/min with the same current. [2 Ω]

3. A 320 V series motor takes 80 A and runs at 1080 rev/min at full load. The armature resistance is 0.2 Ω and the series winding resistance is 0.05 Ω. Assuming the flux is proportional to the field current, calculate the speed when developing full-load torque, but with a 0.15 Ω diverter in parallel with the field winding.

   [1239 rev/min]

22.16 Motor cooling

Motors are often classified according to the type of enclosure used, the type depending on the conditions under which the motor is used and the degree of ventilation required.

The most common type of protection is the **screen-protected type**, where ventilation is achieved by fitting a fan internally, with the openings at the end of the motor fitted with wire mesh.

A **drip-proof type** is similar to the screen-protected type but has a cover over the screen to prevent drips of water entering the machine.

A **flame-proof type** is usually cooled by the conduction of heat through the motor casing.

With a **pipe-ventilated type**, air is piped into the motor from a dust-free area, and an internally fitted fan ensures the circulation of this cool air.

Now try the following exercises

Exercise 138 Short answer questions on d.c. machines

1. A ...... converts mechanical energy into electrical energy

2. A ...... converts electrical energy into mechanical energy

3. What does 'commutation' achieve?

4. Poor commutation may cause sparking. How can this be improved?

5. State any five basic parts of a d.c. machine

6. State the two groups armature windings can be divided into

7. What is armature reaction? How can it be overcome?

8. The e.m.f. generated in an armature winding is given by $E = 2p\Phi nZ/c$ volts. State what p, Φ, n, Z and c represent

9. In a series-wound d.c. machine, the field winding is in ...... with the armature circuit

10. In a d.c. generator, the relationship between the generated voltage, terminal voltage, current and armature resistance is given by $E = $ ......

11. A d.c. machine has its field winding in parallel with the armatures circuit. It is called a ...... wound machine

12. Sketch a typical open-circuit characteristic for (a) a separately excited generator (b) a shunt generator (c) a series generator

13. Sketch a typical load characteristic for (a) a separately excited generator (b) a shunt generator

14. State one application for (a) a shunt generator (b) a series generator (c) a compound generator

15. State the principle losses in d.c. machines

16. The efficiency of a d.c. machine is given by the ratio (......) per cent

17. The equation relating the generated e.m.f., E, terminal voltage, armature current and armature resistance for a d.c. motor is $E = $ ......

18. The torque T of a d.c. motor is given by $T = p\Phi ZI_a/\pi c$ newton metres. State what p, Φ, Z, I and c represent

19. Complete the following. In a d.c. machine
    (a) generated e.m.f. $\propto$ ...... $\times$ ......
    (b) torque $\propto$ ...... $\times$ ......

20. Sketch typical characteristics of torque/armature current for
    (a) a shunt motor
    (b) a series motor
    (c) a compound motor

21. Sketch typical speed/torque characteristics for a shunt and series motor

22. State two applications for each of the following motors:
    (a) shunt   (b) series   (c) compound

In questions 23 to 26, an electrical machine runs at n rev/s, has a shaft torque of T, and takes a current of I from a supply voltage V

23. The power input to a generator is ...... watts

24. The power input to a motor is ...... watts

25. The power output from a generator is ...... watts

26. The power output from a motor is ...... watts

27. The generated e.m.f. of a d.c machine is proportional to ...... volts

28. The torque produced by a d.c. motor is proportional to ...... Nm

29. A starter is necessary for a d.c. motor because the generated e.m.f. is ...... at low speeds

30. The speed of a d.c. shunt-wound motor will ...... if the value of resistance of the shunt field regulator is increased

31. The speed of a d.c. motor will ...... if the value of resistance in the armature circuit is increased

32. The value of the speed of a d.c. shunt-wound motor ...... as the value of the armature current increases

33. At a large value of torque, the speed of a d.c. series-wound motor is ......

34. At a large value of field current, the generated e.m.f. of a d.c. shunt-wound generator is approximately ......

35. In a series-wound generator, the terminal voltage increases as the load current ......

36. One type of d.c. motor uses resistance in series with the field winding to obtain speed variations and another type uses resistance in parallel with the field winding for the same purpose. Explain briefly why these two distinct methods are used and why the field current plays a significant part in controlling the speed of a d.c. motor

37. Name three types of motor enclosure

Exercise 139   Multi-choice questions on d.c. machines
(Answers on page 421)

1. Which of the following statements is false?
   (a) A d.c. motor converts electrical energy to mechanical energy
   (b) The efficiency of a d.c. motor is the ratio input power to output power
   (c) A d.c. generator converts mechanical power to electrical power
   (d) The efficiency of a d.c. generator is the ratio output power to input power
   A shunt-wound d.c. machine is running at n rev/s and has a shaft torque of T Nm. The

supply current is IA when connected to d.c. bus-bars of voltage V volts. The armature resistance of the machine is R_a ohms, the armature current is $I_a A$ and the generated voltage is E volts. Use this data to find the formulae of the quantities stated in questions 2 to 9, selecting the correct answer from the following list:
(a) $V - I_a R_a$ (b) $E + I_a R_a$
(c) VI (d) $E - I_a R_a$
(e) $T(2\pi n)$ (f) $V + I_a R_a$

2. The input power when running as a generator

3. The output power when running as a motor

4. The input power when running as a motor

5. The output power when running as a generator

6. The generated voltage when running as a motor

7. The terminal voltage when running as a generator

8. The generated voltage when running as a generator

9. The terminal voltage when running as a motor

10. Which of the following statements is false?
    (a) A commutator is necessary as part of a d.c. motor to keep the armature rotating in the same direction
    (b) A commutator is necessary as part of a d.c. generator to produce unidirectional voltage at the terminals of the generator
    (c) The field winding of a d.c. machine is housed in slots on the armature
    (d) The brushes of a d.c. machine are usually made of carbon and do not rotate with the armature

11. If the speed of a d.c. machine is doubled and the flux remains constant, the generated e.m.f. (a) remains the same (b) is doubled (c) is halved

12. If the flux per pole of a shunt-wound d.c. generator is increased, and all other variables are kept the same, the speed (a) decreases (b) stays the same (c) increases

13. If the flux per pole of a shunt-wound d.c. generator is halved, the generated e.m.f. at

constant speed (a) is doubled (b) is halved (c) remains the same

14. In a series-wound generator running at constant speed, as the load current increases, the terminal voltage
    (a) increases (b) decreases
    (c) stays the same

15. Which of the following statements is false for a series-wound d.c. motor?
    (a) The speed decreases with increase of resistance in the armature circuit
    (b) The speed increases as the flux decreases
    (c) The speed can be controlled by a diverter
    (d) The speed can be controlled by a shunt field regulator

16. Which of the following statements is false?
    (a) A series-wound motor has a large starting torque
    (b) A shunt-wound motor must be permanently connected to its load
    (c) The speed of a series-wound motor drops considerably when load is applied
    (d) A shunt-wound motor is essentially a constant-speed machine

17. The speed of a d.c. motor may be increased by
    (a) increasing the armature current
    (b) decreasing the field current
    (c) decreasing the applied voltage
    (d) increasing the field current

18. The armature resistance of a d.c. motor is 0.5 Ω, the supply voltage is 200 V and the back e.m.f. is 196 V at full speed. The armature current is:
    (a) 4 A   (b) 8 A
    (c) 400 A   (d) 392 A

19. In d.c. generators iron losses are made up of:
    (a) hysteresis and friction losses
    (b) hysteresis, eddy current and brush contact losses
    (c) hysteresis and eddy current losses
    (d) hysteresis, eddy current and copper losses

20. The effect of inserting a resistance in series with the field winding of a shunt motor is to:
    (a) increase the magnetic field
    (b) increase the speed of the motor

(c) decrease the armature current
(d) reduce the speed of the motor

21. The supply voltage to a d.c. motor is 240 V. If the back e.m.f. is 230 V and the armature resistance is 0.25 Ω, the armature current is:
    (a) 10 A   (b) 40 A
    (c) 960 A   (d) 920 A

22. With a d.c. motor, the starter resistor:
    (a) limits the armature current to a safe starting value
    (b) controls the speed of the machine
    (c) prevents the field current flowing through and damaging the armature
    (d) limits the field current to a safe starting value

23. From Fig. 22.31, the expected characteristic for a shunt-wound d.c. generator is:
    (a) P   (b) Q
    (c) R   (d) S

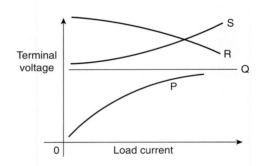

Figure 22.31

24. A commutator is a device fitted to a generator. Its function is:
    (a) to prevent sparking when the load changes
    (b) to convert the a.c. generated into a d.c. output
    (c) to convey the current to and from the windings
    (d) to generate a direct current

Chapter 23

Three-phase induction motors

At the end of this chapter you should be able to:

- appreciate the merits of three-phase induction motors
- understand how a rotating magnetic field is produced
- state the synchronous speed, $n_s = (f/p)$ and use in calculations
- describe the principle of operation of a three-phase induction motor
- distinguish between squirrel-cage and wound-rotor types of motor
- understand how a torque is produced causing rotor movement
- understand and calculate slip
- derive expressions for rotor e.m.f., frequency, resistance, reactance, impedance, current and copper loss, and use them in calculations
- state the losses in an induction motor and calculate efficiency
- derive the torque equation for an induction motor, state the condition for maximum torque, and use in calculations
- describe torque-speed and torque-slip characteristics for an induction motor
- state and describe methods of starting induction motors
- state advantages of cage rotor and wound rotor types of induction motor
- describe the double cage induction motor
- state typical applications of three-phase induction motors

23.1 Introduction

In d.c. motors, introduced in Chapter 22, conductors on a rotating armature pass through a stationary magnetic field. In a **three-phase induction motor**, the magnetic field rotates and this has the advantage that no external electrical connections to the rotor need be made. Its name is derived from the fact that the current in the rotor is **induced** by the magnetic field instead of being supplied through electrical connections to the supply.

The result is a motor which: (i) is cheap and robust, (ii) is explosion proof, due to the absence of a commutator or slip-rings and brushes with their associated sparking, (iii) requires little or no skilled maintenance, and (iv) has self-starting properties when switched to a supply with no additional expenditure on auxiliary equipment. The principal disadvantage of a three-phase induction motor is that its speed cannot be readily adjusted.

DOI: 10.1016/B978-0-08-089056-2.00023-1

23.2 Production of a rotating magnetic field

When a three-phase supply is connected to symmetrical three-phase windings, the currents flowing in the windings produce a magnetic field. This magnetic field is constant in magnitude and rotates at constant speed as shown below, and is called the **synchronous speed**.

With reference to Fig. 23.1, the windings are represented by three single-loop conductors, one for each phase, marked $R_S R_F$, $Y_S Y_F$ and $B_S B_F$, the S and F signifying start and finish. In practice, each phase winding comprises many turns and is distributed around the stator; the single-loop approach is for clarity only.

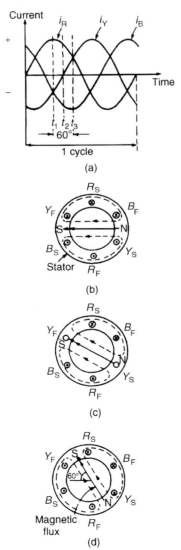

Figure 23.1

When the stator windings are connected to a three-phase supply, the current flowing in each winding varies with time and is as shown in Fig. 23.1(a). If the value of current in a winding is positive, the assumption is made that it flows from start to finish of the winding, i.e. if it is the red phase, current flows from R_S to R_F, i.e. away from the viewer in R_S and towards the viewer in R_F. When the value of current is negative, the assumption is made that it flows from finish to start, i.e. towards the viewer in an 'S' winding and away from the viewer in an 'F' winding. At time, say t_1, shown in Fig. 23.1(a), the current flowing in the red phase is a maximum positive value. At the same time t_1, the currents flowing in the yellow and blue phases are both 0.5 times the maximum value and are negative.

The current distribution in the stator windings is therefore as shown in Fig. 23.1(b), in which current flows away from the viewer, (shown as $\otimes$) in R_S since it is positive, but towards the viewer (shown as $\odot$) in Y_S and B_S, since these are negative. The resulting magnetic field is as shown, due to the 'solenoid' action and application of the corkscrew rule.

A short time later at time t_2, the current flowing in the red phase has fallen to about 0.87 times its maximum value and is positive, the current in the yellow phase is zero and the current in the blue phase is about 0.87 times its maximum value and is negative. Hence the currents and resultant magnetic field are as shown in Fig. 23.1(c). At time t_3, the currents in the red and yellow phases are 0.5 of their maximum values and the current in the blue phase is a maximum negative value. The currents and resultant magnetic field are as shown in Fig. 23.1(d).

Similar diagrams to Fig. 23.1(b), (c) and (d) can be produced for all time values and these would show that the magnetic field travels through one revolution for each cycle of the supply voltage applied to the stator windings.

By considering the flux values rather than the current values, it is shown below that the rotating magnetic field has a constant value of flux. The three coils shown in Fig. 23.2(a), are connected in star to a three-phase supply. Let the positive directions of the fluxes produced by currents flowing in the coils, be ϕ_A, ϕ_B and ϕ_C respectively. The directions of ϕ_A, ϕ_B and ϕ_C do not alter, but their magnitudes are proportional to the currents flowing in the coils at any particular time. At time t_1, shown in Fig. 23.2(b), the currents flowing in the coils are:

i_B, a maximum positive value, i.e. the flux is towards point P; i_A and i_C, half the maximum value and negative, i.e. the flux is away from point P.

These currents give rise to the magnetic fluxes ϕ_A, ϕ_B and ϕ_C, whose magnitudes and directions are as shown

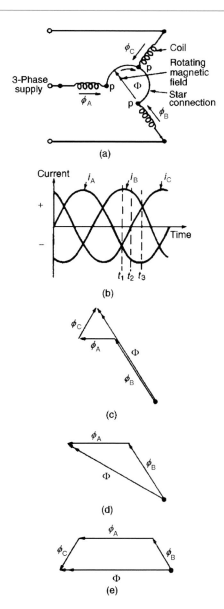

Figure 23.2

The magnetic fluxes and the resultant magnetic flux are as shown in Fig. 23.2(e).

Inspection of Fig. 23.2(c), (d) and (e) shows that the magnitude of the resultant magnetic flux, Φ, in each case is constant and is $1\frac{1}{2}$ × the maximum value of ϕ_A, ϕ_B or ϕ_C, but that its direction is changing. The process of determining the resultant flux may be repeated for all values of time and shows that the magnitude of the resultant flux is constant for all values of time and also that it rotates at constant speed, making one revolution for each cycle of the supply voltage.

23.3 Synchronous speed

The rotating magnetic field produced by three-phase windings could have been produced by rotating a permanent magnet's north and south pole at synchronous speed, (shown as N and S at the ends of the flux phasors in Fig. 23.1(b), (c) and (d)). For this reason, it is called a 2-pole system and an induction motor using three-phase windings only is called a 2-pole induction motor. If six windings displaced from one another by 60° are used, as shown in Fig. 23.3(a), by drawing the current and resultant magnetic field diagrams at various time values, it may be shown that one cycle of the supply

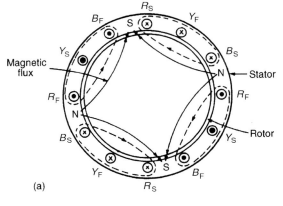

(a)

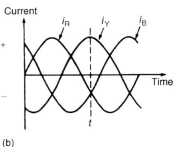

(b)

Figure 23.3

in Fig. 23.2(c). The resultant flux is the phasor sum of ϕ_A, ϕ_B and ϕ_C, shown as Φ in Fig. 23.2(c). At time t_2, the currents flowing are:

i_B, 0.866 × maximum positive value, i_C, zero, and i_A, 0.866 × maximum negative value.

The magnetic fluxes and the resultant magnetic flux are as shown in Fig. 23.2(d).

At time t_3,

i_B is 0.5 × maximum value and is positive

i_A is a maximum negative value, and

i_C is 0.5 × maximum value and is positive.

current to the stator windings causes the magnetic field to move through half a revolution. The current distribution in the stator windings are shown in Fig. 23.3(a), for the time t shown in Fig. 23.3(b).

It can be seen that for six windings on the stator, the magnetic flux produced is the same as that produced by rotating two permanent magnet north poles and two permanent magnet south poles at synchronous speed. This is called a 4-pole system and an induction motor using six phase windings is called a 4-pole induction motor. By increasing the number of phase windings the number of poles can be increased to any even number.

In general, if f is the frequency of the currents in the stator windings and the stator is wound to be equivalent to p **pairs** of poles, the speed of revolution of the rotating magnetic field, i.e. the synchronous speed, n_s is given by:

$$n_s = \frac{f}{p} \text{rev/s}$$

Problem 1. A three-phase 2-pole induction motor is connected to a 50 Hz supply. Determine the synchronous speed of the motor in rev/min.

From above, $n_s = (f/p)$ rev/s, where n_s is the synchronous speed, f is the frequency in hertz of the supply to the stator and p is the number of **pairs** of poles. Since the motor is connected to a 50 hertz supply, $f = 50$.

The motor has a two-pole system, hence p, the number of pairs of poles, is 1. Thus, synchronous speed, $n_s = (50/1) = 50$ rev/s $= 50 \times 60$ rev/min
$$= 3000 \text{ rev/min}.$$

Problem 2. A stator winding supplied from a three-phase 60 Hz system is required to produce a magnetic flux rotating at 900 rev/min. Determine the number of poles.

Synchronous speed,

$$n_s = 900 \text{ rev/min} = \frac{900}{60} \text{rev/s} = 15 \text{ rev/s}$$

Since

$$n_s = \left(\frac{f}{p}\right) \text{ then } p = \left(\frac{f}{n_s}\right) = \left(\frac{60}{15}\right) = 4$$

Hence **the number of pole pairs is 4** and thus **the number of poles is 8**

Problem 3. A three-phase 2-pole motor is to have a synchronous speed of 6000 rev/min. Calculate the frequency of the supply voltage.

Since $n_s = \left(\frac{f}{p}\right)$ then

frequency, $f = (n_s)(p)$

$$= \left(\frac{6000}{60}\right)\left(\frac{2}{2}\right) = \mathbf{100\,Hz}$$

Now try the following exercise

Exercise 140 Further problems on synchronous speed

1. The synchronous speed of a 3-phase, 4-pole induction motor is 60 rev/s. Determine the frequency of the supply to the stator windings.
   [120 Hz]

2. The synchronous speed of a 3-phase induction motor is 25 rev/s and the frequency of the supply to the stator is 50 Hz. Calculate the equivalent number of pairs of poles of the motor.
   [2]

3. A 6-pole, 3-phase induction motor is connected to a 300 Hz supply. Determine the speed of rotation of the magnetic field produced by the stator.
   [100 rev/s]

23.4 Construction of a three-phase induction motor

The stator of a three-phase induction motor is the stationary part corresponding to the yoke of a d.c. machine. It is wound to give a 2-pole, 4-pole, 6-pole, ... rotating magnetic field, depending on the rotor speed required. The rotor, corresponding to the armature of a d.c. machine, is built up of laminated iron, to reduce eddy currents.

In the type most widely used, known as a **squirrel-cage rotor**, copper or aluminium bars are placed in slots cut in the laminated iron, the ends of the bars being welded or brazed into a heavy conducting ring, (see Fig. 23.4(a)). A cross-sectional view of a three-phase induction motor is shown in Fig. 23.4(b).

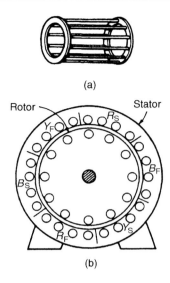

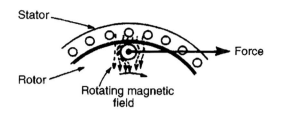

Figure 23.5

Figure 23.4

The conductors are placed in slots in the laminated iron rotor core. If the slots are skewed, better starting and quieter running is achieved. This type of rotor has no external connections which means that slip-rings and brushes are not needed. The squirrel-cage motor is cheap, reliable and efficient. Another type of rotor is the **wound rotor**. With this type there are phase windings in slots, similar to those in the stator. The windings may be connected in star or delta and the connections made to three slip-rings. The slip-rings are used to add external resistance to the rotor circuit, particularly for starting (see Section 23.13), but for normal running the slip-rings are short-circuited.

The principle of operation is the same for both the squirrel-cage and the wound rotor machines.

23.5 Principle of operation of a three-phase induction motor

When a three-phase supply is connected to the stator windings, a rotating magnetic field is produced. As the magnetic flux cuts a bar on the rotor, an e.m.f. is induced in it and since it is joined, via the end conducting rings, to another bar one pole pitch away, a current flows in the bars. The magnetic field associated with this current flowing in the bars interacts with the rotating magnetic field and a force is produced, tending to turn the rotor in the same direction as the rotating magnetic field, (see Fig. 23.5). Similar forces are applied to all the conductors on the rotor, so that a torque is produced causing the rotor to rotate.

23.6 Slip

The force exerted by the rotor bars causes the rotor to turn in the direction of the rotating magnetic field. As the rotor speed increases, the rate at which the rotating magnetic field cuts the rotor bars is less and the frequency of the induced e.m.f.'s in the rotor bars is less. If the rotor runs at the same speed as the rotating magnetic field, no e.m.f.'s are induced in the rotor, hence there is no force on them and no torque on the rotor. Thus the rotor slows down. For this reason the rotor can never run at synchronous speed.

When there is no load on the rotor, the resistive forces due to windage and bearing friction are small and the rotor runs very nearly at synchronous speed. As the rotor is loaded, the speed falls and this causes an increase in the frequency of the induced e.m.f.'s in the rotor bars and hence the rotor current, force and torque increase. The difference between the rotor speed, n_r, and the synchronous speed, n_s, is called the **slip speed**, i.e.

$$\text{slip speed} = n_s - n_r \text{ rev/s}$$

The ratio $(n_s - n_r)/n_s$ is called the **fractional slip** or just the **slip**, s, and is usually expressed as a percentage. Thus

$$\text{slip, } s = \left(\frac{n_s - n_r}{n_s}\right) \times 100\%$$

Typical values of slip between no load and full load are about 4 to 5 per cent for small motors and 1.5 to 2 per cent for large motors.

Problem 4. The stator of a three-phase, 4-pole induction motor is connected to a 50 Hz supply. The rotor runs at 1455 rev/min at full load. Determine (a) the synchronous speed and (b) the slip at full load.

(a) The number of pairs of poles, $p = (4/2) = 2$. The supply frequency $f = 50$ Hz. The **synchronous speed**, $n_s = (f/p) = (50/2) = \mathbf{25 \text{ rev/s}}$.

Section 3

(b) The rotor speed, $n_r = (1455/60) = 24.25$ rev/s.

$$\text{Slip, s} = \left(\frac{n_s - n_r}{n_s}\right) \times 100\%$$

$$= \left(\frac{25 - 24.25}{25}\right) \times 100\%$$

$$= \mathbf{3\%}$$

Problem 5. A three-phase, 60 Hz induction motor has 2 poles. If the slip is 2 per cent at a certain load, determine (a) the synchronous speed, (b) the speed of the rotor, and (c) the frequency of the induced e.m.f.'s in the rotor.

(a) $f = 60$ Hz and $p = (2/2) = 1$. Hence **synchronous speed**, $n_s = (f/p) = (60/1) = \mathbf{60\,rev/s}$ or $60 \times 60 = \mathbf{3600\,rev/min}$.

(b) Since slip,

$$s = \left(\frac{n_s - n_r}{n_s}\right) \times 100\%$$

$$2 = \left(\frac{60 - n_r}{60}\right) \times 100$$

Hence

$$\frac{2 \times 60}{100} = 60 - n_r$$

i.e.

$$n_r = 60 - \frac{2 \times 60}{100} = 58.8\,\text{rev/s}$$

i.e. the rotor runs at $58.8 \times 60 = \mathbf{3528\,rev/min}$

(c) Since the synchronous speed is 60 rev/s and that of the rotor is 58.8 rev/s, the rotating magnetic field cuts the rotor bars at $(60 - 58.8) = 1.2$ rev/s.

Thus the frequency of the e.m.f.'s induced in the rotor bars, is $f = n_s p = (1.2)(\frac{2}{2}) = \mathbf{1.2\,Hz}$.

Problem 6. A three-phase induction motor is supplied from a 50 Hz supply and runs at 1200 rev/min when the slip is 4 per cent. Determine the synchronous speed.

$$\text{Slip, } s = \left(\frac{n_s - n_r}{n_s}\right) \times 100\%$$

Rotor speed, $n_r = (1200/60) = 20$ rev/s and $s = 4$.

Hence

$$4 = \left(\frac{n_s - 20}{n_s}\right) \times 100\% \text{ or } 0.04 = \frac{n_s - 20}{n_s}$$

from which, $n_s(0.04) = n_s - 20$ and
$$20 = n_s - 0.04\,n_s = n_s(1 - 0.04).$$

Hence **synchronous speed**,

$$n_s = \frac{20}{1 - 0.04} = 20.8\dot{3}\,\text{rev/s}$$

$$= (20.8\dot{3} \times 60)\,\text{rev/min}$$

$$= \mathbf{1250\,rev/min}$$

Now try the following exercise

Exercise 141   Further problems on slip

1. A 6-pole, 3-phase induction motor runs at 970 rev/min at a certain load. If the stator is connected to a 50 Hz supply, find the percentage slip at this load. [3%]

2. A 3-phase, 50 Hz induction motor has 8 poles. If the full load slip is 2.5 per cent, determine
    (a) the synchronous speed,
    (b) the rotor speed, and
    (c) the frequency of the rotor e.m.f.'s.
    [(a) 750 rev/min (b) 731 rev/min (c) 1.25 Hz]

3. A three-phase induction motor is supplied from a 60 Hz supply and runs at 1710 rev/min when the slip is 5 per cent. Determine the synchronous speed. [1800 rev/min]

4. A 4-pole, 3-phase, 50 Hz induction motor runs at 1440 rev/min at full load. Calculate
    (a) the synchronous speed,
    (b) the slip, and
    (c) the frequency of the rotor induced e.m.f.'s.
    [(a) 1500 rev/min (b) 4% (c) 2 Hz]

23.7   Rotor e.m.f. and frequency

Rotor e.m.f.

When an induction motor is stationary, the stator and rotor windings form the equivalent of a transformer as shown in Fig. 23.6.

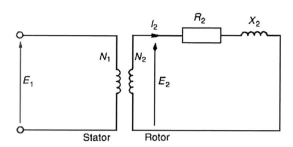

Figure 23.6

The rotor e.m.f. at standstill is given by

$$E_2 = \left(\frac{N_2}{N_1}\right) E_1 \qquad (1)$$

where E_1 is the supply voltage per phase to the stator.

When an induction motor is running, the induced e.m.f. in the rotor is less since the relative movement between conductors and the rotating field is less. The induced e.m.f. is proportional to this movement, hence it must be proportional to the slip, s. Hence **when running**, rotor e.m.f. per phase $= E_r = s E_2$

i.e. rotor e.m.f. per phase $= s\left(\frac{N_2}{N_1}\right) E_1 \qquad (2)$

Rotor frequency

The rotor e.m.f. is induced by an alternating flux and the rate at which the flux passes the conductors is the slip speed. Thus the frequency of the rotor e.m.f. is given by:

$$f_r = (n_s - n_r)p = \left(\frac{n_s - n_r}{n_s}\right)(n_s p)$$

However $(n_s - n_r)/n_s$ is the slip s and $(n_s p)$ is the supply frequency f, hence

$$f_r = sf \qquad (3)$$

Problem 7. The frequency of the supply to the stator of an 8-pole induction motor is 50 Hz and the rotor frequency is 3 Hz. Determine (a) the slip, and (b) the rotor speed.

(a) From equation (3), $f_r = sf$. Hence $3 = (s)(50)$ from which,

$$\textbf{slip, s} = \frac{3}{50} = \textbf{0.06 or 6\%}$$

(b) Synchronous speed, $n_s = f/p = 50/4 = 12.5$ rev/s or $(12.5 \times 60) = 750$ rev/min

$$\text{Slip, } s = \left(\frac{n_s - n_r}{n_s}\right)$$

hence $\qquad 0.06 = \left(\frac{12.5 - n_r}{12.5}\right)$

$$(0.06)(12.5) = 12.5 - n_r$$

and **rotor speed,**

$$\boldsymbol{n_r} = 12.5 - (0.06)(12.5)$$

$$= \textbf{11.75 rev/s or 705 rev/min}$$

Now try the following exercise

Exercise 142 **Further problems on rotor frequency**

1. A 12-pole, 3-phase, 50 Hz induction motor runs at 475 rev/min. Determine
    (a) the slip speed,
    (b) the percentage slip, and
    (c) the frequency of rotor currents.
    [(a) 25 rev/min (b) 5% (c) 2.5 Hz]

2. The frequency of the supply to the stator of a 6-pole induction motor is 50 Hz and the rotor frequency is 2 Hz. Determine
    (a) the slip, and
    (b) the rotor speed, in rev/min.
    [(a) 0.04 or 4% (b) 960 rev/min]

23.8   Rotor impedance and current

Rotor resistance

The rotor resistance R_2 is unaffected by frequency or slip, and hence remains constant.

Rotor reactance

Rotor reactance varies with the frequency of the rotor current. At standstill, reactance per phase, $X_2 = 2\pi f L$. When running, reactance per phase,

$$X_r = 2\pi f_r L$$

$$= 2\pi (sf)L \quad \text{from equation (3)}$$

$$= s(2\pi f L)$$

i.e. $\qquad \boldsymbol{X_r = sX_2} \qquad (4)$

Figure 23.7 represents the rotor circuit when running.

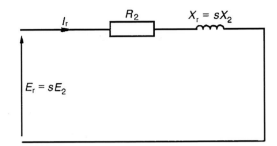

Figure 23.7

Rotor impedance

Rotor impedance per phase,

$$Z_r = \sqrt{R_2^2 + (sX_2)^2} \qquad (5)$$

At standstill, slip $s = 1$, then

$$Z_2 = \sqrt{R_2^2 + X_2^2} \qquad (6)$$

Rotor current

From Fig. 23.6 and 23.7, at standstill, starting current,

$$I_2 = \frac{E_2}{Z_2} = \frac{\left(\dfrac{N_2}{N_1}\right)E_1}{\sqrt{R_2^2 + X_2^2}} \qquad (7)$$

and when running, current,

$$I_r = \frac{E_r}{Z_r} = \frac{s\left(\dfrac{N_2}{N_1}\right)E_1}{\sqrt{R_2^2 + (sX_2)^2}} \qquad (8)$$

23.9 Rotor copper loss

Power $P = 2\pi nT$, where T is the torque in newton metres, hence torque $T = (P/2\pi n)$. If P_2 is the power input to the rotor from the rotating field, and P_m is the mechanical power output (including friction losses)

then

$$T = \frac{P_2}{2\pi n_s} = \frac{P_m}{2\pi n_r}$$

from which,

$$\frac{P_2}{n_s} = \frac{P_m}{n_r} \quad \text{or} \quad \frac{P_m}{P_2} = \frac{n_r}{n_s}$$

Hence

$$1 - \frac{P_m}{P_2} = 1 - \frac{n_r}{n_s}$$

$$\frac{P_2 - P_m}{P_2} = \frac{n_s - n_r}{n_s} = s$$

$P_2 - P_m$ is the electrical or copper loss in the rotor, i.e. $P_2 - P_m = I_r^2 R_2$. Hence

$$\text{slip}, s = \frac{\text{rotor copper loss}}{\text{rotor input}} = \frac{I_r^2 R_2}{P_2} \qquad (9)$$

or power input to the rotor,

$$P_2 = \frac{I_r^2 R_2}{s} \qquad (10)$$

23.10 Induction motor losses and efficiency

Figure 23.8 summarises losses in induction motors. Motor efficiency,

$$\eta = \frac{\text{output power}}{\text{input power}} = \frac{P_m}{P_1} \times 100\%$$

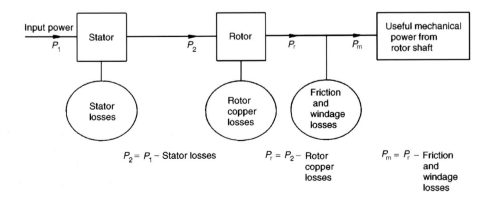

Figure 23.8

Problem 8. The power supplied to a three-phase induction motor is 32 kW and the stator losses are 1200 W. If the slip is 5 per cent, determine (a) the rotor copper loss, (b) the total mechanical power developed by the rotor, (c) the output power of the motor if friction and windage losses are 750 W, and (d) the efficiency of the motor, neglecting rotor iron loss.

(a) Input power to rotor = stator input power
$$- \text{ stator losses}$$
$$= 32 \text{ kW} - 1.2 \text{ kW}$$
$$= 30.8 \text{ kW}$$

From equation (9),

$$\text{slip} = \frac{\text{rotor copper loss}}{\text{rotor input}}$$

i.e. $\qquad \dfrac{5}{100} = \dfrac{\text{rotor copper loss}}{30.8}$

from which, **rotor copper loss** = $(0.05)(30.8)$
$$= \textbf{1.54 kW}$$

(b) Total mechanical power developed by the rotor

$$= \text{rotor input power} - \text{rotor losses}$$
$$= 30.8 - 1.54 = \textbf{29.26 kW}$$

(c) Output power of motor

$$= \text{power developed by the rotor}$$
$$- \text{friction and windage losses}$$
$$= 29.26 - 0.75 = \textbf{28.51 kW}$$

(d) Efficiency of induction motor,

$$\eta = \left(\frac{\text{output power}}{\text{input power}} \right) \times 100\%$$

$$= \left(\frac{28.51}{32} \right) \times 100\%$$

$$= \textbf{89.10\%}$$

Problem 9. The speed of the induction motor of Problem 8 is reduced to 35 per cent of its synchronous speed by using external rotor resistance. If the torque and stator losses are unchanged, determine (a) the rotor copper loss, and (b) the efficiency of the motor.

(a) Slip, $s = \left(\dfrac{n_s - n_r}{n_s} \right) \times 100\%$

$$= \left(\frac{n_s - 0.35 n_s}{n_s} \right) \times 100\%$$

$$= (0.65)(100) = 65\%$$

Input power to rotor = 30.8 kW (from Problem 8)

Since $\qquad s = \dfrac{\text{rotor copper loss}}{\text{rotor input}}$

then **rotor copper loss** = $(s)(\text{rotor input})$

$$= \left(\frac{65}{100} \right) (30.8)$$

$$= \textbf{20.02 kW}$$

(b) Power developed by rotor

$$= \text{input power to rotor} - \text{rotor copper loss}$$
$$= 30.8 - 20.02 = 10.78 \text{ kW}$$

Output power of motor

$$= \text{power developed by rotor}$$
$$- \text{friction and windage losses}$$
$$= 10.78 - 0.75 = 10.03 \text{ kW}$$

Efficiency,

$$\eta = \left(\frac{\text{output power}}{\text{input power}} \right) \times 100\%$$

$$= \left(\frac{10.03}{32} \right) \times 100\%$$

$$= \textbf{31.34\%}$$

Now try the following exercise

Exercise 143   Further problems on losses and efficiency

1. The power supplied to a three-phase induction motor is 50 kW and the stator losses are 2 kW. If the slip is 4 per cent, determine
   (a) the rotor copper loss,
   (b) the total mechanical power developed by the rotor,

(c) the output power of the motor if friction and windage losses are 1 kW, and

(d) the efficiency of the motor, neglecting rotor iron losses.

[(a) 1.92 kW (b) 46.08 kW (c) 45.08 kW (d) 90.16%]

2. By using external rotor resistance, the speed of the induction motor in Problem 1 is reduced to 40 per cent of its synchronous speed. If the torque and stator losses are unchanged, calculate

(a) the rotor copper loss, and

(b) the efficiency of the motor.

[(a) 28.80 kW (b) 36.40%]

23.11 Torque equation for an induction motor

Torque

$$T = \frac{P_2}{2\pi n_s} = \left(\frac{1}{2\pi n_s}\right)\left(\frac{I_r^2 R_2}{s}\right)$$

(from equation (10))

From equation (8), $I_r = \dfrac{s\left(\dfrac{N_2}{N_1}\right)E_1}{\sqrt{R_2^2 + (sX_2)^2}}$

Hence torque per phase,

$$T = \left(\frac{1}{2\pi n_s}\right)\left(\frac{s^2\left(\dfrac{N_2}{N_1}\right)^2 E_1^2}{R_2^2 + (sX_2)^2}\right)\left(\frac{R_2}{s}\right)$$

i.e.

$$T = \left(\frac{1}{2\pi n_s}\right)\left(\frac{s\left(\dfrac{N_2}{N_2}\right)^2 E_1^2 R_2}{R_2^2 + (sX_2)^2}\right)$$

If there are m phases then torque,

$$T = \left(\frac{m}{2\pi n_s}\right)\left(\frac{s\left(\dfrac{N_2}{N_1}\right)^2 E_1^2 R_2}{R_2^2 + (sX_2)^2}\right)$$

i.e.

$$T = \left(\frac{m\left(\dfrac{N_2}{N_1}\right)^2}{2\pi n_s}\right)\left(\frac{sE_1^2 R_2}{R_2^2 + (sX_2)^2}\right) \quad (11)$$

$$= k\left(\frac{sE_1^2 R_2}{R_2^2 + (sX_2)^2}\right)$$

where k is a constant for a particular machine, i.e.

$$\text{torque, } T \propto \left(\frac{sE_1^2 R_2}{R_2^2 + (sX_2)^2}\right) \quad (12)$$

Under normal conditions, the supply voltage is usually constant, hence equation (12) becomes:

$$T \propto \frac{sR_2}{R_2^2 + (sX_2)^2}$$

$$\propto \frac{R_2}{\dfrac{R_2^2}{s} + sX_2^2}$$

The torque will be a maximum when the denominator is a minimum and this occurs when

$$\frac{R_2^2}{s} = sX_2^2$$

i.e. when

$$s = \frac{R_2}{X_2} \quad \text{or} \quad R_2 = sX_2 = X_r$$

from equation (4). Thus **maximum torque** occurs when rotor resistance and rotor reactance are equal, i.e. when $R_2 = X_r$

Problems 10 to 13 following illustrate some of the characteristics of three-phase induction motors.

Problem 10. A 415 V, three-phase, 50 Hz, 4-pole, star-connected induction motor runs at 24 rev/s on full load. The rotor resistance and reactance per phase are 0.35 Ω and 3.5 Ω respectively, and the effective rotor-stator turns ratio is 0.85:1. Calculate (a) the synchronous speed, (b) the slip, (c) the full load torque, (d) the power output if mechanical losses amount to 770 W, (e) the maximum torque, (f) the speed at which maximum torque occurs, and (g) the starting torque.

(a) Synchronous speed, $n_s = (f/p) = (50/2) =$ **25 rev/s** or $(25 \times 60) = $ **1500 rev/min**

(b) Slip, $s = \left(\dfrac{n_s - n_r}{n_s}\right) = \dfrac{25 - 24}{25} = $ **0.04** or **4%**

(c) Phase voltage,

$$E_1 = \frac{415}{\sqrt{3}} = 239.6 \text{ volts}$$

Full load torque,

$$T = \left(\frac{m\left(\dfrac{N_2}{N_1}\right)^2}{2\pi n_s}\right)\left(\frac{sE_1^2 R_2}{R_2^2 + (sX_2)^2}\right)$$

from equation (11)

$$= \left(\frac{3(0.85)^2}{2\pi(25)}\right)\left(\frac{(0.04)(239.6)^2(0.35)}{(0.35)^2 + (0.04 \times 3.5)^2}\right)$$

$$= (0.01380)\left(\frac{803.71}{0.1421}\right)$$

$$= \textbf{78.05 Nm}$$

(d) Output power, including friction losses,

$$P_m = 2\pi n_r T$$
$$= 2\pi(24)(78.05)$$
$$= 11\,770 \text{ watts}$$

Hence, **power output** $= P_m - $ mechanical losses

$$= 11\,770 - 770$$
$$= 11\,000 \text{ W}$$
$$= \textbf{11 kW}$$

(e) Maximum torque occurs when $R_2 = X_r = 0.35\,\Omega$

Slip, $s = \dfrac{R_2}{X_2} = \dfrac{0.35}{3.5} = 0.1$

Hence **maximum torque,**

$$\textbf{T}_\textbf{m} = (0.01380)\left(\frac{sE_1^2 R_2}{R_2^2 + (sX_2)^2}\right) \text{ from part (c)}$$

$$= (0.01380)\left(\frac{0.1(239.6)^2 0.35}{0.35^2 + 0.35^2}\right)$$

$$= (0.01380)\left(\frac{2009.29}{0.245}\right) = \textbf{113.18 Nm}$$

(f) For maximum torque, slip $s = 0.1$

Slip, $s = \left(\dfrac{n_s - n_r}{n_s}\right)$

i.e.

$$0.1 = \left(\frac{25 - n_s}{25}\right)$$

Hence $(0.1)(25) = 25 - n_r$ and
$$n_r = 25 - (0.1)(25)$$

Thus speed at which maximum torque occurs, $n_r = 25 - 2.5 = $ **22.5 rev/s** or **1350 rev/min**

(g) At the start, i.e. at standstill, slip $s = 1$. Hence,

$$\text{starting torque} = \left(\frac{m\left(\dfrac{N_2}{N_1}\right)^2}{2\pi n_s}\right)\left(\frac{E_1^2 R_2}{R_2^2 + X_2^2}\right)$$

from equation (11) with $s = 1$

$$= (0.01380)\left(\frac{(239.6)^2 0.35}{0.35^2 + 3.5^2}\right)$$

$$= (0.01380)\left(\frac{20\,092.86}{12.3725}\right)$$

i.e. **starting torque** $= $ **22.41 Nm**

(Note that the full load torque (from part (c)) is 78.05 Nm but the starting torque is only 22.41 Nm)

Problem 11.   Determine for the induction motor in Problem 10 at full load, (a) the rotor current, (b) the rotor copper loss, and (c) the starting current.

(a) From equation (8), **rotor current**,

$$I_r = \frac{s\left(\frac{N_2}{N_1}\right)E_1}{\sqrt{R_2^2 + (sX_2)^2}}$$

$$= \frac{(0.04)(0.85)(239.6)}{\sqrt{0.35^2 + (0.04 \times 3.5)^2}}$$

$$= \frac{8.1464}{0.37696} = \mathbf{21.61\,A}$$

(b) Rotor copper

$$\text{loss per phase} = I_r^2 R_2$$

$$= (21.61)^2(0.35)$$

$$= 163.45\,\text{W}$$

Total copper loss (for 3 phases)

$$= 3 \times 163.45$$

$$= \mathbf{490.35\,W}$$

(c) From equation (7), starting current,

$$I_2 = \frac{\left(\frac{N_2}{N_1}\right)E_1}{\sqrt{R_2^2 + X_2^2}} = \frac{(0.85)(239.5)}{\sqrt{0.35^2 + 3.5^2}} = \mathbf{57.90\,A}$$

(Note that the starting current of 57.90 A is considerably higher than the full load current of 21.61 A)

Problem 12. For the induction motor in Problems 10 and 11, if the stator losses are 650 W, determine (a) the power input at full load, (b) the efficiency of the motor at full load, and (c) the current taken from the supply at full load, if the motor runs at a power factor of 0.87 lagging.

(a) Output power $P_m = 11.770\,\text{kW}$ from part (d), Problem 10. Rotor copper loss $= 490.35\,\text{W} = 0.49035\,\text{kW}$ from part (b), Problem 11.
Stator input power,

$$P_1 = P_m + \text{rotor copper loss} + \text{rotor stator loss}$$

$$= 11.770 + 0.49035 + 0.650$$

$$= \mathbf{12.91\,kW}$$

(b) Net power output $= 11\,\text{kW}$ from part (d), Problem 10. Hence efficiency,

$$\eta = \frac{\text{output}}{\text{input}} \times 100\% = \left(\frac{11}{12.91}\right) \times 100\%$$

$$= \mathbf{85.21\%}$$

(c) Power input, $P_1 = \sqrt{3}\,V_L I_L \cos\phi$ (see Chapter 20) and $\cos\phi = \text{p.f.} = 0.87$ hence, **supply current**,

$$I_L = \frac{P_1}{\sqrt{3}\,V_L \cos\phi} = \frac{12.91 \times 1000}{\sqrt{3}(415)0.87} = \mathbf{20.64\,A}$$

Problem 13. For the induction motor of Problems 10 to 12, determine the resistance of the rotor winding required for maximum starting torque.

From equation (4), rotor reactance $X_r = sX_2$. At the moment of starting, slip, $s = 1$. Maximum torque occurs when rotor reactance equals rotor resistance hence for **maximum torque**,
$R_2 = X_r = sX_2 = X_2 = \mathbf{3.5\,\Omega}$.

Thus if the induction motor was a wound rotor type with slip-rings then an external star-connected resistance of $(3.5 - 0.35)\,\Omega = 3.15\,\Omega$ per phase could be added to the rotor resistance to give maximum torque at starting (see Section 23.13).

Now try the following exercise

Exercise 144   Further problems on the torque equation

1. A 400 V, three-phase, 50 Hz, 2-pole, star-connected induction motor runs at 48.5 rev/s on full load. The rotor resistance and reactance per phase are $0.4\,\Omega$ and $4.0\,\Omega$ respectively, and the effective rotor-stator turns ratio is 0.8:1. Calculate
   (a) the synchronous speed,
   (b) the slip,
   (c) the full load torque,
   (d) the power output if mechanical losses amount to 500 W,
   (e) the maximum torque,
   (f) the speed at which maximum torque occurs, and
   (g) the starting torque.
   [(a) 50 rev/s or 3000 rev/min (b) 0.03 or 3%
   (c) 22.43 Nm (d) 6.34 kW (e) 40.74 Nm
   (f) 45 rev/s or 2700 rev/min (g) 8.07 Nm]

2. For the induction motor in Problem 1, calculate at full load
    (a) the rotor current,
    (b) the rotor copper loss, and
    (c) the starting current.
                [(a) 13.27 A (b) 211.3 W (c) 45.96 A]

3. If the stator losses for the induction motor in Problem 1 are 525 W, calculate at full load
    (a) the power input,
    (b) the efficiency of the motor, and
    (c) the current taken from the supply if the motor runs at a power factor of 0.84.
                [(a) 7.57 kW (b) 83.75% (c) 13.0 A]

4. For the induction motor in Problem 1, determine the resistance of the rotor winding required for maximum starting torque.   [4.0 Ω]

23.12 Induction motor torque-speed characteristics

From Problem 10, parts (c) and (g), it is seen that the normal starting torque may be less than the full load torque. Also, from Problem 10, parts (e) and (f), it is seen that the speed at which maximum torque occurs is determined by the value of the rotor resistance. At synchronous speed, slip $s = 0$ and torque is zero. From these observations, the torque-speed and torque-slip characteristics of an induction motor are as shown in Fig. 23.9.

The rotor resistance of an induction motor is usually small compared with its reactance (for example, $R_2 = 0.35\,\Omega$ and $X_2 = 3.5\,\Omega$ in the above Problems), so that maximum torque occurs at a high speed, typically about 80 per cent of synchronous speed.

Curve P in Fig. 23.9 is a typical characteristic for an induction motor. The curve P cuts the full load torque line at point X, showing that at full load the slip is about 4–5 per cent. The normal operating conditions are between 0 and X, thus it can be seen that for normal operation the speed variation with load is quite small – the induction motor is an almost constant-speed machine. Redrawing the speed-torque characteristic between 0 and X gives the characteristic shown in Fig. 23.10, which is similar to a d.c. shunt motor as shown in Chapter 22.

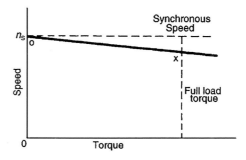

Figure 23.10

If maximum torque is required at starting then a high resistance rotor is necessary, which gives characteristic Q in Fig. 23.9. However, as can be seen, the motor has a full load slip of over 30 per cent, which results in a drop in efficiency. Also such a motor has a large

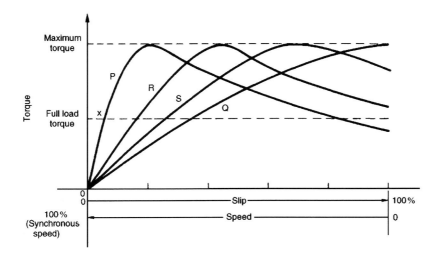

Figure 23.9

speed variation with variations of load. Curves R and S of Fig. 23.9 are characteristics for values of rotor resistances between those of P and Q. Better starting torque than for curve P is obtained, but with lower efficiency and with speed variations under operating conditions.

A **squirrel-cage induction motor** would normally follow characteristic P. This type of machine is highly efficient and about constant-speed under normal running conditions. However it has a poor starting torque and must be started off-load or very lightly loaded (see Section 23.13 below). Also, on starting, the current can be four or five times the normal full load current, due to the motor acting like a transformer with secondary short-circuited. In Problem 11, for example, the current at starting was nearly three times the full load current.

A **wound rotor induction motor** would follow characteristic P when the slip-rings are short-circuited, which is the normal running condition. However, the slip-rings allow for the addition of resistance to the rotor circuit externally and, as a result, for starting, the motor can have a characteristic similar to curve Q in Fig. 23.9 and the high starting current experienced by the cage induction motor can be overcome.

In general, for three-phase induction motors, the power factor is usually between about 0.8 and 0.9 lagging, and the full load efficiency is usually about 80–90 per cent.

From equation (12), it is seen that torque is proportional to the square of the supply voltage. Any voltage variations therefore would seriously affect the induction motor performance.

23.13 Starting methods for induction motors

Squirrel-cage rotor

(i) **Direct-on-line starting**

With this method, starting current is high and may cause interference with supplies to other consumers.

(ii) **Auto transformer starting**

With this method, an auto transformer is used to reduce the stator voltage, E_1, and thus the starting current (see equation (7)). However, the starting torque is seriously reduced (see equation (12)), so the voltage is reduced only sufficiently to give the required reduction of the starting current. A typical arrangement is shown in Fig. 23.11. A double-throw switch connects the auto transformer in circuit for starting, and when the motor is

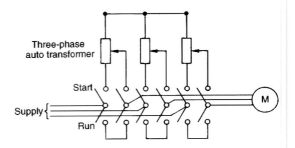

Figure 23.11

up to speed the switch is moved to the run position which connects the supply directly to the motor.

(iii) **Star-delta starting**

With this method, for starting, the connections to the stator phase winding are star-connected, so that the voltage across each phase winding is $(1/\sqrt{3})$ (i.e. 0.577) of the line voltage. For running, the windings are switched to delta-connection. A typical arrangement is shown in Fig. 23.12. This method of starting is less expensive than by auto transformer.

Wound rotor

When starting on load is necessary, a wound rotor induction motor must be used. This is because maximum torque at starting can be obtained by adding external resistance to the rotor circuit via slip-rings, (see Problem 13). A face-plate type starter is used, and as the resistance is gradually reduced, the machine characteristics at each stage will be similar to Q, S, R and P of Fig. 23.13. At each resistance step, the motor operation will transfer from one characteristic to the next so that the overall starting characteristic will be as shown by the bold line in Fig. 23.13. For very large induction motors, very gradual and smooth starting is achieved by a liquid type resistance.

23.14 Advantages of squirrel-cage induction motors

The advantages of squirrel-cage motors compared with the wound rotor type are that they:

(i) are cheaper and more robust

(ii) have slightly higher efficiency and power factor

(iii) are explosion-proof, since the risk of sparking is eliminated by the absence of slip-rings and brushes.

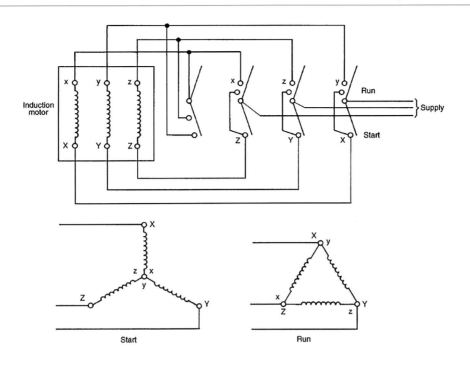

Figure 23.12

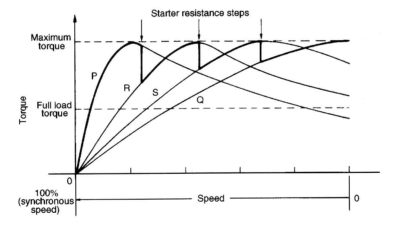

Figure 23.13

23.15 Advantages of wound rotor induction motors

The advantages of the wound rotor motor compared with the cage type are that they:

(i)   have a much higher starting torque

(ii) have a much lower starting current

(iii) have a means of varying speed by use of external rotor resistance.

23.16 Double cage induction motor

The advantages of squirrel-cage and wound rotor induction motors are combined in the double cage induction motor. This type of induction motor is specially constructed with the rotor having two cages, one inside the other. The outer cage has high resistance conductors so that maximum torque is achieved at or near starting. The inner cage has normal low resistance copper conductors but high reactance since it is embedded deep in the iron core. The torque-speed characteristic of the inner cage is that of a normal induction motor, as shown in Fig. 23.14. At starting, the outer cage produces the torque, but when running the inner cage produces the torque. The combined characteristic of inner and outer cages is shown in Fig. 23.14. The double cage induction motor is highly efficient when running.

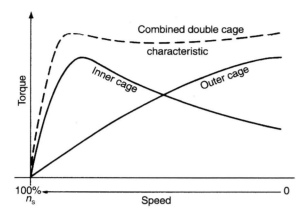

Figure 23.14

23.17 Uses of three-phase induction motors

Three-phase induction motors are widely used in industry and constitute almost all industrial drives where a nearly constant speed is required, from small workshops to the largest industrial enterprises.

Typical applications are with machine tools, pumps and mill motors. The squirrel-cage rotor type is the most widely used of all a.c. motors.

Now try the following exercises

Exercise 145   **Short answer questions on three-phase induction motors**

1. Name three advantages that a three-phase induction motor has when compared with a d.c. motor

2. Name the principal disadvantage of a three-phase induction motor when compared with a d.c. motor

3. Explain briefly, with the aid of sketches, the principle of operation of a 3-phase induction motor

4. Explain briefly how slip-frequency currents are set up in the rotor bars of a 3-phase induction motor and why this frequency varies with load

5. Explain briefly why a 3-phase induction motor develops no torque when running at synchronous speed. Define the slip of an induction motor and explain why its value depends on the load on the rotor

6. Write down the two properties of the magnetic field produced by the stator of a three-phase induction motor

7. The speed at which the magnetic field of a three-phase induction motor rotates is called the ...... speed

8. The synchronous speed of a three-phase induction motor is ...... proportional to supply frequency

9. The synchronous speed of a three-phase induction motor is ...... proportional to the number of pairs of poles

10. The type of rotor most widely used in a three-phase induction motor is called a ......

11. The slip of a three-phase induction motor is given by: $s = \dfrac{......}{...} \times 100\%$

12. A typical value for the slip of a small three-phase induction motor is ... %

13. As the load on the rotor of a three-phase induction motor increases, the slip ......

14. $\dfrac{\text{Rotor copper loss}}{\text{Rotor input power}} = ...$

15. State the losses in an induction motor

16. Maximum torque occurs when ...... = ...

17. Sketch a typical speed-torque characteristic for an induction motor

18. State two methods of starting squirrel-cage induction motors

19. Which type of induction motor is used when starting on-load is necessary?

20. Describe briefly a double cage induction motor

21. State two advantages of cage rotor machines compared with wound rotor machines

22. State two advantages of wound rotor machines compared with cage rotor machines

23. Name any three applications of three-phase induction motors

Exercise 146   Multi-choice questions on three-phase induction motors

(Answers on page 421)

1. Which of the following statements about a three-phase squirrel-cage induction motor is false?
   (a) It has no external electrical connections to its rotor
   (b) *A* three-phase supply is connected to its stator
   (c) *A* magnetic flux which alternates is produced
   (d) It is cheap, robust and requires little or no skilled maintenance

2. Which of the following statements about a three-phase induction motor is false?
   (a) The speed of rotation of the magnetic field is called the synchronous speed
   (b) A three-phase supply connected to the rotor produces a rotating magnetic field
   (c) The rotating magnetic field has a constant speed and constant magnitude
   (d) It is essentially a constant speed type machine

3. Which of the following statements is false when referring to a three-phase induction motor?
   (a) The synchronous speed is half the supply frequency when it has four poles
   (b) In a 2-pole machine, the synchronous speed is equal to the supply frequency
   (c) If the number of poles is increased, the synchronous speed is reduced
   (d) The synchronous speed is inversely proportional to the number of poles

4. A 4-pole three-phase induction motor has a synchronous speed of 25 rev/s. The frequency of the supply to the stator is:
   (a) 50 Hz   (b) 100 Hz
   (c) 25 Hz   (d) 12.5 Hz

Questions 5 and 6 refer to a three-phase induction motor. Which statements are false?

5. (a) The slip speed is the synchronous speed minus the rotor speed
   (b) As the rotor is loaded, the slip decreases
   (c) The frequency of induced rotor e.m.f.'s increases with load on the rotor
   (d) The torque on the rotor is due to the interaction of magnetic fields

6. (a) If the rotor is running at synchronous speed, there is no torque on the rotor
   (b) If the number of poles on the stator is doubled, the synchronous speed is halved
   (c) At no-load, the rotor speed is very nearly equal to the synchronous speed
   (d) The direction of rotation of the rotor is opposite to the direction of rotation of the magnetic field to give maximum current induced in the rotor bars

A three-phase, 4-pole, 50 Hz induction motor runs at 1440 rev/min. In questions 7 to 10, determine the correct answers for the quantities stated, selecting your answer from the list given below:
   (a) 12.5 rev/s   (b) 25 rev/s   (c) 1 rev/s
   (d) 50 rev/s   (e) 1%   (f) 4%
   (g) 50%   (h) 4 Hz   (i) 50 Hz
   (j) 2 Hz

7. The synchronous speed

8. The slip speed

9. The percentage slip

10. The frequency of induced e.m.f.'s in the rotor

11. The slip speed of an induction motor may be defined as the:
   (a) number of pairs of poles ÷ frequency
   (b) rotor speed − synchronous speed
   (c) rotor speed + synchronous speed
   (d) synchronous speed − rotor speed

12. The slip speed of an induction motor depends upon:
    (a) armature current (b) supply voltage
    (c) mechanical load (d) eddy currents

13. The starting torque of a simple squirrel-cage motor is:
    (a) low
    (b) increases as rotor current rises
    (c) decreases as rotor current rises
    (d) high

14. The slip speed of an induction motor:
    (a) is zero until the rotor moves and then rises slightly
    (b) is 100 per cent until the rotor moves and then decreases slightly
    (c) is 100 per cent until the rotor moves and then falls to a low value
    (d) is zero until the rotor moves and then rises to 100 per cent

15. A four-pole induction motor when supplied from a 50 Hz supply experiences a 5 per cent slip. The rotor speed will be:
    (a) 25 rev/s   (b) 23.75 rev/s
    (c) 26.25 rev/s   (d) 11.875 rev/s

16. A stator winding of an induction motor supplied from a three-phase, 60 Hz system is required to produce a magnetic flux rotating at 900 rev/min. The number of poles is:
    (a) 2   (b) 8
    (c) 6   (d) 4

17. The stator of a three-phase, 2-pole induction motor is connected to a 50 Hz supply. The rotor runs at 2880 rev/min at full load. The slip is:
    (a) 4.17%   (b) 92%
    (c) 4%   (d) 96%

18. An 8-pole induction motor, when fed from a 60 Hz supply, experiences a 5 per cent slip. The rotor speed is:
    (a) 427.5 rev/min   (b) 855 rev/min
    (c) 900 rev/min   (d) 945 rev/min

This revision test covers the material contained in Chapters 22 and 23. *The marks for each question are shown in brackets at the end of each question.*

1. A 6-pole armature has 1000 conductors and a flux per pole of 40 mWb. Determine the e.m.f. generated when running at 600 rev/min when (a) lap wound (b) wave wound. (6)

2. The armature of a d.c. machine has a resistance of 0.3 Ω and is connected to a 200 V supply. Calculate the e.m.f. generated when it is running (a) as a generator giving 80 A (b) as a motor taking 80 A. (4)

3. A 15 kW shunt generator having an armature circuit resistance of 1 Ω and a field resistance of 160 Ω generates a terminal voltage of 240 V at full load. Determine the efficiency of the generator at full load assuming the iron, friction and windage losses amount to 544 W. (6)

4. A 4-pole d.c. motor has a wave-wound armature with 1000 conductors. The useful flux per pole is 40 mWb. Calculate the torque exerted when a current of 25 A flows in each armature conductor. (4)

5. A 400 V shunt motor runs at its normal speed of 20 rev/s when the armature current is 100 A. The armature resistance is 0.25 Ω. Calculate the speed, in rev/min when the current is 50 A and a resistance of 0.40 Ω is connected in series with the armature, the shunt field remaining constant. (7)

6. The stator of a three-phase, 6-pole induction motor is connected to a 60 Hz supply. The rotor runs at 1155 rev/min at full load. Determine (a) the synchronous speed, and (b) the slip at full load. (6)

7. The power supplied to a three-phase induction motor is 40 kW and the stator losses are 2 kW. If the slip is 4 per cent determine (a) the rotor copper loss, (b) the total mechanical power developed by the rotor, (c) the output power of the motor if frictional and windage losses are 1.48 kW, and (d) the efficiency of the motor, neglecting rotor iron loss. (9)

8. A 400 V, three-phase, 100 Hz, 8-pole induction motor runs at 24.25 rev/s on full load. The rotor resistance and reactance per phase are 0.2 Ω and 2 Ω respectively and the effective rotor-stator turns ratio is 0.80:1. Calculate (a) the synchronous speed, (b) the slip, and (c) the full load torque. (8)

Three-phase systems:

Star $I_L = I_p$ $V_L = \sqrt{3} V_p$

Delta $V_L = V_p$ $I_L = \sqrt{3} I_p$

$P = \sqrt{3} V_L I_L \cos\phi$ or $P = 3 I_p^2 R_p$

Two-wattmeter method

$P = P_1 + P_2$ $\tan\phi = \sqrt{3} \dfrac{(P_1 - P_2)}{(P_1 + P_2)}$

Transformers:

$\dfrac{V_1}{V_2} = \dfrac{N_1}{N_2} = \dfrac{I_2}{I_1}$ $I_0 = \sqrt{(I_M^2 + I_C^2)}$

$I_M = I_0 \sin\phi_0$ $I_c = I_0 \cos\phi_0$

$E = 4.44 f \Phi_m N$

$\text{Regulation} = \left(\dfrac{E_2 - E_1}{E_2}\right) \times 100\%$

Equivalent circuit: $R_e = R_1 + R_2 \left(\dfrac{V_1}{V_2}\right)^2$

$X_e = X_1 + X_2 \left(\dfrac{V_1}{V_2}\right)^2$ $Z_e = \sqrt{(R_e^2 + X_e^2)}$

Efficiency, $\eta = 1 - \dfrac{\text{losses}}{\text{input power}}$

Output power $= V_2 I_2 \cos\phi_2$

Total loss $=$ copper loss $+$ iron loss

Input power $=$ output power $+$ losses

Resistance matching: $R_1 = \left(\dfrac{N_1}{N_2}\right)^2 R_L$

D.C. Machines:

Generated e.m.f. $E = \dfrac{2p\Phi n Z}{c} \propto \Phi\omega$

($c = 2$ for wave winding, $c = 2p$ for lap winding)

Generator: $E = V + I_a R_a$

Efficiency, $\eta = \left(\dfrac{VI}{VI + I_a^2 R_a + I_f V + C}\right) \times 100\%$

Motor: $E = V - I_a R_a$

Efficiency, $\eta = \left(\dfrac{VI - I_a^2 R_a - I_f V - C}{VI}\right) \times 100\%$

$\text{Torque} = \dfrac{E I_a}{2\pi n} = \dfrac{p\Phi Z I_a}{\pi c} \propto I_a \Phi$

Three-phase induction motors:

$n_S = \dfrac{f}{p}$ $s = \left(\dfrac{n_s - n_r}{n_s}\right) \times 100$

$f_r = sf$ $X_r = s X_2$

$I_r = \dfrac{E_r}{Z_r} = \dfrac{s\left(\dfrac{N_2}{N_1}\right) E_1}{\sqrt{[R_2^2 + (s X_2)^2]}}$ $s = \dfrac{I_r^2 R_2}{P_2}$

Efficiency,

$\eta = \dfrac{P_m}{P_1} = \dfrac{\text{input} - \text{stator loss} - \text{rotor copper loss} - \text{friction \& windage loss}}{\text{input power}}$

Torque,

$T = \left(\dfrac{m\left(\dfrac{N_2}{N_1}\right)^2}{2\pi n_s}\right)\left(\dfrac{s E_1^2 R_2}{R_2^2 + (s X_2)^2}\right) \propto \dfrac{s E_1^2 R_2}{R_2^2 + (s X_2)^2}$

Section 4

Laboratory Experiments

Chapter 24

Some practical laboratory experiments

This chapter contains 10 straightforward practical laboratory experiments to help supplement and enhance academic studies. Copies of these exercises have been made available on line at http://www.booksite.elsevier.com/newnes/bird and may be edited by tutors to suit availability of equipment and components.

The list of experiments is not exhaustive, but covers some of the more important aspects of early electrical engineering studies.

Experiments covered are:

- **Ohm's law** (see Chapter 2)
- **Series-parallel d.c. circuit** (see Chapter 5)
- **Superposition theorem** (see Chapter 13)
- **Thévenin's theorem** (see Chapter 13)
- **Use of CRO to measure voltage, frequency and phase** (see Chapter 14)
- **Use of CRO with a bridge rectifier circuit** (see Chapter 14)
- **Measurement of the inductance of a coil** (see Chapter 15)
- **Series a.c. circuit and resonance** (see Chapter 15)
- **Parallel a.c. circuit and resonance** (see Chapter 16)
- **Charging and discharging a capacitor** (see Chapter 18)

DOI: 10.1016/B978-0-08-089056-2.00024-3

24.1 Ohm's law

Objectives:

1. To determine the voltage-current relationship in a d.c. circuit and relate it to Ohm's law.

Equipment required:

1. D.C. Power Supply Unit (PSU).

2. Constructor board (for example, 'Feedback' EEC470).

3. An ammeter and voltmeter or two Flukes (for example, 89).

4. LCR Data bridge.

Procedure:

1. Construct the circuit shown below with $R = 470\,\Omega$.

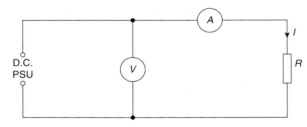

2. Check the colour coding of the resistor and then measure its value accurately using an LCR data bridge or a Fluke.

3. Initially set the d.c. power supply unit to 1 V.

4. Measure the value of the current in the circuit and record the reading in the table below.

5. Increase the value of voltage in 1 V increments, measuring the current for each value. Complete the table of values below.

Resistance $R = 470\,\Omega$
[colour code is]:

Voltage V (V)	1	2	3	4	5	6	7	8
Current I (mA)								

6. Repeat procedures 1 to 5 for a resistance value of $R = 2.2\,\text{k}\Omega$ and complete the table below.

Resistance $R = 2.2\,\text{k}\Omega$
[colour code is]:

Voltage V (V)	1	2	3	4	5	6	7	8
Current I (mA)								

7. Repeat procedures 1 to 5 for a resistance value of $R = 10\,\text{k}\Omega$ and complete the table below.

Resistance $R = 10\,\text{k}\Omega$
[colour code is]:

Voltage V (V)	1	2	3	4	5	6	7	8
Current I (mA)								

8. Plot graphs of V (vertically) against I (horizontally) for $R = 470\,\Omega$, $R = 2.2\,\text{k}\Omega$ and $R = 10\,\text{k}\Omega$ respectively.

Conclusions:

1. What is the nature of the graphs plotted?

2. If the graphs plotted are straight lines, determine their gradients. Can you draw any conclusions from the gradient values?

3. State Ohm's law. Has this experiment proved Ohm's law to be true?

24.2 Series-parallel d.c. circuit

Objectives:

1. To compare calculated with measured values of voltages and currents in a series-parallel d.c. circuit.

Equipment required:

1. D.C. Power Supply Unit (PSU).

2. Constructor board (for example, 'Feedback' EEC470).

3. An ammeter and voltmeter or a Fluke (for example, 89).

4. LCR Data bridge.

Procedure:

1. Construct the circuit as shown below.

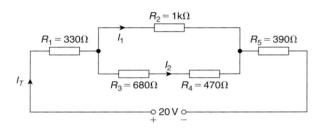

2. State the colour code for each of the five resistors in the above circuit and record them in the table below.

3. Using a Fluke or LCR bridge, measure accurately the value of each resistor and note their values in the table below.

Resistor	R_1	R_2	R_3	R_4	R_5
Colour code					
Exact value					

4. Calculate, using the exact values of resistors, the voltage drops and currents and record them in the table below.

Quantity	Calculated value	Measured value
V_{R_1}		
V_{R_2}		
V_{R_3}		
V_{R_4}		
V_{R_5}		
I_T		
I_1		
I_2		

5. With an ammeter, a voltmeter or a Fluke, measure the voltage drops and currents and record them in the above table.

Conclusions:

1. Compare the calculated and measured values of voltages and currents and comment on any discrepancies.

2. Calculate the total circuit power and the power dissipated in each resistor.

3. If the circuit was connected for 2 weeks, calculate the energy used.

24.3   Superposition theorem

Objectives:

1. To measure and calculate the current in each branch of a series-parallel circuit.

2. To verify the superposition theorem.

Equipment required:

1. Constructor board (for example, 'Feedback' EEC470).

2. D.C. Power Supply Units.

3. Digital Multimeter, such as a Fluke (for example, 89).

4. LCR Data bridge.

Procedure:

1. Construct the circuit as shown below, measuring and noting in the table below the exact values of the resistors using a Fluke or LCR bridge.

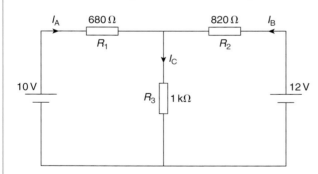

2. **Measure** the values of I_A, I_B and I_C and record the values in the table below.

$R_1\,(\Omega)$	$R_2\,(\Omega)$	$R_3\,(\Omega)$

I_A (mA)	I_B (mA)	I_C (mA)

3. Remove the 12 V source from the above circuit and replace with a link, giving the circuit shown on the next column.

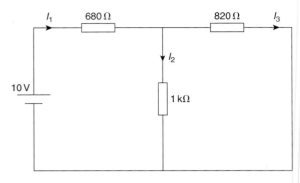

4. **Measure** the values of I_1, I_2 and I_3 and record the values in the table below.

Measured I_1 (mA)	Measured I_2 (mA)	Measured I_3 (mA)

Calculated I_1 (mA)	Calculated I_2 (mA)	Calculated I_3 (mA)

5. **Calculate** the values of I_1, I_2 and I_3 and record the values in the above table.

6. Replace the 12 V source in the original circuit and then replace the 10 V source with a link, giving the circuit shown below.

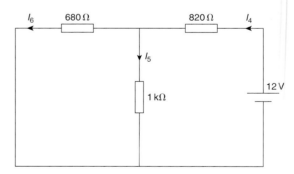

7. **Measure** the values of I_4, I_5 and I_6 and record the values in the table below.

Measured I_4 (mA)	Measured I_5 (mA)	Measured I_6 (mA)

Calculated I_4 (mA)	Calculated I_5 (mA)	Calculated I_6 (mA)

8. **Calculate** the values of I_4, I_5 and I_6 and record the values in the above table.

9. By superimposing the latter two diagrams on top of each other, calculate the algebraic sum of the currents in each branch and record them in the table below.

Measured $I_A = I_1 - I_6$	Measured $I_B = I_4 - I_3$	Measured $I_C = I_2 + I_5$

Calculated $I_A = I_1 - I_6$	Calculated $I_B = I_4 - I_3$	Calculated $I_B = I_2 + I_5$

Conclusions:

1. State in your own words the superposition theorem.

2. Compare the measured and calculated values of I_A, I_B and I_C in procedure 9 and comment on any discrepancies.

3. Compare these values of I_A, I_B and I_C with those measured in procedure 2 and comment on any discrepancies.

4. Can the principle of superposition be applied in a circuit having more than two sources?

24.4 Thévenin's theorem

Objectives:

1. To calculate Thévenin's equivalent of a given circuit.

2. To verify Thévenin's theorem.

Equipment required:

1. Constructor board (for example, 'Feedback' EEC470).

2. D.C. Power Supply Units.

3. Digital Multimeter, such as a Fluke (for example, 89).

4. LCR Data bridge.

Procedure:

1. Construct the circuit as shown below, measuring and noting in the table below the exact values of the resistors using a Fluke or LCR bridge.

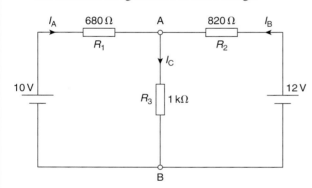

2. **Measure** the values of I_A, I_B and I_C and record the values in the table below.

$R_1(\Omega)$	$R_2(\Omega)$	$R_3(\Omega)$

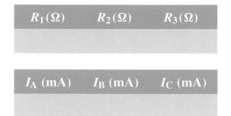

I_A (mA)	I_B (mA)	I_C (mA)

3. Remove the $1\,k\Omega$ resistor from the above circuit and **measure** the open-circuit voltage V_{OC} at the terminals AB. Record the value in the table in the next column.

4. With the $1\,k\Omega$ resistor still removed, remove the two voltage sources replacing each with a link.

Now **measure** the resistance r_{OC} across the open circuited terminals AB and record the value in the table below.

Measured V_{OC} (V)	Measured r_{OC} (Ω)	Calculated V_{OC} (V)	Calculated r_{OC} (Ω)

5. **Calculate** values of V_{OC} and r_{OC} and record the values in the above table.

6. Compare the measured and calculated values of V_{OC} and r_{OC}.

7. Using the calculated values of V_{OC} and r_{OC} calculate and record the current I_C from the circuit below.

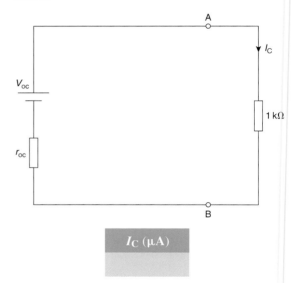

I_C (μA)

8. Compare this value of I_C with that initially measured in the original circuit (i.e. procedure 2).

9. Calculate the voltage V shown in the circuit below, using your calculated value of I_C, and record the value in the table below.

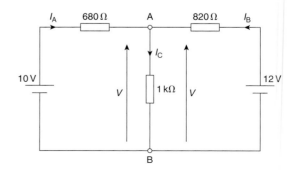

10. The terminal voltage of a source, $V = E - I \times r$. Using this, calculate and record the values of I_A and I_B, i.e. transpose the equations:
$V = 10 - I_A \times 680$ and $V = 12 - I_B \times 820$.

V (V)	I_A (mA)	I_B(mA)

11. Compare these values of I_A and I_B with those initially measured in the original circuit (i.e. procedure 2).

Conclusions:

1. State in your own words Thévenin's theorem.

2. Compare the measured and calculated values of I_A, I_B and I_C and comment on any discrepancies.

3. Can Thévenin's theorem be applied in a circuit having more than two sources?

4. If the $1\,\mathrm{k}\Omega$ resistor is replaced with (a) $470\,\Omega$ (b) $2.2\,\mathrm{k}\Omega$, calculate the current flowing between the terminals A and B.

24.5 Use of a CRO to measure voltage, frequency and phase

Objectives:

1. To measure a d.c. voltage using an oscilloscope.
2. To measure the peak-to-peak voltage of a waveform and then calculate its r.m.s. value.
3. To measure the periodic time of a waveform and then calculate its frequency.
4. To measure the phase angle between two wave-forms.

Equipment required:

1. Cathode ray oscilloscope (for example, 'Phillips' digital Fluke PM3082).
2. Constructor board (for example, 'Feedback' EEC470).
3. Function Generator ('Escort' EFG 3210).
4. D.C. Power Supply Unit.
5. Fluke (for example, 89).

Procedure:

1. Switch on the oscilloscope and place the trace at the bottom of the screen.
2. Set the d.c. power supply unit to 20 V, making sure the output switch is in the off position.
3. Connect a test lead from channel 1 of the CRO to the d.c. PSU.
4. Switch on the output of the d.c. PSU.
5. Measure the d.c. voltage output on the CRO.

d.c voltage

6. Connect up the circuit as shown below.

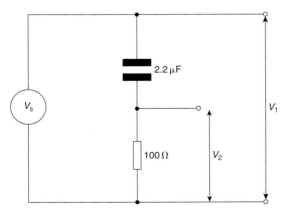

7. Set the function generator to output a voltage of 5 V at 500 Hz.

8. Measure the peak-to-peak voltages at V_1 and V_2 using the CRO and record in the table below.
9. Calculate the r.m.s. values corresponding to V_1 and V_2 and record in the table below.
10. Measure the voltages V_1 and V_2 using a Fluke.
11. Measure the periodic time of the waveforms obtained at V_1 and V_2 and record in the table below.
12. Calculate the frequency of the two waveforms and record in the table below.

Voltage	Peak-to-peak voltage	r.m.s. value
V_1		
V_2		

Voltage	Periodic time	Frequency
V_1		
V_2		

13. Measure the phase angle ϕ between the two waveforms using:

$$\phi = \frac{\text{displacement between waveforms}}{\text{periodic time}} \times 360°$$

$$= \frac{t}{T} \times 360°$$

(For example, if $t = 0.6\,\text{ms}$ and $T = 4\,\text{ms}$, then $\phi = \frac{0.6}{4} \times 360° = \mathbf{54°}$)

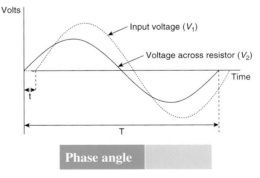

Phase angle

Conclusions:

1. Is a measurement of voltage or current with a Fluke an r.m.s. value or a peak value?
2. Write expressions for the instantaneous values of voltages V_1 and V_2 (i.e. in the form $V = A\sin(\omega t \pm \phi)$ where ϕ is in radians).

24.6 Use of a CRO with a bridge rectifier

Objectives:

1. To measure and observe the input and output waveforms of a bridge rectifier circuit using a CRO.

2. To investigate smoothing of the output waveform.

Equipment required:

1. Cathode Ray Oscilloscope (for example, 'Phillips' digital Fluke PM3082).

2. Constructor board (for example, 'Feedback' EEC470).

3. Transformer (for example, IET 464).

4. Bridge rectifier.

5. Fluke (for example, 89).

Procedure:

1. Construct the circuit shown below with a mains transformer stepping down to a voltage V_1 between 15 V and 20 V.

2. Measure the output voltage V_1 of the transformer using a Fluke and a CRO, noting the value in the table below. Sketch the waveform.

3. Measure the output voltage V_2 of the bridge rectifier using a Fluke and observe the waveform using a CRO, noting the value in the table below. Sketch the waveform.

4. Place a 100 μF capacitor across the terminals AB and observe the waveform across these terminals using a CRO. Measure the voltage across terminals AB, V_3, noting the value in the table below. Sketch the waveform.

5. Place a second 100 μF capacitor in parallel with the first across the terminals AB. What is the effect on the waveform? Measure the voltage across terminals AB, V_4, noting the value in the table below. Sketch the waveform.

V_1 r.m.s.	V_2 d.c.	V_3 d.c.	V_4 d.c.

Conclusions:

1. What is the effect of placing a capacitor across the full-wave rectifier output?

2. What is the total capacitance of two 100 μF capacitors connected in parallel?

3. What is meant by ripple? Comment on the ripple when (a) one capacitor is connected, (b) both capacitors are connected.

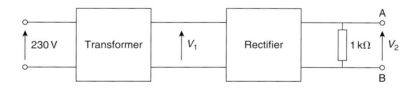

24.7   Measurement of the inductance of a coil

Objectives:

1. To measure the inductance of a coil.

Equipment required:

1. Constructor board (for example, 'Feedback' EEC470).

2. D.C. Power Supply Unit.

3. Function Generator (for example, 'Escort' EFG 3210).

4. Unknown inductor.

5. Digital Multimeter, such as a Fluke (for example, 89).

6. LCR Data bridge.

Procedure:

1. Construct the circuit, with the inductance of unknown value, as shown below.

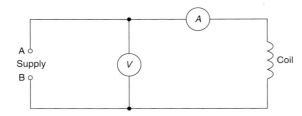

2. Connect a d.c. power supply unit set at 1 V to the terminals AB.

3. Measure the voltage V and current I in the above circuit.

4. Calculate the resistance R of the coil, using $R = \dfrac{V}{I}$ recording the value in the table below.

5. Remove the d.c. PSU and connect an a.c. function generator set at 1 V, 50 Hz to the terminals AB.

6. Measure the voltage V and current I in the above circuit.

7. Calculate the impedance Z of the coil, using $Z = \dfrac{V}{I}$, recording the value in the table below.

8. From the impedance triangle, $Z^2 = R^2 + X_L^2$, from which, $X_L = \sqrt{Z^2 - R^2}$. Calculate X_L and record the value in the table below.

$R\,(\Omega)$	$Z\,(\Omega)$	$X_L = \sqrt{Z^2 - R^2}\,(\Omega)$	$L = \frac{X_L}{2\pi f}\,(\text{H})$

9. Since $X_{\mathrm{L}} = 2\pi f L$ then $L = \dfrac{X_L}{2\pi f}$; calculate inductance L and record the value in the table above.

10. Hence, **for the coil, $L = \ldots$ H** and **resistance, $R = \ldots\ \Omega$.**

11. Measure the inductance of the coil using an LCR data bridge.

12. Using an ammeter, a voltmeter or a Fluke, measure the resistance of the coil.

Conclusions:

1. Compare the measured values of procedures 11 and 12 with those stated in procedure 10 and comment on any discrepancies.

24.8   Series a.c. circuit and resonance

Objectives:

1. To measure and record current and voltages in an a.c. series circuit at varying frequencies.

2. To investigate the relationship between voltage and current at resonance.

3. To investigate the value of current and impedance at resonance.

4. To compare measured values with theoretical calculations.

Equipment required:

1. Cathode Ray Oscilloscope (for example, 'Phillips' digital Fluke PM3082).

2. Constructor board (for example, 'Feedback' EEC470).

3. Function Generator (for example, 'Escort' EFG 3210).

4. Digital Multimeter, such as a Fluke (for example, 89).

5. LCR Data bridge.

Procedure:

1. Construct the series RCL circuit as shown below, measuring and noting the exact values of R, C and L.

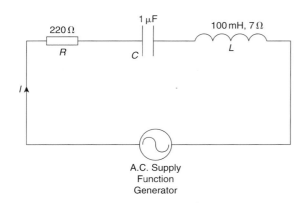

2. Set the a.c. supply (function generator) to 2 V at 100 Hz.

3. Measure the magnitude of the current in the circuit using an ammeter or Fluke and record it in the table on the next column.

4. Measure the magnitudes of V_R, V_C and V_L and record them in the table in the next column.

5. Calculate the values of X_L and X_C and record them in the table below.

6. Using the values of circuit resistance (which is $R+$ resistance of coil), X_L and X_C, calculate impedance Z.

7. Calculate current I using $I = \dfrac{V}{Z}$

8. Repeat the procedures 2 to 7 using frequencies of 200 Hz up to 800 Hz and record the results in the table below. Ensure that the voltage is kept constant at 2 V for each frequency.

Supply voltage V	Measured I (mA)	Measured V_R (V)	Measured V_C (V)	Measured V_L (V)
2V, 100 Hz				
2V, 200 Hz				
2V, 300 Hz				
2V, 400 Hz				
2V, 500 Hz				
2V, 600 Hz				
2V, 700 Hz				
2V, 800 Hz				

Supply voltage V	Calculate X_L (Ω)	Calculate X_C (Ω)	Calculate Z (Ω)	Calculate $I = \dfrac{V}{Z}$ (mA)
2V, 100 Hz				
2V, 200 Hz				
2V, 300 Hz				
2V, 400 Hz				
2V, 500 Hz				
2V, 600 Hz				
2V, 700 Hz				
2V, 800 Hz				

9. Plot a graph of measured current I (vertically) against frequency (horizontally).

10. Plot on the same axes a graph of impedance Z (vertically) against frequency (horizontally).

11. Determine from the graphs the resonant frequency f_r.

12. State the formula for the resonant frequency of a series LCR circuit. Use this formula to calculate the resonant frequency f_r.

13. Set the supply voltage to 2 V at the resonant frequency and measure the current I and voltages V_R, V_C and V_L.

14. Connect a cathode ray oscilloscope such that channel 1 is across the whole circuit and channel 2 is across the inductor.

15. Adjust the oscilloscope to obtain both waveforms.

16. Adjust the function generator from 2 V, 100 Hz up to 2 V, 800 Hz. Check at what frequency the voltage across L (i.e. channel 2) is a maximum. Note any change of phase either side of this frequency.

Conclusions:

1. Compare measured values of current with the theoretical calculated values and comment on any discrepancies.

2. Comment on the values of current I and impedance Z at resonance.

3. Comment on the values of V_R, V_C and V_L at resonance.

4. What is the phase angle between the supply current and voltage at resonance?

5. Sketch the phasor diagrams for frequencies of (a) 300 Hz (b) f_r (c) 700 Hz.

6. Define resonance.

7. Calculate the values of Q-factor and bandwidth for the above circuit.

24.9 Parallel a.c. circuit and resonance

Objectives:

1. To measure and record currents in an a.c. parallel circuit at varying frequencies.
2. To investigate the relationship between voltage and current at resonance.
3. To calculate the circuit impedance over a range of frequencies.
4. To investigate the value of current and impedance at resonance and plot their graphs over a range of frequencies.
5. To compare measured values with theoretical calculations.

Equipment required:

1. Constructor board (for example, 'Feedback' EEC470).
2. Function Generator (for example, 'Escort' EFG 3210).
3. Digital Multimeter, such as a Fluke (for example, 89).
4. LCR Data bridge.

Procedure:

1. Construct the parallel LR–C circuit as shown below, measuring and noting the exact values of R, C and L.

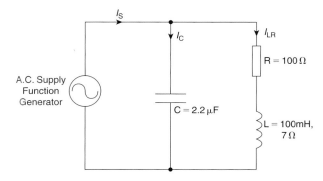

2. Set the function generator to 3 V, 100 Hz using a Fluke.

3. **Measure** the magnitude of the supply current, I_S, capacitor current, I_C, and inductor branch current, I_{LR} and record the results in the table on the next column.

4. Adjust the function generator to the other frequencies listed in the table ensuring that the voltage remains at 3 V. Record the values of the three currents for each value of frequency in the table below.

Supply Voltage V	Measured I_S (mA)	Measured I_C (mA)	Measured I_{LR} (mA)	Calculate $I_C = \dfrac{V}{-JX_C}$
3V, 100 Hz				
3V, 150 Hz				
3V, 200 Hz				
3V, 220 Hz				
3V, 240 Hz				
3V, 260 Hz				
3V, 280 Hz				
3V, 300 Hz				
3V, 320 Hz				
3V, 340 Hz				
3V, 360 Hz				
3V, 380 Hz				
3V, 400 Hz				
3V, 450 Hz				

Supply Voltage V	Calculate $I_{LR} = \dfrac{V}{R+JX_{LR}}$	Calculate $I_S = I_C + I_{LR}$	Calculate $Z = \dfrac{V}{I_S}$
3V, 100 Hz			
3V, 150 Hz			
3V, 200 Hz			
3V, 220 Hz			
3V, 240 Hz			
3V, 260 Hz			
3V, 280 Hz			
3V, 300 Hz			
3V, 320 Hz			
3V, 340 Hz			
3V, 360 Hz			
3V, 380 Hz			
3V, 400 Hz			
3V, 450 Hz			

5. **Calculate** the magnitude and phase of I_C, I_{LR} and $I_S (= I_C + I_{LR})$ for each frequency and record the values in the table on the previous page.

6. **Calculate** the magnitude and phase of the circuit impedance for each frequency and record the values in the table on the previous page.

7. Plot a graph of the magnitudes of I_S, I_C, I_{LR} and Z (vertically) against frequency (horizontally), all on the same axes.

8. Determine from the graphs the resonant frequency.

9. State the formula and calculate the resonant frequency for the LR–C parallel circuit.

Conclusions:

1. Compare measured values of the supply current I_S with the theoretical calculated values and comment on any discrepancies.

2. Comment on the values of current I and impedance Z at resonance.

3. Compare the value of resonance obtained from the graphs to that calculated and comment on any discrepancy.

4. Compare the graphs of supply current and impedance against frequency with those for series resonance.

5. Calculate the value of dynamic resistance, R_D and compare with the value obtained from the graph.

6. What is the phase angle between the supply current and voltage at resonance?

7. Sketch the phasor diagrams for frequencies of (a) 200 Hz (b) f_r (c) 400 Hz.

8. Define resonance.

9. Calculate the values of Q-factor and bandwidth for the above circuit.

24.10 Charging and discharging a capacitor

Objectives:

1. To charge a capacitor and measure at intervals the current through and voltage across it.

2. To discharge a capacitor and measure at intervals the current through and voltage across it.

3. To plot graphs of voltage against time for both charging and discharging cycles.

4. To plot graphs of current against time for both charging and discharging cycles.

Equipment required:

1. Constructor board (for example, 'Feedback' EEC470).

2. D.c. Power Supply Unit.

3. Digital Multimeter, such as a Fluke (for example, 89).

4. LCR Data bridge.

5. Stop watch.

Procedure:

1. Construct the series CR circuit as shown below, measuring the exact values of C and R.

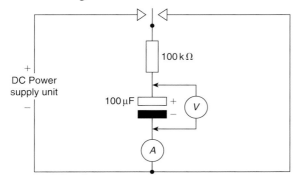

2. Set the D.C. Power Supply Unit to 10 V, making sure the output switch is in the off position.

3. Charge the capacitor, measuring the capacitor voltage (in volts) at 5 second intervals over a period of 60 seconds. Record results in the table on the next column.

4. Discharge the capacitor, measuring the capacitor voltage at 5 second intervals over a period of 60 seconds. Record results in the table on the next column.

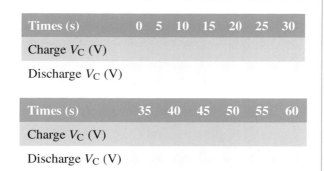

Times (s)	0	5	10	15	20	25	30
Charge V_C (V)							
Discharge V_C (V)							

Times (s)	35	40	45	50	55	60
Charge V_C (V)						
Discharge V_C (V)						

5. Again, charge the capacitor, this time measuring the current (in μA) at 5 second intervals over a period of 60 seconds. Record results in the table below.

6. Discharge the capacitor, measuring the current at 5 second intervals over a period of 60 seconds. Record results in the table below.

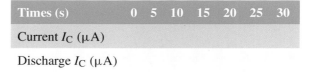

Times (s)	0	5	10	15	20	25	30
Current I_C (μA)							
Discharge I_C (μA)							

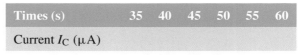

Times (s)	35	40	45	50	55	60
Current I_C (μA)						
Discharge I_C (μA)						

7. Plot graphs of V_C against time for both charge and discharge cycles.

8. Plot graphs of I_C against time for both charge and discharge cycles.

9. Calculate the time constant of the circuit (using the measured values of C and R).

10. Take a sample of the times and calculate values of V_C and I_C using the appropriate exponential formulae $V_C = V(1 - e^{-t/CR})$, $V_C = Ve^{-t/CR}$ and $I_C = Ie^{-t/CR}$.

Conclusions:

1. Compare theoretical and measured values of voltages and currents for the capacitor charging and discharging.

2. Discuss the charging and discharging characteristics of the capacitor.

3. Comment on reasons for any errors encountered.

4. What is the circuit time constant? What does this mean? Approximately, how long does the voltage and current take to reach their final values?

Answers to multiple-choice questions

Chapter 1. Exercise 4 (page 7)

1 (c)	4 (a)	7 (b)	9 (d)	11 (b)
2 (d)	5 (c)	8 (c)	10 (a)	12 (d)
3 (c)	6 (b)			

Chapter 2. Exercise 10 (page 19)

1 (b)	4 (b)	7 (b)	10 (c)	12 (d)
2 (b)	5 (d)	8 (c)	11 (c)	13 (a)
3 (c)	6 (d)	9 (b)		

Chapter 3. Exercise 15 (page 28)

1 (c)	3 (b)	5 (d)	7 (b)	9 (d)
2 (d)	4 (d)	6 (c)	8 (c)	

Chapter 4. Exercise 18 (page 40)

1 (d)	4 (c)	7 (d)	10 (d)	12 (a)
2 (a)	5 (b)	8 (b)	11 (c)	13 (c)
3 (b)	6 (d)	9 (c)		

Chapter 5. Exercise 25 (page 59)

1 (a)	4 (c)	7 (b)	9 (b)	11 (d)
2 (a)	5 (c)	8 (d)	10 (c)	12 (d)
3 (c)	6 (a)			

Chapter 6. Exercise 32 (page 76)

1 (b)	4 (c)	6 (b)	8 (a)	10 (c)
2 (a)	5 (a)	7 (b)	9 (c)	11 (d)
3 (b)				

Chapter 7. Exercise 38 (page 88)

1 (d)	5 (c)	8 (c)	11 (a) and (d),	12 (a)
2 (b)	6 (d)	9 (c)	(b) and (f),	13 (a)
3 (b)	7 (a)	10 (c)	(c) and (e)	
4 (c)				

Chapter 8. Exercise 42 (page 100)

1 (d)	3 (d)	5 (b)	7 (d)	9 (a)
2 (c)	4 (a)	6 (c)	8 (a)	10 (b)

Chapter 9. Exercise 50 (page 112)

1 (c)	4 (b)	7 (c)	9 (c)	11 (a)
2 (b)	5 (c)	8 (d)	10 (a)	12 (b)
3 (c)	6 (a)			

Chapter 10. Exercise 60 (page 141)

1 (d)	7 (c)	13 (b)	19 (d)
2 (a) or (c)	8 (a)	14 (p)	20 (a)
3 (b)	9 (i)	15 (d)	21 (d)
4 (b)	10 (j)	16 (o)	22 (c)
5 (c)	11 (g)	17 (n)	23 (a)
6 (f)	12 (c)	18 (b)	

Chapter 11. Exercise 64 (page 155)

1 (c)	3 (d)	5 (b)	7 (c)	9 (a)
2 (a)	4 (c)	6 (b)	8 (d)	10 (b)

Chapter 12. Exercise 68 (page 175)

1 (b)	5 (a)	9 (b)	13 (b)	17 (c)
2 (b)	6 (d)	10 (c)	14 (b)	18 (b)
3 (c)	7 (b)	11 (a)	15 (b)	19 (a)
4 (a)	8 (d)	12 (b)	16 (b)	20 (b)

Chapter 13. Exercise 76 (page 206)

1 (d)	5 (a)	8 (a)	11 (b)	14 (b)
2 (c)	6 (d)	9 (c)	12 (d)	15 (c)
3 (b)	7 (c)	10 (c)	13 (d)	16 (a)
4 (c)				

Chapter 14. Exercise 82 (page 224)

1 (c)	4 (a)	7 (b)	9 (b)	11 (b)
2 (d)	5 (d)	8 (c)	10 (c)	12 (d)
3 (d)	6 (c)			

Chapter 15. Exercise 90 (page 245)

1 (c)	5 (a)	9 (d)	13 (b)	17 (c)
2 (a)	6 (b)	10 (d)	14 (c)	18 (a)
3 (b)	7 (a)	11 (b)	15 (b)	19 (d)
4 (b)	8 (d)	12 (c)	16 (b)	

Chapter 16. Exercise 98 (page 264)

1 (d)	5 (h)	9 (a)	12 (d)
2 (g)	6 (b)	10 (d), (g), (i) and (l)	13 (c)
3 (i)	7 (k)	11 (b)	14 (b)
4 (s)	8 (l)		

Chapter 17. Exercise 103 (page 276)

1 (d)	4 (c)	7 (b)	9 (d)	11 (d)
2 (b)	5 (c)	8 (a)	10 (b)	12 (c)
3 (a)	6 (a)			

Chapter 18. Exercise 107 (page 293)

1 (c)	5 (g)	9 (a)	13 (c)	16 (c)
2 (b)	6 (e)	10 (d)	14 (j)	17 (a)
3 (b)	7 (l)	11 (g)	15 (h)	18 (a)
4 (g)	8 (c)	12 (b)		

Chapter 19. Exercise 111 (page 309)

1 (c)	3 (b)	5 (a)	7 (d)	9 (c)
2 (b)	4 (d)	6 (b)	8 (a)	10 (c)

Chapter 20. Exercise 117 (page 331)

1 (g)	5 (f)	9 (l)	12 (j)	15 (c)
2 (c)	6 (a)	10 (d)	13 (d)	16 (b)
3 (a)	7 (g)	11 (f)	14 (b)	17 (c)
4 (a)	8 (l)			

Chapter 21. Exercise 130 (page 355)

1 (a)	5 (c)	9 (b)	13 (h)	17 (c)
2 (d)	6 (a)	10 (g)	14 (k)	18 (b) and (c)
3 (a)	7 (b)	11 (d)	15 (j)	19 (c)
4 (b)	8 (a)	12 (a)	16 (f)	20 (b)

Chapter 22. Exercise 139 (page 381)

1 (b)	6 (a)	11 (b)	16 (b)	21 (b)
2 (e)	7 (d)	12 (a)	17 (b)	22 (a)
3 (e)	8 (f)	13 (b)	18 (b)	23 (c)
4 (c)	9 (b)	14 (a)	19 (c)	24 (d)
5 (c)	10 (c)	15 (d)	20 (b)	

Chapter 23. Exercise 146 (page 399)

1 (c)	5 (b)	9 (f)	13 (a)	16 (b)
2 (b)	6 (d)	10 (j)	14 (c)	17 (c)
3 (d)	7 (b)	11 (d)	15 (b)	18 (b)
4 (a)	8 (c)	12 (c)		

Index

Absolute permeability, 80
  permittivity, 64
  potential, 56
A.c. bridges, 136
  generator, 209
  values, 211
Acceptor circuit, 238
Active filter, 266
  power, 242, 247
Advantages of:
  auto transformers, 351
  squirrel cage induction motor, 396
  three-phase systems, 330
  wound rotor induction motor, 397
Air capacitors, 73
Alkaline cell, 31
Alternating voltages and currents, 209
Alternative energy, 39
Aluminium, 145
Ammeter, 12, 116
Amplifier gain, 298, 300
Amplifier, transistor, 168
Amplitude, 123, 211
Analogue instruments, 115
  to digital conversion, 124, 307
Angle of lag, 215
  lead, 215
Angular velocity, 215
Anode, 31, 150
Antimony, 145
Apparent power, 242, 247
Applications of resonance, 256
Armature, 359
  reaction, 360
Arsenic, 145
Asymmetrical network, 266
Atoms, 11, 144
Attenuation, 266
  bands, 266
Attraction-type m.i. instrument, 115
Audio frequency transformer, 341
Auto transformer, 349
Avalanche breakdown, 151
  effect, 148
Average value, 211

Back e.m.f., 368
Balanced network, 267

Band-pass filter, 274
Band-stop filter, 275
Bandwidth, 241, 296
Base, 158
Batteries, 30, 33, 36
  disposal of, 38
B-H curves, 80
Bipolar junction transistor, 157, 158, 160
  characteristics, 161
Block diagram, electrical, 9
BJT characteristics, 164, 165
Boron, 145
Breakdown voltage, 148
Bridge, a.c., 136
  megger, 12
  rectifier, 222
  Wheatstone, 134
Brush contact loss, 367
Buffer amplifier, 302

Calibration accuracy, 138
Camera flash, 286
Capacitance, 63, 66
Capacitive a.c. circuit, 227
Capacitive reactance, 227
Capacitors, 61, 63
  applications of, 61
  charging, 278
  discharging, 75, 283
  energy stored, 72
  in parallel and series, 67
  parallel plate, 66
  practical types, 73
Capacity of cell, 38
Carbon resistors, 21
Cathode, 31, 150
Cell capacity, 38
  fuel, 38
  primary, 30, 35
  secondary, 31, 36
  simple, 31
Ceramic capacitor, 74
Characteristic impedance, 267
Characteristics, transistor, 161
Charge, 4, 11, 63
  density, 64
  force on, 99

Charging a capacitor, 278
  experiment, 419
  of cell, 33
Chemical effects of current, 18
  electricity, 31
Choke, 108
Circuit diagram symbols, 10
CIVIL, 228
Class A amplifier, 170
Closed-loop gain, 298
Coercive force, 87
Collector, 158
Colour coding of resistors, 26
Combination of waveforms, 218
Common-mode rejection ratio, 297
Communications system, 10
Commutation, 359
Commutator, 359, 360
Comparison between electrical and magnetic materials, 87
Complex wave, 130
Composite series magnetic circuits, 83
Compound winding, 360
Compound wound generator, 365
  motor, 374
Conductance, 6
Conduction in semiconductor materials, 145
Conductors, 11, 15, 143
Constant current source, 197
Contact potential, 146, 147
Continuity tester, 12, 119
Control, 98
Cooling of transformers, 341
Copper loss, 344, 366
  rotor, 390
Core loss, 366
  component, 336
Core type transformer, 341
Corrosion, 32
Coulomb, 4, 11, 63
Coulomb's law, 62
Covalent bonds, 145
Cumulative compound motor, 374
Current, 11
  decay in L-R circuit, 288
  division, 49

Current (*continued*)
 gain, in transistors, 163, 164
 growth, L-R circuit, 286
 leakage, 159
 magnification, 256
 main effects, 17
 transformer, 352
Cut-off frequency, 266, 268, 271
Cycle, 210

Damping, 99, 115
D.c. circuit theory, 183, 190
 generator, 362
 characteristics, 362
 efficiency, 367
D.c. machine, 358
 construction, 359
 losses, 366
 torque, 368
D.c. motor, 97, 359, 368
 efficiency, 374
 speed control, 377
 starter, 376
 torque, 369
 types, 370
D.c. potentiometer, 135
D.c. transients, 278
Decibel, 131
 meter, 132
Delta connection, 318, 321
Delta/star comparison, 330
Depletion layer, 146, 147
Derived units, 3
Design impedance, 268
Dielectric, 63, 65
 strength, 72
Differential amplifier, 296, 303, 304
 compound motor, 374
Differentiator circuit, 292
Diffusion, 146
Digital to analogue conversion, 306
Digital multimeter, 118, 119
 storage oscilloscope, 115
Diode characteristics, 148
Disadvantages of auto transformers, 351
Discharging capacitors, 75, 283
 of cell, 33
Disposal of batteries, 38
Diverter, 378
Doping, 145
Double beam oscilloscope, 123
Double cage induction motor, 397
Drift, 11
Dynamic current gain, 163
Dynamic resistance, 255

Earth point, 56
 potential, 57
Edison cell, 36
Eddy current loss, 344
Effective value, 211
Effect of time constant on rectangular
 wave, 291
Effects of electric current, 17
Efficiency of:
 d.c. generator, 367
 d.c. motor, 374
 induction motor, 390
 transformer, 344
Electrical:
 energy, 6, 16
 measuring instruments, 12, 114
 potential, 5
 power, 6, 15
 safety, 215
Electric:
 bell, 93
 cell, 31
 current, 11
 field strength, 62
 flux density, 64
Electrochemical series, 31
Electrodes, 31
Electrolysis, 31
Electrolyte, 31
Electrolytic capacitor, 74
Electromagnetic induction, 101
 laws of, 102
Electromagnetism, 91
Electromagnets, 93
Electromechanical system, 10
Electronic instruments, 118
Electrons, 11, 31, 144
Electroplating, 31
Electrostatic field, 62
E.m.f., 5, 32
 equation of transformer, 337
 in armature winding, 360
 induced in conductors, 103
 of a cell, 32
Emitter, 158
Energy, 4, 6, 16
 stored in:
 capacitor, 72
 inductor, 108
Equivalent circuit of transformer, 341

Farad, 63
Faraday's laws, 103
Ferrite, 87

Field effect transistor, 157, 166
 amplifiers, 168
 characteristics, 166, 168
Filter, 223, 256, 266
 networks, 266
Fleming's left hand rule, 95
Fleming's right hand rule, 102
Fluke, 119
Force, 4
 of attraction or repulsion, 62
 on a charge, 99
 on a current-carrying conductor, 94
Form factor, 212
Formulae, lists of, 179, 312, 402
Forward bias, 147
 characteristics, 148
Forward transconductance, 167
Frequency, 123, 210
Friction and windage losses, 366
Fuel cells, 38
Full wave bridge rectifier, 222
 rectification, 221
Fundamental, 130
Fuses, 18, 215

Gallium arsenide, 145
Galvanometer, 134
Generator: 358
 a.c., 209
 d.c., 358
Geothermal energy, 39
 hotspots, 39
Germanium, 143, 145
Grip rule, 93

Half-power points, 241
Half-wave rectification, 221
Harmonics, 130
Heating effects of current, 18
Henry, 106
Hertz, 210
High-pass filter, 266, 270
Hole, 144, 145
Hydroelectricity, 39
Hydrogen cell, 38
Hysteresis, 87
 loop, 87
 loss, 87, 344

Impedance, 229, 233, 248, 249
 triangle, 229, 233
Impurity, 144
Indium, 145
Indium arsenide, 145
Induced e.m.f., 103

Inductance, 106
  of a coil, 108
Induction motor, 383
  construction, 386
  double cage, 397
  losses and efficiency, 390
  principle of operation, 387
  production of rotating field, 384
  starting methods, 396
  torque equation, 392
  torque-speed characteristic, 395
  uses of, 398
Inductive a.c. circuit, 226
  reactance, 226
  switching, 291
Inductors, 107
Initial slope and three point method, 280
Instantaneous values, 211
Instrument loading effect, 119
Insulated gate field effect transistor
    (IGFET), 166
Insulation and dangers of high current
    flow, 18
  materials, 215
  resistance tester, 12, 119
Insulators, 11, 15, 143
Integrated circuits, 154
Integrator circuit, 291
  op amp, 303
Internal resistance of cell, 33
Interpoles, 359
Intrinsic semiconductors, 146
Inverting amplifier op amp, 298
Ion, 11, 31
Iron losses, 344, 366
Isolating transformer, 351
Iterative impedance, 267

Joule, 4, 6, 16
Junction gate field effect transistor
    (JFET), 166

Kilowatt hour, 6, 16
Kirchhoff's laws, 183

Laboratory experiments, 405
Lamps in series and parallel, 57
Lap winding, 360
Laws of electromagnetic induction, 102
L-C parallel circuit, 250
Lead acid cell, 36
Leakage current, transistor, 159
Leclanché cell, 35
Lenz's law, 102

Letter and digit code for resistors, 27
Lifting magnet, 94
Light emitting diodes, 150, 153
Linear device, 12
  scale, 115
Lines of electric force, 62
  magnetic flux, 78
Lithium-ion battery, 31
Loading effect, 53, 119
Load line, 171
Local action, 32
Logarithmic ratios, 131
Losses:
  d.c. machines, 366
  induction motors, 390
  transformers, 344
Loudspeaker, 95
Low-pass filter, 266, 267
LR-C parallel a.c. circuit, 251

Magnetic:
  applications, 77
  circuits, 77
  effects of current, 18
  field due to electric current, 91
  fields, 78
  field strength, 79
  flux, 78
  flux density, 78
  force, 78
  screens, 83
Magnetisation curves, 80
Magnetising component, 336
Magnetising force, 79
Magnetomotive force, 79
Majority carriers, 146
Mangenese battery, 31
Matching, 347
Maximum efficiency of transformers,
    346
  power transfer theorem, 204
  repetitive reverse voltage, 151
  value, 211
Maxwell bridge, 136
Mean value, 211
Measurement errors, 138
Measurement of inductance experiment,
    414
  power in 3 phase system, 325
Megger, 12, 119
Mercury cell, 35
Mesh connection, 318, 321
Metal oxide resistors, 21
Mica capacitor, 73
Minority carriers, 146

Motor, 358
Motor cooling, 380
Motor, d.c., 97, 358, 368
  cooling, 379
  efficiency, 374
  speed control, 377
  starter, 376
  types, 370
Moving coil instrument, 98
Moving coil rectifier instrument, 116
  iron instrument, 115
Multimeter, 12, 119
Multiples of units, 13
Multiplier, 116
Mutual inductance, 106, 110

Negative feedback, 296
Neutral conductor, 318
  point, 318
Neutrons, 11
Newton, 4, 94
Nickel cadmium cells, 36
Nickel-metal cells, 36
Nife cell, 36
Nominal impedance, 268, 271
Non-inverting amplifier, 300
Non-linear device, 13
  scale, 115
Norton's theorem, 197
Norton and Thévenin equivalent
    circuits, 200
n-p-n transistor, 158
n-type material, 145
Nucleus, 11
Null method of measurement, 134

Ohm, 5, 12
Ohmmeter, 12, 119
Ohm's law, 13
  experiment, 406
Open-circuit characteristic, generator,
    363
Operating point, 172
Operational amplifiers, 295
  differential amplifier, 296, 303, 304
  integrator, 303
  inverting amplifier, 298
  non-inverting amplifier, 300
  parameters, 297
  summing amplifier, 302
  transfer characteristics, 296
  voltage comparator, 303
  voltage follower, 301
Oscilloscope, analogue, 12, 115, 122
  digital, 115, 122, 123

Paper capacitor, 73
Parallel:
    a.c. circuits, 247
    experiment, 417
    connected capacitors, 67
    d.c. circuits, 46
    lamps, 58
    networks, 46
    plate capacitor, 66
    resonance, 252, 254
    applications of, 256
Passbands, 266
Passive filter, 266
Peak factor, 212
    inverse voltage, 151
    value, 123, 211
Peak-to-peak value, 211
Pentavalent impurity, 144, 145
Period, 210
Periodic time, 123, 210
Permanent magnet, 78
Permeability, 80
    absolute, 80
    of free space, 80
    relative, 80
Permittivity, 64
    absolute, 64
    of free space, 64
    relative, 64
Phasor, 215
Phosphor, 145
Photovoltaic cells, 39
Plastic capacitor, 74
Polarisation, 31, 32
Potential:
    absolute, 56
    difference, 5, 11
    divider, 44
    electric, 5
    gradient, 63
Potentiometer, d.c., 44, 53, 135
Power, 4, 15
    active, 242, 247
    apparent, 242, 247
    electrical, 6, 15
    factor, 243, 258
    improvement, 258
    in a.c. circuits, 241, 247
    in 3-phase systems, 323
    measurement in 3-phase systems, 325
    reactive, 242, 247
    transformers, 341
    triangle, 242
p-n junction, 146
p-n-p transistor, 159
p-type material, 145

Practical types of capacitor, 73
Prefixes of units, 3
Primary cells, 30, 35
Principal of operation of:
    d.c. motor, 97
    moving-coil instrument, 98
    3-phase induction motor, 387
    transformer, 334
Protons, 11, 144
Public address system, 9

Q-factor, 137, 239, 256
Q-meter, 137
Quantity of electricity, 11
Quiescent point, 171

Radio frequency transformer, 341
Rating, 334
R-C parallel a.c. circuit, 248
R-C series a.c. circuit, 232
Reactive power, 242, 247
Rectification, 151, 221
Rectifier diodes, 150
Regulation of transformer, 343
Relative permeability, 80
    permittivity, 64
    voltage, 56
Relay, 93
Reluctance, 83
Rejector circuit, 255
Remanence, 87
Remanent flux density, 87
Renewable energy, 39
Repulsion type m.i. instrument, 115
Reservoir capacitor, 222
Resistance, 5, 11, 21
    internal, 33
    matching, 347
    variation, 21
Resistivity, 22
Resistor colour coding, 26
    construction, 21
Resonance:
    applications of, 256
    parallel, 252, 254
    series, 235, 238
Reverse bias, 147
    characteristics, 148
Rheostat, 53, 54
Ripple, 222
R-L-C series a.c. circuit, 234
R-L parallel a.c. circuit, 247
R-L series a.c. circuit, 229
R.m.s. value, 123, 211
Rotation of loop in magnetic field, 105
Rotor copper loss, 390

Saturation flux density, 87
Scale, 115
Schottky diodes, 153
Screw rule, 92, 93
Secondary cells, 31, 36
Selectivity, 241
Self-excited generators, 362
Self inductance, 106
Semiconductor diodes, 143, 150
    materials, 144
Semiconductors, 143, 145
Separately-excited generators, 362
Series:
    a.c. circuits, 226
    experiment, 415
    circuit, 43
    connected capacitors, 68
    d.c. circuits, 43
    lamps, 57
    resonance, 235, 238
    winding, 360
    wound generator, 364
    motor, 372, 378
Series-parallel d.c. circuit experiment,
        407
Shells, 11, 144
Shell type transformer, 341
Short circuits, 57
Shunt, 116
    field regulator, 377
    winding, 360
    wound generator, 363
    motor, 370, 377
Siemen, 6
Silicon, 143, 145
Silicon controlled rectifiers, 152
Silver oxide battery, 31
Simple cell, 31
Sine wave, 210, 211
Single-phase:
    parallel a.c. circuit, 247
    series a.c. circuit, 246
    voltage, 317
S.I. units, 3
Sinusoidal waveform equation, 215
Slew rate, 298
Slip, 387
Smoothing of rectified waveform, 222
Solar energy, 39
    panels, 39
Solenoid, 92
Spectrum analysis, 130
Speed control of d.c. motors, 377
Squirrel-cage rotor induction motors,
        386, 396
    advantages of, 396

Star connection, 318
    point, 318
Star/delta comparison, 330
Stator, 359
Steady state, 279
Stopbands, 266
Stroboscope, 12
Sub-multiples of units, 13
Sub-system, 10
Summing amplifier, 302, 306
Superposition theorem, 187
    experiment, 408
Switched-mode power supplies, 154
Switching inductive circuits, 291
Symbols, electrical, 10
Symmetrical network, 266
Synchronous speed, 384, 385
System, electrical, 9

T-network, 266
Tachometer, 12
Tangent method, 280
Telephone receiver, 94
Temperature coefficient of resistance, 24
    control system, 10
Tesla, 79
Thermal generation of electron-hole
        pairs, 146
Thévenin and Norton equivalent
        circuits, 200
Thévenin's theorem, 192
    experiment, 410
Three-phase:
    induction motor, 383
    power, 323, 325
    supply, 317
    systems, 317
        advantages of, 330
    transformers, 351
Thyristors, 152
Tidal power, 39
Time constant:
    C-R circuit, 279
    L-R circuit, 287

Titanium oxide capacitor, 74
Torque equation:
    for induction motor, 392
    of a d.c. machine, 369
Torque-speed characteristics of
            induction motor, 395
Transfer characteristic, 161, 296
Transformation ratio, 334
Transformers, 333
    audio frequency, 341
    auto, 349
    construction, 341
    cooling, 341
    current, 352
    e.m.f. equation, 337
    equivalent circuit, 341
    isolating, 351
    losses and efficiency, 344
    no-load phasor diagram, 336
    on-load phasor diagram, 339
    power, 341
    principle of operation, 334
    radio frequency, 341
    rating, 334
    regulation of, 343
    three-phase, 351
    voltage, 354
    windings, 341
Transient C-R circuit, 280
    L-R circuit, 286
Transients, 278
Transistor:
    action, 158, 160
    amplifier, 168
    bias, 160
    characteristics, 161
    classification, 157
    connections, 158
    current flow, 160
    leakage current, 159
    operating configuration, 161
    parameters, 162
    symbols, 158
Transistors, 157
Trivalent impurity, 145

True power, 242, 247
Two-port networks, 266

UK supply voltage, 319
Unbalanced network, 267
Unit of electricity, 16
Units, S.I., 3
Use of CRO, experiments, 412, 413

Vacuum, 64
Valence shell, 144
Varactor diodes, 150, 153
Variable air capacitor, 73
Virtual digital storage oscilloscope, 127
    earth, 298
    test and measuring instruments, 126
Volt, 5, 11
Voltage, 11
    comparator, 303, 307
    follower amplifier, 301
    gain, transistor, 173
    magnification at resonance, 239
    regulator, 152
    transformer, 354
    triangle, 229, 232
Voltmeter, 12, 116

Watt, 4, 15
Wattmeters, 12, 119
Waveform harmonics, 130
Waveforms, 210
    combination of, 218
Wave winding, 360
Weber, 78
Wheatstone bridge, 134
Wind power, 39
Wire-wound resistors, 21
Work, 4
Wound rotor induction motor, 387, 396
    advantages of, 397

Yoke, 359

Zener diode, 150, 151
    effect, 148